Fundamentals of

Inhalation therapy

Fundamentals of Inhalation therapy

DONALD F. EGAN, M.D.

Director, Section of Chest Diseases, New Britain General Hospital, New Britain, Connecticut; formerly Director, Department and School of Inhalation Therapy, Yale–New Haven Hospital, New Haven, Connecticut; Associate Clinical Professor, Department of Medicine, Yale University School of Medicine, New Haven, Connecticut

With 148 illustrations

Saint Louis

The C. V. Mosby Company

1969

Printed in the United States of America

Standard Book Number 8016-1501-1

Library of Congress Catalog Card Number 76-85809

Distributed in Great Britain by Henry Kimpton, London

Preface

The purpose of this book is to present what is felt to be minimum knowledge for the safe and effective administration of inhalation therapy. It is intended primarily for the student inhalation therapist and for the working therapist who requires a reference for review. However, the needs of others were considered; thus, chapters dealing with equipment and clinical application are designed as much for the physician who treats patients with respiratory illnesses, for the resident physician, and for the nurse as they are for the therapist. The better the physician understands the fundamentals of the therapy he prescribes, the wiser will be his use and expectations of it.

Three points should be emphasized: First, no text can be all things to all people. This book will serve a purpose for the student in a hospital-based inhalation therapy school that will be different from what it will provide for the student in a junior college. It represents something of a compromise treatment of material required for each of their separate needs. Nevertheless, it is believed that if both these students understand the principles discussed they will be good inhalation therapists. Second, if the text is to be confined as much as possible to its primary subject, the student must be expected to possess a certain amount of previously acquired knowledge. He should have had a basic course in chemistry and, preferably but not necessarily, one in physics, along with a working knowledge of common logarithms and scientific notation. The last two can be taught or reviewed along with anatomy during the initial weeks of an inhalation therapy school curriculum. Skills in these subjects will be put to use early in the text. Third, the sequence of chapters is deliberate, based upon 8 years of writing and experimenting with curricula at the inhalation therapy schools of the Yale–New Haven Hospital, New Haven, Connecticut, and the New Britain General Hospital, New Britain, Connecticut. Each topic is dependent upon the one that precedes it, and the order is that which I have found best suited to guide the student into a solid understanding of the fundamentals of therapy.

Repetition is freely used whenever it is felt necessary to emphasize important topics, especially in overlapping areas or in different contexts. The absolute and relative values of each topic have been carefully weighed, and nothing is included that does not bear on some aspect of inhalation therapy.

Much has been omitted in the interest of time and space economy. Notably absent are sections on emergency resuscitation, because of the excellent available descriptions and training aids; pulmonary function tests, because they warrant publications in their own right; and hyperbaric medicine, because it is not yet a function of inhalation therapy.

It is hoped that the inhalation therapist will be stimulated to explore more deeply on his own many interesting things that have been only touched upon in this book. It is further hoped that other teachers will put their thoughts into therapist-oriented texts so that a significant library will be developed in this important medical technology.

I am indebted to Miss Eleanor Shure, who bore the brunt of typing the many rough drafts as well as the bulk of the manuscript, and Mrs. Henrietta Else, for her assistance in completing the final work. The photographs were prepared by the medical photographer of the New Britain General Hospital, Mr. Albert Spitzer.

Donald F. Egan, M.D.

Contents

Fundamentals of

Inhalation therapy

Chapter 1

Gases, the atmosphere, and the gas laws

A gas, which may not be seen, cannot be felt, and has no inherent confining boundaries, almost invokes an impression of nothingness until we become aware of the tremendous activity of its components and its great flexibility. It can be compressed, can expand, can produce heat, can cool, and can be liquefied. From its behavior, we can infer that a gas consists of much empty space, with its substance in minute particle form, and it is with the general relationship between such space and particles that we will be concerned.

MOBILITY OF GASES

The substance of gases consists of molecular particles, which are in constant motion, called *kinetic activity.* All matter is composed of molecules, some loosely associated and some densely packed together, giving certain characteristics to various types of matter. Substances with a high density of molecules are solids, whereas those with easily mobile molecules are called fluids. Gases and liquids fall in the second group. It should not be supposed that the molecules of solids cannot move, for they respond to such stimuli as vibrations, bending, stretching, and temperature. Fluidity, however, implies the easy flowing of molecules over one another and the ability to conform readily to the confines of a container. Mercury, although a metal, can thus be described as fluid.

Particles that make up the substance of gases are minute in size, within the range of 10^{-8} to 10^{-7} cm in diameter, with weights varying from 10^{-23} to 10^{-20} gm. The kinetic theory tells us that these particles are in *constant rapid* motion, following completely random paths, and that their speed is phenomenal. Hydrogen particles move 1.84×10^5 cm per second (greater than 1 mile per second), and oxygen 4.6×10^4 cm per second ($^1/_3$ of a mile per second).[1] During this intense activity the particles "collide" with one another and with the surface of enclosing containers. Actually, the particles probably repulse one another before physical contact, but the forces involved can best be visualized in the mind as collisions. The average number of collisions per second for each molecule of hydrogen is 1×10^{10}, for oxygen 4.6×10^9, and for carbon dioxide 6.2×10^9. The *mean free path* of gas molecules describes the average distance traveled by the molecules between collisions. Again, for hydrogen this distance is 1.66×10^{-5} cm, for oxygen 8.8×10^{-6} cm, and for carbon dioxide 5.8×10^{-6} cm.[2] Very fine particles of an insoluble substance such as carbon or metal dust suspended in water, if viewed under a microscope, can be seen to move about in an erratic random manner. This is called *Brownian movement* and is produced by the kinetic activity of water molecules striking the suspended material.

To view the phenomenon of kinetic activity in familiar quantitative terms, let us imagine oxygen molecules in a pure sample of that gas to be the size of Ping-Pong balls. We can see them, in the mind's eye, in large numbers bouncing off walls, ceiling, floor, and each other, never stopping and never settling to the floor. Considering the relative sizes of oxygen molecules and Ping-Pong balls, the mean free path, and the average number of collisions of the molecules, the Ping-Pong balls would travel an average distance of 40 feet between collisions. This gives us some concept of the great distance between molecules in relation to their size as well as the mass of "nothingness" that makes up a gas.

PRESSURE OF GASES

All gases exert pressure, whether free in the atmosphere, enclosed in a container, or dissolved in a liquid such as blood. In physiology, this pressure is frequently referred to as the *tension* of a gas. Gas pressure is dependent upon molecular kinetic activity, and is the result of molecular bombardment upon any confining surface, be it a steel cylinder or the earth's surface, and we may consider such pressure as the striking force of molecules attempting to escape. In addition, the force of the earth's gravity by its effect upon the molecular masses of the gas, augments the gas pressure against the dependent confining surface of a gas volume. Thus, in a container of gas, although the travel of molecules is random in all directions, pressure in the bottom of the vessel is somewhat higher than elsewhere, as the force of molecular impingement is aided by gravity. The amount of pressure exerted by a gas depends upon the *number* of particles present and the *frequency* of their collisions. The frequency, in turn, is related to the *velocity* of the gas particles, for the greater the speed of travel, the greater will be the number of collisions per unit of time, the greater the force of collisions, and the greater the gas tension.

Gas particle velocity is not a constant value but is directly related to gas temperature, and as temperature rises the kinetic activity accelerates, molecular collisions increase in number, and the pressure of the gas rises. Conversely, with dropping temperature molecular activity declines, particle velocity and collision frequency drop, and pressure is lowered. The familiar increase in automobile tire pressure while driving on a hot pavement is an example of the relationship between gas tension and temperature. This relationship between molecular activity and temperature can be graphically illustrated by a special temperature scale, which the student will put to practical use when he studies the gas laws. We will describe the concept of *absolute temperature* and the two subscales by which it is calibrated. There is a temperature at which all molecular activity ceases, a theoretical value arrived at by projection and calculation, which, although very closely approximated, has not actually been attained. If we are interested in the relative kinetic behavior of gases at various temperatures, a point of no activity provides a logical zero on which to build a scale. This is called *absolute zero* ($0°_{abs}$) and is the origin of the absolute temperature scale. If it is calibrated in Celsius temperature units, it is called the *Kelvin scale* (K), and if in Fahrenheit units, the *Rankine scale* (R).

Kelvin scale

In Celsius units, molecular activity stops at about −273° C. Therefore, 0° K = −273° C, and 0° C = 273° K since 0° C is 273 temperature units above 0° K. When used as symbols in formulas, Celsius temperatures are often designated by a small t and absolute temperatures by a capital T or a capital K. A simple equation to keep in mind is $°K = t + 273$. In other words, to convert Celsius degrees to Kelvin, add 273. Thus

$$25° \text{ C} = 25 + 273 = 298° \text{ K}$$
$$37° \text{ C} = 37 + 273 = 310° \text{ K}$$
$$-15° \text{ C} = -15 + 273 = 258° \text{ K}$$

Rankine scale

Used frequently in engineering but rarely in medical science, the Rankine scale is based on Fahrenheit units. Since −273° C = −460° F (refer to formulas to convert between Celsius and Fahrenheit scales), then 0° R = −460° F, and $°R = °F + 460$. Fig. 1-1 is a scalar representation of the relation between gase-

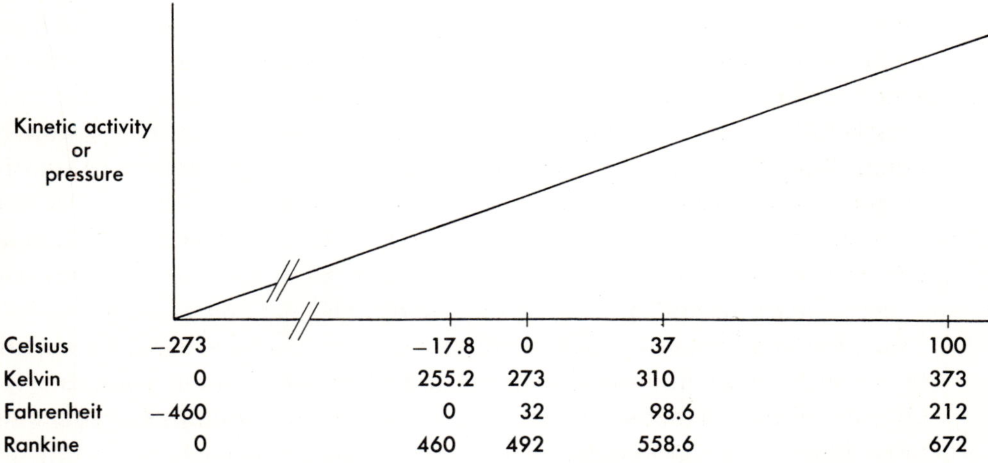

Fig. 1-1. Linear relationship between gas molecular activity, or pressure, and temperature. Comparable readings of the four scales are indicated for five temperature points.

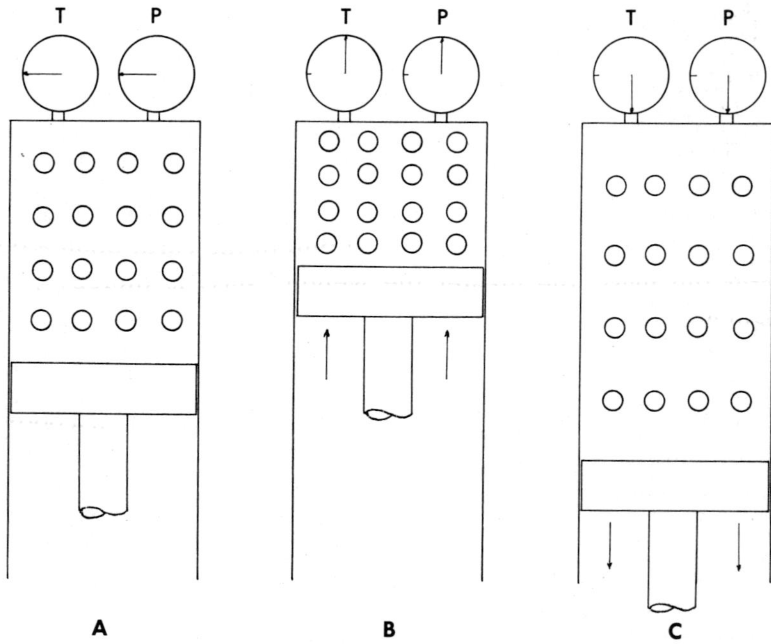

Fig. 1-2. A mass of gas in the resting state exerts a given pressure at a given temperature, in cylinder **A.** In **B,** as the piston compresses the gas, the molecules are crowded closer together, and the increased energy of molecular collisions is reflected in a rise of both temperature and pressure. Conversely, retraction of the piston in **C** allows the gas to expand, and the temperature and pressure drop as molecular interaction decreases.

ous kinetic activity, or pressure, and five commonly used temperatures of the four related scales.

Because of the relatively great distances between molecules, gases possess the quality of *compressibility.* When pressure is exerted on a gas, the molecules can be brought closer together as their intervening spaces are narrowed. Conversely, if the container of a volume of gas enlarges, the gas therein *expands* to accommodate the new volume, and its molecules range further apart. Fig. 1-2 illustrates the relationship between compression and expansion of a given mass of gas molecules and corresponding temperature and pressure changes. Because the tremendous energy of molecular collision is expended as heat, compression of a gas produces *heat* as well as a buildup of pressure among the molecules. As compression brings the molecules closer together, the frequency of collisions increases, and both heat and pressure increase. Thus, the heat of compression may be considered as a means of dissipating the great increase in kinetic energy that accompanies compression. It should be quite apparent that expansion of a gas produces a drop in temperature as molecular collision frequency decreases. Cooling of expansion is utilized in refrigerating systems, and is part of the natural phenomenon of cooling through expansion of large air masses.

DENSITY OF GASES

Before considering the density of gases specifically, we will need some definitions. We must learn the relationship between the widely used physical terms mass, weight, and density. The word *mass* refers to the substance of an object, the quantity of matter it contains, the number and nature of its molecules, and is characterized by having inertia and by being subject to the pull of gravity. *Weight* is the gravitational pull of the earth upon a body, thus the greater the mass, the greater the weight. Mass is thereby proportional to weight and is measured in arbitrary units as weight, against such standards as the kilogram and the pound. It should be noted that weight varies with the position of mass relative to the surface of the earth, decreasing both toward the earth's center and away from its surface. The *inertia* of a body, that quality of mass which requires force to start it in motion from a resting state or to change its velocity once in motion, remains unchanged no matter where it is located.

Density may be defined as the amount of mass per unit volume of a body, the concentration of its molecules, and is usually employed as *weight density*. Density is thus the *weight of a body per unit volume* and in our field of interest is most often described in grams per cubic centimeter for solids and liquids, and grams per liter for gases. Other units, such as pounds per cubic foot, can also be used. A mass weighing 15 gm and measuring 3 cc has a density of 5 gm/cc. A ton of feathers and a ton of bricks weigh the same, but the obvious difference in the volumes of similar weights of these substances makes for widely differing densities. *Specific gravity* is a variation of density measurement whereby the density of solids and liquids is calibrated against the density of water used as a standard of unity, and gases against oxygen or hydrogen. A liquid with a specific gravity of 1.5, for example, has a density half again as great as that of water. Specific gravity values of gases play a negligible role in pulmonary physiology, whereas gas densities are of great importance.

One of the laws of physics and chemistry tells us that weights of all atoms, in grams corresponding to their atomic weights, and weights of all molecules, in grams corresponding to their molecular weights, always contain the same number of their respective particles, 6.02×10^{23}. This is known as *Avogadro's number.* Although these quantities are often referred to as "gram atomic weights" and "gram molecular weights," they are each technically known as a *mole.* To put it another way, any quantity of matter that contains 6.02×10^{23} atoms, molecules, or even ions is called a mole. Further, Avogadro's law states that equal volumes of all gases, at the same temperature and pressure, contain the same number of molecules or, conversely, that at constant temperature and pressure equal numbers of molecules of all gases occupy the same volume. Thus, under standard conditions of a temperature of 0° C and a pressure of 1 atmosphere, moles of all gases (gram-molecular weights, gmw, 6.02×10^{23} molecules) measure *22.4 liters.* Since density equals weight divided by vol-

Table 1-1. *Examples of gas densities (D) under standard conditions*

$$D\ O_2 = \frac{gmw}{22.4} = \frac{32}{22.4} = 1.43 \text{ gm/liter}$$

$$D\ N_2 = \frac{gmw}{22.4} = \frac{28}{22.4} = 1.25 \text{ gm/liter}$$

$$D\ He = \frac{gmw}{22.4} = \frac{4}{22.4} = 0.1785 \text{ gm/liter}$$

$$D\ CO_2 = \frac{gmw}{22.4} = \frac{44}{22.4} = 1.965 \text{ gm/liter}$$

ume, the density of any gas is its *gmw* ÷ *22.4* and is expressed as *grams per liter.* Examples of gas densities are shown in Table 1-1.

Densities of gas mixtures are easily calculated if the percentage composition of the mixture is known. Given the following mixed gases:

Gas A = 10%
Gas B = 60%
Gas C = 30%

$$D = \frac{(0.10 \times \text{gmw A}) + (0.60 \times \text{gmw B}) + (0.30 \times \text{gmw C})}{22.4}$$

Calculate the density of a mixture of 30% HBr and 70% ethylene (C_2H_4):

$$D = \frac{(0.3 \times 81) + (0.7 \times 28)}{22.4} = \frac{43.9}{22.4} = 1.955 \text{ gm/liter}$$

Exercise 1-1. Calculate densities of the following:

(a) C_2H_2 (acetylene)
(b) NH_3 (ammonia)
(c) SiF_4 (silicon fluoride)
(d) CO (carbon monoxide)
(e) SO_2 (sulfur dioxide)
(f) 5% CO_2 + 95% O_2
(g) 80% He + 20% O_2
(h) 70% He + 30% O_2
(i) 25% CH_4 + 75% C_4H_{10}
(j) 3% SO_2 + 15% N_2 + 82% O_2

COMPOSITION OF THE ATMOSPHERE

The atmosphere upon which we, as oxygen-breathing creatures, are completely dependent is a mixture of many gases plus water vapor. The elements composing the atmosphere, with the exception of water vapor, which will be discussed separately later, have the approximate concentrations shown in Table 1-2.

The atmosphere is divided into two major segments, three subsegments, and several layers, each with certain physical and/or chemical properties[3]:

1. The first major segment is the *inner atmosphere,* extending from the earth's surface to an altitude of about 600 miles; it is composed of the following subsegments called spheres:

a. The *troposphere* extends from the earth's surface to an outer border called the tropopause, an average distance of some 8 miles up but varying with the latitude of the earth. It is higher over the equator than over

Table 1-2. *Approximate composition of the atmosphere*

Element	*Percent*	
Nitrogen (N_2)	78.08	
Oxygen (O_2)	20.95	(99.99%)
Argon (Ar)	0.93	
Carbon dioxide (CO_2)	0.03	
Neon (Ne)	1.8×10^{-3}	
Helium (He)	5.0×10^{-4}	
Krypton (Kr)	1.0×10^{-4}	
Hydrogen (H_2)	1.0×10^{-4}	
Xenon (Xe)	1.0×10^{-5}	
Ozone (O_3)	1.0×10^{-5}	
Radon (Rn)	6.0×10^{-18}	

Table 1-3. *Summary of atmospheric divisions*

Atmosphere	*Strata*	*Approximate height in miles*
Free space		Above 1200
Outer	Exosphere	600-1200
	Ionosphere	50-600
	Stratosphere	8-50
Inner	Troposphere	0-8

the poles. The troposphere is characterized by decreasing temperatures with altitude, reaching a low of approximately −55° C (−67° F), and has much turbulence.

b. The *stratosphere* continues from 8 to about 50 miles above the earth. The first layer of the stratosphere, from 8 to 15 miles up, is one of constant temperature around −55° C (−67° F) and has little turbulence. The next layer, from 15 to 30 miles, shows an increase in temperature, reaching a high of 10° C (50° F). The third and last layer of the stratosphere, from 30 to 50 miles, has a sharp temperature drop to −72° C (−100° F) and there is a return of turbulence. At approximately 50 miles of altitude the stratopause separates the stratosphere from the next sphere.

c. The *ionosphere* reaches from a distance of 50 miles outward to a distance of 600 miles. Here, there are several layers of ions, resulting from photochemical reactions between solar ultraviolet radiation and atmospheric molecules. The ionosphere is important as a reflector for the electromagnetic waves of radio communication. Temperatures in this sphere soar up to 2000° C (3600° F), but because the density of the air molecules is so low in this region, such temperatures have little meaning in our usual concept of temperature. As with the other spheres, a boundary called the ionopause delineates the end of the ionosphere.

2. The second major segment is the outer atmosphere, which is also called

the *exosphere.* This region extends from the 600-mile limit to about 1200 miles from earth, where it blends with the vacuum of *free space.* It is a marginal area where molecular collisions become progressively more rare.

The gravitational pull of the earth on atmospheric gas molecules produces the greatest density of molecules close to its surface, a density that decreases steadily outward to the vacuum of free space. It is speculated, however, that despite decreasing density, the percentage composition of the atmosphere, as described earlier, remains fairly constant to a height of at least some *60 miles.* Beyond this limit, with a decrease in mass air movement to keep the gases well mixed, there is a separation of the elements on the basis of their molecular weights. This phenomenon, called diffusion separation, disrupts the composition of the air as we know it on earth.

MEASUREMENT OF AIR PRESSURE

In cardiopulmonary physiology and therapy of cardiopulmonary diseases, we are constantly dealing with the principles of gas pressure, and it is vitally important that the student clearly understand this aspect of gas physics. Pressure, in any context, is defined as a *force* applied to a specific *surface area.* For

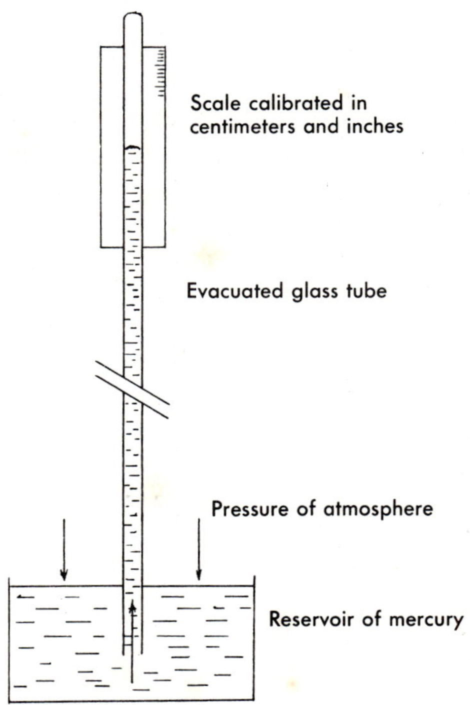

Fig. 1-3. The major components of a mercury barometer include a mercury reservoir, into which is inverted the open end of an evacuated glass tube, and a scale, by which the height of the mercury column can be read in inches and centimeters. The atmospheric pressure, acting on the surface of the mercury reservoir, is balanced by the weight of the column of mercury in the tube.

our purposes such force is usually expressed as grams per square centimeter (gm/cm^2) or pounds per square inch (lb/in^2) (psi). The force exerted by gases is a result of their kinetic molecular bombardment already discussed, and in a mixture of gases such as air this force is the sum of molecular activity of all the constituent gases. If we visualize the atmospheric mantle enveloping the earth, described above, we can understand that the molecular activity of atmospheric gases will exert a force against the surface of the earth. To view it another way, we can see that the many miles of atmosphere rest upon the earth as an object rests upon a table, exerting a force of pressure upon the earth's surface. It is of physiologic as well as meteorologic importance to be able to measure the force exerted by the air upon the earth.

Air pressure is measured indirectly by means of a barometer (*baros*, Greek, "weight"; *metron*, "measure"). Basically, a barometer consists of an evacuated glass tube approximately 37 inches tall with an inside diameter of 0.25 inch, closed at the top, and with its lower end immersed in a reservoir of mercury in a flexible container. The pressure of the atmosphere on the mercury reservoir forces the mercury up the vacuum tube, a distance relative to the atmospheric force, and the height of the column of mercury in the glass tube is measured in both inches and centimeters (Fig. 1-3). This procedure balances the pressure of the atmosphere against a column of mercury in a vacuum, and if the weight per surface area of the mercury can be calculated, this value will equal the pressure of the air.

A principle of physics tells us that the *pressure* exerted by a column of fluid is equal to the height of the column times the density of the fluid. Thus:

(1) Pressure (P) in gm/cm^2 = Height in cm × Density in gm/cm^3

$$P = cm \times \frac{gm}{cm^3}$$

$$= gm/cm^2$$

or

(2) Pressure (P) in lb/in^2 = Height in in × Density in lb/in^3

$$P = in \times \frac{lb}{in^3}$$

$$= lb/in^2$$

Because of shifting air currents and the mobility of huge masses of air, atmospheric density varies over different areas of the earth's surface and is reflected in constantly changing pressures as measured at the surface. Nevertheless, it has been demonstrated that at sea level the average atmospheric pressure will support a column of mercury 76 cm (760 mm), or 29.9 inches high. If we also know that mercury has a density of *13.6 gm/cm³* (i.e., is 13.6 times as heavy as water), or *0.491 lb/in³*, then we can easily calculate the atmospheric pressure (P_B) by the formulas given above.

(1) P in $gm/cm^2 = 76 \times 13.6 = 1034\ gm/cm^2$
(2) P in $lb/in^2 = 29.9 \times 0.491 = 14.7\ lb/in^2$

These two values, 1034 gm/cm^2 and 14.7 lb/in^2, are used as standards and are *called 1 atmosphere of pressure* (1 atm). It is evident, however, that for recording air pressure, there is no need to calculate the actual gm/cm^2 or lb/in^2 but only to record the height of the mercury column. Thus, pressure might be reported as 77.2 cm (772 mm) or 30.4 inches of Hg. In effect, this means that the atmospheric pressure is of such a magnitude that it is able to hold up a column of mercury 772 mm or 30.4 inches high. Their dynamic implications are exactly the same as actual force per surface area values of 1050 gm/cm^2 and 14.9 lb/in^2.

Mercury is used as the agent for measuring the air pressure because its density is such that at ordinary pressures it assumes a height which is easy and convenient to read. It would be possible, although not practical, to construct a barometer of water. At 1 atm pressure (76 cm Hg, or 29.9 in Hg) water, which is 13.6 times lighter than mercury, would rise to a height of *33.9 feet.* However, when very small pressures are being measured, expressing the pressure in terms of *centimeters of water* may be more convenient than in centimeters or millimeters of mercury. For example, a pressure of 2 cm Hg *(20 mm Hg)* is the same as 27.2 cm H_2O (2 × 13.6). A pressure gauge calibrated in centimeters of water would be easier to read than one calibrated in centimeters or millimeters of mercury. In physiologic work, the student will become accustomed to thinking and speaking in terms of both millimeters of mercury and centimeters of water. Inches of mercury or water are rarely used.

To complete the study, we should consider that method of measuring pressure which uses the *dyne,* frequently encountered in meteorology and physics. A dyne is defined as a unit of *force* that, when acting upon a 1 gm mass, gives to the mass an *acceleration of 1 cm/sec/sec,* or *1 cm/sec*^{2}. It is a fact of basic physics that a freely falling 1 gm mass (under the influence of gravity) will accelerate, or continuously pick up speed, 980.7 cm per second for every second it falls. It thus accelerates 980.7 cm/sec/sec, or 980.7 cm/sec^2. This can be thought of as a force of 1 gm acting on itself (1 gm force acting on 1 gm mass), producing an acceleration of 980.7 cm/sec^2, and therefore an acceleration of 1 cm/sec^2 of a 1 gm mass would be produced by a force of 1/980.7 of a gram. A dyne is thus equal to a force exerted by 1/980.7 gm, or 1.02×10^{-3} gm, and this is practically the equivalent of a milligram. For easy visualization, then, a dyne can be considered as the amount of force that would be exerted by a *milligram weight.*

The meteorologist often expresses air pressure in dynes, using his own terms of "barye," "bar," and "millibar" (mb). To understand this system, note the following relationships:

$$1 \text{ atm} = \text{Height of Hg} \times \text{Density of Hg} = 76 \times 13.6 = \mathit{1034\ gm/cm^2}$$

or

$$1 \text{ atm} = 1034 \text{ gm/cm}^2 \div 1.02 \times 10^{-3} \text{ (or } 1034 \times 980.7) = \mathit{1.014 \times 10^6\ dynes/cm^2}$$

The meteorologic units of pressure are defined as follows:

1 barye = 1 dyne/cm^2
1 bar = 10^6 baryes = 10^6 dynes/cm^2
1 millibar (mb) = 10^{-3} bar = 10^3 baryes = 10^3 dynes/cm^2

Thus, 1 standard atmosphere of pressure = 1034 gm/cm^2 = 1.014 × 10^6 dynes/cm^2 = 1.104 bars = 1014 millibars. In meteorology, atmospheric pressure is most frequently expressed as *millibars.* Millibars can be approximately converted to gm/cm^2 by multiplying by 1.02. In summary, then, the pressure of 1 atmosphere can be expressed as follows:

760 mm (76 cm) Hg
29.9 in Hg
33.9 ft H_2O
1034 gm/cm^2
14.7 lb/in^2
1.014 × 10^6 dynes/cm^2
1014 millibars

Exercise 1-2. Calculate the following pressures to the nearest tenth:

(a) 752 mm Hg, in gm/cm^2
(b) 31.4 in Hg, in lb/in^2
(c) 766 mm Hg, in lb/in^2
(d) 28.4 in Hg, in gm/cm^2
(e) 30.7 in Hg, in ft H_2O
(f) 1022 gm/cm^2, in mm Hg
(g) 15.2 lb/in^2, in in Hg
(h) 15 cm H_2O, in mm Hg
(i) 1018 mb, in mm Hg
(j) 766 mm Hg, in mb

In cardiopulmonary physiology the effect of gases is frequently considered in terms of their partial pressures. *Dalton's law of partial pressures* tells us that the total pressure of a gaseous mixture is equal to the sum of the partial pressures of the constituent gases and that the partial pressure of each gas in the mixture is the pressure it would exert if it occupied the entire volume alone. Thus, each gas contributes its share of the total pressure of a mixture in proportion to its percentage of the mixture. A gas that comprises 25% of a mixture of gases, therefore, will exert a partial pressure of 25% of the total pressure. To simplify an illustration, *dry* air may be considered to consist of but two major gases, O_2 at 21% and N_2 at 79%. Assuming a normal atmospheric pressure of 760 mm Hg, we can show individual partial pressures as follows:

$$
\begin{aligned}
P_B \text{ (dry)} &= 760 \text{ mm Hg} \\
P_{O_2} &= 760 \times 0.21 = 160 \text{ mm Hg} \\
P_{N_2} &= 760 \times 0.79 = \underline{600 \text{ mm Hg}} \\
& \qquad\qquad\qquad\;\; 760 \text{ mm Hg}
\end{aligned}
$$

HYPOBARISM AND HYPERBARISM

Hypobarism and *hyperbarism* refer to air pressures significantly below and above, respectively, the sea level normal of 760 mm Hg, or 1034 gm/cm^2. They are of great importance in man's excursions into outer space and into the sea. Indeed, one aspect of medicine under current investigation is that of hyperbaric medicine, in which the patient is subjected to the effects of several atmospheres of pressure.

It is obvious that with increasing altitude, there is decreasing atmospheric pressure. At any point above the earth, there is less air beyond it to exert pressure than there is on the earth's surface. Conversely, as one descends into the earth, there is a longer column of air exerting pressure on every square centimeter or square inch of surface area, demonstrated by a rising barometric pressure. Increasing pressure is most dramatically exemplified by descent into the sea. Here, water pressure rather than air pressure surrounds the immersed body; but when man invades deep water for a prolonged stay, he must surround himself with protective air at a pressure sufficient to balance that of the water. Because water is heavy and not compressible, a state of hyperbarism is reached much more quickly than is hypobarism above the earth. As a guide, each 33 feet of seawater represents a pressure of 1 atmosphere.

Since we are ultimately interested in the amount of oxygen available to the body cells and will soon learn of the relation between this availability and the pressure of oxygen partial pressure, let us consider the effect of changing atmospheric pressure on oxygen partial pressure. Assume a concentration of oxygen in dry air of 20.95% (this is expressed as the F_{O_2}, or fractional concentration of O_2). At a P_B of 760 mm Hg, the $P_{O_2} = 760 \times 0.2095 = 159$ mm Hg. Although the F_{O_2} of air at 25,000 feet is still 0.2095, the P_B is but 282 mm Hg and the P_{O_2} is thus 59 mm Hg. The important point to note is that, although the F_{O_2} at sea level and at 25,000 feet is the same, the kinetic activity of oxygen at the high altitude is equal to that of a mixture containing only 7.8% oxygen on the ground. In contrast, at a depth of 66 feet into the sea the weight of water exerts a pressure equal to that of 3 atmospheres, or 2280 mm Hg. Air breathed by a diver at this depth would also be subjected to this same pressure, and its P_{O_2} would be 20.95% of 2280, or 477 mm Hg.

Appendix 3 is a table that compares some of the characteristics of dry air at altitudes up to 300,000 feet and, when subjected to pressure at various depths in the sea, to a low of 297 feet. Sea level values are outlined at *0*, with altitudes above and sea depths below. The air density values (gm/liter) assume a sea level temperature of 15° C, at which temperature air has a density of 1.250 gm/liter. The relationship between gas density and temperature will be dealt with in detail later. The column *Atm* indicates the fraction or multiple of 1 atm pressure found at the various levels of altitude and depth. *%O₂ Equiv* refers to percentages of oxygen in breathing mixtures at sea level that would have oxygen partial pressures equal to those recorded in the P_{O_2} column. The student is not expected to memorize this table but to study it so that he will understand the wide environmental variation to which the body is subjected when it ventures from the surface of the earth. Some of the principles illustrated in the table will have important clinical meaning later.

Exercise 1-3. Assuming a F_{O_2} of 0.2095, calculate the following:

(a) The P_{O_2} of dry air at a P_B of 752 mm Hg

(b) The P_{O_2} of dry air at 1068 mb, in mm Hg
(c) The P_B in mm Hg with a P_{O_2} of 140 mm Hg
(d) The P_{O_2} of dry air at 50 ft of seawater
(e) The seawater depth with an O_2 equivalent of 100%

HUMIDITY

The discussions so far have been concerned only with dry gases, but it is now time to consider the important role played by water in gas physics. Invisible moisture is present in the atmosphere in the form of a vapor, assuming the state and characteristics of a gas, and is sometimes referred to as "molecular water" to distinguish it from visible gross "particulate water," such as mist. In this state water particles are subjected to the same kinetic activity as other gases and, like them, exert their own partial pressure, called *vapor pressure.* Atmospheric conditions vary the amount of water vapor in the air, but molecular water is constantly entering the air whenever air is exposed to a water surface.

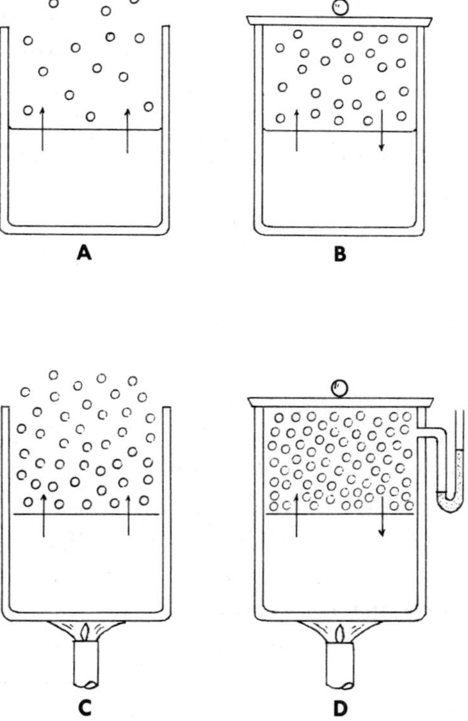

Fig. 1-4. The factors influencing vaporization of water are shown in these four sketches. In **A,** the kinetic activity of molecules at the surface carries the molecules into the surrounding air, and evaporation gradually reduces the reservoir. If the container is covered, as in **B,** vaporization does not stop but a state of equilibrium is reached when the air trapped in the container becomes saturated. At this point, water molecules leave and return to the reservoir in equal numbers. If the open container is heated, **C,** the increased molecular activity speeds the rate of vaporization. When the container is both covered and heated, **D,** more vapor will crowd into the trapped air, raising the vapor pressure as indicated by the attached manometer.

Water enters the atmosphere by vaporization. A volume of water, like a gas, is in constant molecular activity. The energy of some molecules near the surface causes them to escape into the surrounding air, just as long as there is room for them in the air mixture. Thus, a steady flow of air across the water surface accommodates a continuing flow of escaping water molecules, and *evaporation* progressively reduces the water reservoir (Fig. 1-4, *A*). Another principle of physics provides that heat is required to produce the change in state from liquid to gas that occurs in vaporization; this heat is taken from the air immediately adjacent to the water supply, thereby cooling the air. It is this cooling of vaporization that is responsible for the summer cooling effects of large bodies of water. However, should a cover be placed over the water volume, the air thus trapped over the surface will be filled with all the water vapor molecules it can hold and will be described as *saturated with water vapor.* At this point, vaporization does not stop, but a state of equilibrium is established, in which for every molecule escaping from the water another molecule returns to the reservoir from the overlying saturated air (Fig. 1-4, *B*).

Two factors that influence vaporization are temperature and pressure. Vaporization is directly related to temperature, and this relationship can be viewed from two different directions. First, the warmer the air, the more vapor it can hold. In other words, the *capacity* of air for water vapor increases with temperature. Thus, if warm air passes over a water surface, its greater capacity will permit an increased escape of molecules from the water per unit of time, and evaporation will be hastened. Second, if heat is applied to the volume of water, the kinetic activity of water molecules will be increased and more will escape the surface per unit of time (Fig. 1-4, *C*). If, in this instance, a cover is placed over the heated water, the increased kinetic energy of escaping molecules will force more of them into the trapped air, increasing the saturation of the air with a greater number of molecules under an increased pressure (Fig. 1-4, *D*). Water content of air, or any gas, and its degree of saturation are thus a function of temperature. The influence of pressure on vaporization is an inverse one and is mediated through its action at the water surface. It is convenient to visualize vaporization as the escape of water molecules from the surface against the opposition of adjacent air molecules. As the surrounding air pressure increases or decreases, vaporization will be correspondingly retarded or augmented.

The amount of water in a given mass of air (or any gas) can be recorded in one of three ways.

Absolute humidity. This is a measurement of the content or actual weight of water present in a given volume of air expressed in grams per cubic meter (or pounds per cubic foot or yard). Water may be physically extracted from a known air volume by an absorbing agent and weighed, or it may be computed by meteorologic data according to the techniques of the United States Weather Bureau.[4]

Relative humidity. Frequently used is a comparison of the content of water in a volume of air (absolute humidity) and the amount of water the air can hold at a given temperature if saturated, or its *capacity.* The ratio *content/capacity* is the *relative humidity* (RH) and is reported as a percent. If air contains half the water, at a given temperature, that it has the capacity to contain, the RH equals 50%. Thus, at room temperature, air has a capacity of approximately 18 gm/m^3. If the water content is computed as 12 gm/m^3, the air is thus 67% saturated and its RH equals 67%. Instruments called *hygrometers* allow direct and simple measurement of RH without the necessity of extracting and weighing water content of air samples.

Water vapor pressure. In contrast to other gases in a mixture, partial pressure of water vapor does not depend upon its fractional concentration in the mixture but entirely upon temperature and relative humidity. Actual measurements of water vapor pressure in saturated air have been made over a wide range of temperatures, and their values are available in handbooks of chemical data. The vapor pressure in gas less than saturated is the product of its tension, at a given temperature, times the relative humidity, which must be specified. Thus, at a stated temperature, vapor tension of a gas with 50% RH is one half that of saturated gas. It is important to understand that for specific conditions of humidity and temperature, water vapor pressure is an absolute value, regardless of the concentrations of other gases present. Therefore, the partial pressure of other gases is calculated as the product of their fractional concentrations × [total atmospheric pressure – water vapor pressure (which must be computed first)]. In pulmonary physiology, for the most part, gases are considered to be dry, with no water vapor pressure, or saturated. Appendix 4 is the reproduction of a part of a large table that lists the water vapor tensions of saturated gas within the usual physiologic range of our interest. The column to the right represents, at given temperatures, that portion of any atmospheric pressure due solely to water vapor. Thus, at 25° C, in a gas saturated with water and regardless of other gas concentrations, 23.8 mm Hg of the total P_B is due to the action of water molecules. This principle will be used extensively in the next section.

The *dew point* of air is that temperature at which the air becomes saturated with its contained water vapor. Imagine a water content of air sufficient to comprise a relative humidity of 90% at a given temperature. Should the air temperature drop, the RH with the same content of water will increase since, at lower temperatures, the water *capacity* of the air lessens. A temperature can be reached at which the water content now fully saturates the air, with a RH of 100%; at this point excess water vapor, which the air cannot hold, begins to condense as visible droplets on small objects such as blades of grass. This temperature is the dew point. This phenomenon is frequently observed on cooling iced beverage glasses in warm humid weather. As the temperature of the glass drops, the air adjacent to the glass also cools and finally at the dew point water in the air begins to condense on the glass surface.

When an air mass near the earth's surface reaches its dew point, excess water often precipitates as very fine but visible water particles, so light they remain suspended in air as mist or fog. When larger air masses at higher altitudes are chilled by cold air currents, excess water usually falls out as rain or snow. Urban and industrial contamination of air has produced a mixture of fog and smoke or other vapors, called *smog*, which has important public health significance. Smogs may be held close to the ground by a natural phenomenon called a *temperature inversion* when the air, instead of showing a progressive cooling from the ground up, contains a layer of warm air at heights of from 300 to 3000 feet. In such a state, the air is very quiet, with little or no currents to carry away its contaminants.

To prepare for the specific use (in physiologic calculations) of the characteristics of pressure and humidity just covered, the student must understand some conventions adopted in the interest of uniformity. The following definitions should be learned:

1. Standard temperature and pressure (STP) means 0° C and 760 mm Hg.
2. Body temperature (BT) means 37° C.
3. Ambient temperature or pressure (A) means the existing environmental temperature or pressure (as opposed to standard).
4. Saturated gas (S) means a volume of gas with a relative humidity of 100% at a given temperature.
5. Dry gas (D) means a volume of gas with *no* vapor in it.

The various abbreviations are usually grouped, the following being typical examples frequently used:

1. STPD means a volume of dry gas, at a temperature of 0° C and a P_B of 760 mm Hg.
2. BTPS means a volume of gas saturated with water vapor, at 37° C and the ambient environmental P_B.
3. ATPS means a volume of gas saturated with water vapor at ambient temperature (room temperature) and pressure.

When reporting data on gases for physiologic evaluation, we use the following general rules:

1. Volumes of gases as they exist in the lungs are recorded as BTPS.
2. Gases that undergo chemical reaction in the body, such as those measured in blood samples, are recorded as STPD.
3. If saturated gas volumes are to be used in physiologic calculation, they are first corrected to what their volumes would be if dry, then after the calculation are corrected back to the saturated value. Techniques of such manipulation will be learned in the following pages.

THE GAS LAWS

The physics of the natural laws governing gas behavior is a study of considerable depth, invoking many principles and theories that are beyond the scope of our needs in inhalation therapy. Our prime concern will be consideration of the so-called *gas laws*, which describe the relationships between the interdependent variables of temperature, pressure, volume, and mass of gases. These relationships are often referred to as the *ideal behavior* of gases because they are based on theoretical principles that are valid under limited conditions. Fortunately, however, these limitations apply to the usual physiologic ranges with which we have to contend. The *real behavior* of gases concerns deviations from those relationships that we would expect on the basis of the gas laws, under conditions outside the physiologic range. We will first describe the principles and use of the ideal gas laws and then consider some real characteristics of gases when they are exposed to extremes of temperature and pressure.

The ideal gas laws are widely used in chemistry, physics, and pulmonary physiology and in the latter are most frequently concerned with changes in gas volumes brought about by changes in temperature and pressure. The role played by humidity, we will see, is mediated through its effect on pressure. Clinical pulmonary physiology is vitally interested in various segments of lung volumes and what happens to these volumes with environmental or pathologic changes. It is essential that an effective technician, whether he works in a laboratory or in clinical medicine, understand the fundamentals of the gas laws. In the following definitions and applications of the laws, "temperature" *always* means *absolute temperature* (T, or K, as described earlier).

Boyle's law. If temperature (T) and mass (n, for number of molecules) remain constant, volume (V) varies *inversely* with the pressure. This means that, at a constant temperature and mass, as increasing pressure is applied to a given volume of gas, the volume decreases. Obviously, there must be a limit to the shrinkage of the gas volume, for the mass of gas cannot simply disappear as the pressure increases. Actually, the increments in volume reduction become smaller as the units of pressure increase, until a point is reached at which this reciprocal relationship between pressure and volume no longer exists. At this point, the ideal behavior of the gas ceases, and physical changes in the characteristics of the matter of the gas occur, which will be described later as the real behavior referred to above. It is apparent that the converse response of a volume of gas will accompany a reduction in pressure applied to it. These inverse relationships can be expressed as $PV = k$ (a constant), since for the product to remain stable, if one factor changes, the other must change proportionately in the opposite direction. The illustrations of Fig. 1-2 would depict Boyle's law if we employed some means of maintaining the cylinders at a constant temperature.

Charles' law. If pressure (P) and mass (n) remain constant, volume (V) varies *directly* with changes in the absolute temperature (T). This means that, if a mass of gas is kept under a constant pressure, as the absolute temperature of the gas is increased or decreased, its volume will increase or decrease accordingly. Again, as in Boyle's law, the mass of gas cannot be cooled into nothingness, and at a certain point the ideal behavior ceases and other factors come into play. This direct relationship between temperature and volume can be expressed as $V/T = k$, since for the quotient to remain stable, if one value changes, the other must change proportionately in the same direction.

Gay-Lussac's law. If volume (V) and mass (n) remain constant, the pressure (P) exerted by a gas varies *directly* with the absolute temperature (T) of the gas. This means that, if the volume of a mass of gas is kept unchanged, as the absolute temperature of the gas is increased or decreased, its pressure will increase or decrease accordingly. The linear relationship in Fig. 1-1 shows that, theoretically, with no pressure exerted by a gas at 0° K, changes in pressure are proportional to changes in absolute temperature values and are expressed as $P/T = k$. As might be expected, this relation is valid only in the limited *ideal* range.

The relationship between all three variables can be illustrated in one simultaneous expression by combining PV with V/T and P/T into the single

$$PV/T = k$$

It is evident that the above gas laws apply to a given mass of gas; but we will now consider the effects upon P, V, and T of changes in the number of gas molecules that represent either *weight* (absolute number of molecules), or *density* (number of molecules per unit of volume):

1. If volume and temperature are kept constant, pressure must vary *directly* with a change in number of molecules, a relationship expressed as $P/n = k$.
2. If pressure and temperature are kept constant, volume will also vary *directly* with the number of molecules, as $V/n = k$.
3. If pressure and volume are kept constant, temperature and number of molecules must vary inversely with one another. Thus, since both T and n are directly related to P and V,
   a. An increase in n (more molecules for the same volume, or increased density and weight) will need to be compensated for by decreasing the temperature.
   b. A decrease in n (less molecules for the same volume, or decreased density and weight) will have to be compensated for by increasing the temperature.

Thus, the relationship between temperature and number of gas molecules can be expressed as $Tn = k$. The student can work out for himself a mental picture of the effect of a change in n on P, V, and T individually and will recognize that all the four interacting variables can be combined into the one general equation:

$$\frac{PV}{Tn} = k$$

THE COMBINED GAS LAWS

When gas is subjected to changes in P, V, T, and n, singly or in combination, the total product-quotient of PV/Tn remains unchanged. In effect, these variables represent the *matter* of the gas which is neither increased nor decreased, but rather "redistributed" among the variables. This can be stated as follows:

$$\frac{P_1V_1}{T_1n_1} = \frac{P_2V_2}{T_2n_2}$$

The subscript 1 indicates a *before* value, and 2 an *after*. Thus, the products and quotients of the gas variables before a change in one or more of them must be the same after.

In pulmonary physiology, most of the time we will wish to know how much change there will be in a gas volume if it is subjected to changes in pressure and/or temperature. Since the total mass of gas will not be affected, the quantity *n* can be eliminated from the gas equation, but careful analysis of gas problems is necessary to determine whether such a shortened version of the equation can be used. When the equation is now written as

$$\frac{P_1V_1}{T_1} = \frac{P_2V_2}{T_2}$$

it is apparent that, knowing five of the six factors, we can calculate the sixth by simple algebraic rearrangement to equate the unknown with the known data. We will know the original volume (V_1), the original pressure (P_1), the original temperature (T_1); we will also know the new pressure (P_2) and the new temperature (T_2). We will then rearrange the equation so that our unknown, the new volume (V_2), will equal all of our known values. Thus:

$$V_2 = \frac{V_1 \times P_1 \times T_2}{P_2 \times T_1}$$

By putting the known values in their places in the equation and carrying out the indicated arithmetic, we can easily solve the equation. This procedure is called *correcting* a gas volume for changes in pressure and temperature.

This is the form of the *combined gas laws* that is the basis for most of the gas volume calculations, and it should be *learned* well, not by rote memory but through an understanding of what the equation means. If we examine the equation, we see that the new or corrected gas volume (V_2) is a *proportion* of the original volume (V_1) according to changes in P and T. In fact, the equation as written actually demonstrates Boyle's law:

$$V_1 \times \frac{P_1}{P_2}$$

and Charles' law:

$$V_1 \times \frac{T_2}{T_1}$$

the two gas laws dealing with volume change. We know, from Boyle's law, that if pressure on a gas is increased its volume will decrease. In such an instance, P_2 will be greater than P_1, and in the above equation, since V_1 will be multiplied by a fraction *less* than 1 $\left(\frac{P_1}{P_2}\right)$, V_2 will be reduced. The student can see that the converse is also true and can in a similar manner see how the combined gas laws also uphold Charles' law.

Exercise 1-4. Set up the combined gas laws to solve for the following: (a) P_2, (b) T_1, (c) V_1, (d) T_2, (e) n_2

CORRECTION OF DRY GAS VOLUMES

The following technique is suggested for the student to use in all gas volume calculations to avoid mistakes of omission. When proficiency has been reached, shortcuts to suit individual needs can be employed.

Problem 1. Given 100 ml of dry gas measured at 37° C and 760 mm Hg P_B, what would be its volume at 60° C?

Solution:

$V_1 = 100$	$V_2 = ?$
$P_1 = 760$	$P_2 = 760$
$t_1 = 37$	$t_2 = 60$
$T_1 = 37 + 273 = 310$	$T_2 = 60 + 273 = 333$

$$V_2 = \frac{V_1P_1T_2}{P_2T_1} = \frac{100 \times 760 \times 333}{760 \times 310} = 107.4 \text{ ml}$$

(*Note:* Since $P_1 = P_2$, both *could* have been eliminated from the equation, but it is better for the beginner to include all data.)

Problem 2. Given 100 ml of dry gas measured at 37° C and 760 mm Hg P_B, what would be its volume at 800 mm Hg?

Solution:

$V_1 = 100$	$V_2 = ?$
$P_1 = 760$	$P_2 = 800$
$t_1 = 37$	$t_2 = 37$
$T_1 = 37 + 273 = 310$	$T_2 = 37 + 273 = 310$

$$V_2 = \frac{V_1P_1T_2}{P_2T_1} = \frac{100 \times 760 \times 310}{800 \times 310} = 95 \text{ ml}$$

Problem 3. Given 100 ml of dry gas at 37° C and 760 mm Hg, what would be its volume at 60° C and 800 mm Hg?

Solution:

$V_1 = 100$	$V_2 = ?$
$P_1 = 760$	$P_2 = 800$
$t_1 = 37$	$t_2 = 60$
$T_1 = 310$	$T_2 = 333$

$$V_2 = \frac{V_1P_1T_2}{P_2T_1} = \frac{100 \times 760 \times 333}{800 \times 310} = 102 \text{ ml}$$

Exercise 1-5. Convert the following dry gas volumes, as indicated (to 3 digits):

(a) 150 ml at 25° C and 752 mm Hg, to 0° C
(b) 2.5 liters at 18° C and 762 mm Hg, to 748 mm Hg
(c) 325 ml at 20° C and 770 mm Hg, to 37° C and 760 mm Hg
(d) 22.4 liters at 15° C and 730 mm Hg, to 5° C and 755 mm Hg
(e) 95 ml at 28° C and 784 mm Hg, to 20° C and 768 mm Hg

CORRECTION OF GAS VOLUMES CONTAINING WATER VAPOR

Most physiologic gas volume calculations involve gases saturated with water vapor and require correction of volumes from the saturated state to the dry, or the reverse. The student will find it helpful to keep in mind that, since water vapor is in essence a space-occupying gas in a mixture of gases, its removal from a gas volume will shrink the volume and its addition will increase the volume. Thus, in the examples and exercises to follow, whenever a volume of gas saturated with water vapor is to have its volume calculated to what it would be in the dry state (corrected from saturated to dry), the dry volume will be smaller, *unless* other conditions of pressure and temperature counteract the shrinkage. Conversely, correcting from dry to saturated will give a larger volume.

It is emphasized that, in gas volume calculations, the *amount* of water vapor in saturated gas is thought of in terms of the partial pressure it exerts at a given temperature rather than its fractional concentration. The partial pressure of water vapor exerts its influence on gas volumes through its effect on the total gas pressure and slightly modifies the application of Boyle's law. Consider a pressure of 760 mm Hg being exerted on (or by) a volume of dry air and a volume of saturated air. The pressure of 760 mm Hg is actually the *sum* of the partial pressures of the air gases plus that of water vapor. In dry air, the air gases represent the total pressure of 760 mm Hg, whereas in saturated air, the air gases represent the total pressure *minus* the partial pressure of water vapor at the ambient temperature. For convenience, we might refer to atmospheric pressure as being corrected for water vapor and designate it as P_c. Thus, $P_c = (P - P_{H_2O} \text{ at } t)$, where P is the total atmospheric pressure, t the ambient temperature, and P_{H_2O} the value in the right column of the table in Appendix 4. Boyle's law can now be expressed as follows:

$$V_2 = \frac{V_1 \times (P_1 - P_{1H_2O} \text{ at } t_1)}{(P_2 - P_{2H_2O} \text{ at } t_2)} = \frac{V_1 \times P_{1c}}{P_{2c}}$$

Study of this form of Boyle's law will demonstrate that, if V_1 is dry gas, V_2 is saturated gas, and pressure and temperatures remain unchanged, P_{1c} will be larger than P_{2c}, thus making V_2 larger than V_1. This is *expected*, since it is the same as adding moisture to a volume of gas, then calculating the new volume. Use of the *corrected pressure* in Boyle's law simultaneously adjusts for changes in both pressure and humidity. The format for arranging data as demonstrated above will be modified a bit to accommodate water vapor effect:

V_1	= initial volume	V_2	= final volume
P_1	= initial pressure	P_2	= final pressure
t_1	= initial temperature	t_2	= final temperature
P_{1H_2O}	= partial pressure of water vapor at t_1	P_{2H_2O}	= partial pressure of water vapor at t_2
P_{1c}	= corrected initial pressure $= P_1 - P_{1H_2O}$	P_{2c}	= corrected final pressure $= P_2 - P_{2H_2O}$
T_1	$= t_1 + 273$	T_2	$= t_2 + 273$

$$V_2 = \frac{V_1 \times P_{1c} \times T_2}{P_{2c} \times T_1}$$

The following examples illustrate the ease with which the combined gas laws can make corrections for changes in any or all of the variables of pressure, temperature, and water vapor.

Problem 1. Given 100 ml of saturated gas at 760 mm Hg and 25° C, what would be its volume if dry at the same pressure and temperature?

Solution:

$V_1 = 100$		$V_2 = ?$
$P_1 = 760$		$P_2 = 760$
$t_1 = 25$		$t_2 = 25$
$P_{1H_2O} = 23.8$		$P_{2H_2O} = 0$
$P_{1c} = 736.2$		$P_{2c} = 760$
$T_1 = 298$		$T_2 = 298$

$$V_2 = \frac{V_1 P_{1c} T_2}{P_{2c} T_1} = \frac{100 \times 736.2 \times 298}{760 \times 298} = 96.8 \text{ ml}$$

Problem 2. Given 100 ml of saturated gas at 760 mm Hg and 25° C, what would be its volume saturated at the same pressure and 37° C?

Solution:

$V_1 = 100$		$V_2 = ?$
$P_1 = 760$		$P_2 = 760$
$t_1 = 25$		$t_2 = 37$
$P_{1H_2O} = 23.8$		$P_{2H_2O} = 47$
$P_{1c} = 736.2$		$P_{2c} = 713$
$T_1 = 298$		$T_2 = 310$

$$V_2 = \frac{V_1 P_{1c} T_2}{P_{2c} T_1} = \frac{100 \times 736.2 \times 310}{713 \times 298} = 107.5 \text{ ml}$$

Problem 3. Given 100 ml of saturated gas at 754 mm Hg and 20° C, what would be its volume as dry gas at 764 mm Hg and 37° C?

Solution:

$V_1 = 100$		$V_2 = ?$
$P_1 = 754$		$P_2 = 764$
$t_1 = 20$		$t_2 = 37$
$P_{1H_2O} = 17.5$		$P_{2H_2O} = 0$
$P_{1c} = 736.5$		$P_{2c} = 764$
$T_1 = 293$		$T_2 = 310$

$$V_2 = \frac{V_1 P_{1c} T_2}{P_{2c} T_1} = \frac{100 \times 736.5 \times 310}{764 \times 293} = 102.1 \text{ ml}$$

Problem 4. Given 100 ml of saturated gas at 754 mm Hg and 20° C, what would be its volume saturated at 764 mm Hg and 37° C?

Solution:

$V_1 = 100$		$V_2 = ?$
$P_1 = 754$		$P_2 = 764$
$t_1 = 20$		$t_2 = 37$
$P_{1H_2O} = 17.5$		$P_{2H_2O} = 47$
$P_{1c} = 736.5$		$P_{2c} = 717$
$T_1 = 293$		$T_2 = 310$

$$V_2 = \frac{V_1 P_{1c} T_2}{P_{2c} T_1} = \frac{100 \times 736.5 \times 310}{717 \times 293} = 108.5 \text{ ml}$$

Exercise 1-6. Correct the following gas volumes:

(a) 250 ml, saturated at 750 mm Hg and 20° C, to saturated at 764 mm Hg and 25° C
(b) 1.75 liters, dry at 752 mm Hg and 26° C, to saturated at 770 mm Hg and 33° C
(c) 58 ml, saturated at 748 mm Hg and 21° C, to dry at 730 mm Hg and 30° C

(d) 430 ml BTPS at 766 mm Hg, to STPD
(e) 2.28 liters, saturated at 1006 mb and 72° F, to saturated at 1022 mb and 90° F

CORRECTION OF BAROMETRIC READING

Because the barometer is composed of brass, it reacts by expansion and contraction to ambient temperature changes. Even more important, the column of mercury not only responds to atmospheric pressure changes but, like a large thermometer, is significantly affected by temperature. Thus, when we read the mercury level of a barometer, we see the effects of both pressure and temperature. For accuracy in assessing the effects of pressure on gas volume, we must correct our *observed* reading for changes in the mercury column due to temperature. A formula based upon expansion coefficients of brass and mercury at given temperatures is the basis for a table of correction factors prepared by the United States Weather Bureau and reproduced in part in Appendix 5 for the pressures and temperatures most frequently encountered. The table values are *subtracted* from the observed reading. At 30° C, an observed barometric reading of 750 mm Hg would be corrected for temperature by subtracting 3.66 from 750 for a corrected reading of 746.34, rounded off usually to 746.3 or even 746, depending upon degree of accuracy desired. For P_B's between those tabulated, interpolation is used. The correction factor for 764 mm Hg at 25° C is 3.09 + 0.4 of the difference between 3.09 and 3.13, or 3.11 rounded off. From a practical point of view, under usual circumstances the only temperature variations effecting barometric reading are those of the room housing the barometer. Since it is unlikely that the temperature of the average laboratory would exceed seasonal ranges of 60° F to 80° F (16° C to 27° C), or the P_B range 740 to 780 mm Hg, the correction factors would usually be between 1.9 and 3.4.

When given a problem in gas volume correction, the student may assume the barometric value to be a corrected one unless the data specify an *observed* reading. In fact, in any circumstance in which P_B is not specified, it is taken to be 760 mm Hg. However, suppose we are asked to correct a volume of a patient's exhaled air, at an *observed* P_B of 753 mm Hg, with a room temperature of 21° C, to STPD. Our *first* step is to correct the observed pressure for room temperature effect and to record the corrected pressure as P_1 in our listed data. The 760 mm Hg of the STPD needs no correction, because it is a *stated* value, not observed. Thus our data would read:

V_1	=	V_2	=
P_1	= 751.8	P_2	= 760
t_1	= 21	t_2	= 0
P_{1H_2O}	= 18.7	P_{2H_2O}	= 0
P_{1c}	= 733.1	P_{2c}	= 760
T_1	= 294	T_2	= 273

On the other hand, to make a somewhat exaggerated example, if a volume of gas were collected under one set of observed P_B and ambient temperature and we were asked to calculate its volume at a different observed P_B and temperature, both P_1 and P_2 would be corrected values for their respective temperatures. If the principles of correction are understood, the student can reason out the proper calculation procedure for any combination of data, no matter how bizarre.

Exercise 1-7. Set up the final formula to correct V_1 to V_2 according to the following conditions of observed pressures (correct P_B to one decimal place only):

(a) Dry, 730 mm Hg, 30° C to saturated, 730 mm Hg, 30° C
(b) Saturated, 750 mm Hg, 24° C to saturated, 760 mm Hg, 24° C
(c) Saturated, 744 mm Hg, 20° C to dry, 744 mm Hg, 25° C
(d) Dry, 756 mm Hg, 15° C to saturated 738 mm Hg, 22° C
(e) Dry, 766 mm Hg, 24° C to dry, 738 mm Hg, 30° C

THE USE OF FACTORS IN GAS VOLUME CALCULATIONS

Factors are constant values, such as the product-quotients of data that are always present in a certain calculation. Thus, instead of doing the individual arithmetic for each calculation, we use prepared factors. In gas volume determinations, three frequently encountered computations are (1) correction from ATPS to BTPS, (2) correction from ATPS to STPD, and (3) correction from STPD to BTPS. For each of these there are factors available that materially reduce the amount of arithmetic needed, and because the student should understand the derivation of these shortcut agents, they will be described individually.

Factors to correct volumes from ATPS to BTPS. The values in the first column of Appendix 4, when multiplied by V_1, will, in one simple step, correct a gas volume from ATPS to BTPS. Actually, the factors give a very close approximation because, as the footnote to the table explains, all the factors are based on a P_B of 760 mm Hg. Although the answer obtained using a factor might differ from one derived from detailed calculations, the discrepancy is usually small. Derivation of the factors can be illustrated by an example. Let us correct a volume of gas (V_1) saturated at 760 mm Hg and 25° C, to saturated at 760 mm Hg and 37° C (ATPS to BTPS).

V_1	=	V_2	=
P_1	= 760	P_2	= 760
t_1	= 25	t_2	= 37
P_{1H_2O}	= 23.8	P_{2H_2O}	= 47
P_{1c}	= 736.2	P_{2c}	= 713
T_1	= 298	T_2	= 310

$$V_2 = \frac{V_1P_{1c}T_2}{P_{2c}T_1} = \frac{V_1 \times 736.2 \times 310}{713 \times 298} = V_1 \times 1.075$$

Note that the product-quotient for the pressure, temperature, and humidity corrections equals 1.075, the same value found in Appendix 4 corresponding to a gas temperature of 25° C. The student is urged to work out one or two more of these factors in a similar manner, to fix the principle in his mind. If, in the example above, P_1 were 752 mm Hg and P_2 were 758 mm Hg and the calculation were done by the detailed method, the value by which V_1 would be multiplied would be *1.066*. The decision whether to sacrifice accuracy for expediency is usually determined by each individual or laboratory according to needs and objectives.

Factors to correct volumes from ATPS to STPD. Factors of Appendix 6, when multiplied by V_1, will correct V_1 from ATPS to STPD. It is emphasized that the barometric readings of the left column are *observed* values, *not* corrected for temperature. In other words, to use this table, we must use the direct reading from the barometer since the factors *include* temperature adjustment. Let us correct a saturated gas volume at an observed P_B of 770 mm Hg and a room temperature of 20° C to dry gas at 760 mm Hg and 0° C. The first step is to correct 770 mm Hg for 20° C to 767.5 mm Hg. Our data are thus:

$$
\begin{array}{ll@{\qquad}ll}
V_1 & = & V_2 & = \\
P_1 & = 767.5 & P_2 & = 760 \\
t_1 & = 20 & t_2 & = 0 \\
P_{1H_2O} & = 17.5 & P_{2H_2O} & = 0 \\
P_{1c} & = 750 & P_{2c} & = 760 \\
T_1 & = 293 & T_2 & = 273
\end{array}
$$

$$V_2 = \frac{V_1 P_{1c} T_2}{P_{2c}} = \frac{V_1 \times 750 \times 273}{760 \times 293} = V_1 \times 0.919$$

The tabular factor for 770 mm Hg and 20° C is likewise 0.919.

Factors to correct volumes from STPD to BTPS. Factors for this conversion are given in Appendix 7. With ambient pressure as the only variable to consider, the factor for correction to an ambient pressure of 750 mm Hg is derived as follows:

$$
\begin{array}{ll@{\qquad}ll}
V_1 & = & V_2 & = \\
P_1 & = 760 & P_2 & = 750 \\
t_1 & = 0 & t_2 & = 37 \\
P_{1H_2O} & = 0 & P_{2H_2O} & = 47 \\
P_{1c} & = 760 & P_{2c} & = 703 \\
T_1 & = 273 & T_2 & = 310
\end{array}
$$

$$V_2 = \frac{V_1 P_{1c} T_2}{P_{2c}} = \frac{V_1 \times 760 \times 310}{703 \times 273} = V_1 \times 1.227$$

The tabular factor for 750 mm Hg is likewise 1.227.

CALCULATIONS INVOLVING WEIGHT AND DENSITY OF GAS

Gas problems dependent upon variations in weight and density of gases are frequently encountered in chemistry and physics, although rarely in pulmonary physiology. Still, the student should learn how to use the general gas laws equation to solve such problems. It was indicated earlier that the *n* in the gas laws equation refers to numbers of gas molecules, representing gas weight or density. When analyzing a problem involving weight or density, the student will find it helpful to remember that at P_B of 760 mm Hg and 273°K, 1 gmw of a gas occupies 22.4 liters. With a little practice, he will learn how to combine his data to get the desired information. The following examples will illustrate the handling of a few simple, typical problems.

Problem 1. If the density of oxygen is 1.43 gm/liter at 0° C and 1 atm, what is its density at 20° C and 720 mm Hg? (*Note:* Although volume is not mentioned, it is implied in the use of the term *density*, gm/liter. Thus, $V_1 = V_2$ and need not be considered.)

Solution:

$V_1 =$ | $V_2 =$
$P_1 = 760$ | $P_2 = 720$
$T_1 = 273$ | $T_2 = 293$
$n_1 =$ 1.43 gm/liter | $n_2 =$? gm/liter

$$n_2 = \frac{n_1 \times P_2 \times T_1}{P_1 \times T_2} = \frac{1.43 \times 720 \times 273}{760 \times 293} = 1.26 \text{ gm/liter}$$

Problem 2. What volume will be occupied by 2.35 gm of SO_2 at 25° C and 750 mm Hg? (*Note:* The *before* values will be the volume occupied by 1 gmw at STP, to permit the setting of a ratio.)

Solution:

$V_1 =$ 22.4 liters | $V_2 =$? liters
$P_1 = 760$ | $P_2 = 750$
$T_1 = 273$ | $T_2 = 298$
$n_1 =$ 64 gm | $n_2 =$ 2.35 gm

$$V_2 = \frac{V_1 \times P_1 \times T_2 \times n_2}{P_2 \times T_1 \times n_1} = \frac{22.4 \times 760 \times 298 \times 2.35}{750 \times 273 \times 64} = 0.910 \text{ liter}$$

Problem 3. How many grams of air will a 500 liter tank hold if it is filled to 3 atm at 15° C? Assume the gmw of air to be 29. (*Note:* $n_1 =$ density $\times 500 = [29/22.4] \times 500 = 647$ gm)

Solution:

$V_1 =$ 500 liters | $V_2 =$ 500 liters
$P_1 = 1$ | $P_2 = 3$
$T_1 = 273$ | $T_2 = 288$
$n_1 =$ 647 gm | $n_2 =$? gm

$$n_2 = \frac{n_1 \times P_2 \times T_1}{P_1 \times T_2} = \frac{647 \times 3 \times 273}{1 \times 288} = 1840 \text{ gm}$$

In the interest of economizing on time and space, a detailed description of the *molar gas constant* will not be undertaken here. It is a numerical value of the constant of the ratio $PV/nT = k$, where n is in number of moles of gas and V is 22.4 liters at 1 atm and 273° K. For respiratory physiologic use of the gas laws, the molar gas constant is less meaningful than is the tabular system explained on the preceding pages. Once the present technique is mastered, however, the student may find it of interest to study the molar constant and increase his breadth of knowledge of this aspect of physics.

PROPERTIES OF GASES AT EXTREME TEMPERATURES AND PRESSURES

Having covered the ideal gas laws in some detail, we understand the theoretical response of gases to changes in pressure, volume, temperature, and density; we will now consider variations from such relationships as gases are subjected to both low temperatures and high pressures, revealing their *real* characteristics. This will prepare the student for his exposure to the commercially prepared gases with which he will treat patients.

We are familiar with the tremendous kinetic activity of gaseous molecules, a force that permits a mass of gas to distribute itself in an increasing volume of space or, lacking the freedom of mobility, to keep up a steady pressure in its restraint. Opposing the kinetic action of the molecules is another force, called *van der Waals force,* which consists of an attraction between the molecules, tending to draw them together. Although it is independent of temperature, the effectiveness of van der Waals forces is related to both temperature and pressure. For example, at a high temperature the increased kinetic molecular activity far overshadows the van der Waals energy, rendering the latter relatively impotent, whereas at very low temperatures the resulting decrease in kinetic action makes the molecules much more responsive to mutual attraction. By the same token, low pressures exerted on a gas permit the molecules to move freely of their own kinetic volition with little influence by attractive forces, in contrast to the molecular crowding of high pressures, which permits greater increase in the van der Waals effect. In addition to the attractive force between gas molecules, another factor that influences the relation between pressure and volume is attributed to the space occupied by the molecules themselves. Under moderate to low pressures exerted on a given container full of gas, the total mass of matter of the wide-ranging molecules is but a negligible fraction of the total volume of the gas. As the volume is reduced by increasing pressure, however, the resulting molecular density, which is not compressible, comprises a proportionately larger portion of the overall gas volume, disturbing the volume response to pressure predicted by the ideal gas laws.

We can summarize these observations by generalizing that at very low temperatures and/or very high pressures gases deviate in their behavioral patterns as predicted by the classical gas laws, because of the influence of the van der Waals intermolecular attractive force and the volume of compressed gas molecules. Our purposes do not justify pursuing the details of such phenomena further since, in clinical practice, the simple ideal gas laws are sufficiently accurate. For those scientists and technicians whose work requires maximum precision, there is available a modification of Boyle's law that includes correction for the van der Waals effect and density of molecules; and handbooks of chemistry and physics have prepared tables of constants to facilitate such calculations for a wide variety of gases. We will, however, be interested in the effects of excessive temperatures and pressures on the *state* of gases, since those we use may be in liquid or solid forms as well as gaseous. The most familiar example of the three states of matter is that of water, which we know as a solid (ice), gas (vapor), and liquid. Before discussing the state of matter in relation to therapeutic gases, we must deviate slightly to describe and define some physical terms that will make it easier to understand the interesting characteristics of prepared gases. Although we are familiar with the concepts of gas pressure and temperature as functions of kinetic activity, we have not learned the physical units by which heat (energy) is expressed.

Units of heat

Calorie (cal). The quantity of heat required to raise the temperature of 1 gm of water from 14.5° C to 15.5° C is used as the standard and is called a *calorie*. In general use the definition simply describes the amount of heat necessary to raise the temperature of 1 gm of water 1° C. For convenience, in dealing with large quantities, the term "large calorie (Cal)" is sometimes used and is equal to 1000 calories. If it is desired to calculate the heat produced by a chemical reaction, for example, the ingredients are placed in the reaction chamber of an instrument called a *calorimeter.* The heat of the chemical reaction is absorbed by a carefully weighed mass of water surrounding the reaction chamber, and the temperature change in the water is precisely measured. The weight of water in grams multiplied by the Celsius rise in temperature calculates the total calories produced, which can then be expressed as so many calories per unit of weight of the reacting substances. The exact structure of a calorimeter is dependent upon the use to which it is put, but the principle always involves the transfer of heat to a measured mass of water.

British thermal unit (Btu). This is the English measurement system counterpart of the calorie and is the amount of heat required to raise the temperature of 1 lb of water 1° F. One Btu is equal to 252 calories. Generally, science uses the calorie unit of heat expression, consistent with the use of other metric measurements, but engineering and commerce employ the Btu along with other elements of the English system. This unfortunate dichotomy of standards places a burden on the inhalation therapist, who must be familiar with both systems, for his work involves contact with scientific data and the metric system, on the one hand, and commercial gases and other equipment standardized in the English system, on the other.

Heat capacity. This refers to the number of calories required to raise the temperature of 1 gm of a substance 1° C, or 1 lb of a substance 1° F. By definition, the heat capacity of water is 1 calorie in the metric system and 1 Btu in the English system.

Specific heat. This value is a *ratio* between the amount of heat required to raise the temperature of 1 gm of a substance 1° C, or 1 lb of a substance 1° F, at a specific temperature, and the amount of heat required to raise the temperature of 1 gm of water 1° C, or 1 lb of water 1° F, at the specified temperature. Numerically, specific heat is equal to heat capacity, in either of the systems, but because it is a ratio, it is a pure number with no inherent dimensions and has the same meaning in any system of units.

For example, the specific heat of hydrogen, measured at 1 atm and 21° C (70° F) is 3.41. This means that:

$$\frac{\text{Heat required to raise 1 gm } H_2 \text{ 1° C, or 1 lb } H_2 \text{ 1° F, at a given temperature}}{\text{Heat required to raise 1 gm } H_2O \text{ 1° C, or 1 lb } H_2O \text{ 1° F, at a given temperature}} = 3.41$$

Thus, it takes 3.41 times as much heat to elevate the gas temperature as that of the water—3.41 calories for 1 gm of gas as against 1 calorie for 1 gm of water, or 3.41 Btu per pound of gas as against 1 Btu for 1 lb of water.

Because specific heat is among the data frequently provided for medical and commercial gases, special mention should be made of the two ways in which it can be measured. First, the specific heat can be calculated by heating a *constant volume* of a gas, in which case the heat energy applied is transformed into increasing molecular energy. Second, the heated gas may be kept at a *constant pressure,* as in a flexible container, and in this instance, because the expanding gas performs work (uses up heat) in displacing the surrounding atmosphere, more energy is required to bring the gas to the specific temperature. Thus, a gas has two specific heats, that of constant pressure (C_p) being larger than that of constant volume (C_v). In the example of hydrogen, cited above, 3.41 is the constant pressure value, whereas at constant temperature its specific heat is 2.40.

Finally, among the specifications of a given gas, the specific heat may be listed as Btu/(lb-mole)(°F), or less frequently as cal/(gm-mole)(°C). This merely gives the heat value for a pound-molecular weight, or a gram-molecular weight, instead of the value for a pound or a gram. If we wish to convert the figure to a simpler pound or gram relation, it need only be divided by the molecular weight of the gas. Expressed as pound mole or gram mole specific heat, hydrogen would be 6.89 or 3.41 times 2.02 (molecular weight of hydrogen).

Change of state

Because all matter can change its state under certain conditions, theoretically it should be considered as nonspecific or labile in its physical characteristics. However, our familiarity with the usual forms of matter, as we encounter them in daily activities, endows them with a fixed physical state. In inhalation therapy we deal with the so-called *permanent gases,* because in our contact with them they are in the gaseous state. Yet, these same gases can just as well be liquid or solid, depending upon the pressures or temperatures to which they are exposed, and in the interest of economy and ease of transportation and storage, it is often convenient to transform an otherwise "permanent" gas into the liquid or solid state. The therapist should understand the basic thermodynamics of changes of state of those substances he uses as therapeutic gases as well as he understands the function and performance of his mechanical equipment. This means that he must understand the terms and expressions used to describe the specifications of commercially prepared gases, so we will start with a basic term that will lead us into a sequential discussion of the thermal and pressure characteristics of the various states of matter.

If we were to consider the three states of a given substance and on the same graph were to plot individually the various combinations of temperature, in °C, and pressure, in atmospheres, at which the liquid form of the substance and its vapor could transform, one into the other—the solid and the liquid, and the solid and the vapor (sublimation)—three lines would be generated that would intersect at one point. This plot of temperature and pressure is called the *triple point.* The significance of this point is that it is the only combination of temperature and pressure that allows the solid, liquid, and vapor forms of a given substance to exist in equilibrium with one another. Every substance has its own triple point, but Fig. 1-5 is a schematic noncalibrated example of the triple point of water. AB plots the boiling points of water at various pressures or, to look at it another way, the saturated vapor pressure at different temperatures. This emphasizes the relationship between increasing pressure and increasing boiling points of water. AB terminates at the so-called *critical point,* which will be described below. Segment AD represents the conditions for water to *sublime,* or pass directly from the solid state (ice) to vapor, or back. AC relates the transition points between ice and liquid water, the melting (or freezing) points. The steepness of AC indicates the relatively small effect exerted by pressure on melting or freezing points. At any plot of pressure and temperature that falls within the confines of CAB, water can exist *only* as a liquid. Similarly, below DAB, pressures are too low for water to be anything other than gaseous. However, it should be noted that if the temperature is above the triple point an elevation of pressure would transform the vapor into a liquid, and if below this point, directly into ice. DAC delineates the pressure-temperature conditions necessary for the formation of ice. Thus, at all points along each line, two phases of matter exist in complete equilibrium, but only at the triple point do all three equilibrate

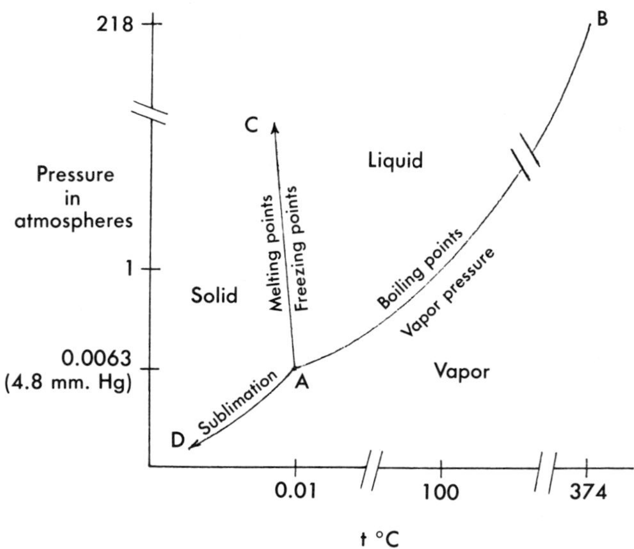

Fig. 1-5. The intersection of the three lines at *A* represents the *triple point* of water. Thus, at a temperature of 0.01° C and a pressure of 4.8 mm Hg, the three states of water (ice, liquid, and vapor) exist in equilibrium. The graphs show the temperature-pressure relationships of boiling, freezing, and sublimation of water.

simultaneously. It should be noted that if the pressure on a volume of water is reduced from 1 atm (760 mm Hg) to 0.0063 atm (4.8 mm Hg) the boiling point of water will drop from 100° C to almost 0° C; but because the reduced pressure slightly alters the melting point of ice (freezing point of water), the lines intersect at 0.01° C. Therefore, at a pressure of 4.8 mm Hg and a temperature of 0.01° C, ice, water, and water vapor coexist in equilibrium, not in a static state but actively, as molecules of the substance (water) transform themselves from one form to the other forms. To appreciate the wide variation in range of triple points, note that the value for Freon-14 is −184° C and 0.88 mm Hg whereas that of krypton is −157° C and 548 mm Hg.

We will now consider the following specific changes in state: solid to liquid and reverse, liquid to vapor and reverse, and solid to vapor and reverse. The student must always bear in mind that such changes are made only at the expense of energy, this energy being supplied by heat that is either given or taken by the matter undergoing change.

Solid to liquid and liquid to solid. A solid will convert to its liquid form at a given temperature known as its *melting point.* The range of melting points is vast, as carbon has a melting point in excess of 3500° C and helium less than −272.2° C. Melting is little affected by pressure, as noted in the example of water, in Fig. 1-5. In order to energize molecules from the fixed immobile (but not motionless) state of a solid into the more freely mobile fluid state, heat is required, which may be applied to the substance or may be extracted by the substance from its surroundings. Thus, with a melting point high above ambient, much heat must be applied to melt a mass of lead, but ice will extract heat from the atmosphere to fuel its transformation into liquid.

The heat needed to melt a substance is referred to as the *heat of fusion* (sometimes called the latent heat of fusion) and is defined as the calories required to change 1 gm of the substance, or the Btu to change 1 lb of the substance, from the solid to the liquid state without changing its temperature. It is called *latent* because at a specific temperature, the melting point, the energy of the applied heat is utilized to effect the molecular change from solid to fluid and does not change the temperature of the mass. Only after the change of state has taken place does continued heat elevate the temperature of the newly formed liquid. Fig. 1-6 depicts the melting point of a solid mass to which heat is being applied. The solid is heated from A to B, with a simultaneous rise in temperature, but at B liquefaction begins and from B to C the temperature of the matter does not vary as the heat energy is utilized in the physical change. After melting is complete, at C, continued heat raises the temperature of the liquid from C to D. The temperature at BC is the melting point of the substance. Although pressure has little influence on melting, for the sake of uniformity scientific tables often report heats of fusion at the triple points. Thus the latent heat of fusion of ice is 80 cal/gm, calcium chloride 54 cal/gm, oxygen 3.3 cal/gm, and argon 6.7 cal/gm, to give some idea of the diversity of energy needed for this change in state.

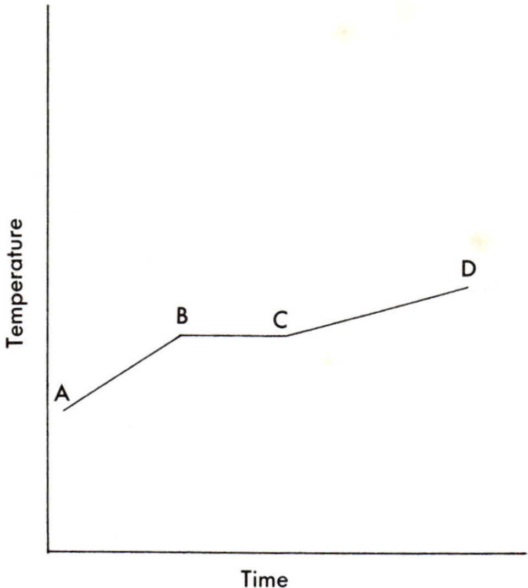

Fig. 1-6. *Heat of fusion* is illustrated by the temperature-time graph. Heat applied to a solid raises its temperature from *A* to *B;* at *B*, the solid begins to liquefy (melt). From *B* to *C*, the applied heat is utilized to accomplish the change in state, and the temperature of the substance does not rise further until liquefaction is complete, *C* to *D*.

Freezing is the reverse of melting, with the conversion of a liquid form into solid. Because considerable energy is utilized in transforming a solid into liquid, this "stored" energy is released during the process of freezing, so that, in a sense, freezing is a heating process in that the freezing liquid must give up heat (by being exposed to cold) as its molecules assume the stable configuration of a solid mass. Thus, for pure substances freezing and melting points are concurrent. In common usage, the transition point between solid and liquid forms is called the freezing point, for matter that is usually in liquid state, and the melting point, for matter that is usually in solid state; i.e., water freezes at 0° C, whereas lead melts at 327° C.

Liquid to vapor and vapor to liquid. These interchanges of physical states are the most relevant to our interest in therapeutic gases, and we have already considered in some detail the mechanism of simple evaporation as the escape of molecules from a liquid surface to mix with the ambient gases immediately adjacent to the surface. Maximum change of state from liquid to vapor (vaporization), however, occurs through the phenomenon of boiling, which differs significantly from evaporation. In the latter, water molecules diffuse into and become a part of ambient gases, whereas the vapor released by boiling escapes with sufficient force to displace, by pushing back, the surrounding gas. Also, whereas simple evaporation is purely a surface activity, boiling produces large bubbles of vapor throughout the depth of the liquid, which rise to the surface to escape. Boiling occurs at the *boiling point,* a temperature at which the vapor pressure of a liquid equals the pressure exerted on the liquid by the ambient gases, and it is influenced by two important factors. First, the boiling point is directly related to the pressure exerted on the surface of the liquid. The greater the pressure applied by ambient molecules, the greater must be the kinetic energy of the fluid molecules to escape against the pressure, energy that can only come from increasing heat. On the other hand, lower ambient pressures allow the easier escape of molecules, and boiling can occur at much lower temperatures. Second, dissolved substances exert a cohesive force that increases the bonding among the molecules so that greater heat energy is required to free them into the vapor state, elevating the boiling point. Although we are accustomed to associate the phenomenon of boiling with high temperatures, such as water at 100° C (212° F), the boiling points of the liquid state of substances we call gases have exceedingly low values. For example, whereas tungsten boils at 5900° C, neon boils at −246° C, ozone at −112° C, and oxygen at −183° C.

Just as energy is needed to liquefy a solid, so is it required to vaporize a liquid, and this energy is called the *heat of vaporization* (sometimes the latent heat of vaporization, or simply the latent heat). It is defined as the calories required to vaporize 1 gm of a liquid, or the Btu to vaporize 1 lb of a liquid, at its normal boiling point. When water is put on a stove to boil, its temperature rises steadily until the boiling point is reached, and then it maintains a constant temperature even though heat continues to enter it. This undetectable or "latent" heat reflects the energy necessary to release the forces holding together water molecules, freeing them to become vapor. It is interesting to note that the heat of vaporization for water is 540 cal/gm, at 100° C, considerably higher than the heat of fusion of ice. This pointedly demonstrates that more energy is required to free water molecules into the vapor state than to rearrange them from the solid to the liquid state.

The therapist will often see the latent heat (of vaporization) listed in the specifications of commercial gases as Btu/lb-mole. For example, the latent heat of methane (CH_4, mol wt 16.04) is given as 3519 Btu/lb-mole, at its normal boiling point of −258.6° F (−126° C). This means that to convert 16.04 lbs of methane (1 lb-mol wt) from a liquid to a gas, 3519 Btu of heat must be supplied, and since *latent heat* refers to the heat required to change 1 lb or 1 gm of substance, the above value can be reduced to the basic units of both the English and metric systems as follows:

(1) $\frac{\text{Btu/lb-mole}}{\text{gmw}} = \text{Btu/lb}$ $\qquad \frac{3519}{16.04} = 219\ \text{Btu/lb}$

(2) Because 1 Btu = 252 calories and 1 lb = 454 gm:

$$\frac{\text{Btu/lb-mole} \times 252}{454} = \text{Btu/lb-mole} \times 0.554$$

$$= \text{cal/gm-mole} \qquad 3519 \times 0.554 = 1950\ \text{cal/gm-mole}$$

(3) $\frac{\text{Btu/lb-mole} \times 0.554}{\text{gmw}} = \text{cal/gm}$ $\qquad \frac{3519 \times 0.554}{16.04} = 122\ \text{cal/gm}$

For every liquid there is a temperature above which the kinetic energy of the molecules is so great that the attractive forces cannot maintain them in a liquid state. This temperature is called the *critical temperature*. Because above this temperature there is no pressure able to maintain the molecules of the matter in a liquid state, the critical temperature is the highest temperature at which a substance can exist as a liquid. If an evacuated sealed tube partially filled with liquid is heated, vapor will escape into the vacuum. The density of the vapor will steadily increase as that of the liquid substance decreases, and when the critical temperature of the liquid is reached, the densities of both vapor and the remaining liquid will be equal and the two phases of matter will become identical without a line of demarcation between them. Further elevation of the temperature will transform the entire mass into vapor. The pressure exerted by the vapor within the evacuated tube at the critical temperature is the *critical pressure*, and on a plotted vapor pressure–temperature curve, the two values identify what is known as the *critical point*. Each substance has its own critical point, at which the gas phase is in equilibrium with the liquid phase and the two are not visibly separated. Attention is drawn to point B on the graph of the triple point, Fig. 1-5. This represents the critical point of water, at a pressure of 218 atm and a temperature of 374° C. Here, the densities of the liquid and vapor phases are indistinguishable, the two are in equilibrium, and beyond this temperature no pressure alone can revert the mass to liquid. Compare the high values for water with the critical values of the gases in Table 1-4.

From a point of view of academic interest only, we can use the concept of critical temperature to differentiate between the terms *gas* and *vapor*, although in practice we use them synonymously. Gas may be considered to be a substance with a critical temperature so low, or a critical pressure so high, that at usual ambient conditions it cannot exist as a liquid with a surface exposed to the atmosphere. On the other hand, a vapor may be described as molecular emanations from a substance with a critical temperature so high that it exists in liquid form at atmospheric pressure. The first group is composed of those substances that we have been referring to as *permanent gases*.

Although we have described the critical points of matter in terms of the stability of liquids, it should be evident that they apply as readily to the transition of gas to liquid. To effect a change of state from gas to liquid, we must cool the gas below its critical temperature and then compress it. Theoretically, it is possible to liquefy a gas by cooling alone, dropping its temperature below

Table 1-4. *Critical points of three gases*

	°C	°F	*atm*
Helium	−267.9	−450.2	2.3
Oxygen	−118.8	−181.1	49.7
Carbon dioxide	31.1	87.9	73

the substance's boiling point, but under no circumstance is it possible to liquefy it by pressure alone if its temperature is above its critical point. The further below its critical temperature a gas can be cooled, the less pressure is needed to liquefy it. Thus, it can be seen that any gas whose critical temperature is above ambient can be liquefied by pressure alone, because allowing the gas to equilibrate with ambient temperature actually keeps it below its critical temperature. Carbon dioxide has a critical temperature slightly above normal room temperature, 31° C, with a corresponding critical pressure of 73 atm, but at room temperature of 21.5° C, less than 60 atm of pressure are needed to convert the gas to liquid.

To maintain a gas in the liquid state for everyday use at ambient temperatures, we must raise its critical temperature above room temperature and must keep the gas under hyperbaric conditions in a strong storage cylinder. The anesthetic gases cyclopropane and nitrous oxide, along with carbon dioxide, are commercially supplied as tanked liquids, and Table 1-5 compares their critical points with the approximate pressures at which they are kept at room temperature to maintain their liquid state. There are many industrial gases that are converted to the liquid state for ease of mass transportation, and with critical temperatures above ambient, they need only be kept under sufficient pressure to assure their liquid form. With release of pressure, the liquid reverts immediately to gas.

Oxygen presents a more complicated problem, but because of its widespread medical and industrial use, carriage and storage are greatly facilitated by keeping it in the liquid state. In contrast to the three gases illustrated above, oxygen has a low critical temperature of −118.8° C (−181.1° F), and we know that no pressure will be able to keep it in liquid form above that value. In the manufacture of oxygen, large quantities of filtered air are subjected to tremendous pressures of up to 200 atm. This, of course, produces much heat, and the compressed gas is passed through heat exchangers and then subjected to a pressure drop of 5 atm. The rapid cooling brings the oxygen in the air below its boiling point of −183° C (−297° F) and it liquefies. If oxygen can be kept in an insulated container so that its temperature does not exceed its boiling point, it will remain liquid at atmospheric pressure. Should higher temperatures be necessary, then it must be subjected to increasing pressures; but at no time can it be allowed to exceed its critical temperature of −118.8° C,

Table 1-5. *Pressures needed to maintain liquid state of gases at room temperature*

Gas	*Critical temperature*		*Critical pressure*		*Approximate pressure in commercial cylinder at room temperature*	
	°C	°F	*atm*	*psi*	*atm*	*psi*
Cyclopropane	125	257	54.2	797	5.4	79
Nitrous oxide	36.5	97.7	71.8	1054	50.6	745
Carbon dioxide	31.1	87.9	73.0	1071	57.0	838

for then it will convert immediately to gas. Reference will again be made to this fact in the discussion of therapeutic gases.

Solid to vapor and vapor to solid. Although it may not be readily apparent, solid matter, as well as liquid, can vaporize, and at any given temperature solids have definite vapor pressures. The strong odor given off by naphthalene (mothballs) is ample evidence of the escape of vapor from a solid. The direct transition from the solid to the gaseous state is called *sublimation*, and because a change of state is involved, energy is transferred. The heat, in calories per gram or Btu per pound, required to convert 1 gm or 1 lb, respectively, of a solid into its vapor is called the *heat of sublimation.* Sublimation somewhat resembles boiling because it occurs when the vapor pressure of the solid equals that of the opposing ambient pressure and because increasing and lowering the ambient pressure directly displaces the subliming point. If temperature is below the melting point of a substance, a drop in pressure causes it to sublime; if the temperature is above the melting point, pressure drop produces boiling. At exactly 0° C, the vapor pressure over ice is 4.6 mm Hg, and if a vacuum less than this pressure is applied to the ice, the ice will sublime directly into water vapor.

Carbon dioxide is an interesting example of sublimation. If the gas is cooled to its critical point of −57° C, it will freeze and the vapor will equilibrate with the solid at a pressure of 5.1 atm, an unusually high level as compared to other permanent gases, most of which are considerably subatmospheric. When solid carbon dioxide is exposed to the atmosphere, the drop in pressure from 5.1 to 1 atm causes the solid state to sublime directly into vapor. We are all familiar with the behavior of commercially prepared solid carbon dioxide, popularly called "dry ice," as it gradually disappears when exposed to ambient conditions, leaving no trace of moisture. On the other hand, if solid carbon dioxide is subjected to pressures in excess of 5.1 atm and allowed to warm above −57° C, it will melt into a liquid without boiling.

It is possible to produce carbon dioxide snow by suddenly releasing the compressed liquid from a commercial tank. A rush of very cold vapor will emerge, carrying with it fine snowlike particles of solidified carbon dioxide. The rapid vaporization of the liquid in the tank requires heat, and in a sense, the liquid steals this heat from itself, freezing part of the material so that the remainder may vaporize.

We can relate the heat energy involved in sublimation to the energies of fusion and vaporization, already described, in the following way: Consider that a given mass of matter is progressing through changes of state from solid to liquid to vapor. We know that the step from solid to liquid utilizes energy, which we call heat of fusion; the conversion of liquid to vapor requires heat of vaporization. Even though the direct transformation from solid to vapor eliminates the liquid phase, the same total energy is required, and the heat of sublimation is thus equal to the sum of heats of fusion and vaporization.

In summary, we can say that all matter can theoretically exist in three physical states or forms, depending upon specific conditions of pressure and temperature. Those substances that we commonly refer to as gases are in the vaporous state because ambient pressure and temperature cannot maintain them as liquids or solids, and we have discussed the physical conditions that permit their conversion to the latter forms. It should be evident now why the ideal gas laws are not applicable to conditions of extreme pressure and temperature. The clear-cut relationships between pressure, temperature, and volume described by the laws break down as the factors of intermolecular force, molecular mass, and change of state influence the behavior of gases subjected to these extremes. This does not diminish the practical clinical value of the gas laws, but understanding the deviations from the laws permits us to see how matter can be manipulated and modified to serve specific purposes. The table in Appendix 8 compares some of pressure-temperature characteristics of a few selected gases and water so the student can see the tremendous range of values that distinguish one type of matter from another. In all probability, data such as this will play no direct role in the therapist's clinical duties, but it is hoped that, knowing something of the nature of the substances that he handles in his daily activities, his work will be a bit more meaningful.

Chapter 2

Solutions and ions

An understanding of some of the characteristics of solutions and ions is necessary to appreciate many of the chemical phenomena of physiology. In turn, to understand the composition of solutions, we must know the systems of measuring quantities of substances that go into solutions, especially systems based on molecular, equivalent, and milliequivalent weights. Familiarity with these terms will make more meaningful many frequently encountered expressions in clinical medicine. It is assumed that, through previous exposure to basic sciences, the student is acquainted with the names of elements, atomic weights, valence, and simple chemical reactions. Material covered in the previous chapter made use of principles of moles and gram-molecular weights. However, unless the student has had more than the usual basic experience in chemistry, he probably has no more than a vague understanding of the meaning of equivalent weights. Because of the latter's important relationship to solutions and to clinical medicine, we will take time to discuss equivalents and milliequivalents. Appendix 9 lists some of the common elements and radicals.

GRAM EQUIVALENTS

The gram-equivalent weight (gew) (gm-equivalent) (equivalent-wt) of an *element or radical* is the number (or fraction) of its gram-atomic weights (gaw) that can combine with or replace, in a chemical reaction, 1 gaw of hydrogen or other monovalent element. In the compound HCl, 1 atom (1 gaw) of Cl combines with 1 atom (1 gaw) of H; therefore the gew of Cl is its gaw of 35.5 gm. In the compound H_2S, 1 atom (1 gaw) of S combines with 2 atoms of H; thus, in combining power, *0.5* gaw of S combines with 1 atom of H, and its gew is one half its gaw, or 16 gm. Although these examples illustrate the technical definition of an equivalent weight, they also show us that the gew of an element or radical is simply its *gaw divided by its valence,* disregarding the sign of the valence. When an element has more than one valence, the valence must be specified or be apparent from chemical combining properties. With a valence of +1, the gew of Na is its gaw; the gew of Cu^{++} is the gaw divided by 2; of $Br^{\equiv}$, its gaw divided by 3.

The gram-equivalent weight of an *acid* is the gram weight of the acid that contains *1 gm-atom of replaceable hydrogen.* For example, in the chemical reaction $HCl + Na \rightarrow NaCl + H$, 1 (the only one) atom of H is replaced by Na from 1 gmw of HCl. Thus 1 gmw of HCl contains 1 replaceable H atom and is the gew of the acid, 36.5 gm. By contrast, sulfuric acid, H_2SO_4, has 2 replaceable H atoms, and its gew is one half its gmw. All of the H atoms in some acids are not completely replaceable, but for our purposes the only one of major importance is *carbonic acid,* H_2CO_3. Usually only *1* H atom is replaceable, as $H_2CO_3 + Na \rightarrow NaHCO_3 + H$. One H atom remains "bound." Thus, the gew of H_2CO_3 is its gmw rather than half of it. Nevertheless, for most acids, the *gew is the gmw of the acid divided by the number of H atoms in its formula.*

As might be expected, the gram-equivalent weight of a *base* is the gm-weight of the base that contains 1 gm-atom of replaceable OH. Except for those bases in which all OH radicals are not replaceable, the *gew is the gmw* of the base divided by the number of OH radicals in its formula.

Exercise 2-1. Assuming complete replaceability of H and OH, calculate the equivalent weights of the following:

(a) HBr	(f) KOH
(b) H_3PO_4	(g) $Zn(OH)_2$
(c) NHO_2	(h) $Al(OH)_3$
(d) H_3AsO_4	(i) NH_4OH
(e) H_2S	(j) $Mg(OH)_2$

The gram-equivalent weight of a *normal salt* is its gram weight, which contains the number of atoms of the negative radical that will react with 1 atom of H. It is conveniently calculated by dividing the gmw of the salt by the *total* number of *either* positive or negative valence charges (valence × subscript). The gew of $NaCl = 58.5$ gm; of $Fe_2O_3 = 159.8 \div 6 = 26.6$ gm.

Finally, the gram-equivalent weight of a *complex salt,* such as an acid, basic, or double salt, must be calculated in terms of a specific element or radical of the salt. The gmw of the salt is divided by the *total* valence of the specific element or radical. For the acid salt sodium dihydrogen phosphate, NaH_2PO_4, the gew's of its elements and radical would be:

For Na^+	gmw of salt ÷ 1
For H^+	gmw of salt ÷ 2
For $PO_4^{\equiv}$	gmw of salt ÷ 3

Exercise 2-2. Calculate the gew's of the following:

(a) MgF_2
(b) $CaCl_2$
(c) Na_3PO_4
(d) $Ca_3(PO_4)_2$
(e) $Al(OH)_2Cl$

To determine the number (or fraction) of gram equivalents in a given weight of a substance, we divide the gram weight of the substance by its gram-equivalent weight. Thus, 58.5 gm of NaCl divided by its gew of $58.5 = 1$ gew, whereas 29.25 gm divided by $58.5 = 0.5$ gew. Or, 510 gm of $AgNO_3 = 510 \div 170 = 3$ gew.

Exercise 2-3. Calculate the number of gew's in the indicated quantities of the following compounds:

(a) 62 gm MgF_2
(b) 50 gm $CaCl_2$
(c) 120 gm $Na_3(PO_4)$
(d) 10 gm $Ca_3(PO_4)_2$
(e) 1.5 kg $CuCl_2$

MILLIGRAM EQUIVALENTS

Now that we have covered the basic definitions, we can introduce another term intimately related to gram-equivalent weight, the *milligram-equivalent weight* (meq) (milliequivalent) (mg-eq). A milliequivalent is 0.001 of a gram equivalent, is expressed in milligrams instead of grams, and is used only as a matter of convenience for small quantities. The relation between milliequivalents and gram equivalents can be shown by the example of NaCl. A gew of NaCl is 58.5 gm; its meq value is 58.5 *mg*. Thus, if we wish to refer to 58.5 mg of NaCl, instead of calling it 0.001 gew (0.585 gm ÷ 58.5 gm = 0.001 gew), we would say 1 meq. As a rule, if the weight of a substance is given in milligrams, its equivalent weight is expressed in milliequivalents, and if a gram equivalent is less than 0.5, it is multiplied by 1000 and expressed as milliequivalents. This is not a restrictive rule but is intended only as a practical guide.

Exercise 2-4. Convert the following to the proper corresponding weights or equivalents:

(a) 5.3 gm Na_2CO_3
(b) 6.8 mg $CaSO_4$
(c) 1.2 gm $CuCl_2$
(d) 2.3 meq $AlBr_3$
(e) 9.5 meq $AgNO_3$

IMPORTANCE OF EQUIVALENTS

The *equivalent* of a substance is the chemically reacting quantitative unit of the substance. Thus, if substance A reacts chemically with substance B, exactly 1 gew or 1 meq of A will react exactly with 1 gew or 1 meq of B, to produce gew's or meq's of their products. Identical multiples or fractions of gew's and meq's react to produce the same multiples or fractions of gew's and meq's of their products. In the following reaction, note how the sum of the equivalent weights (gew or meq) of the two reactants equals the sum of the equivalent weights of the two products. This is referred to as the *balance* of the equation.

HCL +	NaOH →	NaCl +	HOH
36.5	40	58.5	18
gm or mg	gm or mg	gm or mg	gm or mg

In this equation, if we knew only the weight in grams of one of the reactants, by determining how many equivalents this represented, we could determine the weight of the other reactant needed for a quantitatively exact reaction.

Thus, given 20 mg of NaOH, which is 0.5 meq, we would need 18.25 mg, or 0.5 meq, of HCl to produce exactly 0.5 meq of NaCl and HOH. Similarly, if we desired a specific amount of one of the products, we could determine the amounts of reactants needed.

In medicine it has become customary to refer quantitatively to certain essential substances that are highly reactive in the body in terms of their equivalent weights. This is especially true of such elements as sodium, potassium, and chlorine and the bicarbonate radical (HCO_3^-), which are in small enough quantities to be measured in milliequivalents. To the physiologist, the number of chemically reactive units (meq's) present in the blood is more meaningful than just bulk weight in milligrams. Since the therapist will have occasion to note certain laboratory data of his patients, the method of reporting the above elements by the laboratory should be explained.

In the hospital clinical laboratory, the above blood chemicals (also referred to as *electrolytes,* to be described later) are quantitatively analyzed and measured in blood samples as *milligrams per 100 ml of blood,* or mg%. These values are then converted by the technician into the corresponding *equivalent weights* and reported as so many equivalents (milliequivalents) per *liter* of blood, or *meq/liter.* Transposition between meq/liter and mg% is easily accomplished as follows:

$$(1)\ \text{meq} = \frac{\text{mg}}{\text{equiv wt}}$$

$$\text{meq/liter} = \frac{\text{mg\%} \times 10}{\text{equiv wt}}$$

$$(2)\ \text{mg} = \text{meq} \times \text{equiv wt}$$

$$\text{mg\%} = \frac{\text{meq/liter} \times \text{equiv wt}}{10}$$

Thus, if in a blood sample there were 322 mg% of Na, it would be reported as

$$\frac{322 \times 10}{23} = 140\ \text{meq/liter}$$

As a check, 140 meq/liter $= \dfrac{140 \times 23}{10}$ or 322 mg%.

Exercise 2-5. Convert the following to the corresponding meq/liter, or mg%:

(a) 296 mg% Na
(b) 82 meq/liter Cl
(c) 23 mg% K
(d) 9 mg% Ca
(e) 26 meq/liter HCO_3

DEFINITION OF A SOLUTION

A solution is an intimate mixture of two substances, with one so evenly dispersed throughout the other that the mixture is homogeneous. The substance being dissolved, or going into solution, is called the *solute* and the medium in which it is dissolved is called the *solvent.* The ease with which a solute mixes with a solvent is a measure of its solubility. The four factors influencing solubility are as follows.

1. **NATURE OF THE SOLUTE.** The degree to which all substances go into solution in a given solvent is a physical characteristic of matter, with wide variability.
2. **NATURE OF THE SOLVENT.** As with solutes, solvents vary widely in their ability to incorporate substances into solutions.
3. **TEMPERATURE.** In general, the solubility of most solid solutes increases with temperature; the solubility of gases, however, varies inversely with temperature.
4. **PRESSURE.** Solubility varies directly with pressure.

A solution is described as *dilute* if it has a relatively small amount of solute in proportion to solvent. Fig. 2-1 shows three different states of a solution. In *A*, the solution is considered dilute because it has relatively few solute particles. A *saturated* solution is one with the maximum amount of solute that can be held by a given volume of solvent at a constant temperature, in the presence of an excess of solute. In such a mixture the dissolved solute is in equilibrium with the undissolved solute. Saturated solutions are usually prepared by adding a known excess of solute to the solvent, allowing the excess to remain in contact with the solution. In Fig. 2-1, *B* is a saturated solution and the excess solute is depicted as an undissolved mass at the bottom of the container. Although there is more solute in contact with solvent than the latter can accommodate at a fixed temperature, the excess must not be thought of as completely inert. Molecules of solvent in solution precipitate into the solid state at the same rate that new molecules leave the supply of solute and go into solution. This is the state of equilibrium that characterizes a saturated solution. A solution is said to be *supersaturated*, when it contains more solute in solution than does a saturated solution at the same temperature and pressure. If a saturated solution is heated, upsetting the solute equilibrium and allowing more solute to go into solution, and the remaining undissolved sol-

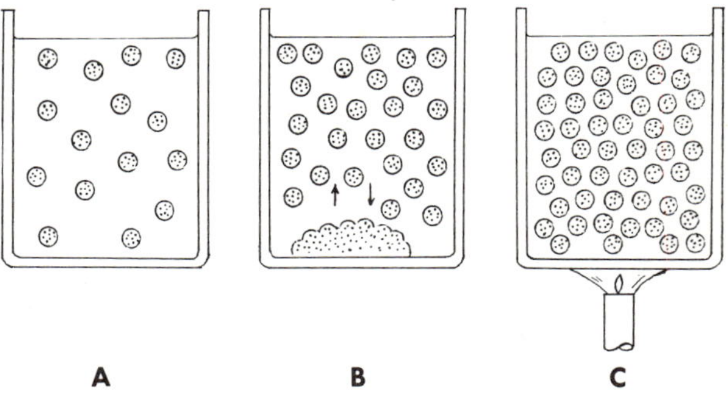

Fig. 2-1. In the dilute solution, **A**, the solute particles are relatively few in number, whereas in the saturated solution, **B**, the solvent contains all the solute it can hold in the presence of an excess of solute. Heating the solution, **C**, dissolves more solute particles, which may remain in solution if gently cooled, creating a state of supersaturation.

ute is filtered and the solution allowed to cool gently, then the solution will contain an excess of dissolved solute. Solution *C*, in Fig. 2-1, can be considered the result of applying heat to solution *B*, driving the remainder of the excess solute into solution. The additional dissolved particles may remain in solution, even after cooling to the temperature of the original saturated state, if extreme care is taken. Such a supersaturated solution is unstable, and the excess of dissolved solute may be precipitated out of solution by such physical stimuli as shaking or vibrating, or by adding to the solution a small amount the solid solute.

Most of the solutions of physiologic importance in the body are *dilute* in nature, and it is of interest that solutes in dilute solution demonstrate many of the properties of gases. This behavior is due to the relatively large distances between the molecules of solute in dilute concentrations, and it is hoped that the student may be stimulated to learn, through independent study, how the principles of the gas laws apply to liquids. We will concern ourselves only with brief descriptions of four of the major characteristics of weak solutions.

1. **VAPOR PRESSURE DEPRESSION.** The vapor pressure of a solution is less than that of the pure solvent. This is attributed to interference with the escape of solvent molecules by solute molecules, at the liquid surface.
2. **BOILING POINT ELEVATION.** The boiling point of a solution is higher than that of the pure solvent, and its elevation is directly proportional to the number of solute particles in a given weight of solvent.
3. **FREEZING POINT DEPRESSION.** The freezing point of a solution is lower than that of the pure solvent, and its depression is directly proportional to the number of solute particles in a given weight of solvent.
4. **OSMOTIC PRESSURE.** This will be discussed separately, a few paragraphs later.

QUANTITATIVE CLASSIFICATION OF SOLUTIONS

Ratio solution. The relationship of the solute to the solvent is expressed as a proportion (1:100, parts per thousand, etc.). This is used quite frequently in describing concentrations of pharmaceuticals.

Weight per volume solution (W/V). Often erroneously referred to as a "percent solution," the W/V solution is the one most commonly used in pharmacy and medicine for solids dissolved in liquids. It is calibrated in *weight of solute per volume of solution as grams of solute per 100 ml of solution.* Thus, although 50 gm of glucose in 1 liter of solution is not a true percent relationship, for a weight cannot be a percent of a volume, it is customarily called a 5% (W/V) solution. In contrast, a liquid dissolved in a liquid is measured as volumes of solute to volumes of solution.

Percent solution (%). Used in chemistry, a percent solution is calibrated as *weight of solute per weight of solution.* Thus, 5 gm of glucose dissolved in 95 gm of water is true percent solution, since the glucose is 5% of the total solution weight of 100 gm.

Molal solution (m). Less frequently used in physiologic chemistry than the following two types, a molal solution contains *1 mole of solute per kilogram of solvent.* Thus, a 1 m solution of NaCl contains 58.5 gm (gmw) dissolved in *1000 gm of solvent.* It is of value when precise concentrations of moles or molecules are desired over a wide temperature range. Since volumes of liquids vary with temperature as do gases, a molal solution, with its solvent measured in weight, is independent of temperature, and at all temperatures a given weight of solvent will contain the same number of moles or molecules.

Example. What is the molality of a solution with 162.1 gm of $FeCl_3$ dissolved in 500 gm of water? 162.1 gm/500 gm = 324.2 gm/1000 gm. The gmw of $FeCl_3$ is 162.1 gm. Thus, 324.2 ÷ 162.1 = 2 gmw dissolved in 1000 gm of water, a 2 molal solution.

Molar solution (M). Chemically and physiologically, the molar solution and the normal solution, to be described next, are the most important types of solutions. A molar solution is defined as *1 mole of solute per liter of solution* (or 1 millimole, mM, per milliliter of solution). A 1 M solution of NaCl contains 58.5 gm (gmw) *per liter of solution;* a 0.5 M solution has 29.25 gm per liter of solution; a 2M solution, 117 gm per liter, etc. The chemical importance of the molar solution lies in the fact that equal volumes of solutions of equal *molarity* contain the same number of moles and equal number of molecules.

Example. What is the molarity of a solution containing 1.07 gm NH_4Cl in 100 ml of solution? 1.07 gm/100 ml = 10.7 gm/liter. The gmw of NH_4Cl is 53.5 gm. 10.7 gm ÷ 53.5 gm = 0.2 gmw. Thus, 1.07 gm of NH_4Cl/100 ml is the same as 10.7 gm/liter, or 0.2 gmw/liter, and the molarity is 0.2 M.

Normal solution (N). Widely used in chemistry and biochemistry, a normal solution has *1 gram-equivalent weight of solute per liter of solution* (or 1 milligram-equivalent weight of solute per milliliter of solution). Thus 1 gmw of HCl, ½ gmw of H_2SO_4, ⅓ gmw of AlF_3, and ⅙ gmw of $Al_2(SO_4)_3$ each in 1 liter of solution make a 1 N solution. In all instances in which gram-equivalent weight is the same as gram-molecular weight, the normal solution is also the molar solution. Fractions of equivalent weights in solution constitute corresponding fractional normalities. The importance of normal solutions lies in the fact that equal volumes of solutions of equal normality, which react chemically, react completely.

Example. What is the normality of a solution with 39.75 gm of Na_2CO_3 dissolved in 250 ml of solution? 39.75 gm/250 ml = 159 gm/liter. The gew of Na_2CO_3 is 53 gm (gmw ÷ 2). 159 gm ÷ 53 gm = 3 gew. Thus, 39.75 gm Na_2CO_3/250 ml is the same as 159 gm/liter, or 3 gew/liter, and the normality is 3 N.

Exercise 2-6. Calculate the following:

(a) How many grams of solute are there in 300 ml of a 3% (W/V) solution?
(b) What volume will contain 70 mg of solute of a 7% (W/V) solution?

(c) How many grams of solute and solvent are needed for 250 gm of a 10% solution?
(d) What weight of water is needed to dissolve 13 gm of $BaCl_2$ to make a 0.25 m solution?
(e) What is the molarity of a solution with 16 gm of CH_3OH (methyl alcohol) in 200 ml of solution?
(f) How many milliliters of 0.1 M $AgNO_3$ solution contain 8.5 gm of solute?
(g) How many grams of $C_{12}H_{22}O_{11}$ (cane sugar) are there in 50 ml of a 3 M solution?
(h) What is the normality of a solution with 13.25 gm of Na_2CO_3 in 500 ml of solution?
(i) How many milliliters of 2 N solution of $AlCl_3$ contain 8.89 gm?
(j) How many milligrams of $Al_2(SO_4)_3$ are there in 10 ml of 0.2 N solution?

OSMOTIC PRESSURE

One of the physical characteristics of solutions that has great physiologic significance is *osmotic pressure*. This is a measurable force produced by mobility of the solvent particles under certain conditions. Imagine a thin porous sheet so constructed as to permit the passage through it of molecules of solvent but not solute. Such a structure is called a *semipermeable membrane*. Should such a membrane be placed so as to divide a solution into two com-

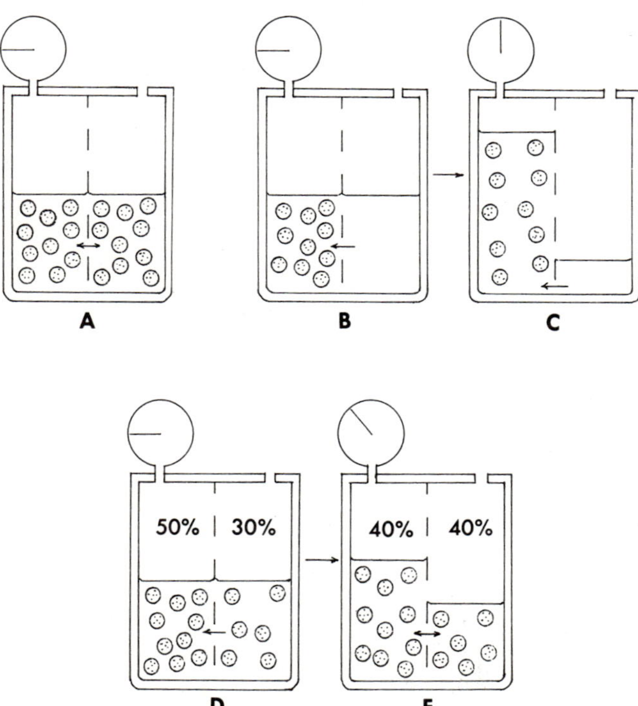

Fig. 2-2. Osmotic pressure is illustrated by the solutions in the above five containers. The containers are divided into two compartments by semipermeable membranes that permit the passage through them of solvent molecules but not solute (dotted circles). The numbers of solute particles represent relative concentrations of the solutions, and since they are fixed in number and are confined by the membranes, volume changes are a function of the diffusible solvent, movements of which are indicated by the arrows through the membranes. The arrows between containers **B** and **C**, and **D** and **E**, indicate progressive sequences of osmotic pressure. See text for further description.

partments, molecules of solvent would pass freely through it from one side to the other (Fig. 2-2, *A*). However, the number of molecules that pass (or diffuse) in one direction must be equaled by the number passing in the opposite, to maintain an equal ratio between solute and solvent particles (which determines the concentration of the solution) on both sides of the membrane.

Let us now put a solution on one side of the semipermeable membrane and pure solvent on the other. Solvent molecules will move through the membrane, but only in one direction, from the pure solvent to the solution and will continue to move until the supply of solvent is exhausted. The force driving the solvent molecules through the membrane is termed *osmotic pressure* and can be measured by connecting the expanding column of the solution to a manometer (Fig. 2-2, *B* and *C*). This pressure can be considered as a force that tries to distribute solvent molecules so there will be the same ratio between solute and solvent particles, thus the same concentration, on both sides of the membrane. Or it may be convenient to visualize osmotic pressure as the attractive force of solute particles in a concentrated solution for more solvent particles from a less concentrated solution. If we modify the conditions by placing a 50% solution on one side of the membrane and a 30% solution on the other, again the solvent molecules will penetrate the barrier, from the dilute to the concentrated side, (Fig. 2-2, *D* and *E*). The greater number of solute particles per solvent molecules in the concentrated solution attract solvent molecules away from the smaller concentration of solute particles in the dilute solution, and migration of solvent molecules will continue until the attractive force (osmotic pressure) of solute is equal on both sides of the membrane. Such an equilibrium implies an equal ratio of solute/solvent particles in both compartments, or an equal concentration of 40%. At this point, solvent particles move equally in both directions.

Osmotic pressure is directly proportional to the concentration of solute and will be twice as strong in a 2% solution as in a 1%. Thus, for a given *amount* of solute, the osmotic pressure is inversely proportional to the volume, an application of Boyle's law to liquids. Also, osmotic pressure varies directly with temperature, increasing $1/273$ for each degree Celsius.

Body cell walls are semipermeable membranes, and through the action of osmotic pressure the direction of water throughout the body is kept within physiologic ranges. The term *tonicity* refers to the relative degree of osmotic pressure exerted by a solution. In a very general way, the average body cellular fluid has a tonicity equal to that of a 0.9% NaCl solution, often referred to as physiologic (or normal) saline. For comparative purposes, any other solution with similar tonicity is called *isotonic*, one with greater tonicity *hypertonic*, and one with less *hypotonic*. Some cellular walls possess *selective permeability*, allowing the passage not only of water, but of specific solutes, and through this mechanism nutrients and physiologically active substances are distributed throughout the body.

DILUTION CALCULATIONS

Often it is necessary to make a dilute solution from a stock preparation, and this can be done accurately if the concepts of solution concentrations are understood. Such dilution problems usually involve medications and are based on the pharmacologic weight/volume percent principle defined earlier. Diluting a solution increases its volume without changing the *amount* of solute it contains but reduces its concentration. Therefore, the amount of solute in a given sample after dilution is the same as was present in the smaller original volume. It should be clear that the amount of solute present in a sample of a solution can be expressed as *volume* × *concentration*. For example, the amount of solute in 50 ml of a 10% solution (10 gm/100 ml) is 5 gm. $50 \times 0.1 = 5$. In diluting a solution, then, the initial volume times the initial concentration equals the final volume times the final concentration. This may be simplified as

$$V_1C_1 = V_2C_2$$

and when three of the data are known, the fourth can be calculated.

1. Given 10 ml of a 2% solution, dilute to a concentration of 0.5%. This requires finding the new volume.

$$V_1C_1 = V_2C_2$$

$$V_2 = \frac{V_1C_1}{C_2} = \frac{10 \times 2}{0.5} = 40 \text{ ml}$$

Thus, 30 ml added to 10 ml of 2% solution make 40 ml of 0.5% solution.

2. If 50 ml of water are added to 150 ml of a 3% solution, calculate the new concentration.

$$V_1C_1 = V_2C_2$$

$$C_2 = \frac{V_1C_1}{V_2} = \frac{150 \times 3}{200} = 2.25\%$$

3. Given 50 ml of $\frac{N}{3}$ solution, dilute it to $\frac{N}{10}$ concentration. Here, concentration is given as normality, but it can be used as well as percent.

$$V_1C_1 = V_2C_2$$

$$V_2 = \frac{V_1C_1}{C_2} = \frac{50 \times 0.333}{0.1} = 167 \text{ ml}$$

Exercise 2-7. Calculate the following:

(a) To what volume would 15 ml of 6% solution be diluted to make a 4% solution?
(b) How much water would be added to 65 ml of a 3% solution to make 2.5%?
(c) What was the concentration of 25 ml of solution, if the addition of 14 ml of water produced a 6.5% solution?
(d) How much 3 M solution is needed to make 12 ml of 0.2 M solution?
(e) If 92.75 mg of Na_2CO_3 are dissolved in 0.5 ml of water, what would be the normality of the solution after the addition of 0.67 ml of water?

OTHER "SOLUTIONS"

Two types of liquid mixtures that are considered with solutions but which do not have specific characteristics of solutions are *colloids* and *suspensions.* Colloids (sometimes called *dispersions* or *gels*) consist of large molecules, or clumps of molecules, that are able to attract and hold large numbers of water molecules. Egg white, glue, soap, and gelatin are common examples. Colloid solutions are cloudy or opalescent, exert only slight osmotic pressure, and have little effect upon boiling or freezing points. *Suspensions*—of which clay in water is a typical example—consist of large particles that are merely suspended in a liquid vehicle without the intimate relationship between solvent and solute found in solutions. Dispersion of the suspended particles depends upon physical agitation, and when the mixture is allowed to stand, the particles settle out.

ELECTROLYTES

One of the most important cardiopulmonary functions is the stability of acid-base balance, to be discussed in detail later; but to understand its fundamentals, the student must first understand the principles of electrolytes and ions. Indeed, the mechanism for regulation of acidity and alkalinity of the body and the transportation of respiratory gases to and from the tissues are so intimately related that neither can be fully intelligible without knowledge of the other. We will now consider some of the terms to be used later in our study of physiology.

Any substance in *aqueous* solution that can carry an electric current is called an *electrolyte.* Nonconductors are called *nonelectrolytes.* In general, most of the common chemically active inorganic elements and compounds, such as sodium chloride and sulfuric acid are strong electrolytes. In contrast, organic compounds are usually relatively poor conductors of electricity and are considered to be weak electrolytes.

Although all dissolved substances *increase the boiling point of water, decrease the freezing point of water,* and *produce osmotic pressure,* electrolytes do so to a much greater degree than do nonelectrolytes. The quantitative difference in these physical properties can be analyzed as follows:

1. Avogadro's principle tells us that gram-molecular weights of all substances dissolved in the same amount of solution have the same number of molecules per unit of volume.
2. A solution that contains half as many molecules as another will, quantitatively, exert half the effects listed above. Thus, these effects must be due to the *number* of particles in solution, not to the kind or size.
3. Solutions of electrolytes, however, with the *same number of molecules* as nonelectrolytes exert a greater effect than do nonelectrolytes.
4. Molecules of electrolytes, therefore, must break down further into a *larger number* of *smaller particles.* These small, submolecular particles are electrically charged and are called *ions.* The breakdown of elec-

trolyte molecules into the smaller ions in aqueous solution is called *electrolytic dissociation*, or *ionization*.

IONS

Ions are responsible for the transmission of current through solutions and may be either positively or negatively charged, but their sum is neutral. The degree of ionic dissociation varies with substances, their concentration, and temperature; it ranges from a fraction of 1% to over 90%. Ions are designated by the appropriate chemical symbol with a positive or negative superscript, i.e., Na^+, Cl^-. Positive ions are called *cations*, and negative ions, *anions*.

Ionization of acids, bases, and salts gives us the following definitions, which, although not technically precise or complete according to current chemical theories, are suitable for our limited purpose:

1. An *acid* is a compound that yields H^+ in aqueous solution.

$$HCl \rightleftharpoons H^+ + Cl^-$$
$$HNO_3 \rightleftharpoons H^+ + NO_3^-$$
$$H_2SO_4 \rightleftharpoons 2H^+ + SO_4^{=}$$

   a. Some acids, with more than one replaceable H ion, may dissociate in stages as dilution increases:

$$(1)\ H_3PO_4 \rightleftharpoons H^+ + H_2PO_4^-$$
$$(2)\ \rightleftharpoons H^+ + H^+ + HPO_4^{=}$$
$$(3)\ \rightleftharpoons H^+ + H^+ + H^+ + PO_4^{\equiv}$$

   b. H^+ does not exist free in solution but attaches itself to a water molecule to form the *hydronium ion* (H_3O^+), with a single positive electric charge. Thus, in an aqueous solution, the ionization of HCl as it reacts with the water would properly be written as:

$$HCl + H_2O \rightleftharpoons H_3O^+ + Cl^-$$

   The hydronium ion represents the hydrogen ion and, for the sake of simplicity, is often omitted, the H^+ being indicated alone.

   c. The more H^+ present, the more acid is the solution.

2. A *base* is a compound that yields OH^- in aqueous solution.

$$NaOH \rightleftharpoons Na^+ + OH^-$$
$$KOH \rightleftharpoons K^+ + OH^-$$
$$Ca(OH)_2 \rightleftharpoons Ca^{++} + 2OH^-$$

   The more OH^- present, the more alkaline is the solution.

3. A *salt* is a compound formed by replacing, in whole or in part, the hydrogen of an acid with a metal or positive radical.

$$NaCl \rightleftharpoons Na^+ + Cl^-$$
$$KNO_3 \rightleftharpoons K^+ + NO_3^-$$
$$NaHCO_3 \rightleftharpoons Na^+ + HCO_3^-$$

MEASUREMENT OF ELECTROLYTIC DISSOCIATION

The physiologically active chemical compounds of the body are, for the most part, weak electrolytes, and their ionic behavior is described in the electrolytic dissociation theory, which states that:

1. A proportion of the molecules in an aqueous solution of a *weak* electrolyte dissociate into ions, and the remainder of the molecules persist undissociated. At a given temperature and concentration, balance (equilibrium) is maintained between dissociated (ionized) and undissociated (un-ionized) molecules.
2. After equilibrium has become established, the *product* of the *molar* concentration (moles per liter) of the *ions or dissociated molecules* divided by the *molar* concentration of the *undissociated molecules* is a *constant* value at a given temperature. This is called the *dissociation constant*, or *K*.

The wide difference in the percentage of molecules that dissociate into ions, between three strong and three weak electrolytes, is illustrated in Table 2-1.

Let us make a quantitative comparison between a 0.1 M solution of HCl with 90% ionization and a 0.1 M solution of H_2CO_3 with 0.17% ionization. One liter of each solution will contain 0.1 mole, or 0.1 gmw, of its respective acid solute. Ninety percent of the HCl molecules, or 0.90 of 0.1 mole, 0.09 of a mole, dissociate into ions. 0.01 of a mole or gmw remains as intact molecules. Since each dissociating molecule produces one cation and one anion, the concentration, or number per liter of each, is the same as the concentration of the dissociating molecules. Thus, we can summarize the ionic and molecular concentrations of the 0.1 M HCl solutions:

Concentration of H ions = 0.09 mole (or gm-ion) per liter
Concentration of Cl ions = 0.09 mole (or gm-ion) per liter
Concentration of HCl molecules = 0.01 mole (or gm-mole) per liter

Of the 0.1 M solution of H_2CO_3, which dissociates into H^+ and HCO_3^- (bicarbonate) ions, 0.0017 of 0.1 of a mole, 0.00017 mole, of the acid dissociates into ions; 0.9983 of 0.1 mole, 0.09983 of a mole, remains undissociated. Thus:

Concentration of H ions = 0.00017 mole (gm-ion) per liter
Concentration of HCO_3 ions = 0.00017 mole (gm-ion) per liter
Concentration of H_2CO_3 molecules = 0.09983 mole (gm-mole) per liter

Further, a 0.1 M solution contains $6.02 \times 10^{23} \times 0.1$, or 6.02×10^{22} molecules

Table 2-1. *Percent molecular dissociation of 0.1 M solutions at 25° C*

NaOH	90%	CH_3COOH	1.33%
HCl	90%	H_2CO_3	0.17%
HNO_3	90%	H_3BO_3	0.01%

per liter. Therefore, on the basis of the known percentage of molecules that dissociate into ions, the actual number of ions and molecules per liter can be computed as shown in Table 2-2.

Examples of the electrolytic dissociation theory can be expressed in one equation, relating the dissociated and undissociated molecules with the constant. It must be remembered that this relationship holds only for weak electrolytes. The numerators of the following equations are in *molar* concentrations (moles or gram-ionic weights per liter) of ions, and the denominators are in molar concentrations (moles or gram-molecular weights per liter) of undissociated molecules of solute.

(1) Symbolic representation of an acid, HA:

$$\frac{H^+ \times A^-}{HA} = K$$

(2) Symbolic representation of a base, BOH:

$$\frac{B^+ \times OH^-}{BOH} = K$$

(3) Acetic acid:

$$\frac{H^+ \times CH_3COO^-}{CH_3COOH} = 1.8 \times 10^{-5}$$

(4) Carbonic acid:

$$\frac{H^+ \times HCO_3^-}{H_2CO_3} = 4.3 \times 10^{-7}$$

(5) Boric acid:

$$\frac{H^+ \times H_2BO_3^-}{H_3BO_3} = 5.8 \times 10^{-10}$$

The actual calculation of a dissociation constant will be demonstrated, using acetic acid (CH_3COOH). At 25° C, 1.33% of a 0.1 M solution of the acid undergoes ionization, and thus 98.67% of the molecules do not dissociate. Slight though it is, the dissociation of acetic acid is $CH_3COOH \rightleftarrows H^+ + CH_3COO^-$.

1. Since 0.1 M solution of acetic acid contains 0.1 gmw of acid per liter, of which 1.33% ionizes, then 0.1×0.0133 or 0.00133 of a mole of acid per liter produces ions, and 0.1×0.9867 or 0.09867 of a mole per liter remains un-ionized.
2. Each molecule that ionizes produces 2 ions, H^+ and CH_3COO^- (acetate

Table 2-2. *Concentrations of ions and molecules in 0.1 M HCl and 0.1 M H_2CO_3*

	H^+ *per liter*	*Anions per liter*	*Molecules per liter*
0.1 M HCl	5.428×10^{22}	5.428×10^{22}	6.02×10^{21}
0.1 M H_2CO_3	1.0234×10^{20}	1.0234×10^{20}	6.0099×10^{22}

ion), and the concentration of *each* is thus the same as that of the ionizing molecules, 0.00133 of a mole of ions per liter. Accordingly, the concentration of undissociated molecules is 0.09867 of a mole of ions per liter.

3. By definition, K is equal to the ratio between the product of the molar ion concentrations and the molar concentration of the undissociated molecules, or:

$$\frac{H^+ \times CH_3COO^-}{CH_3COOH} = K$$

$$\frac{0.00133 \times 0.00133}{0.09867} = K$$

$$K = 1.8 \times 10^{-5}$$

Exercise 2-8. Calculate the K of the following symbolic acid and base:

(a) 0.1 M HA, with 2.5% ionization
(b) 0.05 M BOH, with 1.9% ionization

The ionization of *water* is the basis for a system of calibrating acidity and alkalinity that will be discussed below. Pure water dissociates into the two ions H^+ and OH^-, and although its degree of ionization is very minute, it has an important disocciation constant. In a sense, water consists of an aqueous solution of H^+ and OH^-, or it may be thought of as a solution of these two ions dissolved in molecular water. Its ion/molecule ratio can be expressed in the usual manner:

$$\frac{H^+ \times OH^-}{HOH} = K$$

However, the degree of ionization of water is so small, and the concentration of un-ionized molecules is proportionally so large, that any small change in the degree of ionization would not produce a detectable reciprocal change in the concentration of the undissociated molecules. If one stood on a sandy beach, holding a dozen grains of sand in one hand, the exchange of a few grains between those in the hand and those on the beach would be significant to the concentration in the hand but would be unnoticed on the beach. Thus, the concentration of molecular water can be considered as another constant in the ratio, which can be rewritten as:

$$\frac{H^+ \times OH^-}{K_2} = K_1$$

and

$$H^+ \times OH^- = K_1K_2 = K_w$$

The dissociation constant of water, K_w, had been determined to be 1×10^{-14}. Therefore, if

$$H^+ \times OH^- = 10^{-14}$$

then, because there is one H^+ for each OH^-, the concentration of each ion is *10^{-7} moles or gram ions per liter.* Pure water is as much acid as it is alkaline and is thus *neutral* in reaction.

DESIGNATION OF ACIDITY AND ALKALINITY

For convenience, concentrations of H and OH ions in this section will be symbolized by cH^+ and cOH^-. We have seen that pure water is neutral in its reaction, with equal cH^+ and cOH^-. Using this as a reference point, we can state that any solution having a *greater cH^+* than that of water is acid in its reaction or any solution with lesser *cOH^-* than that of water is also acidic. Similarly, a solution with a greater cOH^-, or a lesser cH^+, than that of water is basic in reaction. By agreement, the *hydrogen ion concentration* (cH^+) of pure water has been adopted as the standard by which to compare reactions of other solutions. Electrochemical techniques are used to measure the cH^+ of unknown solutions and the degree of their acidity or alkalinity determined by variation of their cH^+ above or below 1×10^{-7}. Thus, a solution with a cH^+ of 8.2×10^{-4} has a *higher* cH^+ than water and is acid; one with a cH^+ of 3.6×10^{-8} has less H ions than water and is alkaline. There are two related techniques for recording acidity and alkalinity of solutions, using the cH^+ of water as the neutral standard:

The first method reports simply the actual measured molar concentration of H ions, which can then be compared to that of water. We know the cH^+ of water is 1×10^{-7} of a mole per liter, but this is an awkward expression to verbalize. Written as a decimal, it would be 0.0000001, or one ten-millionth of a mole, also awkward. Being smaller than a millionth, a ten-millionth falls into the next thousandth increment of the decimal system, the billionth (prefixed *nano*). Thus, one ten-millionth equals 100 billionths, and the H ion concentration of water can be designated as 100 nanomoles (nM) per liter. With this as a reference, any solution having a cH^+ of 100 nM/liter is neutral, greater than 100 nM/liter acid, and less than 100 nM/liter alkaline. The degree of acidity or alkalinity is proportional to the distance of a given cH^+ from the 100 nM/liter reference. This system of nomenclature is very limited in its use because of the tremendous range of possible cH^+, from the very acid to the very alkaline. It is not feasible to convert all cH^+ values to nanomoles, for this does not eliminate all awkward numbers. The system is applicable to needs of cardiopulmonary physiology, however, because the range of H ion concentrations is very narrow and seldom exceeds values of 20 to 100 nM/liter.

Second, to simplify acid-base comparisons, the principle of *pH* was developed. pH is the "hydrogen ion exponent," *the negative log of the hydrogen ion concentration, used as a positive number.* It is derived by converting the entire value for cH^+ to a single negative exponent of 10 by calculating its logarithm. The cH^+ of water is 1×10^{-7}, and since the log of 1×10^{-7} is -7, the pH of water is 7. Note the equations at the top of the following page.

(1) cH^+ of 8.2×10^{-4}
$pH = \log 8.2 \times 10^{-4} = \bar{4}.914 = -3.086 = \mathit{3.09}$
(2) cH^+ of 4.0×10^{-8}
$pH = \log 4.0 \times 10^{-8} = \bar{8}.602 = -7.398 = \mathit{7.40}$
(3) cH^+ of 6.7×10^{-11}
$pH = \log 6.7 \times 10^{-11} = \overline{11}.826 = -10.174 = \mathit{10.17}$

It is obvious that any solution with a pH of 7 is neutral, corresponding to the cH^+ of pure water. As the pH value *decreases* numerically below 7, because it is in reality a negative log, it represents an actual cH^+ greater than 7 and therefore is acid. Conversely, pH values greater than 7 represent lower cH^+ and are alkaline. The pH scale represents this graphically:

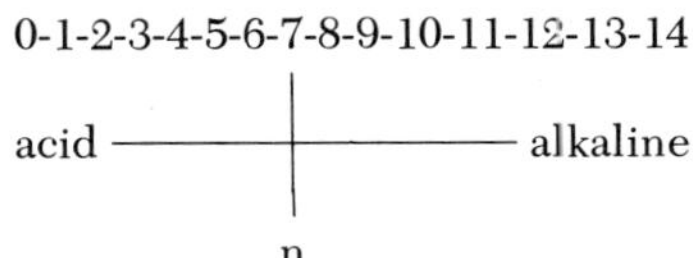

The compactness of the pH scale is nicely illustrated if we compare its midpoint and two extremes with corresponding molecular concentrations of H ions:

pH	*cH*
0	10^{0} or 1.0 M/liter
7	10^{-7} or 100 nM/liter
14	10^{-14} or 10^{-5} nM/liter

Exercise 2-9. Calculate the pH of the following (to 2 decimals):

(a) $cH^+ = 7.6 \times 10^{-5}$
(b) $cH^+ = 3.04 \times 10^{-2}$
(c) $cH^+ = 5.16 \times 10^{-12}$
(d) $cH^+ = 1.01 \times 10^{-8}$
(e) $cH^+ = 8.66 \times 10^{-10}$

Exercise 2-10. Calculate the cH^+ of the following:

(a) pH = 3.21
(b) pH = 8.92
(c) pH = 5.01
(d) pH = 10.26
(e) pH = 6.66

Chapter 3

Ventilation

The terms *ventilation* and *respiration* are frequently used interchangeably for they are generally synonymous, but to many there is a subtle difference between them. Ventilation may be considered as the mechanical movement of air into and out of the lung in a cyclic fashion, whereas respiration often refers to the exchange of oxygen and carbon dioxide in the lung and at the body cell. The primary function of the lung is respiration, to supply the body with oxygen and to remove the waste product of metabolism, carbon dioxide; but to fulfill this function, the lung must have adequate ventilation. Thus, we will begin our study of cardiopulmonary physiology with a consideration of the first need—aeration of the lung.

Ventilation is a cyclic activity, both automatic and voluntary, and consists of two components—an inward flow of air, called *inhalation* or inspiration, and an outward flow, called *exhalation* or expiration. The physical forces responsible for this air movement constitute the mechanics of ventilation. The inhalation-exhalation cycle moves a volume of gas into and out of the respiratory tract, the *tidal volume* (V_T). As the student observes his own ventilatory pattern, he will note that both tidal volume and *rate of breathing* (f, for frequency per minute) vary with physical activity. The product of these two factors, and a physiologically important parameter to evaluate, is the *minute volume* ($\dot{V}_E$). This is the amount of gas moved per minute, and although theoretically it should equal the tidal volume times the frequency, for practical reasons it is defined as the volume *exhaled* per minute (indicated by its symbol) and is measured by time-collecting exhaled respiratory gas. The relationships between tidal volume, minute volume, frequency, the nature of the airways through which the gas flows, and the physical forces responsible for gas movement are critical in determining the effectiveness of ventilation, and some of the important factors influencing them will be defined and discussed.

DEAD SPACE

It is of utmost importance that the inhalation therapist understand the concept of *dead space* and the role it plays in ventilation. Dead space (V_D) is defined as that portion of the respiratory tract which is *ventilated but not perfused by the pulmonary circulation.* It should be recalled that *perfusion* refers to the end point in arterial blood flow, where capillaries and tissue cells come into intimate contact for mutual exchange of contents. A review of anatomy will remind the student that the respiratory tract is supplied by two circulations, the systemic and the pulmonary. The conducting airways of the bronchial tree are served by the systemic circulation, and the bronchial and bronchiolar cells (as any other body tissue) are perfused by branches of the bronchial arteries to maintain their viability and function. The alveoli, however, are perfused by capillaries of the pulmonary circulation, and it is here that pulmonary arterial blood bathes the alveolar cells and is but a fraction of a micron away from alveolar air. Only at this level can oxygen and carbon dioxide pass between air and blood. By definition, then, ventilatory dead space consists of the conducting airways down to the level of gas exchange and *any alveoli* that, for one reason or another to be considered later, receive less than their normal pulmonary capillary perfusion. It is thus evident that dead space does not contribute to respiration but constitutes a volume which must be filled by ventilation before air can reach perfused alveoli.

Dead space is of three types: *anatomic* (V_D ant), *alveolar* (V_D alv), and *physiologic* (V_D phys). These are diagramatically illustrated in Fig. 3-1.

1. *Anatomic dead space* consists of the purely conducting airways of the nose and mouth, pharynx, larynx, trachea, bronchi, and bronchioles to the respiratory level.

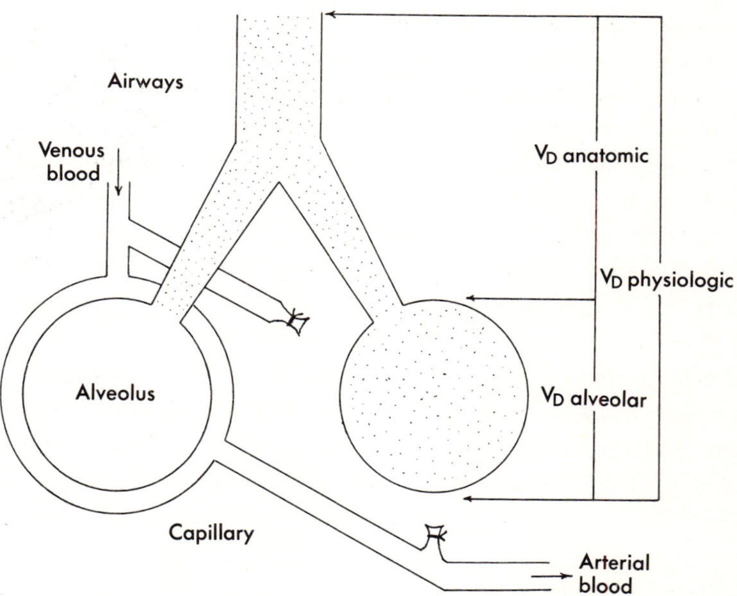

Fig. 3-1. The three types of dead space are shown in this sketch, which schematically represents two alveoli, their supporting airways, and capillaries. One alveolus is normally perfused and ventilated; but the capillary to the other is shown as if it were tied off and removed, so that the alveolus is freely ventilated but not perfused. The relationships of the dead spaces are indicated, as defined in the text.

2. *Alveolar dead space* is a less well-defined volume that consists of a variable number of alveoli whose perfusion is reduced or absent due, among other causes, to gravitational shifts in pulmonary blood flow distribution in the normal subject, and to impaired flow in the diseased.
3. *Physiologic dead space* is the sum of the anatomic and alveolar dead spaces, and its description as "physiologic" implies that it is the functional dead space of ventilation.

Measurement of dead spaces can be performed in the cardiopulmonary laboratory by techniques that will not be discussed here. In theory, all alveoli should be perfused, with no alevolar dead space. Therefore, physiologic and anatomic dead spaces should be identical and, as a rough guide, in the average adult should measure approximately between 150 and 160 ml. Should there be some alveoli with inadequate perfusion, a small alveolar dead space will exist that will increase the physiologic dead space.

CLASSIFICATION OF VENTILATION

Types of ventilation may be classified according to the two categories of physiologic and clinical. *Physiologically,* we can consider *total ventilation,* or *minute volume* ($\dot{V}_E$), *dead space ventilation* ($\dot{V}_D$), and *alveolar ventilation* ($\dot{V}_A$). For safe and effective management of patients in ventilatory failure, the inhalation therapist must clearly understand the differences between and the importance of each of these types:

1. *Total ventilation* refers to the amount of air moved into and out of the entire respiratory tract in liters per minute in the resting state. Normally ranging from 5 to 10 liters per minute, this volume gives but a rough estimation of ventilatory efficiency since it does not indicate how much air is reaching alveoli.
2. *Dead space ventilation* is the minute volume in liters that ventilates the physiologic dead space.
3. *Alveolar ventilation* is the minute volume in liters that ventilates all the perfused alveoli and obviously is the difference between the total and dead space ventilation. Usually it is between 4 and 5 liters per minute.

Functionally, only the alveolar ventilation is of importance since it determines how much air will be available for gas exchange. Perhaps it is already evident that a patient's breathing pattern can be so disturbed that, with a rapid rate and a small tidal volume, a large total volume of air may be moved which does little more than ventilate the dead space, leaving but a small amount to reach the alveoli.

Clinically, in the resting state, we note *normal ventilation, hypoventilation,* and *hyperventilation:*

1. *Normal ventilation* is that amount of minute ventilation which provides adequate alveolar ventilation, at a normal rate, and with a minimum of effort. We will see later that disruption of easy ventilation by disease,

even with satisfactory alveolar aeration, can produce some of man's most serious physical disability.

2. *Hypoventilation* is that state of impaired breathing whereby the alveoli are inadequately ventilated to fulfill the body's gas exchange needs. Hypoventilation may be the result of either a *pathologic increase in the dead space* or a *reduction in tidal volume.* Table 3-1 illustrates theoretical examples of each, with volumes measured in milliliters. To compensate for an increased V_D, the patient must increase either rate or tidal volume, and in each instance the additional muscular effort is disabling. The only compensation for a decreased tidal volume is an increase in rate. Again, this is possible only to a certain degree and is also physically strenuous. We will see later that the patient with this defect, by virtue of his underlying disease, is usually unable to compensate at all. The inhalation therapist will find that the treatment of hypoventilation will be one of his most demanding responsibilities.
3. *Hyperventilation* is an overaeration of the alveoli beyond physiologic needs due to an increase in tidal volume or rate or both and may be voluntary or involuntary. It can upset respiratory stability and impair circulation, but it is especially important for the therapist to note that hyperventilation is often induced by certain inhalation therapy procedures, a point that will be strongly emphasized later during discussions on techniques.

Table 3-1. *Types of hypoventilation and their compensation*

	Normal	*Hypoventilation due to increased V_D*	*Compensation*	
V_T	450	450	450	600
V_D	150	300	300	300
f	15	15	30	15
V_E	6750	6750	13,500	9000
$\dot{V}_D$	2250	4500	9000	4500
$\dot{V}_A$	4500	2250	4500	4500

	Normal	*Hypoventilation due to reduced tidal volume*	*Compensation*
V_T	450	225	225
V_D	150	150	150
f	15	15	60
$\dot{V}_E$	6750	3375	13,500
$\dot{V}_D$	2250	2250	9000
$\dot{V}_A$	4500	1125	4500

ACTION OF VENTILATORY MUSCLES[5,6,7]

Movements of the thoracic cage

At this time, the student should review the anatomy of the thorax, paying particular attention to the relationships between the skeletal parts, the shape of the ribs, and the thoracic musculature. The thorax is somewhat like a cone, with a wide base bounded by the diaphragm and a narrow opening at the top called the *operculum.* The latter is bounded by the first ribs and the manubrium of the sternum. For purposes of discussion, the ribs are grouped into three categories—the *first rib,* the *vertebrosternal ribs* (2 to 7), and the *vertebrochondral ribs* (8 to 10):

1. The *first rib* moves about the axis of its neck, raising and lowering the sternum. Although the motion is slight, it produces some increase in the anteroposterior (A-P) diameter of the chest. During quiet breathing this action is not utilized, but it becomes important under conditions of stress.
2. The six *vertebrosternal ribs* (2 to 7) play an important role in ventilation. In contrast to the first rib, these move about two axes simultaneously, the axis of the rib neck and the axis between the angle of the rib and its sternal junction (Fig. 3-2). As they rotate about the axes of their necks (A, in Fig. 3-3), their sternal ends rise and fall, thus increasing the

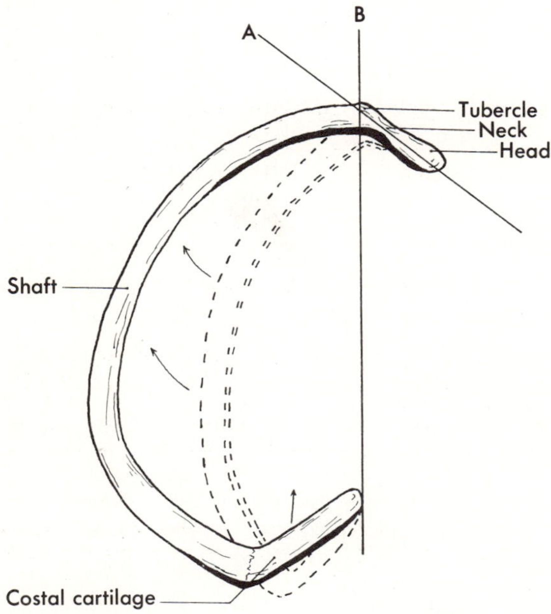

Fig. 3-2. The two axes about which the vertebrosternal ribs rotate during ventilation are indicated by lines *A* and *B*. The former passes through the length of the rib head and neck; the latter follows an A-P direction from the tip of the costal cartilage to the tubercle. The rib undergoes a compound movement from its starting position (dotted outline), the shaft swinging upward and laterally about axis *B*, and the anterior end moving upward about axis *A*.

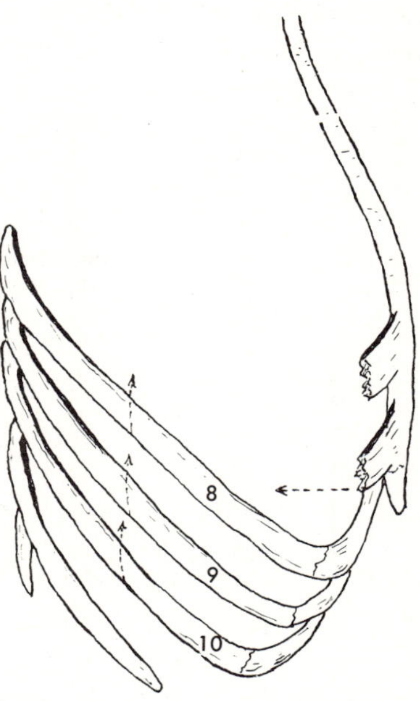

Fig. 3-3. The vertebrochondral ribs, *8* to *10*, have laterosuperior movement like ribs 2 to 7, but elevation of their anterior ends retracts the lower end of the sternum, shortening the A-P diameter of the thorax in that plane.

A-P thoracic diameter. This action is referred to as the "pump handle motion." At the same time, these ribs move about the longer axes from their angles to the sternum (B, in Fig. 3-2), leading to an up-and-down motion of the middle segments of the ribs. This, called a "bucket handle" motion, produces an increase and decrease in the transverse diameter of the chest. Thus, the compound action of these ribs increases and decreases both A-P and transverse diameters smoothly and synchronously.

3. The *vertebrochondral ribs* (8 to 10) have rotation patterns similar to the vertebrosternal group. However, elevation of the anterior ends of these ribs produces a backward movement of the lower end of the sternum, with *reduction* in thoracic A-P diameter (Fig. 3-3). Outward rotation of the middle portions of the ribs increases the transverse diameter, as do the vertebrosternal ribs.

There are some who do not believe the ribs rotate about their neck axes but rather *abduct* by a sliding motion. Ribs 11 and 12 are not included in any of the above groups since they do not participate in changing the contour of the chest but instead act as muscular insertion points.

The diaphragm

The diaphragm is one of the two major ventilatory muscles, which, by its location and action, is best able to vary the volume of the thorax to produce the pressure changes needed for ventilation. It arises from three locations, the lumbar vertebrae, the costal margin, and the xiphoid, its fibers converging to interlace into a broad connective tissue sheet called the *central tendon*. The configuration of this muscle is that of a tent or a dome, dividing the chest from the abdomen. It is pierced by several structures, such as the esophagus, the aorta, many nerves, and the vena cava and receives its motor innervation from the *phrenic nerves*. Although the diaphragm is a single anatomic structure, the union of its central tendon with the fibrous pericardium functionally divides its dome into two "leaves." For convenience, these are often referred to as the right and left diaphragms, or hemidiaphragms. With the liver immediately below it, the right dome is about 1 cm higher than the left, in the resting position, at the end of a quiet exhalation; and although the movements of both leaves are usually synchronous, because each has its own nerve supply, each may function independently of the other.

The mechanical action of the diaphragm is twofold:

1. Contraction draws down the central tendon, flattening its contour, increasing the volume of the thorax, and lowering intrathoracic pressure. As the diaphragm descends, intra-abdominal pressure increases and the muscles of the abdominal wall relax, allowing the upper abdomen to balloon outward. Splinting or rigidity of the abdominal wall interferes with diaphragmatic descent.
2. Contraction of the costal fibers of the diaphragm *raises* and *everts* the costal margin, if the dome is intact and intra-abdominal pressure is normal. As the abdominal pressure increases during inspiration, this pressure acts as a fulcrum against which continued contraction of the diaphragmatic fibers pulls up and out on the costal margin. In Fig. 3-4, the descending diaphragm is opposed by increasing intra-abdominal pressure. This pressure finally stabilizes the central portion of the diaphragm so that the force of continued contraction is expended as traction on the costal attachments of the diaphragm. Because of the spring-like tension of the ribs and the contour of the thorax at this level, the costal margin is pulled upward and outward, increasing the lateral diameter of the chest.

During inhalation therefore, as the diaphragm contracts, its dome descends and the costal margin of the chest moves outward so that the thorax enlarges both vertically and transversely. It is important to understand and visualize this combined action, for the action is easily disturbed in pulmonary disease. Thus, if the diaphragm is abnormally low in position, not only is there a diminished vertical excursion (with a resulting reduction in tidal volume), but contraction of the costal fibers, instead of elevating the costal margin, may even pull in the lower chest boundary and narrow the thorax laterally. Illustration *B*, in Fig. 3-4, shows an abnormal diaphragm, low in position and relatively flat in contour. Because of its starting position, it can descend very little on contraction, and with loss of its domed shape, contraction tends to

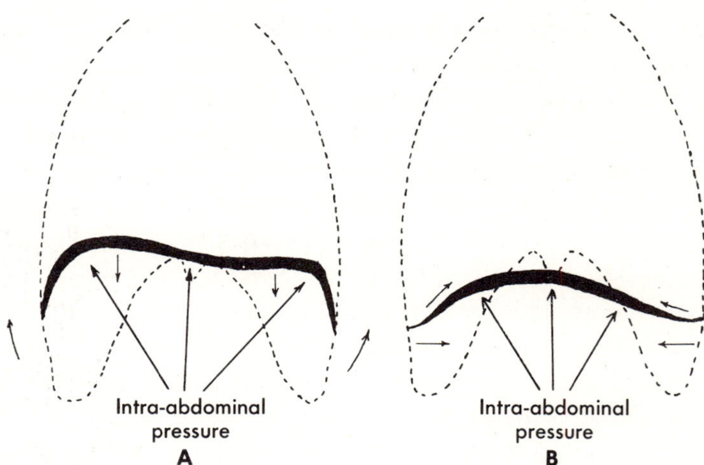

Fig. 3-4. A, As the normal diaphragm contracts, it descends, gradually building up pressure in the abdomen until the intra-abdominal pressure acts as a fulcrum against which continued contraction everts the costal margin, enlarging the thorax further. **B,** Contraction of the diaphragm, which is abnormally low at the start of inspiration, can only pull in the costal margin, reducing the lower thoracic diameters.

pull its fibers centrally on a horizontal plane. This pulls in the costal margin and reduces the diameter of the chest. Much of the little gain in vertical diameter from the limited mobility of the diaphragm is negated by the simultaneous lateral shortening. The diaphragm takes no active part in exhalation and returns to its inspiratory resting position during the passive recoil of the thorax, to be explained later. During forced exhalation, as against resistance, the diaphragm does expel gas from the lung as it is pushed upward by intra-abdominal pressure generated by contracting abdominal muscles.

At rest, the normal tidal movement of the diaphragm is about 1.5 cm, and with deep breathing 6 to 10 cm. With quiet breathing the excursions of both leaves of the diaphragm are about equal, but with a deep inspiration, the right diaphragm may move more than the left. In the supine position, the total diaphragmatic movement is the same as in the erect position. In a head-down, 45-degree supine tilt, however, the resting level of the diaphragm rises about 6 cm, causing a reduction of the functional residual capacity and the expiratory reserve volume. When the subject lies in a lateral position, his lower diaphragm tends to rise into the chest. Although the diaphragm is the principal ventilatory muscle and the only one used in normal quiet breathing, it is not essential for survival, as adequate ventilation is possible even when the diaphragm is completely paralyzed. It is estimated that, in the normal adult, each centimeter of vertical movement moves 350 ml of air; thus an excursion of 1.5 cm would effect a tidal volume of 525 ml. This figure does not include the additional increase in thoracic volume from expansion of the lower thorax, which, of course, would increase the tidal volume. It has also been suggested that the diaphragm contributes about 75% of the vital capacity although much of its movement may be the result of abdominal muscle contraction, forcing the diaphragm passively into the chest.

Affected by paralysis, the diaphragm (either or both leaves) tends to stay at the normal level at rest. During deep inhalation, however, it *rises* as other ventilatory muscles or one normal hemidiaphragm produce a fall in intrathoracic pressure. In quiet breathing the paralyzed leaf may remain immobile or move in either direction. The inspiratory balance of pressure above and below the diaphragm tends to make the paralyzed leaf rise, whereas outward movement of the lower ribs tends to stretch and flatten it, and its final course is the resultant of these two forces.

Finally, it should be noted that the diaphragm performs important functions other than ventilation. Because it is able to aid in generating high intra-abdominal pressure by remaining fixed while the abdominal muscles contract, the diaphragm greatly facilitates defecation, vomiting, coughing and sneezing, and parturition.

The intercostal muscles

The intercostals, the second of the major ventilatory muscles, consist of two sets of muscles filling the gaps between the ribs; they are designated as *internal* and *external:*

1. The *external intercostal muscles* arise from the inferior edge of each rib from the rib tubercle to its costochondral junction. The fibers pass inferiorly and anteriorly to insert into the superior edge of the rib below. These muscles are thicker posteriorly than anteriorly and are thicker than the internal intercostals.
2. The *internal intercostal muscles* are located beneath the external intercostals and arise from the inferior edge of each rib from the anterior end of the intercostal space to the rib angles. The fibers pass inferiorly and posteriorly to insert into the superior edge of the rib below. This muscle group is divided into two functional parts:
   a. *Interosseous* portion, located between the sloping parts of the ribs
   b. *Intercartilaginous* portion, located where the costal cartilages slope superiorly and anteriorly

Although there is considerable controversy as to the exact mechanism by which the intercostal muscles function, it is well established that by contraction they elevate the ribs, thereby increasing the inspiratory chest volume. This function has been documented by noting its absence during paralysis of muscles. In addition, the muscles solidify and stabilize the chest wall and prevent intercostal bulging or retraction during intrathoracic pressure changes. It is felt that most of the ventilatory effect of the intercostals is produced by the external intercostals and the intercartilaginous portion of the internal intercostals. These muscles contract during inhalation and maintain contraction into early exhalation, by this action elevating the ribs. In the presence of flow rates up to 40 liters/min the intercostals are quiet during most of exhalation. However, with flow rates in excess of 50 liters/min the intercostals of the lower spaces contract toward the end of exhalation and also do the same during voluntary maximum exhalation. This action probably gives stability to the chest in the presence of powerful abdominal contraction. As noted above, intercostal contraction continues into early exhalation during quiet breathing, but it then fades as expiratory airflow rises to its maximum. This is not a true exhalation act of the intercostals, for if it were, the peak expiratory airflow would occur at once while lung recoil was also maximal. It is believed that this function of the intercostals is to retard airflow during early exhalation and to facilitate a smoother and less turbulent exhalation. Finally, it appears that contraction of the interosseous portion of the internal intercostals *depresses* the ribs; but the exact role they play in normal ventilation is not clear.

The scalene muscles

The *anterior, medial,* and *posterior* scalene muscles, although individual structures, are considered as a functional unit. Primarily skeletal muscles of the neck, they are also *accessory muscles of ventilation* and play an important role in breathing. The scalenes arise from the transverse processes of the lower five cervical vertebrae and insert into the upper surface of the first rib (anterior and medial scalenes) and the second rib (posterior scalene).

Although the scalenes give support to the neck, we are interested in their ventilatory action. Basically, they elevate and fix firmly the first and second ribs. Their most important function is to aid inhalation under conditions of stress when the diaphragm and intercostals are inadequate to fulfill respiratory needs; this may occur in normal subjects undergoing severe exertion or in patients with pulmonary disease. In a normal subject, *static* inspiratory efforts (against a closed glottis or other obstruction, with no movement of air) bring the scalenes into play as intra-alveolar pressure drops; and when this pressure reaches −10 cm H_2O, scalenes are active in all subjects. During expiratory efforts the scalenes are inactive until intra-alveolar pressure reaches 40 cm H_2O, at which point they contract. It is felt that the expiratory function of the scalenes is to fix the ribs against the contraction of the abdominal muscles and to prevent herniation of the apex of the lung during coughing.

The sternomastoid muscle

Designed to rotate the head and support it, the sternomastoid is another accessory ventilatory muscle of importance. It arises by two heads from the manubrium of the sternum and the medial end of the clavicle. The heads fuse into a single body that courses superiorly and slightly posteriorly to insert into the mastoid process and occipital bone of the skull. This muscle is usually prominent on each side of the neck of most subjects and is especially noticeable with rotary movements of the head.

When functioning to mobilize the head, the sternomastoid pulls from its sternoclavicular origin, rotating the head to the opposite side and turning it slightly upward. As a ventilatory muscle, however, when the subject fixes the head and neck with other skeletal muscles, the sternomastoid pulls from its skull insertions and elevates the sternum, increasing the A-P diameter of the chest. In all subjects it contracts when intra-alveolar pressures reach −10 cm H_2O but has no action during exhalation. In the supine position, most subjects during normal free breathing can attain a volume of 2.5 liters and a flow rate of 60 liters/min without use of the sternomastoids. An interesting discrepancy should be noted. During natural, free breathing, normal subjects can move about 2.5 liters of air at intra-alveolar pressures varying from −25 to −50 cm H_2O with the diaphragm and intercostals alone, and yet under static conditions an intra-alveolar pressure of −10 cm H_2O brings the sternomastoid into play. This is not clearly understood.

In chronic pulmonary disease, the sternomastoid becomes active in inhalation when the thorax becomes so inflated (elevated resting level) that the low diaphragm loses its efficiency. As the sternomastoids contract and pull up on the sternum, the ribs rotate about their neck axes but not about the rib angle–sternal junction axes. This produces an up-and-down motion with little side expansion. In extreme cases, A-P expansion of the thorax may cause the lower ribs to become indrawn, partially negating the increase in chest volume.

The pectoralis major muscle

The third most important accessory ventilatory muscle, the pectoralis major is a powerful bilateral anterior chest muscle with the primary function of pulling the upper arms into the body in a hugging motion. It is a large, fan-shaped muscle arising from the medial half of the clavicle, the anterior surface of the sternum and the first six costal cartilages, and a fibrous sheath enclosing muscles of the abdominal wall. The muscle fibers converge into a thick tendon that inserts into the upper part of the humerus. It is the pectoralis major that forms the anterior fold of the axilla, and in a muscular individual its outlines are plainly visible beneath the skin.

Like the other accessory ventilatory muscles, the pectoralis pulls in a direction opposite to that of its primary function. If the arms and shoulders are fixed, as by leaning on the elbows or firmly grasping a table, the pectoralis can use its insertion as an origin and pull with great force on the anterior chest, lifting up ribs and sternum and increasing thoracic A-P diameter. The inhalation therapist will soon become accustomed to seeing patients with chronic pulmonary disease assume characteristic poses for maximum use of their pectoralis. In advanced cases, most of the air moved may be the result of the action of this powerful muscle. It aids inhalation only, taking no part in exhalation.

The abdominal muscles

Several muscles make up the abdominal wall, with the obvious purpose of providing support and safety to the abdominal contents. Some of them, however, play an indirect but important role in ventilation and can thus be considered as accessory ventilatory muscles. Four of these will be briefly identified:

1. The *external oblique* arises from the lower eight ribs; posterior fibers insert into the iliac crest, and the rest course obliquely down and forward to insert into a fibrous sheath (aponeurosis) with their counterparts from the other side; the lower edge forms the inguinal ligament in the groin.
2. The *internal oblique* arises from the iliac crest and the inguinal ligament; posterior fibers pass upward to insert into the last three ribs; the rest slope upward and forward to a fibrous aponeurosis.
3. The *transverse abdominal* arises from the costal cartilages of the lower ribs, iliac crest, and lateral part of inguinal ligament; it passes horizontally forward to an aponeurosis.
4. The *abdominal rectus* arises from the pubic bones, passes upward in a sheath formed by the aponeuroses described above, and inserts into costal cartilages 5 to 7; it is often well defined in a muscular individual.

The abdominals are expiratory muscles with two important actions—to increase intra-abdominal pressure and to draw the lower ribs down and medially. In the relaxed supine position, the abdominals are inactive during quiet breathing; and they are often inactive in the erect position. With increasing ventilation, the abdominals come into play when the expiratory flow rate reaches 40 liters/min. At this level of gas velocity or in the presence of significant resistance to exhalation, or if exhalation is required beyond the preinspiratory resting level (as in inflating a balloon), the elastic recoil of the thorax does not have adequate force to remove enough air in the allotted time. In such circumstances, contraction of the powerful abdominals builds up strong intra-abdominal pressure and drives the diaphragm, like a piston, into exhalation. Contraction of these muscles also occurs at the end of voluntary maximum *inhalation* and is a factor limiting the extent of inhalation. In chronic pulmonary disease, especially in the presence of airway obstruction, effective use of the abdominals is often lost, and without this powerful generator of force to push the diaphragm into expiratory action, the patient is at a great disadvantage.

Summary of ventilatory muscle action

There are other muscles that play varying roles in assisting ventilation and thus can qualify as accessory ventilatory muscles. Most of them are concerned with stabilizing the body to provide better leverage for muscles directly concerned with air movement. However, if the therapist thoroughly understands the function of the muscles described above, he will have an adequate foundation for learning some of the therapeutic techniques to be taken up later. In summary, the function of the ventilatory muscles may be tabulated as follows:

1. *Quiet ventilation*
   a. Inspiration
      (1) Diaphragm in all subjects
      (2) Intercostals in most subjects
      (3) Scalenes in some subjects
   b. Expiration
      Some persistence of contraction of inspiratory muscles early in expiration
2. *Moderately increased ventilation*
   a. For flow rates up to 50 liters/min, same as above
   b. For flow rates between 50 and 100 liters/min, sternomastoid action toward end of inspiration; increased abdominals and intercostals toward end of expiration
3. *Greatly increased ventilation*
   Above 100 liters/min, all inspiratory accessories active, and abdominals throughout expiration

CONTROL OF VENTILATION

Central control of ventilation

Until fairly recently, the central control of ventilation was believed to rest in a single *respiratory center* located in the medulla of the brain, and the mechanism of this center was felt to be quite simple and straightforward. It was believed that, as arterial blood perfused the highly specialized cells of the center, the partial pressure of its contained carbon dioxide was sensed by the cells. If the P_{CO_2} was higher than normal, impulses from the center traveled the vagus nerve to the ventilatory muscles and increased activity of the latter blew off excess of the gas. Conversely, low values of P_{CO_2} restrained ventilatory activity, allowing CO_2 to be retained in the body until normal blood values were reached. Recognition of this process was the first step toward identifying the many feedback systems that we now know exist in the body. However, continued study of ventilatory control makes it clear that the mechanism is far more complex than originally thought, and although there is much yet unknown and there are many differences of opinion on the subject, we will review simply what is now the most probable basic mechanism for ventilatory control.

Instead of one respiratory center, there are at least three, two located in the pons and one in the medulla. In addition, there is a less well-localized area in the medulla. We will discuss in sequence, the *medullary center,* the *apneustic center,* the *pneumotaxic center,* and the *chemoreceptor area*[8]:

The *medullary center,* from its name obviously located in the medulla of the brain, functionally is considered to consist of two parts—an inspiratory center and an expiratory center. These structures receive signals from many sources of the body indicating the nature of ventilation needed to satisfy the body's needs at any given moment. They respond by sending impulses to the ventilatory muscles to set up a suitable rhythmic sequence of inhalation and exhalation. This medullary center is the one originally considered to be the sole regulator, responding to P_{CO_2}, but it has been determined that CO_2 levels do not act in this region. The medullary center can be considered, for simple visualization, as the final coordinator of all the regulatory mechanisms and as the dispatcher of the definitive signals to the ventilatory muscles. It thus responds to the other centers as well as to the higher brain centers of voluntary action.

The *apneustic center* is located in the lower portion of the pons and is thereby known as a pontine center. Apneusis is a condition in which ventilation stops in the inspiratory position. In such instances, the resting level is end-inspiratory, rather than end-expiratory, although the apneustic level is at the end of *full* inspiration. The apneustic center, if unrestrained, promotes deep and prolonged inspiration but normally is controlled by the *pneumotaxic center* and *inflation reflexes* (Hering-Breuer) from the lung, which will be described later. Disease of the pons causing abnormal stimulation of the apneustic center can produce apneustic breathing, a gasping type of ventilation with maximal inspiration.

The *pneumotaxic center* is another pontine center, located slightly higher than the apneustic. As noted above, it controls the effect of the apneustic center and encourages a rhythmic ventilation. It has been suggested that the pneumotaxic center receives inspiratory impulses from the medullary center and in turn sends impulses to the medullary expiratory center, thus limiting the extent of inhalation.

The *chemoreceptor area* is a more diffusely distributed group of specialized cells in the medulla than is the medullary center and thus cannot be designated as a center. A chemoreceptor cell is one that has the ability to differentiate between concentrations or pressures of naturally occurring chemicals perfusing it. The area with which we are concerned identifies and monitors partial pressure of arterial carbon dioxide. Actually, it is believed that the chemoreceptor cells respond to the hydrogen ion concentration, rather than to the actual P_{CO_2} itself, although the latter determines the former.[9] Because of this, these cells have recently come to be called *central hydrogen ion receptors*, as well as central chemoreceptors. These receptors send their impulses to the medullary center, where they are added to all the other information being received by the center to determine the net total ventilatory needs of the body.

Peripheral control of ventilation

In addition to those structures located in the brain, there are a host of other areas in the body that influence ventilation by stimulating the higher centers by way of *reflexes*. A familiar example is the sudden hyperventilation that accompanies the application of cold water to the skin. As these reflex mechanisms are remote from the brain, they are referred to as peripheral. It would be impractical as well as inappropriate to attempt to describe each individually, but we will, however, consider two important peripheral regulators of ventilation, the *carotid and aortic* bodies and the *inflation reflex:*

The *carotid and aortic bodies* will be considered together since, in our field of interest, their function is the same.[10] These are small nodular structures composed of chemoreceptor cells, one group located in the fork where each common carotid artery divides into the external and internal carotids and the other clustered in the wall of the ascending arch of the aorta. These structures are in intimate contact with arterial blood through small arteries branching from their large supporting arteries. The function of these bodies is to monitor the amount of *oxygen* perfusing them, in contrast to the function of the central chemoreceptors described above. There is also one other difference. Whereas the central chemoreceptors respond to partial *pressure* of CO_2, the peripheral chemoreceptors are more sensitive to changes in the *amount* of oxygen supplied to them, since they will be stimulated by a low blood flow even though the P_{O_2} is normal. We can thus say that the stimulus energizing the carotid and aortic bodies is a low oxygen supply to their cells. Again, in contrast to the central receptors, high concentrations of oxygen do not affect them. The bodies are not very sensitive reactors, however, and the oxygen supply must drop to a low level before they will be stimulated. In a sense, these structures function as a last-minute defense against oxygen lack, after the oxygen has fallen critically low. We may correlate the action of the central and peripheral chemoreceptors as follows: The central receptors are important in contributing to the instant-by-instant ventilatory needs of the body, by informing the medullary center of changes in ventilation required to maintain a stable level of CO_2. Should the central receptors fail through disease or in the presence of a normal P_{CO_2} should severe oxygen deprivation ensue, then the peripheral receptors will be activated to stimulate the medullary centers for increased ventilation. Much reference will be made to this mechanism throughout the remainder of the study of inhalation therapy, for it is one of the most important physiologic concepts for the therapist to learn.

The *inflation reflex,* commonly called the Hering-Breuer reflex (not entirely accurate, since Hering and Breuer recognized other reflexes), carries impulses from the lung to the brain through the vagus nerve. Sensory receptors in the lung respond to the stretch of the distending lung and relay inhibitory impulses to the central controls, interfering with the function of the latter and limiting further inflation. By restricting unnecessary inhalation, the inflation reflex assists the respiratory system in moving a volume of air adequate to supply the alveoli with a minimum of energy expenditure.

Let us summarize, briefly, the interaction of the many factors that control ventilation. The medullary center functions somewhat as a sorting device of the many afferent nerve impulses reaching it and from this data determines the most suitable ventilatory pattern for the body's needs for a given moment. Although automatic in its response, the center is subject to voluntary override from the higher brain areas of the cerebral cortex. Respiratory information reaches the medullary center from many parts of the body; but of these, three are of outstanding importance: (1) The general breathing pattern is determined by the CO_2 partial pressure of the arterial blood, which is sensed by central chemoreceptors in response to changes in hydrogen ion concentrations. (2) Should these receptors fail, the reserve peripheral chemoreceptors of the aortic and carotid bodies, responsive to low concentrations of O_2, stimulate the medullary center. (3) To facilitate efficient ventilation with the minimal use of energy, stretch reflexes in the lung limit the extent of inhalation and encourage the medullary center to establish a smooth and easy combination of tidal volume and rate. In the background, as it were, is the apneustic center of the pons with its inherent ability to produce a full and sustained inhalation, acting as a sort of guarantee against failure of the lung to expand. The pneumotaxic center, also in the pons, keeps the apneustic function in check and, in addition, appears to correlate inspiratory and expiratory impulses of the medullary center and to help maintain a rhythmic ventilation. It must be understood that this summary is oversimplified and, since much is yet unknown about ventilatory control, may even be incorrect in some details; but it permits a practical view of the major forces involved as a foundation for understanding effects of pulmonary disease and the rationale of therapy.

LUNG-THORAX RELATIONSHIP

Effective ventilation depends upon cooperative but reciprocal action between the lung and the thorax, a relationship crudely illustrated by the balloon-in-a-box model as shown in Fig. 3-5, the box representing the thorax, and the balloon the lungs. A review of anatomy will recall that, between the pleura-lined thoracic wall and the pleura-covered lung, there exists the *pleural* or *intrapleural space.* Although in the living subject, the approximation of the two pleural surfaces, separated by only a thin film of moisture, makes the space more potential than real, it plays an important role in ventilation and for purposes of illustration is depicted in sketches as a true space.

The resting level or resting position of the chest is the configuration that it assumes at the end of a quiet effortless exhalation and is often referred to as the *end-expiratory position,* less frequently as the *preinspiratory level.* In sketch *A* of Fig. 3-5, the relations of the lung and thorax are shown at the resting level. The airtight thoracic box encloses a small partial vacuum of about -4 cm H_2O, as indicated by the attached manometer, maintained by opposing elasticity of the lungs and thorax, to be described in more detail below. The pulmonary balloon is suspended in the box, and because it is exposed to and in equilibrium with atmospheric pressure, the surrounding subatmospheric intrathoracic pressure keeps it partially filled with air. Thus, at the end of exhalation there is still a considerable amount of air in the lungs. The inspiratory flow of air into the lung is brought about by enlargement of the thoracic

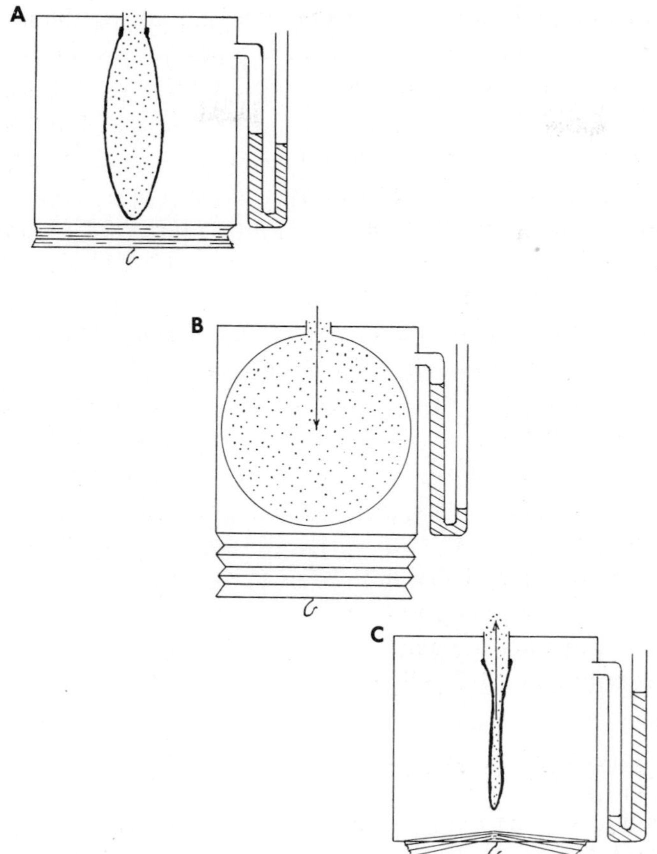

Fig. 3-5. Balloon-in-a-box model of the lung-thorax. **A,** In the resting position, a small negative pressure in the box keeps the balloon slightly distended with air. **B,** As the box expands by dropping its floor, its cavity becomes more negative, and air flows into the balloon. **C,** If the floor of the box is pushed higher than its usual resting level, positive pressure develops in the box, expressing additional air from the balloon but not emptying it.

box through the effort of ventilatory muscles. Sketch *B* of Fig. 3-5 shows the accordion-like bottom of the box dropping, enlarging the volume of the box, and simulating the action of the diaphragm. The living thorax, a flexible structure, also expands laterally as muscles act upon the ribs. Intrathoracic pressure drops further with this increase in volume of the sealed container, the pressure drop is transmitted into the balloon across its flexible wall, intra-balloon (intra-alveolar) pressure momentarily becomes subatmospheric, and air flows into it. This difference between the higher atmospheric and lower alveolar pressures is called a *pressure gradient* (ΔP). It is a "head of pressure" that allows fluid to flow from the high end of the gradient to the low. The concept of gradients is of great importance in cardiopulmonary physiology and will be extensively used as we progress. During quiet inhalation intrapleural pressure drops only to about −6 cm H_2O, but a strong inspiratory effort against an obstruction, such as a closed glottis, can drop the pressure to −50 cm H_2O. Exhalation is a passive recoil of the elastic stretch of the lung balloon, made possible by a relaxation of the muscular forces acting on the thoracic box. Air flows from the lung until the resting level is reached to terminate the cycle. Exhalation can be continued below the resting level by bringing into play positive expiratory muscular forces. Principally, this invokes strong contractions of the abdominal muscles to force the diaphragm into the thorax, as illustrated in sketch *C* of Fig. 3-5. With this maneuver, the resting negative intrathoracic pressure is replaced by a positive pressure that, against strong resistance, may reach 70 cm H_2O.[11] Although more air is forced from the lungs, the latter can never be completely emptied.

We have described, in general terms, the basic factors responsible for airflow into and out of the lungs and will now consider some of the forces that both initiate and limit air movement. As referred to above, the ventilatory cycle is the net sum of the action of the opposing forces of the chest and lung, and we will use a different model to illustrate these points, emphasizing that we are not talking about another subject but viewing the same from a slightly different angle. The thorax (which in our context includes the diaphragm) consists of flexible ribs and muscles; and through the intrinsic elastic forces of its tissues, it tends to expand and enlarge, much as a bent bow is under stress to spring straight. Counteracting these chest forces are forces of the lung, whose elastic tissues are stretched and tend to contract and shrink. To understand how these two systems of elastic energy relate to one another, consider the lung-thorax complex as consisting of one set of *bowed flat* springs

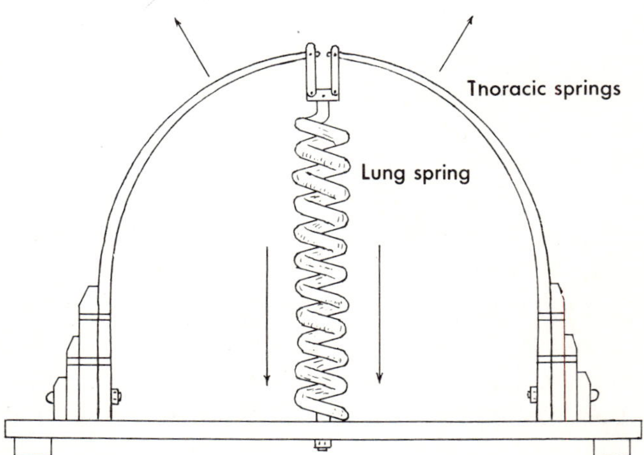

Fig. 3-6. The counteracting forces of the lungs and thorax are schematically represented by two sets of springs. In the resting position, the bowed flat thoracic springs are shown as held under bent tension by the coiled lung spring, itself partially stretched by the action. Arrows indicate the direction each spring tends to move to reach its own position of rest. From the lung-thorax resting position, the thorax can expand or contract, depending upon the action of the ventilatory muscles. These muscles can assist the thoracic springs to overcome the restraint of the lung spring, or they can compress the thoracic springs and assist the recoil of the lung spring.

(thorax) exerting an expansile force tied to a *stretched coiled* spring (lungs) exerting a contractile force, each holding the other in check (Fig. 3-6). At the resting level, the chest and lung forces are equal in opposite directions, momentarily in perfect balance, as each prevents the other from following its natural inclination. Although we refer to this brief static period as "resting," it must not be thought that expenditure of energy is wanting, any more than a temporary stalemate in a rope-pull contest can be considered free of physical activity. Indeed, in the airtight balloon-in-a-box structure of the lung-thorax, at the resting position each force is pulling against the other with power equal to that exerted by a 4 cm column of water, developing in the intervening intrapleural "space" a partial vacuum of the same magnitude.

Inhalation can occur only when the resting level balance between the forces of the lung and thorax is broken by the addition of muscular energy to the elasticity of the thorax. In addition to the effect of diaphragmatic contraction on chest expansion, the intercostal and accessory ventilatory muscles, in a sense, take hold of the bowed "flat springs" of Fig. 3-6 and pull them outward to help them overcome the "coiled spring" of the lung. It is easy to imagine that the depth of inspiration is determined by the amount of chest force applied to overcome lung stretch and that this effort, in turn, is regulated by the mechanism of ventilatory control already discussed. At the end-inspiratory level necessary to satisfy immediate body gas needs, airflow stops and the chest and lung forces are again in momentary balance. At this point the muscles activating the thorax relax, and the elasticity of the stretched lung, along with the increased intra-abdominal pressure, passively returns the lung-thorax system to the resting level. Exhalation against resistance such as obstructive airway disease, in which pulmonary passive recoil lacks the force to move air at a suitable rate, or exhalation below the resting level, as noted above and shown in sketch *C*, Fig. 3-5, principally utilizes the abdominal muscles to generate the power necessary to deflate the lung. By employing a little imagination, we can visualize this effort as a force bowing the flat springs of Fig. 3-6. Against obstruction, this active expiratory force helps the coiled spring return the expanded thorax to the resting position. To expel air below the resting level, this force helps the coiled spring to flex the increasing resistance of the flat springs. Details of other factors influencing the function of the lung-thorax system, such as surface tension and bronchopulmonary diseases, will be discussed in the following sections.

This is an advantageous point at which to introduce the subject of lung volumes, for they are dependent upon the lung-thorax relationship. Fig. 3-7 illustrates the volumetric divisions of the total capacity of the lung, and it should be observed that a designated capacity consists of two or more volumes. The lower dashed line identifies the end-expiratory resting level, and the upper, the *tidal volume* (V_T) end-inspiration. Because the chest forces limit collapse of the lung at the end-expiratory resting level, air remains in the lung at this point and is called the *functional residual capacity* (FRC).

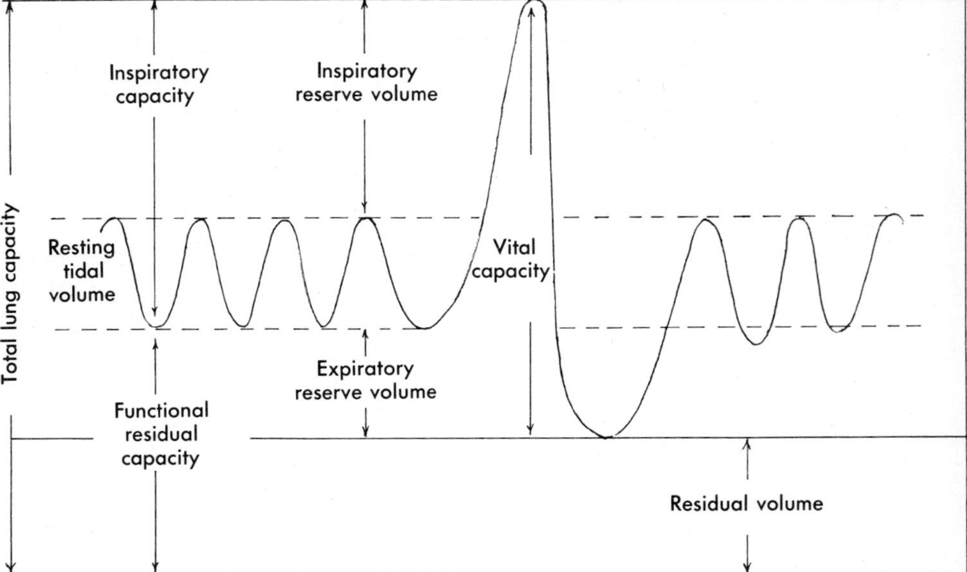

Fig. 3-7. Lung capacities and volumes. Volumetric divisions of the total gas capacity of the lungs. A capacity consists of two or more volumes. See text for description.

Forced exhalation, as described above, can remove air below the resting level by "dipping into" the FRC. This extra air, so expelled, is the *expiratory reserve volume* (ERV). Even after the most strenuous expiratory effort, air still remains in the lung and cannot be removed voluntarily; this is known as the *residual volume* (RV). Thus, the FRC is the sum of the ERV and the RV. If a subject inhales *maximally* from the resting level, then exhales *maximally*, he will move a quantity of air known as the *vital capacity* (VC), so called because all his ventilation is within its limits. Note that the VC consists of three volumes, the ERV, the V_T, and the *inspiratory reserve volume* (IRV). The last represents the available expansion of the lung-thorax, beyond resting needs, for exertion or any other demand for deep breathing. The *inspiratory capacity* (IC) measures the total inhalation potential from the resting level. Finally, the sum of the VC and the RV comprises the *total lung capacity* (TLC). All these values can be measured in the cardiopulmonary laboratory, by direct or indirect methods, and, although our current interest in them will be confined to their relationship to physiology and disease, some rough guides to their actual values should be of interest to the student. There is great variability in lung volume measurements among individuals, depending upon size and physical conditioning, and between health and disease; but Table 3-2 will give some quantitative visualization for average normal adults.

In the illustration of Fig. 3-6, if we separate the sets of springs, it is apparent that each set will follow its natural tendency—the thoracic flat springs will spring outward and the lung coiled spring will contract. The same phe-

Table 3-2. *Normal lung volumes*

Vital capacity	2.5 to 5.0 liters
Expiratory reserve volume	0.8 to 1.2 liters
ERV/VC ratio	0.25 to 0.40
Functional residual capacity	1.5 to 2.7 liters
Residual volume	0.8 to 1.5 liters
Total lung capacity	3.3 to 6.5 liters
RV/TLC ratio	0.25 or less

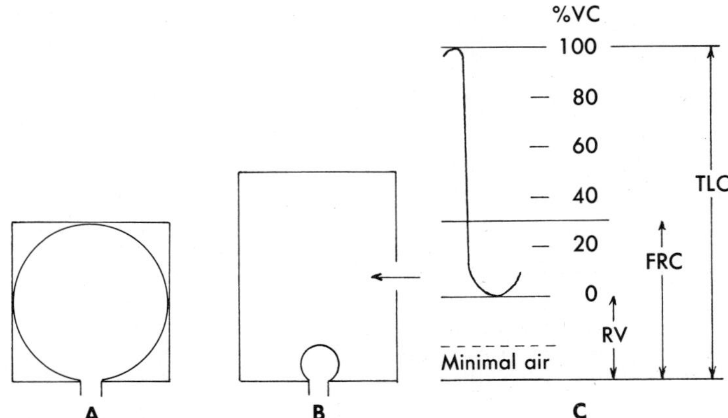

Fig. 3-8. The resting levels of the intact lung-thorax and the separated lung and thorax are plotted against the total lung capacity. In **A**, the intact system at its resting level contains the *FRC* and is expanded to about 30% of the *VC*. In **B**, the arrow indicates a break in the thoracic wall, exposing the lung to atmosphere and destroying the lung-thorax seal. The lung, containing the *minimal air*, collapses to a new resting level, which is about 40% of the *RV*, and the thorax expands to its own unopposed level of about 50% of the *VC*.

nomenon will occur if we break the vacuum-sealed intrapleural space, letting it equilibrate with the atmosphere. If the thorax (either side or both) is opened, it will actually expand to a larger volume and assume its own *thoracic resting position*. At the same time, the lung, freed from its suction adherence to the thoracic wall, will collapse to a smaller volume than the RV of the intact system; but even when exposed to atmospheric pressure, the lung does not become completely airless and still contains a small amount of air called *minimal air*. Fig. 3-8 diagrammatically illustrates the effect of breaking the seal between thorax and lung. In *A*, the lung-thorax is at the resting level, where the lung contains the FRC. *B* depicts the results of equilibrating the intrathoracic space with atmospheric pressure by opening the intact thorax. The lung collapses to its smallest size, the minimal air volume, while the thorax enlarges to its unopposed thoracic resting position. *C* is a plot of the TLC against *A* and *B*, breaking the VC into increments of 20% each. The normal lung-thorax resting position is seen to be at approximately 30% of the VC whereas, with disruption of the system, the minimal air level of the lung is about 40% of the RV and the thorax expands to its resting level of some 50% of the VC.

Finally, aiding the synchronous movement of lung and thorax is the force of *pleural traction.* In the normal intact lung-thorax complex, both visceral and parietal pleura are in contact during the entire breathing cycle, separated only by the thin film of fluid covering the pleural surfaces, mentioned above. The cohesive force of this fluid layer, working with the intra-alveolar pressure gradient, helps to hold together the pleural surfaces so that, as the thorax expands and contracts, the lung accompanies it smoothly. In a sense, the lung is partially "dragged" into inflation by the thorax and is held firmly against the inner thoracic wall during exhalation.

SURFACE TENSION AND VENTILATION

So far, the collapsing tendency of the lung springs has been attributed only to the elastic fibers in its structure. Augmenting this elastic recoil, however, is another factor that has assumed clinical importance—*surface tension* (ST); a brief review of the principles of surface tension will expedite understanding its role in ventilation.[12-14] Surface tension may be defined as the force exerted by molecules moving away from the surface and toward the center of a liquid, tending to make a sphere or a curved surface smaller. It occurs at an *interface* or junction between two substances, as liquid and air, and is best illustrated in a relatively small drop of fluid. Molecules in the mass of a liquid are subjected to physical forces of mutual attraction and are so

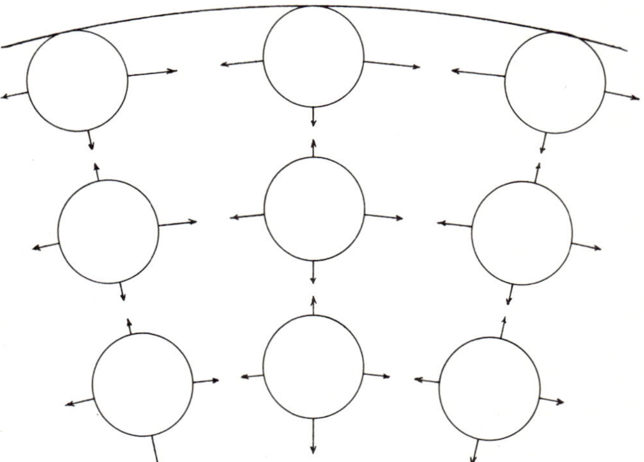

Fig. 3-9. The force of surface tension in a drop of liquid is shown by the action of its fluid molecules. Those molecules within the substance of the drop are mutually attracted to one another (arrows) and can move about randomly in a state of balance. Mass attraction can pull the molecules of the outermost layer inward only, creating a centrally directed force, called surface tension, which tends to contract the liquid into a sphere. Pressure within the drop is raised above atmospheric and is expressed by the formula of Laplace, described in the text.

balanced that they can freely move in all directions. Those molecules on the surface, however, can be attracted only inwardly by their fellow molecules, and the pressure they exert can be likened to an elastic film tending to contract into a sphere. Fig. 3-9 illustrates the force of mass attraction between liquid molecules. Those molecules at the fluid-air interface have no molecules distally to attract them but are pulled only centrally. This tension over the surface of a drop of liquid keeps it intact in a spherical shape while falling in space or resting on a surface. Surface tension is measured in *dynes per linear centimeter across the surface* and may be visualized as the force (in dynes) necessary to produce a tear 1 cm long in the surface layer of a liquid, if one could grasp the surface in the hands and stretch it like a thin rubber sheet until it split. ST is a demonstrable phenomenon that permits an insect to walk on the surface of a pond and enables a needle to float in a glass of water. Surface tensions vary widely between substances and for the same substance vary inversely with temperature. Table 3-3 lists some examples of surface tension values.

The force of ST, like a fist compressing a ball, produces an increase in pressure within a drop of liquid above the ambient. Thus, a pressure gradient, or difference in pressure (ΔP), exists across the surface of the drop. The P within the drop, dependent upon the specific ST and the radius of the drop, is expressed by the formula of Laplace as:

$$P = \frac{2\ ST}{r}$$

where ST is in dynes/cm, r is the radius in centimeters, and P is in dynes/cm^2. The derivation of this formula is explained in any standard text of physics. Given a drop with a radius of 2 mm and a ST of 60 dynes/cm, calculate the pressure inside the drop:

$$P = \frac{2 \times 60}{0.2\ \text{cm}} = \frac{120}{0.2} = 600\ \text{dynes/cm}^2$$

or

$$P = \frac{600\ \text{dynes/cm}^2}{980} = 6.13 \times 10^{-1}\ \text{g/cm}^2$$

Table 3-3. *Examples of surface tension*

Substance	°C	*ST in dynes/cm*
Water	20	73
Water	37	70
Tissue fluid	37	50
Whole blood	37	58
Plasma	37	73
Ethyl alcohol	20	22
Mercury	17	547

or

$$P = Ht \times D$$

$$\therefore Ht = \frac{P}{D} = \frac{6.13 \times 10^{-1}}{1} = 6.13 \times 10^{-1} \text{ cm } H_2O$$

More pertinent to our interests is the effect of surface tension on a bubble, which, for purposes of description, can be considered as a spherical volume of gas enclosed in a thin film of fluid. Fig. 3-10 shows that, thin though it is, the liquid film has surface tension which exerts pressure on its enclosed gas molecules. Indeed, because ST is found only at an interface and the film has two surfaces, the force of ST in a bubble is *twice* that exerted on a spherical drop of the same size and substance. Thus, the ST's of the two surfaces act together to compress the gas bubble. The pressure gradient across a bubble wall can also be expressed by Laplace's law, with a modification:

$$P = \frac{4\ ST}{r}$$

where ST is the surface tension of the liquid in which the bubble is immersed and r is the radius of the bubble in centimeters. It is apparent that if the example in the preceding paragraph were a bubble instead of a drop the pressure would be double the calculated value.

From the foregoing it can be seen that for a given liquid the *smaller* the drop or bubble the *greater* will be the pressure from surface tension. When inflating a balloon, we must use maximum force to *start* inflation, to overcome the initial resistance, then progressively less, up to the capacity of the balloon. Similarly, it would require more pressure to inflate a small bubble than a large one because of the increased pressure of ST in the former. Fig. 3-11 illustrates changes in pressure in bubbles accompanying changes in size and in ST. As the size of bubble *A* increases to *B*, the pressure drops, according to Laplace's law. Bubble *C* demonstrates that the pressure can remain unchanged if the ST is somehow lowered. Or, to view it differently, Fig. 3-12 shows that if two

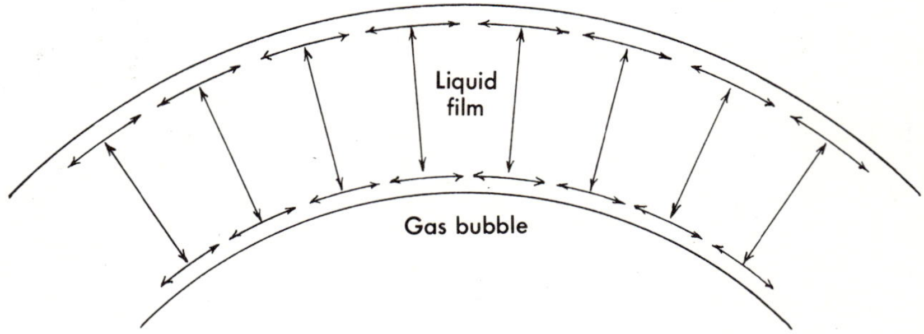

Fig. 3-10. A bubble is a volume of gas enclosed by a thin film of fluid, which has two surfaces. Thus, the forces of surface tension on both surfaces produce a pressure within the bubble twice that in a liquid drop of the same substance and radius.

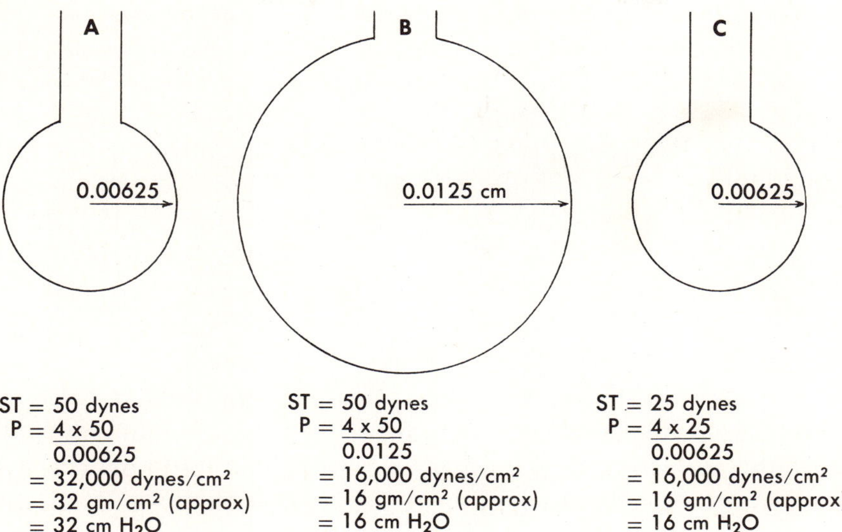

Fig. 3-11. The internal pressure of a bubble varies with the size of the bubble and the surface tension of its liquid film. An increase in radius from **A** to **B** drops the pressure, but **C** shows that the same pressure drop can accompany a reduction in surface tension, without changing bubble size.

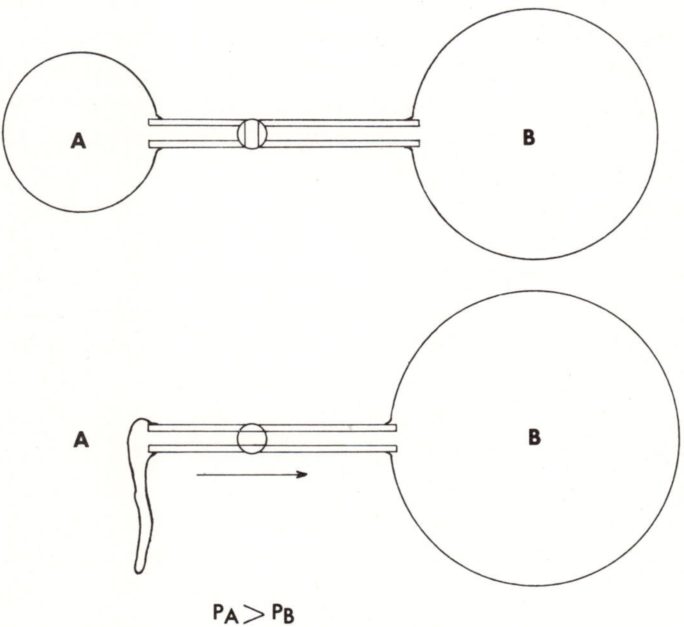

Fig. 3-12. When two bubbles of different sizes, **A** and **B**, but with the same surface tension, are allowed to communicate, the greater pressure in the smaller causes it to empty into the larger.

bubbles of different sizes are allowed to communicate the smaller will empty into the larger because of the greater pressure in the former.

The ability to alter surface tension is a physical phenomenon of great importance to pulmonary physiology, and the principle involved will be discussed before we relate it to function. Certain substances can lower ST on contact with fluid surfaces, and are called *surfactants*. Soaps and detergents are the most common examples. These agents weaken the molecular bonds at the surface, thus reducing the surface tension and lowering intrabubble pressure. Sketch *C*, Fig. 3-11, illustrates this effect. An air bubble in water shrinks and finally disappears under the stress of ST pressure, but the addition of soap to the water, by lowering ST, prolongs or stabilizes the bubble. On the other hand, a surfactant such as a detergent, by reducing ST, disrupts and disperses small drops of water, making the water "wetter" and increasing its ability to penetrate deeper into fabrics and minute crevices for better removal of dirt.

Let us recall the microscopic structure of the lung, with its millions of alveoli, each one of which is in intimate contact with a thin film of intercellular fluid, and let us view it as a mass of tiny bubbles in interstitial fluid. It is easy now to imagine each of these "alveolar bubbles" as being subjected to forces of tissue fluid surface tension; and indeed, experimental and clinical evidence indicates that ST is an important factor in the mechanics of ventilation. The passive exhalation recoil of the "lung springs" to the resting position is due to alveolar ST acting with the elastic fibers of the lung. The effect of lung ST is to produce alveolar collapse, and reinflation by inhalation against the ST pressure would be very difficult were it not for the presence in the alveoli of a natural surfactant.

Pulmonary surfactant exists as a single molecule-thick film lining the alveolar walls. Chemically, it is a phospholipid, composed of fatty acids bound to lecithin, and it functions in a most remarkable fashion. Apparently there is a fixed amount of surfactant in each alveolus, and its ability to lower ST is dependent upon a quantitative ratio between it and alveolar surface area. At the ventilatory resting level, because the alveoli are partially deflated, there is a relatively large amount of surfactant in relation to alveolar surface area. Surface tension is lowered, intrapulmonary pressure is lowered, and the alveoli can be easily inflated. As the alveoli distend with inhaled air, their stretched walls present an increasing surface area. At the same time, the surfactant film becomes stretched and thinned, the ratio of surfactant to surface area falls, and the effect of surfactant decreases. ST increases until a point is reached at which the forces of ST and lung elasticity prevent further distention and cause the alveoli gradually to deflate, and the cycle repeats. The "half-life" of surfactant is measured in hours (the length of time it takes for half a given mass to disappear in the metabolic process of deterioration), and if its natural replacement is impaired or it is pathologically destroyed faster than it can be replaced, alveolar collapse (atelectasis) rapidly develops.[63] Were it not for the action of pulmonary surfactant, inflating partially collapsed alveoli would require great physical effort and inhalation would be seriously handicapped. Indeed, in disease states characterized by absence of surfactant, the work of breathing is at times insurmountable.

Exercise 3-1. Calculate the following:

(a) At the resting level, if lung ST is 30 dynes/cm, how many centimeters of water pressure are needed to start inflation of an alveolus with a diameter of 90μ?
(b) With a ST of 70 dynes/cm, what is the diameter of a bubble that can be maintained by an inflating pressure of 9 mm Hg?

ELASTIC RESISTANCE TO VENTILATION

When discussing the "springs" of the lung and thorax, we were describing the characteristic of *elasticity*, whereby an object that is stretched by a force tends to recoil to its original shape or position upon release of the force. The elasticity of the lung-thorax presents a resistance that must be overcome during inhalation, a resistance that often increases in disease. A measurement of elasticity, called *compliance*, can be made to evaluate the work of breathing; it gives an estimate of the "stiffness" of the lungs and thorax. Compliance is defined as the *volume change in the lung per unit of pressure change*, and its units are liter per centimeter of water. Measurements must be made under *static* conditions, or at points of *no airflow*, to eliminate such other factors as airflow resistance, etc. It is evident that as the lungs *lose* their elasticity and become less compliant, or stiffer, the value of this ratio decreases. For a simple analogy, if a balloon contained 1 liter of air under a pressure of 15 cm H_2O and it expanded to 1.5 liters after the pressure was raised to 20 cm H_2O, its compliance equals $\Delta V \div \Delta P$, or $0.5 \div 5$, or 0.1 liter/cm H_2O. The pressure-volume relationship of a simple spring is illustrated in Fig. 3-13, where there is a

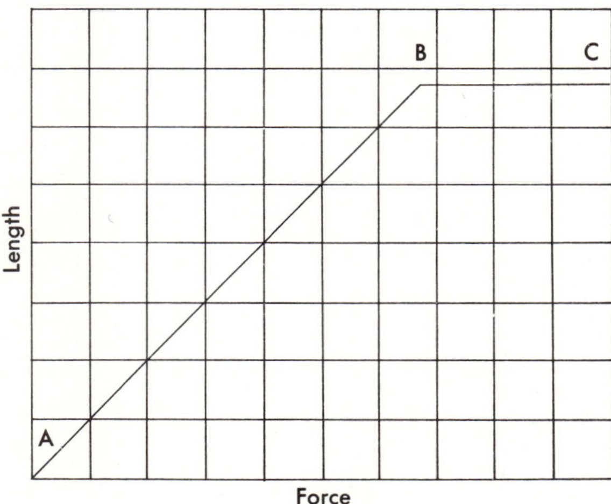

Fig. 3-13. The graph demonstrates compliance of a simple spring (increase in length/increase in force). With increasing force, the spring lengthens in a linear manner, from *A* to *B*, but at the point of maximum stretch further force produces no additional increase in length, *B* to *C*.

linear response of spring distance to force, up to the limit of stretch. The human ventilatory system, however, is composed of two sets of springs as previously illustrated in Fig. 3-6, and the lung-thorax compliance is obviously the net resultant of each. Thus, ventilatory compliance can be considered as a triad of total compliance of lung and thorax (C_{LT}), compliance of the lung alone (C_L), and compliance of the thorax alone (C_T). It should be noted that the compliance of the lung-thorax is *less* than that of either lung or thorax alone; and the student who is acquainted with electrical terminology will recognize that the relationship between total compliance and its two constituents is expressed in the same inverse manner as electrical resistors in parallel:

$$\frac{1}{C_{LT}} = \frac{1}{C_L} + \frac{1}{C_T}$$ [15]

Lung-thorax compliance (C_{LT}) can be measured in one of three general ways: (1) The subject, completely relaxed voluntarily or from anesthesia or disease, is placed in a body respiratory with his head outside at ambient pressure, and ventilation is controlled by the application of negative pressure to the surface of the body (Fig. 3-14). With the subject exhaling into a measuring device such as a spirometer and by varying the negative pressure and correlating this with the volume of air moved, the flexibility of the combined lungs and thorax in terms of liters of air moved per centimeter H_2O pressure exerted can be calculated.[16] (2) A cuffed endotracheal tube placed in an anesthetized subject allows ventilation of the lungs at various delivered *positive* pressures. These values, with their corresponding tidal volumes measured in a spirometer, provide compliance data. Normal C_{LT} by both these methods is about *0.1 liter/cm H_2O.* (3) A slightly different technique is the construction of a *relaxation-pressure curve.*[17] With a small pressure-transmitting plastic tube attached to a recording device and placed in his nose, the subject inhales a measured amount of air from a spirometer. Then, with tightly closed nose and mouth, he relaxes his ventilatory muscles, and the elastic recoil of lung and

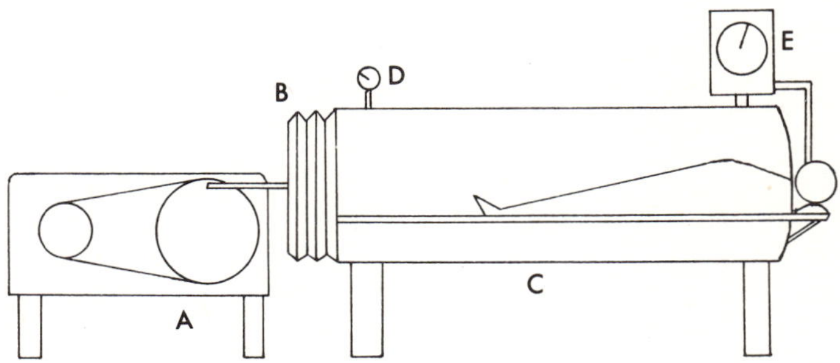

Fig. 3-14. This is a schematic representation of a subject in a body respirator. The motor, *A*, operates bellows, *B*, to create a rhythmic subatmospheric pressure in the cylindrical respirator, *C*, which is recorded by gauge, *D*. As the subject is ventilated by negative pressure applied to his body, his exhaled air is collected and measured in a meter, *E*. Volume change of the lung-thorax per unit of pressure applied can be determined.

thorax produces an alveolar pressure recorded by the nasal tube. Repeated at different V_E levels, a curve is produced. Compliance by this method is a bit higher than by the above two methods, about *0.12 liter/cm H_2O*. It should be noted that whether the ventilatory pressure is positive or negative makes no difference; for compliance depends upon the *absolute* pressure change for each volume change.

Pulmonary compliance (C_L) is calculated by measuring the *intrapleural pressure* at different levels of end-inspiratory volumes and plotting a pressure-volume curve that is generally linear in the ranges used. Since it is hazardous to invade the pleural cavity, a balloon-tipped catheter is swallowed until the balloon is at a midchest position. The balloon is attached to a pressure-recording device, and the soft-walled esophagus readily transmits surrounding intrapleural pressure to the balloon. The subject inhales to several different levels from a volume recorder (spirometer), and at the peak of each tidal volume (momentarily a static state with no airflow) the corresponding pressure is noted. From this data, liters per centimeter H_2O can be calculated. An intraesophageal tube records negative intrapleural pressure of a spontaneously breathing subject, but the lungs of a relaxed unconscious or anesthetized subject can be inflated with a positive pressure and the same data obtained. Fig. 3-15 schematically represents the record of three breaths with their corresponding intraesophageal pressures, demonstrating a normal lung compliance of 0.2 liter/cm H_2O.

Thoracic compliance (C_T) is determined indirectly, by using the inverse relationship described above. If lung-thorax and lung compliances are determined simultaneously, their values can be used to calculate C_T. Thus if $C_{LT}=$ 0.1 liter/cm H_2O and $C_L = 0.2$ liter/cm H_2O, then:

$$\frac{1}{C_{LT}} = \frac{1}{C_L} + \frac{1}{C_T} \qquad \frac{1}{C_T} = \frac{1}{0.1} - \frac{1}{0.2}$$

$$\frac{1}{0.1} = \frac{1}{0.2} + \frac{1}{C_T} \qquad C_T = 0.2 \text{ liter/cm } H_2O$$

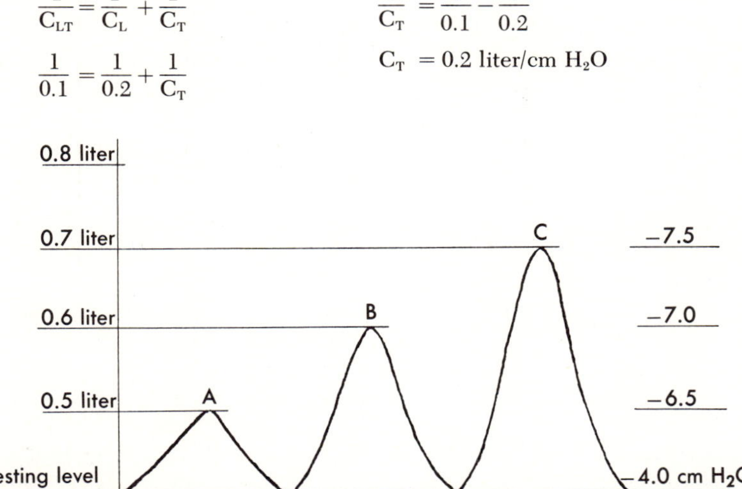

Fig. 3-15. From the resting level with an intrapleural pressure of −4 cm H_2O, to the static end-inspiratory point *A*, 0.5 liter of air moves with a pressure change of 2.5 cm H_2O. The same p-v relationships exist at *B* and *C*. Compliance calculated between any two points is 0.2 liter/cm H_2O.

***Exercise* 3-2.** Calculate the thoracic compliance in the following example:

Given: $C_{LT} = 0.072$ liter/cm H_2O
$C_L = 0.12$ liter/cm H_2O
Calculate: C_T

NONELASTIC RESISTANCE TO VENTILATION

The forces of ventilation must overcome not only elastic tissue tension but also the resistance offered by nonelastic tissue, such as muscle, cartilage, fat, abdominal contents, and the movement of large blood vessels and airways over one another. The inertia of these structures corresponds to the retarding effect of *friction* in any mobile system and modifies the ideal pressure-volume relationship previously described. The work involved in overcoming tissue friction can be illustrated simply as in Fig. 3-16, graphing the stretch of a spring hampered by friction. The uninhibited length response to increasing pressure without friction is recorded as a dashed line (similar to Fig. 3-13), whereas the response slowed by friction follows the solid line. The latter is curved, as a result of the drag of friction. Area 1 represents the amount of work done to overcome elasticity, and Area 2 the additional work to overcome friction.[18]

Fig. 3-16 demonstrates another important characteristic of nonelastic resistance. The tension of elasticity is *continuously* present, once force has been applied to a spring, whether the force is static or changing. In the lung-thorax, once distention has started, elasticity is present whether air is flowing or the

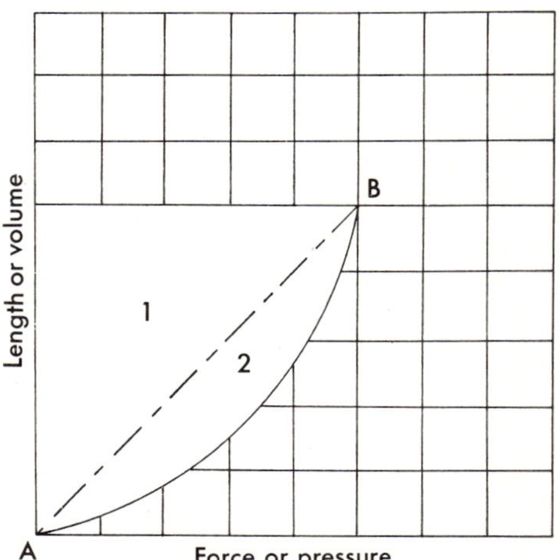

Fig. 3-16. Point *A* is the resting level, and *B* is end-inspiration. Dashed *A-B* represents the pressure-volume relationship of pure elastic resistance, and curved *A-B* the "drag" added by nonelastic friction. At *B*, where airflow momentarily ceases, nonelastic resistance is inactive because it is dependent upon movement. The curved line thus disappears, leaving only the elastic resistance of stretch. Areas *1* and *2* represent the work of overcoming elastic and nonelastic resistance, respectively.

lung is at a static breath-holding position. Nonelastic resistance is present *only* during movement, as when force is moving the spring or air is flowing in the lung, and is absent at static positions of no airflow. In Fig. 3-16, point A represents the resting position of no airflow and no distention of the lung; point B is the end-inspiratory pause with distention but no airflow. At B, therefore, only elastic resistance is active. The maximum effect of nonelastic resistance is noted where the two lines are most divergent, the period of greatest rate of airflow.

AIRWAY RESISTANCE TO VENTILATION

Flow of gas through the airways produces resistance to ventilation that varies with characteristics of the gas, the nature of the flow, and the condition of the conducting passages. This resistance is a ratio between the driving pressure responsible for gas movement and the flow rate of the gas per second; it is calibrated in centimeters H_2O/liter/sec. The pressure involved is the so-called *transairway* pressure, or the *gradient* between the mouth (atmospheric) and the alveolar pressures, responsible for the flow of gas. Remember, it makes no difference whether the driving pressure is negative (below ambient atmospheric), producing a negative gradient as in spontaneous breathing, or positive, as in mechanical ventilation. The sign of the pressure is unimportant because we are interested only in the absolute difference between atmospheric and alveolar tensions. During inhalation, alveolar pressure drops below atmospheric, and air flows into the lung, with reverse mechanics during exhalation. Thus:

$$R \text{ (in cm } H_2O\text{/liter/sec)} = \frac{\Delta P \text{ (in cm } H_2O)}{\dot{V} \text{ (in liters/sec)}}$$

The normal airway resistance ranges from *0.6 to 2.4 cm H_2O/liter/sec*, measured at a standard flow rate of *0.5 liter/sec.* Suppose pulmonary disease so alters airways by partial obstruction that, to overcome the resistance, strong inspiratory efforts are needed, dropping the alveolar pressure to lower values and widening the mouth-alveolar gradient. The following examples compare the data of such a condition with the normal and illustrate the increase in resistance that such a gradient implies:

$$\textit{Normal:} \quad R = \frac{\Delta P}{\dot{V}} = \frac{1}{0.5} = 2 \text{ cm } H_2O\text{/liter/sec}$$

$$\textit{Abnormal:} \quad R = \frac{\Delta P}{\dot{V}} = \frac{5}{0.5} = 10 \text{ cm } H_2O\text{/liter/sec}$$

Specialized laboratory equipment is available to supply the data needed to calculate airway resistance. Flow rates are measured with a sensitive apparatus called a *pneumotachograph*, which converts gas velocity into pressure and transmits this pressure to a calibrated recorder, either photographic or electronic, from which final measurements are made. Precise alveolar pressures are best determined by a *body plethysmograph*, an airtight box in which the subjects sits or reclines. As he breathes, the pressure changes in his alveoli are reciprocated in the space about him in the box and relayed to a suitable recorder.

Airway resistance is the result of friction between molecules of flowing gas and between the molecules and the wall of the conducting tube. The two physical gas characteristics contributing to resistance are *density* and *viscosity.* The former has been adequately described earlier, and we will now define and discuss the latter. Viscosity of a gas (or liquid) corresponds to friction of a moving solid and varies with individual gases, directly with temperature. The more viscous a gas, the more resistive it is to motion or change of form. It can be visualized as a time-related force exerted by a moving plane surface over a stationary plane surface, expressed in dyne-seconds per square centimeter. A frictional force of 1 dyne over an area of 1 cm^2 for a distance of 1 cm and a period of 1 second is called a *poise.* It should be apparent that viscosity of liquids is greater than that of gases and the values for both are small enough that they are expressed as fractions of poises. Viscosity of liquids is usually recorded as *centipoises* (10^{-2} poises), and of gases as *micropoises* (10^{-6} poises). A few examples in Table 3-4 illustrate the ranges of these values.

Although the student is not expected to be familiar with the details of this aspect of gas physics, analysis of the formula by which gas viscosity is calculated will reveal some relationships of great importance to the inhalation therapist. *Poiseuille's law* tells us that when gas flows through a tube:

$$n = \frac{\Delta P \pi r^4}{8l\dot{V}}$$

where n is viscosity, ΔP is a pressure gradient in dynes per square centimeter between the two ends of the tube, r is the tube radius in centimeters, l is the tube length in centimeters, $\dot{V}$ is gas flow rate in cubic centimeters per second, and $\pi/8$ is a constant.

The importance of this formula to the general topic of ventilation is the information it gives when manipulated to our purposes. First, let us rearrange the equation and equate the two important kinetic ventilatory factors, *pressure* and *flow rate*, to the others. (*Note:* Unless otherwise specified, our use of the

Table 3-4. *Examples of viscosity measurements*

	Substance	°C	*Poises*
Liquids	Water	20	1.005×10^{-2}
	Alcohol, ethyl	20	1.2×10^{-2}
	Glycerine	20	1490×10^{-2}
	Oil, castor	10	2420×10^{-2}
Gases	Air	18	182.7×10^{-6}
	CO_2	20	148×10^{-6}
	O_2	19	201.8×10^{-6}
	He	20	194.1×10^{-6}

term "pressure" means a pressure recorded on a gauge or other device that measures the pressure as above or below ambient atmospheric. Since this implies a "gradient," it is not necessary to use the symbol ΔP, but merely P.)

$$P = \frac{n8l\dot{V}}{\pi r^4} \qquad \dot{V} = \frac{P\pi r^4}{8ln}$$

If we are not interested in quantitative relationships but only in the general effects of changes in these parameters, one on the other, we can modify the equations by eliminating those factors that would not change significantly under our specified conditions. Pi and 8 are obvious constants; in a given subject the tubing length, l, representing the airways, is also generally a constant; since a subject breathes but one gas at a time, for any given circumstance gas viscosity is constant. It is important to note that tube radius, r, is not a constant because, in disease, airway patency is often a critical variable. Thus, the above two equations can be rewritten as simple *proportionalities:*

$$P \cong \frac{\dot{V}}{r^4} \qquad \dot{V} \cong Pr^4$$

Finally, these two can be combined into a single expression that clearly shows the reciprocal relationships between the three important variables:

$$\frac{Pr^4}{\dot{V}}$$

In clinical pulmonary physiology, one of the most frequently encountered conditions is that which involves narrowing of the airways through disease. The above ratio tells us that:

1. If the delivery pressure of gas ventilating the lung remains constant, the flow rate of the gas will vary directly with the *fourth power* of the radius of the airway. We see how a small change in bronchial caliber can effect a tremendous change in the amount of gas reaching alveoli.
2. If the flow rate of the ventilating gas is to remain constant, then the delivery pressure must vary inversely with the fourth power of the airway radius. Thus, to maintain stable ventilation in the presence of narrowing airways, we may need great increases in driving pressure.

In the respiratory tract there are three types of airflow patterns that are related to gas viscosity and density—*laminar, turbulent,* and *tracheobronchial* flow, illustrated in Fig. 3-17:

Laminar flow is a smooth unobstructed flow of gas through a tube of relatively uniform diameter, with few directional changes, and is found mostly in the trachea and main bronchi. Laminar flow is influenced principally by *viscosity* of the gas being moved, at low to moderate flow rates, and thus the relationships outlined above are pertinent in terms of the amount of air moved per unit of time or the pressure needed to move it. In respiratory physiology significant changes in inhaled gas viscosity are rarely of clinical importance. However, uniform narrowing of an airway reduces flow rate in proportion to the fourth power of the new radius or requires a similar increase

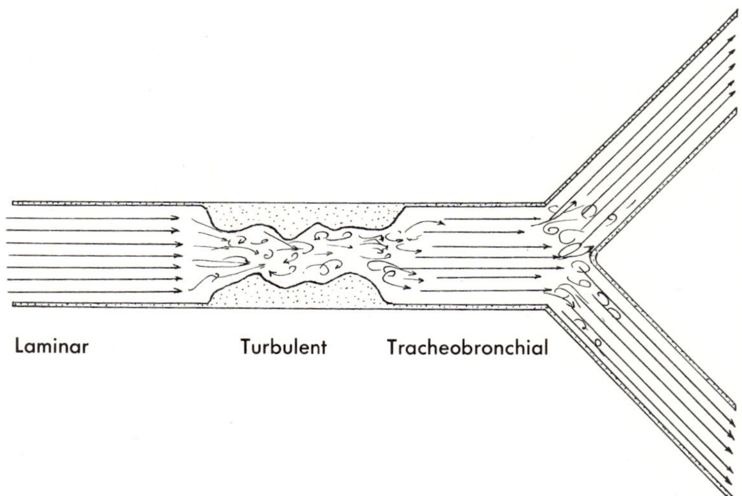

Fig. 3-17. Three patterns of airflow are found in the respiratory tract. *Laminar* flow is straight and unobstructed, found in the large air passages. *Turbulent* flow is rough and swirling, the result of obstruction and sudden directional changes. *Tracheobronchial* flow is a combination of the two, found in the constantly branching and continuously narrowing airways. (After Comroe, J. H., Jr., et al: The lung, Chicago, 1962, Year Book Medical Publishers, Inc.)

in driving pressure to maintain a steady flow. Inspiratory airflow is maintained at a fairly steady rate, but because normal airways gradually narrow, there is a pressure drop from mouth to alveoli. The therapist must always remember that the pressure he measures at the patient's mouth is not the pressure delivered to the lung.

Turbulent flow is rough, with much eddy formation, like that of a stream running over a tortuous, rocky bed, and in the airways is generated by sudden changes in direction or acute reduction in diameter. Flow can also be turbulent, even in smooth passages, at high velocity. Ninety percent of the turbulence in the normal respiratory tract occurs in the irregular passages between the nose and trachea, but it is also found in the distal branchings of the small bronchi and bronchioles.[19] It is a factor of great clinical importance in all airways damaged by disease, especially where abnormal secretions, mucosal edema, or structural changes produce abrupt narrowing.

The influence of turbulence on ventilation is best explained by the *Bernoulli effect* (Daniel Bernoulli, 1700-1782), a natural phenomenon widely evident in our daily lives and the functional basis for much of the equipment used in inhalation therapy. Fig. 3-18, *A*, shows the fundamental relationships between pressure, gas flow rates, and air passage restriction. Fig. 3-18, *B*, illustrates a modification of the Bernoulli effect found in a *venturi* (Giovanni Venturi, 1746-1822). The venturi includes a dilatation of the gas passage just distal to an obstruction, and if the angulation of the funnel is not over 15 degrees, the gas pressure will be restored nearly to its prerestriction level.

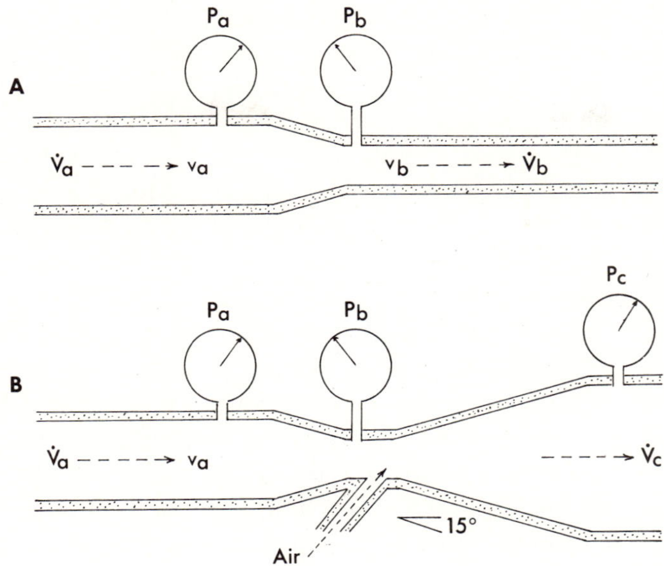

Fig. 3-18. A, The Bernoulli effect demonstrates that the pressure exerted by a steady flow of gas or liquid in a conducting tube varies *inversely* as the *velocity* of the fluid. With an abrupt narrowing of the passage, since the volume of fluid per unit of time leaving ($\dot{V}_b$) must equal the time-volume entering the tube ($\dot{V}_a$), the linear motion of the fluid per unit of time (velocity, v) must increase as it traverses the stricture ($v_b > v_a$). Thus there is a pressure drop distal to the restriction ($P_b < P_a$). **B,** The Venturi principle states that the pressure drop distal to a restriction can be closely restored to the prerestriction pressure if there is a dilatation of the passage immediately distal to the stenosis, with an angle of divergence not exceeding 15 degrees. Thus, P_c approximately equals P_a. The venturi is a widely used device to entrain a second gas to mix with the main-flow gas. The subambient pressure distal to the restriction draws in the second gas just past the restriction, and the increased outflow ($\dot{V}_c > \dot{V}_a$) is accommodated by the widened distal passage.

Widely used in fluid mechanics, venturis in inhalation therapy equipment are designed to draw in or "entrain" a second gas to mix with the main-flow gas. Such entrainment takes place at the point of low pressure, the distal widening not only permitting pressure restoration but also providing ample space for the increased volume of the mixed gases. Reference will be made later to both the Bernoulli phenomenon and the venturi during discussions of equipment.

A distinction should be made here, between the terms *flow rate* and *velocity*. Flow rate is a measure of the movement of a fluid *volume* per unit of time, and velocity is a measure of *linear* movement of a fluid per unit of time. For example, in two conducting tubes with different capacities, gases may move at the same velocity but at widely different flow rates. However, it should be evident that, in a given conducting system operating under a constant delivery pressure, changes in a flow rate entering the system will elicit corresponding qualitative changes in gas velocities through the system. To this limited degree flow rate and velocity are directly related, but Fig. 3-18, *A*, shows us that the introduction of a restriction in the system necessitates an increase in postobstruction velocity to maintain a steady flow rate. We shall use these relationships shortly as we explore in more detail the mechanics of fluid flow.

A moving fluid exerts two kinds of energy—*pressure energy* and *kinetic (or velocity) energy* (KE). Pressure energy is produced by the driving pressure of the fluid, which can be gravitational (a column of liquid or gas, or an elevated reservoir) or compressive (a pump or compressed gas). Kinetic energy is the result of the velocity of the fluid movement. Briefly, kinetic energy is the amount of work performed by matter in motion against a resistive force and is measured in a unit called a *joule*. For our purposes, however, it is not necessary to be quantitatively specific, for we are interested only in the general relationship between such energy and gas flow. Thus, in terms of pressure, kinetic energy can be expressed as *0.5 (density of the fluid) (square of the velocity of the fluid)*, or 0.5 (Dv^2). The derivation of this expression can be found in any standard textbook of physics. Now, the Bernoulli theorem for a continuous fluid flow states that the sum of the pressure and kinetic energies at any one point in the stream will equal the sum of these energies at any other point.[20] This is symbolized in the following equation, relating points a and b in Fig. 3-18, *A*, where P = pressure energy and $0.5Dv^2$ = kinetic energy:

$$P_a + 0.5\ Dv_a^2 = P_b + 0.5\ Dv_b^2$$

To make this equation more applicable to our needs in pulmonary physiology, we can alter it and rewrite it as a proportionality. If we assume we are dealing with a single gas, density will be a constant and can be dropped, giving us the following proportional expression:

$$P_a - P_b \cong v_b^2 - v_a^2$$

Since the velocity at point b is greater than at point a, the delivered pressure at b must be less than the driving pressure at a. This means that as gas flows through a stricture its velocity *increases* and its pressure *decreases* and the magnitude of the pressure drop across the obstruction is proportional to the increase in the *square* of the velocity. Simply, the additional energy expended by the increased velocity reduces the amount of energy available to exert pressure. The implication of this effect is extremely important to the inhalation therapist. If therapeutic gas is applied to the airways of a patient with obstructive disease, the higher the flow rates delivered at a constant pressure, the greater will be the velocities; and with increasing flows, the difference between the squares of the pre- and postobstruction velocities will be widened. The pressure inflating the alveoli will drop in proportion to this difference, or the delivery pressure will have to be increased accordingly to maintain a fixed alveolar pressure. To look at this semiquantitatively, let us simulate, in Table 3-5, the effect of airway obstruction by substituting, in the above proportionality, arbitrary values for v_a (velocity of applied flow rate) and v_b (velocity through the restriction) so that v_b is always one unit greater than v_a. We see

Table 3-5. *Diminishing final pressure with increasing flow rate*

v_b	v_a	$v_b^2 - v_a^2$	$P_a - P_b$
2	1	$4 - 1$	3
3	2	$9 - 4$	5
4	3	$16 - 9$	7

that, with increasing applied flow rates (velocities at point a) at a fixed driving pressure, delivered pressures gradually diminish. The clinical application of this principle will be dealt with in some detail in later chapters.

There is yet another valuable clinical aspect to the Bernoulli phenomenon. Let us rewrite the above proportionality to include the density factor (eliminating the 0.5 as a constant):

$$P_a - P_b \cong D\,(v_b^2 - v_a^2)$$

Inspection shows that, with a given increase in velocity, the pressure drop across a restriction will be lessened if the gas density is reduced. Thus, with obstructed airways, where the Bernoulli effect can be expected to exert a strong influence on the effectiveness of ventilation, distal pressure loss will be minimized with the use of low-density gases. This knowledge makes available to us a very valuable therapeutic tool, and we will see a practical use of the material just discussed when we consider the clinical use of helium.

Tracheobronchial flow is a descriptive term given to the mixture of laminar and turbulent flows found in the normal respiratory tract. Smooth gas flow through short segments of the tract is increasingly broken by the continuous branching of the airways, and even the relatively straight segments become progressively narrower with deeper penetration. Ventilation is thus the net sum of both laminar and turbulent flows, and effective alveolar pressure is related to the gas flow rate and tube radius in the laminar areas and the square of the gas velocity in the turbulent areas. The body's apparatus for moving air into and out of the lungs is designed to function against a normal balance of these resistances, but when they are increased by disease, the disability that results often requires the skilled services of inhalation therapy.

This is a good place to tie together the related factors of compliance, ventilatory frequency, flow rate, and airway resistance, which we have been describing individually. If his knowledge of these parameters is to have useful clinical meaning, the therapist must see the role played by each in reference to the others. Since the basic function of ventilation is the movement of air, the amount of air moved per unit of energy or pressure exerted will determine the efficiency of the system. This, we have already learned, is the description of compliance and is a measure of the elastic resistance of the lung-thorax system. However, we also know that the amount of air moved is dependent upon the state of the airways, the degree of their resistance to airflow. Thus, although the elastic resistance determines the pressure necessary to generate a given volume change, flow resistance determines the pressure needed for a given flow rate. From a practical point of view, then, the overall functional or *measured* lung-thorax compliance is really the net sum of the *actual* compliance of the system and the airway resistance. We can say that the general quality of airflow throughout the lungs is dependent upon the *uniformity of distribution* of both the elastic properties (actual compliance) in all areas of the lung and the flow-resistive properties (airway resistance) among all the airways. More specifically, it has been determined that, when flow rates are low, pulmonary air distribution is dependent upon lung elasticity and, when flow rates are high, upon airway resistance.[15]

Of clinical importance is the observation that, in normal healthy subjects, measured compliance does not vary as much with increased breathing rates as in patients with chronic bronchopulmonary disease, in whom measured compliance progressively drops as frequency increases. Thus, the patient with obstructive disease needs increasing effort to move a given volume of air as he breathes at higher rates. Although his *actual alveolar compliance may be normal* (a possibility, even in diseased states), his measured compliance, or the volume of air he moves per unit of pressure, is depressed. Fig. 3-19

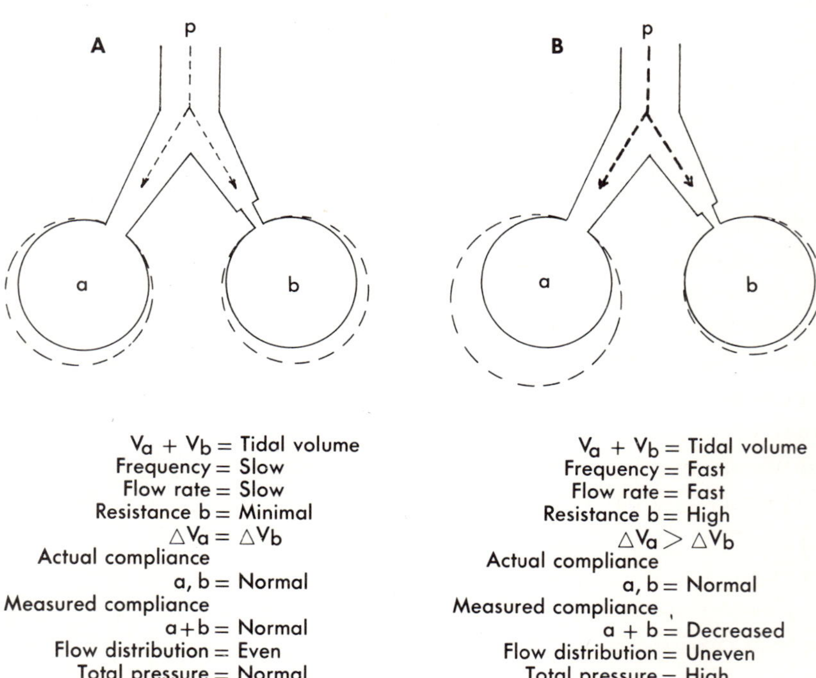

Fig. 3-19. The effect of airway resistance on measured total compliance is shown in sketches where one of each pair of alveoli, with normal actual compliance, is obstructed. The solid-line alveoli are at the resting level, the broken-line at end-tidal inspiration. *P* designates ventilatory pressure. In **A**, with a slow rate, the obstruction has little effect on total ventilation, for the volume changes in the alveoli are equal. In **B**, the increased flow rate reduces the ventilation of alveolus *b*, while *a* compensates by hyperinflating. The increased ventilatory pressure, which attempts to overcome the resistance, lowers the measured, apparent, total compliance.

shows the reason for this. For a given volume of air per breath (tidal volume), as the frequency of breathing increases so does the flow rate, since the volume must be moved faster with each ventilatory excursion. At low frequencies, with low flow rates, the effect of resistance is minimal and air is equally distributed between two alveoli because the actual compliance of the two pulmonary units determines the distribution of the air. With an increase in breathing frequency, as flow rate increases, the accompanying flow resistance of the obstruction causes a wide discrepancy in the distribution of flow to the alveoli, while increasing the total pressure needed to move the air. It can be deduced that for the overall functional compliance to remain unchanged in the presence of variable rates of breathing, the distribution of flow must remain unchanged. This requires that the elastic properties and the flow-resistive properties of all the pathways of the lung be distributed in a specific manner, one that is apparently found only in normal lungs. This state can be described briefly. In any pathway of the lung, the product of compliance and resistance is the unit of time[21]:

$$\text{Compliance} \times \text{Resistance} = \text{Time}$$

because

$$\frac{\text{Volume}}{\text{Pressure}} \times \frac{\text{Pressure}}{\text{Volume/Time}} = \text{Time}$$

This product is called the *time-constant*, and if it is the same for all pathways in the lung, then the flow distribution is independent of frequency and overall compliance is independent of rate. It is also obvious that, since "time" is a constant, resistance and compliance must vary indirectly, one with the other. Although this may appear to be a somewhat abstract and academic description of the related functions, if the therapist can assimilate it into his total knowledge of ventilatory mechanics, it will explain to him some of the difficulties that he will encounter in the field of mechanical ventilation as he attempts to correlate pressures, flow rates, and time factors in clinical situations. Also, this view of *compliance* gives a more realistic picture of the relation between volumes and pressures than did the simpler, more classical definition described earlier.

EXHALATION MECHANICS

Because of its clinical importance, the mechanics of exhalation deserves special consideration. It will be emphasized later that disturbances in exhalation produce some of the most frequent and severe examples of pulmonary disability. Whereas inhalation is a function of the active contraction of the several muscle groups described earlier, quiet exhalation is the result of *passive recoil* of elastic tissue of the lung, aided by the force of surface tension. At end-inspiration, ventilatory muscles "let go," allowing the lung-thorax to return to the resting level. Under conditions of stress, or in response to airflow obstruction, exhalation may be active through abdominal muscle action, forcing the diaphragm upward for more rapid emptying of the lung. Of critical importance in determining the passivity or activity of exhalation is the element of *time*. If the body's gas exchange needs, for a given level of physical exertion, can be satisfied by an effortless passive exhalation before the succeeding inhalation is triggered, then supplementary muscular activity will not be needed; but if there is an increased gas exchange need, or if disease of the respiratory tract is impeding gas flow or uptake, or there has been loss of lung-thorax elasticity, the body may require additional expiratory effort to move enough air from the lungs in *time* to satisfy the need. This effortful exhalation may be so energy consuming as to produce marked disability.

It should be evident that airway resistance to exhalation and loss of elasticity are important factors in determining ventilatory patterns. During quiet breathing, airway resistance to inhalation and exhalation in healthy subjects is about the same, even though the negative intrathoracic pressure of inhalation dilates and elongates the bronchioles and the rising pressure of exhalation narrows and shortens them. Forced exhalation, on the other hand, does increase resistance, and if exhalation is forced through normally patent airways and against negligible resistance, as in unobstructed hyperventilation, the high velocity of exhaled air creates its own resistance due to turbulence, but the expiratory muscular effort responsible is adequate to maintain smooth airflow. However, many pulmonary diseases damage and weaken the walls of the bronchioles. In such circumstances, should airway obstruction or loss of elasticity necessitate a strong expiratory effort to overcome resistance, the excessive positive pressures generated in the thorax may collapse the weakened bronchioles before the alveoli they drain are emptied. This condition of *air trapping* is a common complication of chronic bronchopulmonary disease, often posing a management problem for the inhalation therapist, and will be dealt with more fully later.

With prolonged airway resistance or loss of elasticity, structural changes may occur in the chest. A major consequence of these disturbances is the gradual elevation of the resting level of the chest, as air trapping and/or inadequate recoil force prevent the lung-thorax from returning to its original, normal end-expiratory position. As shown in Fig. 3-20, this produces an increase in both the functional residual capacity and the residual volume. If uncorrected over a sufficient period of time, there is a progressive increase in the size of the thorax, especially in its anteroposterior diameter, the deformity descriptively called a "barrel chest." This is a remarkable phenomenon, since it most frequently occurs after the middle years, when the skeleton is well fixed, but it attests to the force exerted by the distended lung, coupled with the traction of accessory ventilatory muscles, to be described later. Because of the elevated resting level, the affected subject gives the appearance of holding his chest in the inspiratory position, a condition frequently seen in pulmonary emphysema.

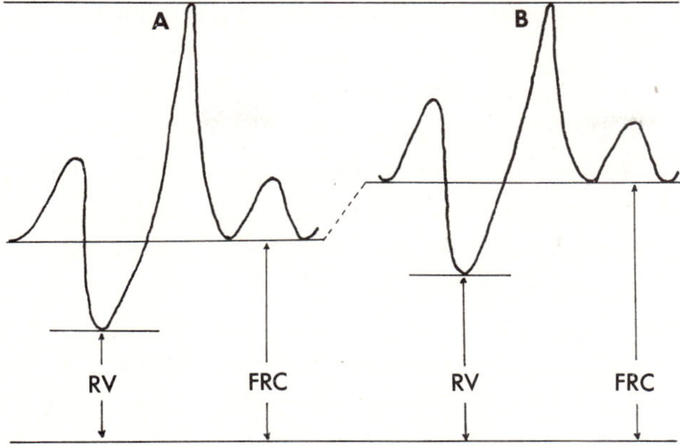

Fig. 3-20. Sketch **A** shows the resting level before, and **B** after, the effect of long-standing airway resistance and/or loss of lung elasticity, as the expansile thoracic springs dominate the pulmonary. Both functional residual capacity and residual volume enlarge. As disease progresses, loss of pulmonary flexibility decreases the expiratory reserve volume, further enlarging the residual volume, and continuing distention may depress the diaphragm to expand the total lung capacity.

SUMMARY

The importance of the material covered in this chapter justifies a brief summary to emphasize a few clinical points of interest to the inhalation therapist. In good health, the complex integrated respiratory control system is able to assure the body of a maximally effective ventilation, with a minimum of effort for any given level of need. Indeed, except under conditions of physical stress, we are generally unaware of the easy rhythmicity of our own breathing, until it becomes impaired. Although we have not yet considered details of internal physiologic derangement of blood gas exchange that can upset the normal pattern of breathing, we should be impressed with the multitude of physical factors that influence ventilation and wonder at the ease with which it is accomplished.

The effective inhalation therapist must be observant. He must be able to judge, at least grossly, the general efficiency of his patient's ventilation on the basis of clinical observation. This means that he must have a clear mental picture of a *normal* breathing pattern for a given individual. He will note, for example, the rate and depth of tidal air exchange and attempt to determine whether the patient is hypoventilating or hyperventilating. He will evaluate the patient's work of breathing by looking for evidence of the use of accessory muscles of ventilation, the resting end-expiratory chest level, signs of inspiratory epigastric retraction or retraction of the costal margins, and evidence of expiratory abdominal contraction. He will observe the time relations between inspiration and expiration to see whether the normal inspiration-longer-than-expiration pattern is reversed. Such information will aid him in carrying out, most efficiently and comfortably, his assigned treatment. Many times, of course, effortful breathing is obvious and the great effort to breath is apparent at once. Such a patient can be described as short of breath at rest or at any specified level of activity. The therapist will frequently hear the term *dyspnea* used, and he should understand its real meaning. Dyspnea is a symptom, a subjective feeling experienced only by the patient, not objectively observed by someone else. If a patient states that he is having difficulty breathing, then he is dyspneic. It means that he is uncomfortably aware of the need to work to breathe, and the therapist will be surprised at the number of patients who are obviously breathing with effort but who do not complain of it.

Although there are many pathologic aberrations in ventilatory patterns, there is one type with which the therapist should be familiar because of its frequency. This is referred to as "periodic breathing," and although there are variations of it, the most common is known as *Cheyne-Stokes respiration.* It is characterized by alternating periods of hyperventilation and apnea. Tidal volume excursions get progressively deeper with each breath, reach a maximum, gradually get smaller in amplitude, and then cease completely. Each period of ventilation and apnea can last up to 20 seconds.[22] The "waxing and waning" pattern is characteristic and makes this disorder easy to recognize, even when the apnea may not be quite complete. Cardiovascular rather than respiratory factors are usually responsible for Cheyne-Stokes breathing, which is basically the result of cerebral oxygen want due to a reduced circulatory output of the left ventricle associated with obstructive cerebrovascular disease that reduces blood flow to the brain. Despite the apneic intervals, average blood carbon dioxide levels are usually low because of the hyperventilation. We are not concerned with the treatment of this condition, but the therapist should be on the watch for it and call it to the attention of attending medical or nursing personnel whenever he notes it.

A less commonly encountered periodic pattern is *Biot's respiration.* This is somewhat similar to Cheyne-Stokes, except that the hyperventilatory phases are abrupt in onset and termination, without the crescendo-decrescendo character of Cheyne-Stokes. The respiratory efforts may vary in intensity, and the intervening apneic periods may be unequal and irregular. Biot's breathing is usually the result of severe brain damage, and although the exact mechanism is not known, many feel that there may be a reduced inhibitory action of the higher brain centers on the inspiratory function of the respiratory center, allowing periodic breakthrough of excessive inspiratory efforts.[23]

Chapter 4

Blood gases and acid-base balance

The natural mechanisms of ventilation in good health, and the techniques of inhalation therapy in the treatment of disease, are designed to provide the circulating blood with sufficient oxygen for general cellular needs and to remove excess carbon dioxide. The sequence of the discussions so far has been purposely arranged to consider the more important and influential factors concerned with reaching these objectives, in an orderly and progressive manner. In this chapter, we will review the principles governing the actual movement of the respiratory gases into and out of the circulation and the transportation systems that carry the gases between lung and body cells. However, the respiratory gases, in addition to their participation in cellular metabolic needs, strongly influence the stability of the acid-base balance of the body, and we must include this aspect of physiology as an integral part of the overall study of blood gases. We will start with a discussion of the physical dynamics of alveolar blood diffusion and conclude with the physiologic and clinical aspects of acid-base balance.

MECHANICS OF DIFFUSION

Our study of the physiology of the respiratory tract has now brought us to that critically vital structure, the perfused alveolus. So far we have been concerned with factors responsible for the mass movement of air from the atmosphere into the conducting airways. With air in the alveoli, we will now consider the mechanisms by which oxygen is extracted and made available to the body in exchange for carbon dioxide. For this we will have to think microscopically, for we will be dealing with gases at the molecular level and with the physical and chemical reactions in which they take part in their travels to and from body cells. We will first review the manner in which the respiratory gases overcome the boundary between the "inside" and the "outside" of the body, the alveolar wall, by the process of diffusion.

Diffusion is the movement of gas molecules from an area of relatively high partial pressure of the gas to one of low partial pressure. As all motion requires some driving force, so diffusion depends upon a pressure gradient. In our realm of interest, the two gases with which we will be concerned, oxygen and carbon dioxide, not only must diffuse from one anatomic area to another but must also move through formidable obstructions—the alveolar wall–pulmonary capillary barrier (sometimes called the alveolar-capillary [A-C] membrane) and the body cell wall–systemic capillary barrier.[24] Thus, for gases to pass between the alveoli and the pulmonary capillary blood, there must exist a pressure gradient for each gas across this barrier, and the production and magnitude of these gradients will be of great concern to us from here on. Fig. 4-1 schematically illustrates the nature and structure of the A-C barrier, and if we keep in mind the minuscule size of a molecule of gas, we must be impressed with the task facing it in making the obstacle-ridden trip between alveolus and blood, and blood and tissue cell.

Since the A-C membrane is essentially a fluid barrier, the ability of gases to diffuse through it depends upon two physical laws governing the passage of gas through liquid:

1. *Henry's law* states that the weight of a gas dissolving in a liquid at a given temperature is proportional to the partial pressure of the gas. The amount of gas that can be dissolved by 1 ml of a given liquid at standard pressure and specified temperature is called its *solubility coefficient* and varies *inversely* with the temperature. The solubility coefficient of oxygen in plasma, at 37° and 760 mm Hg pressure, is 0.023 ml, and for carbon dioxide is 0.510 ml.

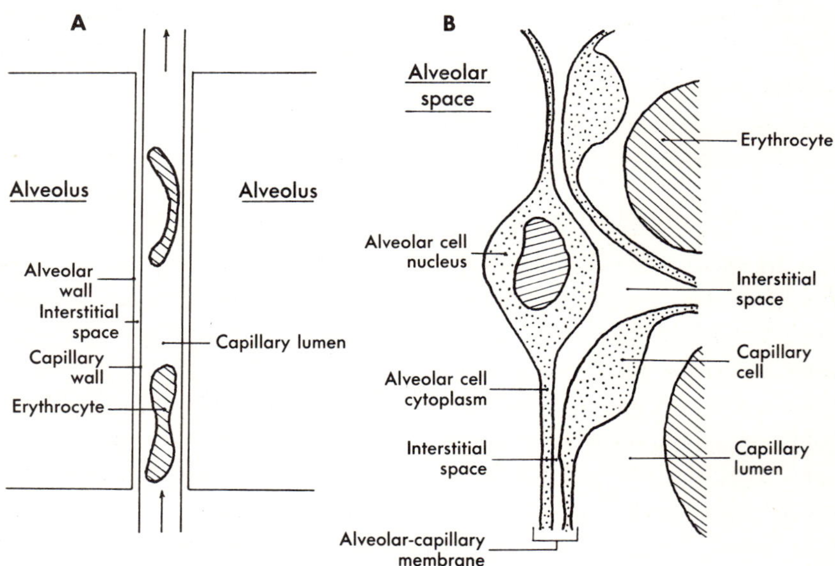

Fig. 4-1. Sketch **A** diagrams the relationship between the components of the alveolar-capillary (A-C) membrane, and **B** is a magnification sketch of a section through the structure. The *alveolar wall* is a cytoplasmic extention of the alveolar epithelial cells; it is separated from the adjacent capillary epithelial cells by a space, which may be real or potential, called the *interstitial* or intermembranous space. This space may contain tissue fibrils, and the accumulation of fluid here is of great clinical importance. The thickness of the A-C membrane varies from 0.4μ to 2.0μ, depending upon the contents of the space. (After Divertie, M. D., and Brown, A. L., Jr.: The fine structure of the normal human alveocapillary membrane, JAMA **187**:938, 1964.)

2. *Graham's law* states that the rate of diffusion (D) of a gas through liquid is directly proportional to its solubility coefficient and inversely proportional to the square root of its density (or gram-molecular weight). The number of milliliters of a gas that will diffuse a distance of 0.001 mm (1μ), over a square centimeter surface per minute, at 1 atm of pressure, is the *diffusion coefficient* of the gas.

Combining the above two properties, we can say that the relative rates of diffusion of two gases are directly proportional to the ratio of their solubilities and inversely proportional to the ratio of the square roots of their densities or gram-molecular weights. To illustrate this, let us compare the relative diffusibility of carbon dioxide with oxygen or, to state it another way, determine how much more or less diffusible is carbon dioxide than oxygen:

$$\text{Diffusibility of } CO_2 \cong \frac{\text{Sol coef } CO_2 \times \sqrt{\text{gmw } O_2}}{\text{Sol coef } O_2 \times \sqrt{\text{gmw } CO_2}}$$

$$\cong \frac{0.510 \times \sqrt{32}}{0.023 \times \sqrt{44}}$$

$$\cong \frac{0.510 \times 5.657}{0.023 \times 6.663}$$

$$\cong \frac{19}{1}$$

In other words, carbon dioxide is 19 times as diffusible as oxygen.

Exercise 4-1. Given the following data, what is the diffusibility of gas B compared to gas A?

	Gas A	*Gas B*
Sol coef	0.25	0.65
gmw	30	50

In cardiopulmonary physiology, knowledge of the diffusing capacity of the lung is sometimes helpful in evaluating pathologic conditions. Discussion of the laboratory techniques for measuring this function is not relevant here, but with the general concepts of diffusion just discussed in mind, we can relate its use to pulmonary evaluation. The expression *diffusion capacity of the lung* (D_L) is defined as the number of milliliters of a specific gas that diffuse from the lung across the A-C membrane into the bloodstream each minute, for each mm Hg difference in the pressure gradient across the membrane. The two most common gases used to measure this function are low concentration carbon *monoxide* (CO) and oxygen, and in reporting values obtained we must identify the gas used. Thus, average normal values are $D_{L_{CO}}$ = 17 ml/min/mm Hg and $D_{L_{O_2}}$ = 20 ml/min/mm Hg.[25]

Disease of the lung, if it modifies diffusion at all, always reduces diffusion. This implies that some absormality has made it difficult for gas molecules to cross the A-C membrane in a reasonable period of time, in response to a normal pressure gradient. The clinical implications of this fact will be discussed further in Chapter 6.

DIFFUSION GRADIENTS

The pressure gradient across the A-C membrane, so essential for gas diffusion, is dependent upon the concentrations of the gases in the inspired air and alveoli, as well as in the blood, and we will consider some of the physiologic normals. Since there is a continuous interchange in the alveoli of oxygen and carbon dioxide, each diluting the other, the alveolar concentrations of these gases are considerably different from their atmospheric concentrations. Table 4-1 presents some average normal values for *dry* inspired, alveolar, and exhaled air.

Correcting for the saturated state of these gases in the alveoli, we note that their alveolar partial pressures (P_A) at 1 atm are about:

O_2	CO_2	N_2	H_2O
100 mm Hg	40 mm Hg	573 mm Hg	47 mm Hg

At the circulatory end of the gradient, the respiratory gases in the blood also exert their own partial pressures. Although we have not yet discussed the transportation and utilization of the gases, we know that venous blood returning to the lung has less oxygen and more carbon dioxide than does arterial blood. Therefore, the partial pressures will differ between the types of blood. The average normal venous (P_v) and arterial (P_a) partial pressures are shown in Table 4-2.

An explanation is in order for the 90 to 100 mm Hg range of arterial oxygen tension listed above. The average $P_{a_{O_2}}$ of a large number of normal subjects would probably fall at about 95 *mm Hg*, in a range that would extend from 90 mm Hg to perhaps 103 mm Hg. If the lung were a "perfect" organ, every alveolus would have exactly the same P_{O_2} and the arterial blood leaving each alveolus would, through the process of diffusion to be described below, have exactly the same P_{O_2} as each alveolus, about 100 mm Hg. We will see later, however, that the lung is not perfect and normally there are slight discrep-

Table 4-1. *Composition of dry inspired, alveolar, and exhaled air*

	$\%O_2$	$\%CO_2$	$\%N_2$, *etc.*[26]
Inspired air	20.95	0.03	79.02
Alveolar air	14.0	5.6	80.4
Exhaled air	16.3	4.5	79.2

Table 4-2. *Gas partial pressures in venous and arterial blood*

$P_{v_{O_2}}$	40 mm Hg
$P_{v_{CO_2}}$	46 mm Hg
$P_{a_{O_2}}$	90-100 mm Hg
$P_{a_{CO_2}}$	40 mm Hg

ancies between the ratios of ventilation to perfusion among the many A-C units. As a result, a sample of mixed arterial blood (blood from all areas of the lung returning to the heart for distribution through the systemic circulation) often has an oxygen tension less than that of an air sample taken from the lungs as a whole. In this text, for the sake of uniformity, mixed arterial blood will be assumed to have an oxygen tension of 95 mm Hg, the 5 mm Hg difference between it and alveolar oxygen tension constituting a normal *alveolar-arterial oxygen tension gradient.* This term will be used again later, with both normal and abnormal connotations. However, when describing physiologic events at the level of a single alveolus and its capillary, we will assume, in the interest of simplicity, that the A-C unit is "perfect" unless otherwise specified and that the local capillary-arterial oxygen tension is 100 mm Hg.

It should be noted that blood values for nitrogen partial pressure were not included. This by no means indicates that such a pressure does not exist. However, as far as the physiology of respiration is concerned, nitrogen is an *inert* gas in that it takes no part in metabolic gas exchange. It can be considered as a filler, taking up whatever space is not used by the two respiratory gases. Nitrogen diffuses readily between alveoli and blood, and the partial pressure it exerts is the difference between (a) the sum of the respiratory gas pressures and the atmospheric pressure and (b) the water vapor pressure. Nitrogen is of medical importance under certain circumstances and will be discussed further when indicated.

We can now correlate the above data on partial pressures and show how they make up gradients to promote a continuous and relatively smooth diffusion of respiratory gases. Consider the alveolus as a small pump that is constantly drawing in oxygen (air) and expelling carbon dioxide, thus maintaining alveolar partial pressures at *average* levels as described above. At any given moment the pressures in the alveolus will vary according to the time of the ventilatory cycle (or cycling of the alveolar pump), but samples of alveolar air over many cycles determine these average partial pressures. Two pressure gradient systems are established, one between alveolar oxygen (100 mm Hg) and venous oxygen (40 mm Hg) and a smaller one between venous carbon dioxide (46 mm Hg) and alveolar carbon dioxide (40 mm Hg). Oxygen, with its partial pressure maintained through the alveolar pump, diffuses from the alveolus into the pulmonary blood, *equilibrating* the P_{O_2} of the blood with that of the alveolus. As the blood flows past the alveolus, it thus takes up oxygen and leaves the capillary as *arterialized* blood, with a P_{O_2} in equilibrium with the alveolar oxygen, around 100 mm Hg. Simultaneously, CO_2 flows from the pulmonary capillary with its P_{CO_2} of 46 mm Hg into the alveolus with its average P_{CO_2} of 40 mm Hg. Again, the alveolar pump, by the regulated exhalation of CO_2, maintains the gradient until the capillary blood has equilibrated with the alveolus, and the arterialized blood leaves the capillary with a P_{CO_2} of 40 mm Hg. Fig. 4-2 illustrates the "perfect" diffusion gradients across the A-C membrane and the manner in which venous blood becomes arterialized.

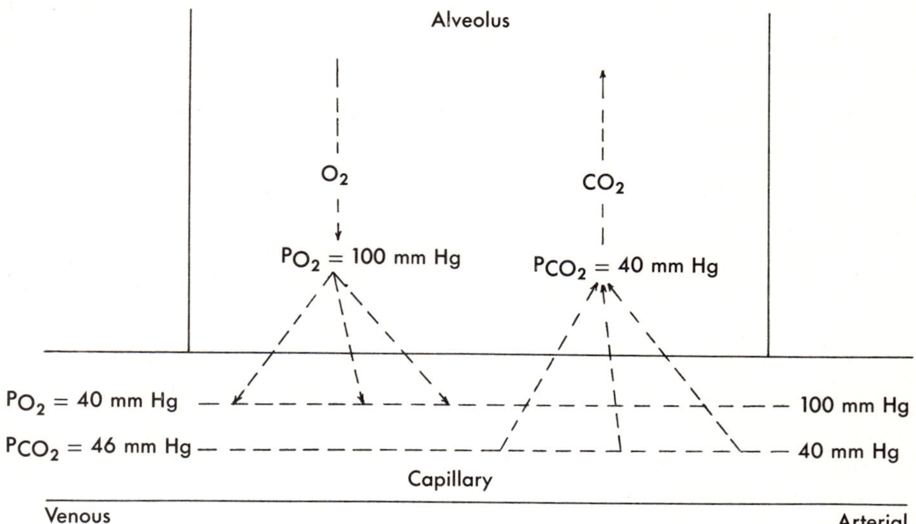

Fig. 4-2. Ventilation maintains the mean alveolar gas tensions as noted in the sketch. As blood enters the venous end of the pulmonary capillary, it loses its CO_2 and takes up O_2, until these two gases are in equilibrium with the mean alveolar tensions, and it leaves the capillary as arterial blood.

We should note that the element of time is a critical factor in the diffusion of oxygen although it is not directly related to the ability of the A-C membrane to exchange the gas. For blood to leave the pulmonary capillary adequately oxygenated, not only is the integrity of the membrane important, but the blood must spend sufficient time in contact with the membrane to permit maximum diffusion. In the normal subject at rest, it takes about 0.75 sec for a given point in the bloodstream to traverse the pulmonary capillary, and with the increased velocity of heavy exercise, about 0.34 sec.[27] Most oxygen diffusion occurs at the beginning of the capillary; thus it would require a very severe diffusion defect to be solely responsible for inadequate oxygenation. However, since such pathologic conditions as fever, acute blood loss, and certain cardiac irregularities, to mention a few, can increase the cardiac output and blood velocity, it is reasonable to suppose that, when associated with sufficient pulmonary disease, the rapid flow of blood through the pulmonary capillaries might be a significant contributing factor to incomplete oxygenation.

Our discussion of gradients so far has centered about the A-C membrane, but for a clear picture of diffusion we must include the equally important gradients at the tissue cellular level, for it is to service the cells that the ventilation-transportation system exists. The respiratory gas gradients at the cell can be visualized as the reverse of those in the lung. As the metabolism of the cell depletes its store of oxygen, the intracellular P_{O_2} drops below that of the blood entering the arterial end of the systemic capillary, and oxygen diffuses into the cell. At the same time, the carbon dioxide diffuses from its higher pressure level in the cell into the capillary blood, and the blood becomes venous, returning to the lung to repeat its circuit. In a sense we are dealing with two sets of gradients (alveolar-blood and blood-cell, for both O_2 and CO_2) that provide gas transportation between the extremes of the two wider gradients of alveolus-cell for O_2 and cell-alveolus for CO_2.

OXYGEN TRANSPORTATION

The mechanism by which oxygen is carried between the alveolus and the body cell will be discussed first, to be followed by a description of the transportation of carbon dioxide; but it must be clearly understood that these two processes occur simultaneously and it is only for convenience and clarity that we are separating them. Both gases are carried in the blood by virtue of their abilities to dissolve in blood or to combine with some of the elements of blood. An understanding of basic principles of gas transportation is essential for the safe and intelligent treatment of cardiopulmonary defects. Oxygen is carried in the blood in two so-called "compartments." One is the blood plasma, in which oxygen is dissolved in very small but important amounts, and the other is the hemoglobin of the erythrocyte, which carries the bulk of the load.

DISSOLVED OXYGEN

As oxygen molecules diffuse into the blood, some go directly into solution in the plasma, and when this compartment is filled, the rest continue into the erythrocytes. The amount of oxygen that dissolves is dependent upon the solubility coefficient of oxygen in plasma at body temperature. Thus, for every 760 mm of pressure Hg, 0.023 ml of oxygen dissolve in each milliliter of plasma. In pulmonary physiology, it is customary to refer to dissolved blood gases in terms of *volume percent* (vol%), which means so many *milliliters of gas* per *100 ml of plasma.* Therefore, for every 760 mm Hg pressure there are 2.3 vol% of dissolved oxygen, and this can be reduced to the basic factor of 0.003 vol% for *each* millimeter of mercury P_{O_2}. Calculation of the amount of oxygen that dissolves in plasma at any P_{O_2} is simply: $Vol\% = P_{O_2} \times 0.003$. In average normal arterial blood, with its $P_{a_{O_2}}$ of 95 to 100 mm Hg, the dissolved oxygen equals 0.3 ml of oxygen for each 100 ml of plasma. However, the $P_{a_{O_2}}$ of a subject breathing pure oxygen theoretically could reach 673 mm Hg, with dissolved oxygen of 2.02 vol%. The value of 673 is reached as follows: Recalling that physiologic gases are calculated in the dry state and assuming complete alveolar-arterial equilibrium with no P_{O_2} gradient, we can calculate that the alveolar gases of a subject breathing pure oxygen at 1 atm have a pressure of $760 - 47 = 713$ mm Hg. After a person has breathed 100% oxygen for several minutes, nitrogen that was in the alveoli during air breathing is completely washed out, leaving only oxygen and carbon dioxide. With a CO_2 tension of 40 mm Hg, alveolar (and presumably arterial) oxygen tension equals $713 - 40$, or 673 mm Hg. A method of estimating $P_{A_{O_2}}$ at any concentration of inhaled oxygen employs the *alveolar air equation,* which will not

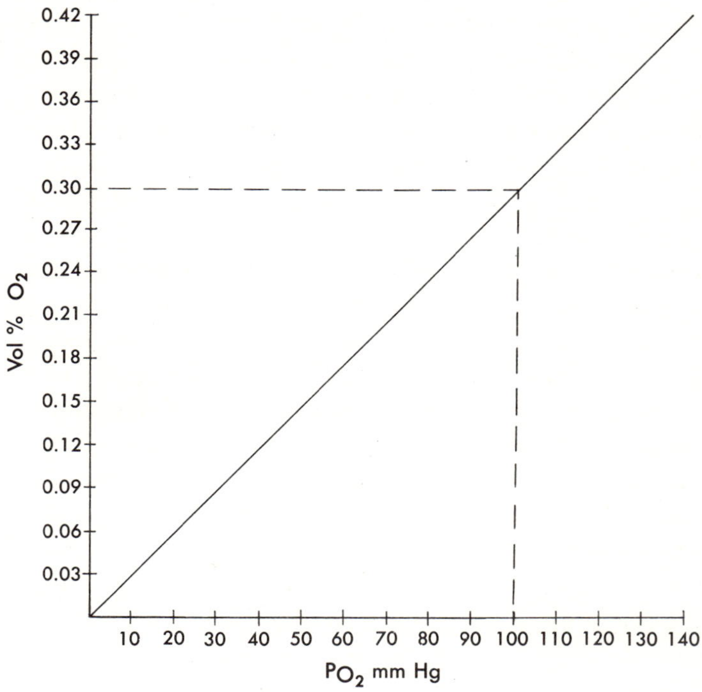

Fig. 4-3. The relationship between the number of milliliters of oxygen dissolved in blood and its consequent partial pressure is linear. Each 0.003 ml of O_2 dissolved in 100 ml of blood (vol% of O_2) exerts a pressure of 1 mm Hg. The dashed line emphasizes the fact that arterial blood, with an average P_{O_2} of 100 mm Hg, has 0.3 ml of O_2 dissolved in each 100 ml.

be considered at this time. Fig. 4-3 illustrates, by graph, the linear relationship between partial pressure of oxygen and vol% of oxygen dissolved in the plasma.

COMBINED OXYGEN

Most of the oxygen in the body is carried physically bound to or combined with the *hemoglobin* (Hb) of the erythrocytes. Hemoglobin is the "red stuff" of the blood, giving to blood its characteristic colors, and except in abnormal conditions, it is always confined to the erythrocyte. Should disease or disturbed physiology produce rupture of the red cells, the spillage of hemoglobin into the plasma is referred to as *hemolysis* of the cell with subsequent *hemoglobinemia.* Hemoglobin is a protein, *globin,* combined with an iron-containing compound called *heme.* It is a large and heavy molecule with a *physical* molecular weight of 66,700, but in its respiratory function its *physiologic* molecular weight is considered to be but 16,700. There are many different kinds of hemoglobin, designated by letters, i.e., A, C, E, F, G, H, I, J, K, S. Some of these types are variants of the normal; others are clinically pathologic. The differences in the hemoglobin types lie in the structure of the globin portion, which is made up of many amino acids derived from diet.

We will soon see that the transportation of oxygen and the transportation of carbon dioxide in the erythrocyte are mutually dependent upon one another since they alternate in using hemoglobin as a carrier; but first we will consider oxygen alone and then relate the two systems. Venous blood leaving the body cells still contains some oxygen, enough to maintain a partial pressure of about 40 mm Hg, but because of its depleted oxygen supply, most of its hemoglobin is called *reduced hemoglobin.* This is often symbolized simply as *Hb* or, since it has acquired a hydrogen ion in its participation in the transport of carbon dioxide from the cells (to be described and illustrated shortly), more properly as *HHb.* In the pulmonary capillaries, immediately upon release of carbon dioxide, the HHb converts to the potassium salt, *KHb.* In this form hemoglobin combines with oxygen molecules diffusing into the erythrocytes, becoming *oxyhemoglobin,* Hb_{O_2}, or better, KHb_{O_2}. One gram-molecular weight of oxygen, 32 gm, can combine with 16,700 gm of hemoglobin, and it is this factor that determines the physiologic molecular weight of hemoglobin as noted above. Because

$$\frac{1 \text{ mole } O_2}{16{,}700 \text{ gm Hb}} = \frac{22{,}400 \text{ ml } O_2}{16{,}700 \text{ gm Hb}} = \frac{1.34 \text{ ml } O_2}{\text{gm Hb}}$$

each gram of hemoglobin is able to take up and carry 1.34 ml of oxygen. If we assume a normal hemoglobin concentration of 15 gm per 100 ml of blood, then the combined oxygen *capacity* is $1.34 \times 15 = 20.1$ ml O_2 per 100 ml of blood, or *20.1 vol%,* and is directly related to the amount and quality of available hemoglobin.

However, the quantity of oxygen actually carried, or the content, is dependent upon the hemoglobin *saturation.* This refers to the amount of oxygen combined with hemoglobin in proportion to the amount of oxygen the hemoglobin is capable of carrying if it has its full load, and it is expressed as a percentage from the ratio content/capacity. Although the capacity can be calculated as above, if the presence of abnormal or inactive hemoglobin is suspected, in the laboratory the oxygen content can be chemically analyzed in vol%; then by exposing the sample to air to allow it to combine maximally with oxygen, we can determine its capacity. If the content is one half the capacity, the saturation is reported as 50%. Because the lung is not a "perfect" organ, as described above, in the normal subject breathing room air at 1 atm pressure, the average saturation of mixed arterial blood ($S_{a_{O_2}}$) is about 97%, and the average saturation of mixed venous blood entering the lung through the pulmonary circulation ($S_{v_{O_2}}$) is about 70% to 75%. Further details of the cause of the arterial deficiency will be considered in Chapter 6. *Unsaturation* is the converse of saturation and refers to the degree to which blood is not saturated. Thus, normal arterial blood may be considered to be 3% unsaturated, and venous blood 30% unsaturated. Since saturation = content/capacity, then content = capacity × saturation, and the amount of oxygen combined with hemoglobin in average normal arterial blood with 15 gm% Hb equals:

$$1.34 \times 15 \times 0.97 = 19.5 \text{ vol\%}$$

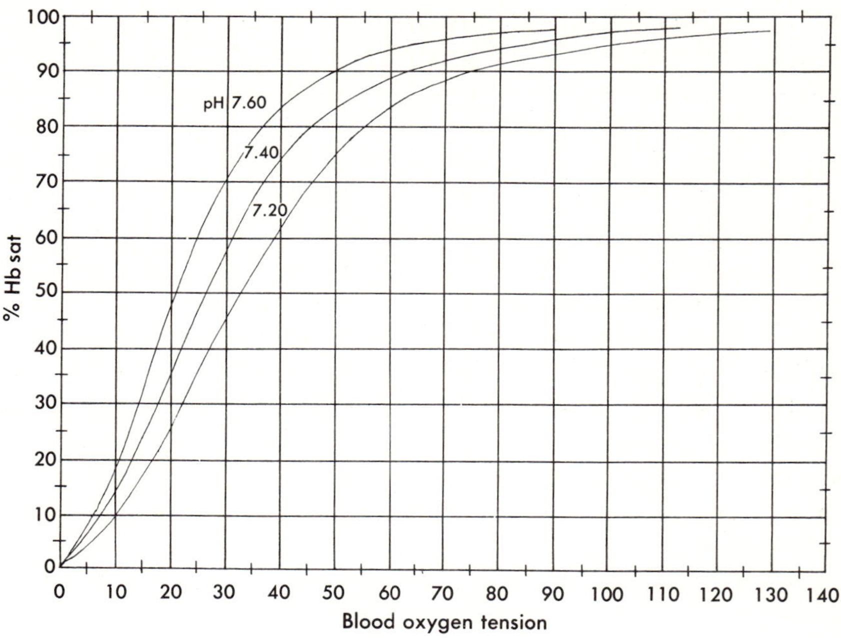

Fig. 4-4. O_2 dissociation curve of blood at 37° C, showing variations at three pH levels. For a given O_2 tension, the higher the blood pH, the more the hemoglobin holds onto its O_2, maintaining a higher saturation.

Let us now consider those factors that are responsible for determining the degree of arterial oxygen saturation—*partial pressure of arterial oxygen, chemical reaction of the blood* (pH), and *body temperature.* One of the most important fundamentals of pulmonary physiology is the relationship between oxygen saturation and these three factors, graphically illustrated in the oxygen dissociation curves, which indicate the physiologic conditions under which oxygen combines with or dissociates from its hemoglobin carrier. When all the elements of ventilation, pulmonary air distribution, ventilation/perfusion ratio, and alveolar diffusion are able to achieve a P_{O_2} of 100 mm Hg in arterial blood with a normal pH of 7.40 at body temperature, the arterial oxygen saturation will be approximately 97%. Fig. 4-4 is the dissociation curve of blood at 37° C, showing the important relationship between $P_{a_{O_2}}$ and $S_{a_{O_2}}$ at three pH values. Note that the dissociation curve is not linear like that of the dissolved oxygen graph but is doubly curved. The upper end of the curve slopes gently downward to the left for a distance and then becomes steep in its middle segment, a characteristic of great physiologic importance. Note that the line at $P_{a_{O_2}}$ of 100 mm Hg meets the normal pH 7.40 curve at a point corresponding to a $S_{a_{O_2}}$ of 97%. Again note that even if some abnormality reduced the $P_{a_{O_2}}$ to 65 mm Hg arterial blood would still be 90% saturated, but if the curve were linear the $S_{a_{O_2}}$ would be only about 64%. The relatively flat upper part of the curve prevents wide fluctuations in saturation (and thus in content) in the presence of oxygen tension drop due to disease or environ-

Table 4-3. *Oxygen content of arterial and venous blood*

	Vol% arterial O_2	*Vol% venous O_2*
Combined O_2 (1.34 × 15 × Sat)	19.5	14.7
Dissolved O_2 (P_{O_2} × 0.003)	0.3	0.1
Total O_2 content	19.8	14.8

mental abnormalities, but below $P_{a_{O_2}}$ of 50 mm Hg, the drop in saturation becomes precipitous.

When arterial blood perfuses body tissues and equilibrates with the oxygen-poor cells, its P_{O_2} drops to the venous level of about 40 mm Hg and its saturation to approximately 73%, but on its return to the lung, where it equilibrates with the alveolar $P_{A_{O_2}}$ of about 100 mm Hg, it again becomes 97% saturated. This portion of the curve, between P_{O_2} of 100 mm Hg and 40 mm Hg, represents the loading and unloading of oxygen in the lung and at the body cell. If we stipulate a hemoglobin content of 15 gm%, assume complete O_2 equilibration between blood and both lung and tissue cell, and assume that the pH remains at 7.40 (actually there is a slight shift of about 0.03 pH units as blood varies between venous and arterial), we can calculate the total volumes percent of oxygen (combined plus dissolved) in both arterial and venous blood, as in Table 4-3.

This arterial-venous (a-v) difference of 5 vol% represents the amount of oxygen given up to tissue cells and is referred to as the *average oxygen uptake*. Obviously, the uptake of all body cells at one time is not the same, but the blood reflects the mean of the body as a whole. It should be apparent that when physiologic abnormalities cause a low $P_{a_{O_2}}$ breathing room air the resulting drop in arterial saturation can often be corrected by so elevating the alveolar P_{O_2} with high oxygen concentrations that the $P_{a_{O_2}}$ will rise toward the upper end of the dissociation curve. Because of the continuing flattening of the upper curve, increasing $P_{a_{O_2}}$ values produce reducing increments of increase in saturation of hemoglobin, and 100% saturation is finally reached at $P_{a_{O_2}}$ of about 340 mm Hg.

The mechanism and clinical significance of blood pH changes will be discussed later, but it should be noted here that the normal dissociation curve *shifts* to the left with increasing pH and to the right with decreasing pH. Given a $P_{a_{O_2}}$ of 50 mm Hg, there is a difference of 15% saturation between a pH of 7.2 and one of 7.6. Variations in blood pH alone, with no change in oxygenation, are able to modify the oxygen content/capacity ratio of hemoglobin; or, to put it another way, the affinity of hemoglobin for oxygen is dependent upon the pH of the blood. A clinically important observation can be made from the effects of the pH shifts of the dissociation curve. For a given $P_{a_{O_2}}$, because the blood is able to maintain a higher oxygen saturation in a state of alkalosis than in acidosis, alkalosis might seem to be a distinct advantage to the body economy and suggest the desirability of that state as a preventative of oxygen want. However, let us compare the performances of both the pH 7.60 and pH 7.20 dissociation curves in a hypothetical situation. We will again assume a hemoglobin concentration of 15 gm%, and complete oxygen equilibration at $P_{a_{O_2}}$ of 100 mm Hg and 40 mm Hg, for arterial and venous blood, respectively. From the dissociation curves we read oxygen saturations of 98% for arterial blood and 84% for venous blood at pH of 7.60 and corresponding saturations of 94% and 62% at pH of 7.20. We can now compute the a-v oxygen difference between the alveoli and tissue cells for each abnormal pH value, comparing them with the normal, as outlined in Table 4-4.

There is less than 1 vol% of oxygen difference between alkalotic and acidotic arterial blood, but after tissue perfusion, the a-v oxygen difference of acidotic blood is more than double that for alkalotic. The important inference here is that alkalotic blood does not dissociate readily but rather holds onto its oxygen, making the oxygen less available to body cells than does normal or acidotic blood. This does not mean that acidosis is beneficial just because

Table 4-4. *a-v oxygen difference at three pH levels*

	Total vol% arterial O_2	*Total vol% venous O_2*	*a-v vol% O_2*
pH 7.60	20.0	17.0	3.0
pH 7.40	19.8	14.8	5.0
pH 7.20	19.2	12.6	6.6

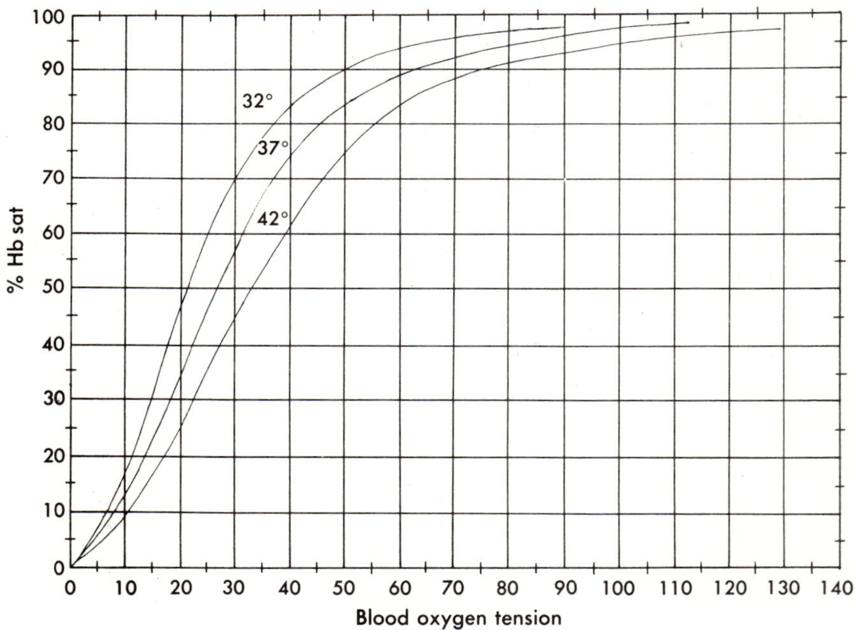

Fig. 4-5. O_2 dissociation curve of blood at a pH of 7.40, showing variations at three temperatures. For a given O_2 tension, the lower the temperature, the more the hemoglobin holds onto its O_2, maintaining a higher saturation.

it releases oxygen more freely, for we will see that the acidotic state is generally a very unwholesome condition for the entire body physiology. Close inspection of the dissociation curves shows that, if the arterial blood has a very low oxygen tension (40 to 50 mm Hg), the oxygen uptake difference between alkalotic and acidotic blood, at venous levels of 10 to 20 mm Hg P_{O_2}, is much less than at normal arterial values, but acidotic blood still releases more oxygen. The therapist will soon learn that the objective of treatment is to restore physiology as close to normal as possible.

Fig. 4-5 illustrates the influence of body temperature on arterial oxygen saturation and dissociation. Many combinations of pH and temperature can produce a host of possible curves. The therapeutic use of low body temperature (hypothermia) employs the principle of reduced oxygen need and utilization under conditions of cooling. This effect is evident in the lower a-v oxygen differences shown on the low temperature dissociation curve. (Compare with pH effect described above.)

CARBON DIOXIDE TRANSPORTATION

As oxygen diffuses from the blood into the body cells, carbon dioxide moves from cells to blood and is transported to the lung for excretion, but we

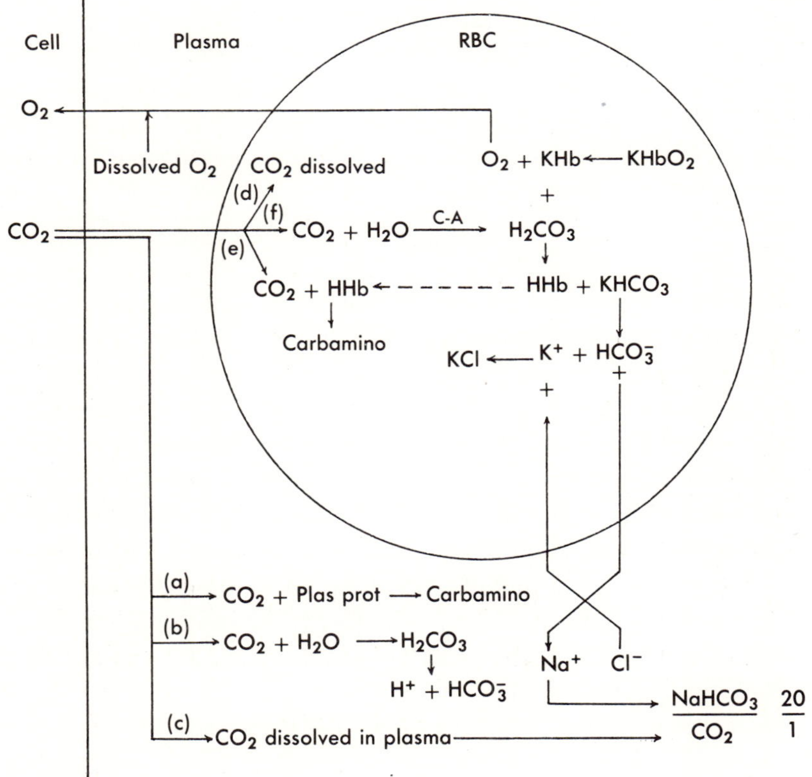

Fig. 4-6. Blood gas exchange at the body cell. See text for explanation.

must remember that all of the carbon dioxide carried in venous blood to the lung is not removed, enough remaining to exert a partial pressure of 40 mm Hg in the arterial blood. The mechanics of CO_2 transportation is more complicated than that of oxygen, but it must be understood clearly, for the amount of CO_2 in transit is one of the major determinants of the acid-base balance of the body. Fifty to sixty volumes percent of carbon dioxide are carried in two plasma and three erythrocyte compartments: *in plasma*—bound to protein, dissolved in plasma; *in erythrocytes*—dissolved in erythrocyte water, combined with hemoglobin, and as carbonic acid. Fig. 4-6 is a simplified composite diagram of the total CO_2 transport system and illustrates the simultaneous functioning of its components, along with some elements of oxygen carriage. Letter notations in the following text refer to the diagrammatic representation in Fig. 4-6 of the reaction under discussion.

Plasma transport of carbon dioxide[28-30]

Bound to protein. A very small amount of CO_2 combines with plasma protein to form a complex called a *carbamino compound* (a). This fraction of the CO_2 in blood is relatively insignificant, comprising but 1.12 vol% of the total.

Dissolved in plasma. Some 5% of the total CO_2 dissolves in the plasma water. Of this, a small amount reacts with the plasma water and through the process of hydrolysis produces carbonic acid (H_2CO_3) (b), the rest remaining in physical solution (c). The dissolved fraction is about 1000 times as great as that which hydrolyzes, a proportion that remains remarkably constant. The carbonic acid that does form dissociates into H^+ and HCO_3^-. That which remains dissolved is physiologically important because it is responsible for determining the pH of the blood.

Erythrocyte transport of carbon dioxide

Dissolved in erythrocyte. Another insignificant portion of CO_2, after it has diffused through the erythrocyte membrane, goes into physical solution in the erythrocyte water and is noted here only for completeness (d).

Combined with hemoglobin. A larger fraction of the gas combines with the *reduced* hemoglobin made available by the release of oxygen to the tissues and, because hemoglobin is a protein, forms carbamino-hemoglobin (e), somewhat similar to its combination with plasma protein. This is a very rapid reaction and, since the combining power of reduced hemoglobin with carbon dioxide is greater than that of oxyhemoglobin, the gas is readily picked up at the cell and discharged at the lung. The carbamino-Hb constitutes from 8% to 10% of the total CO_2 transported but 20% to 25% of the CO_2 released in the lung.

As carbonic acid. The major portion of the transported CO_2 is hydrated in the red cell to H_2CO_3, a normally slow process that is speeded up by an enzyme catalyst called *carbonic anhydrase* (f). The following sequence of steps then takes place: The carbonic acid immediately ionizes, as it does in the plasma. Oxy-Hb, as the potassium salt $KHbO_2$, releases its oxygen to the tissue cell, converting to KHb, which reacts with the newly formed H_2CO_3 to produce potassium bicarbonate, $KHCO_3$, and reduced acid hemoglobin, HHb. As soon as the $KHCO_3$ is formed, it ionizes and the HCO_3^- *diffuses out of the erythrocyte* into the plasma, as part of an interesting maneuver known as the "chloride shift," or the Hamburger phenomenon. To maintain ionic equilibrium, if one ion leaves the red cell, another must enter to replace it. Large amounts of NaCl are present in plasma, and as the bicarbonate ions leave the red cell, chloride ions enter in exchange. The sodium of the plasma NaCl then combines with the bicarbonate from the red cell to form $NaHCO_3$, and the released potassium in the erythrocyte combines with the shifted chloride from the plasma to produce KCl.

In summarizing the respiratory gas transportation, let us always keep in mind that the many processes described do not take place in intermittent stages but occur rapidly, simultaneously, and continuously. The close correlation between oxygen and carbon dioxide transportation is evidenced by the fact that, as soon as oxy-Hb has released oxygen, reduced Hb is available to participate in CO_2 transport. When blood reaches the lung, all reactions are reversed and the diagram of Fig. 4-6 applies but with the direction of the arrows turned about.

Most of the CO_2 is carried in the plasma but must pass through the erythrocyte as HCO_3^- by the chloride shift mechanism. Of critical importance is the relationship between the CO_2 that is carried as the compound $NaHCO_3$ and that which is in physical solution in the plasma. The former is referred to as the *bound* CO_2, and the latter as the *dissolved.* Under normal conditions the ratio of the bound to the dissolved CO_2 is remarkably constant at 20:1. It will be seen in the next few pages that such a ratio is essential to maintain normal acid-base balance of the blood. It was noted above that the amount of physically dissolved CO_2 is directly proportional to the amount of CO_2 that is hydrolyzed in the plasma to H_2CO_3; thus the dissolved CO_2 represents the amount of this acid present in plasma. The 20:1 proportion of combined to dissolved CO_2 is therefore a ratio between an *acid salt* and a *weak acid,* an important concept of buffering to be discussed with acid-base balance.

Because the carriage of CO_2 involves chemical reactions, the chemical quantitative expression of *millimoles per liter* (mM/liter) is more frequently

Table 4-5. *CO_2 content of venous and arterial blood*

	Venous		*Arterial*	
	Vol%	*mM/liter*	*Vol%*	*mM/liter*
Total CO_2	63.9	28.6	56.3	25.2
Combined CO_2	60.5	27.1	53.5	24.0
Dissolved CO_2	3.4	1.5	2.8	1.2
P_{CO_2}	46 mm Hg		40 mm Hg	

used than vol% to indicate amounts of the gas in the blood. The calibration is 1 gmw $\times 10^{-3}$ of CO_2 per liter of plasma. The actual measurement of blood CO_2 in the laboratory is done as vol% but is converted to mM/liter according to the following principle: (These calculations contain an exception to earlier teaching, in that 1 gmw of CO_2 is considered to occupy 22,300 liters).[31]

(1) Volumes% = ml CO_2/100 ml plasma
(2) 1 mM CO_2 = 1 gmw CO_2/1000 = 22,300 ml/1000 = 22.3 ml
(3) 1 mM CO_2/liter = 22.3 ml CO_2/1000 ml plasma = 2.23 ml CO_2/100 ml plasma
(4) Therefore, *mM* CO_2*/liter* = *vol%* $\div$ *2.23*

Average values for CO_2 content of venous and arterial blood are listed in Table 4-5.

ACID-BASE BALANCE

For optimum function of the body cells, the chemical reactions of their environment (body fluids and blood) must remain within a specific narrow range. Deviations of body pH above and below the normal range interfere with cellular metabolism and at extreme levels cause death of the cells. Survival is unlikely when pH drops below 7.0 and probably when it exceeds 7.80. The net result of all the interreactions of substances in the body should produce a hydrogen ion concentration (cH^+) to maintain a blood pH of 7.35 to 7.45, with an average normal of *7.40 for arterial blood*, just slightly alkaline. The pH is influenced by food, drink, and disease, but the body has a great capacity for maintaining a normal reaction in the face of factors that would change it. Maintaining a normal acid-base balance is one of the body's more important functions and one in which respiration plays a major role. Should the blood pH fall below the normal range, becoming *less* alkaline, a state of *acidosis* is said to exist; should it rise above the range, becoming more alkaline, *alkalosis* exists.

Both acidosis and alkalosis fall into two categories. If, because of respiratory disease, ventilation is unable to excrete enough carbon dioxide and abnormal amounts of this gas are retained in the blood, there will be an increase in the blood H_2CO_3. This will increase the total cH^+ of the blood, making it less alkaline and producing *respiratory acidosis.* However, if some abnormal stimulation to ventilation should cause excess carbon dioxide to be eliminated, there would be a concomitant drop in blood H_2CO_3, reducing cH^+ and leaving the blood with an excess alkalinity as *respiratory alkalosis.* The body contains many "fixed acids," such as lactic acid, sulfuric acid, phosphoric acid, hydrochloric acid, to list a few, which are the result of the body's metabolic processes and which exist in fairly regular concentrations. In addition, systemic or so-called *metabolic* diseases may produce abnormal organic acids as well as an increase in the amounts of the normal fixed acids. A disease, such as diabetes, for example, builds up large amounts of abnormal acids in the blood, elevating the blood cH^+ to produce *metabolic acidosis.* Vomiting, on the other hand, can cause such a loss of normal hydrochloric acid in the vomitus that the body cH^+ will drop, with *metabolic alkalosis*. To stabilize the pH, the blood contains an alkaline reserve, referred to as the blood base, for neutralization of fixed and abnormal acids. The base concerned is primarily sodium but also includes potassium, calcium, and magnesium, mostly bound as bicarbonate salts. These compounds are the bulwark of the buffer systems of the body, without which cH^+ could not be maintained at a level value. We will discuss these buffers next and then describe how the buffers are affected by pulmonary and metabolic disease as well as the manner in which both respiratory and renal systems help to keep the buffers in proper supply.

BUFFERS AND THE HENDERSON-HASSELBALCH EQUATION

A "buffer system" is a combination of a *weak* acid and a *salt* of that acid, and when introduced into a chemical reaction, it limits or buffers large changes in hydrogen ion concentration to prevent wide swings in pH. Although the industrial use of buffers is extensive, we are interested only in a few biologic systems, among which the following are worth identifying:

(1) *In plasma*

Carbonic acid/Sodium bicarbonate	$H_2CO_2/NaHCO_3$
Sodium *acid* phosphate/Sodium *alkaline* phosphate	$NaH_2PO_4/NaHPO_4$
Acid proteinate/Sodium proteinate	HProt/NaProt

(2) *In erythrocytes*

Acid hemoglobin/Potassium hemoglobin	HHb/KHb
Potassium *acid* phosphate/Potassium *alkaline* phosphate	KH_2PO_4/K_2HPO_4

The $H_2CO_3/NaHCO_3$ is by far the most important of all the buffers and will be used exclusively in the following to describe the detailed function of a buffer.

If a *strong* acid is added to a buffer pair, the chemical reaction will yield a *weak* acid and a neutral salt, and a *strong* alkali will yield a *weakly* alkaline salt and water. Thus, if HCl is added to the carbonic acid/sodium bicarbonate mixture, the strong acid will react with the bicarbonate of the buffer:

$$\frac{H_2CO_3}{HCl + NaHCO_3} \rightarrow H_2CO_3 + NaCl$$

This converts the strong acidity of HCl to the relatively weak acidity of H_2CO_3, and the increase in cH^+ is slight. Similarly, if NaOH is added to the same buffer, it will react with the H_2CO_3 of the mixture:

$$NaOH + \frac{H_2CO_3}{NaHCO_3} \rightarrow NaHCO_3 + HOH$$

The strong alkalinity of NaOH is "buffered" into the relatively weak alkalinity of $NaHCO_3$. It is evident that eventually the buffer will be used up but in the meantime the cH^+ of the reaction, and thus the pH, will change gradually rather than abruptly.

In a buffer pair, the weak acid is very slightly ionized, whereas its accompanying salt is practically completely ionized, and the cH^+ of the buffer system is proportional to the ratio between the concentration (in moles per liter) of the free acid and the acid "bound" by base as the salt. The cH^+ and pH of any buffer pair can be calculated if the concentration composition of the mixture and the dissociation constant of the weak electrolyte (the acid) are known. Using the simple expression for the dissociation of a weak acid, we will demonstrate how it can be modified to determine the reaction of the buffer. The dissociation of carbonic acid (written as $HHCO_3$) is:

$$HHCO_3 \rightleftharpoons H^+ + HCO_3^- \quad \text{(very slight ionization)}$$

thus

$$\frac{H^+ \times HCO_3^-}{HHCO_3} = K_{ac}$$

and

$$H^+ = K_{ac} \times \frac{HHCO_3}{HCO_3^-}$$

In this buffer mixture, since most of the acid is un-ionized (cH^+ is very minute), the molar concentration of the un-ionized acid in the numerator of the above ratio for all practical purposes is the same as the known acid concentration that was used to prepare the buffer. On the other hand, because the salt, $NaHCO_3$, is almost completely ionized:

$$NaHCO_3 \rightleftharpoons Na^+ + HCO_3^- \quad \text{(complete ionization)}$$

the value of HCO_3^- in the above denominator is approximately the same as the total molar concentration of the salt used in the buffer. Thus, the above dissociation equation for a weak acid can be rephrased to express the dissociation of a buffer system, of which it is a part, by substituting molar concentration of the buffer *salt* in place of the bicarbonate ion:

$$\text{Molar concentration } H^+ = K_{acid} \times \frac{\text{Molar concentration } HHCO_3}{\text{Molar concentration } NaHCO_3}$$

From the above is derived the *Henderson-Hasselbalch equation,* which is a cornerstone of the clinical application of the principles of acid-base balance. Since pH is the negative log of the hydrogen ion concentration used as a positive number, the buffer ionization equation can be rewritten to allow calculation of the pH:

$$H^+ = K_{ac} \times \frac{\text{M/liter Acid}}{\text{M/liter Salt}}$$

$$\log H^+ = \log \left[K_{ac} \times \frac{\text{M/liter Acid}}{\text{M/liter Salt}}\right]$$

$$\log H^+ = \log K_{ac} + \log \left[\frac{\text{M/liter Acid}}{\text{M/liter Salt}}\right]$$

$$pH = -\log K_{ac} - \log \left[\frac{\text{M/liter Acid}}{\text{M/liter Salt}}\right]$$

$$\text{pH} = \text{pK} + \log\left[\frac{\text{M/liter Salt}}{\text{M/liter Acid}}\right]$$

$$\text{pH} = \text{pK}_{ac} + \log\left[\frac{\text{M/liter NaHCO}_3}{\text{M/liter H}_2\text{CO}_3}\right]$$

Note the use of the term *pK*. Similarly to pH, pK means the *negative log of the dissociation constant of the acid component of the buffer system*, used as a positive number. Because laboratory techniques make it easier to determine the amount of *dissolved* CO_2 in the blood than the H_2CO_3 content and because the dissolved CO_2 is directly proportional to the blood H_2CO_3, the concentration of dissolved CO_2 is used in the equation in place of the *Acid*, with a compensatory change in the dissociation constant. Under physiologic conditions, the carbonic acid dissociation, K, has a value of 7.85×10^{-7}, which is easily converted by calculation into a pK of *6.1*. Also, the importance of the numerator of the equation, usually referred to as "base" rather than salt, lies in the HCO_3 ion since it represents and includes "bound" acid. Finally, because of the small quantities involved, it is more convenient to calibrate concentrations as millimoles per liter than moles per liter. The Henderson-Hasselbalch equation, as it applies to the $H_2CO_3/NaHCO_3$ buffer system for determination of blood pH, can be summarized as follows:

$$\text{pH} = 6.1 + \log\left[\frac{\text{mM/liter of Bicarbonate}}{\text{mM/liter of Dissolved CO}_2}\right]$$

APPLICATION OF THE H-H EQUATION

Since carbon dioxide, both dissolved in solution and combined as bicarbonate, is intimately involved in acid-base balance, it is easy to see why ventilation is so important in regulating this balance and why a clear understanding of this relationship is necessary for those treating respiratory diseases. We will discuss in some detail those factors involved in the acid-base equation and learn to use the equation for better understanding of acid-base physiology. For our purpose the term *acid-base balance* refers to the ratio between carbonic acid and its salt, the base sodium bicarbonate. In evaluating this balance, we can measure in the laboratory certain blood values which we then apply to the equation for whatever information we desire. So first we must be acquainted with some of the terms used. *Total CO_2 content* means all the CO_2 that can be chemically extracted and measured from a blood sample. This includes the *sum* of the combined CO_2 (as bicarbonate) and the dissolved CO_2; and it is measured as volumes percent and converted to mM/liter as described earlier. The *dissolved CO_2* is that fraction of the blood gas which is in solution in the blood plasma. The *combined CO_2*, also called *bound CO_2*, *base*, and *bicarbonate*, refers to that portion of the total CO_2 which is contained in the blood bicarbonate. This can be measured directly by chemical analysis or can be computed as the difference between the total and the dissolved CO_2.

Laboratory technology makes it easy and quick to measure directly the partial pressure of CO_2 in a blood sample. The P_{CO_2} can be converted in mM/liter very simply by a factor, the derivation of which is outlined below:

(1) 1 Mole $CO_2 = 22{,}300$ ml at 760 mm Hg pressure
(2) 1 mM $CO_2 = 22.3$ ml
(3) Sol coef CO_2 at 760 mm Hg $= 0.51$ ml CO_2/ml plasma
(4) Thus, the ml CO_2/ml plasma at any $P_{CO_2} = \dfrac{P_{CO_2} \times 0.51}{760}$

(5) The ml CO_2/liter plasma $= \dfrac{P_{CO_2} \times 0.51 \times 1000}{760}$

(6) mM CO_2/liter plasma $= \dfrac{P_{CO_2} \times 0.51 \times 1000}{760 \times 22.3}$

$= P_{CO_2} \times 0.03014$

The normal arterial P_{CO_2} value of 40 mm Hg, multiplied by the factor 0.03 gives a concentration of dissolved CO_2 of *1.2 mM/liter.*

Let us assume that an arterial blood sample yields a total CO_2 content of 56.3 vol%, which converts to a concentration of 25.2 mM/liter, and the P_{CO_2} is 40 mm Hg, or 1.2 mM/liter. The bicarbonate value is the *difference* between these, or 24 mM/liter. The H-H equation can now be used to determine the arterial pH:

$$\begin{aligned} pH &= 6.1 + \log \left[\frac{24}{1.2}\right] \\ &= 6.1 + \log 20 \\ &= 6.1 + 1.301 \\ &= 7.40 \end{aligned}$$

A critical point to learn here is that the blood pH is dependent upon the *ratio* of the bicarbonate to dissolved CO_2 rather than on the absolute value of each. As long as the ratio is 20:1, the pH will always be 7.40. The values could be 12:0.6 or 48:2.4 or any other combination to yield 20. Reference was made to this in the discussion of CO_2 transportation and the student should now be getting to understand the true meaning of "acid-base balance."

Of the three variables in the H-H equation, any one obviously can be calculated if the other two are known. In actual cardiopulmonary practice, compact equipment now available makes it convenient to measure pH, P_{CO_2}, (and P_{O_2}) on the same blood sample, a procedure much easier than the chemical analyses of total CO_2 and HCO_3. Nomograms and charts are also available to show the relation between the various factors. However, to understand fully these relationships, the student should know how to use the H-H equation to solve for an unknown, given two known data. For practice in performing such exercises, equations involving calculation of four different CO_2 values are listed below:

(1) Dissolved CO_2 in mM/liter $= 0.03 \times P_{CO_2}$

(2) $P_{CO_2} = \dfrac{\text{Total } CO_2 \text{ in mM/liter}}{0.03 \times [1 + \text{antilog (pH-6.1)}]}$

(3) Total CO_2 in mM/liter $= 0.03 \times P_{CO_2} \times [1 + \text{antilog (pH-6.1)}]$

(4) HCO_3 in mM/liter = Total CO_2 in mM/liter − Dissolved CO_2 in mM/liter

Equations no. 1 and 4 need no amplification, and no. 3 is a rearrangement of no. 2. The derivation of equation no. 2 is outlined in Appendix 10. Following are examples of acid-base calculations:

1. *Given:* Arterial P_{CO_2} = 52 mm Hg, and total arterial CO_2 content = 62 vol%

   Calculate: Arterial pH

Solution:

Dissolved $CO_2 = 0.03 \times 52 = 1.56$ mM/liter
Total $CO_2 = 62 \div 2.23 = 27.8$ mM/liter
$HCO_3 = 27.8 - 1.56 = 26.24$ mM/liter

$$pH = 6.1 + \log\left[\frac{26.24}{1.56}\right] = 6.1 + 1.225$$

$$pH = 7.33$$

2. *Given:* Arterial pH = 7.24, and arterial P_{CO_2} = 56 mm Hg

   Calculate: Dissolved CO_2, total CO_2, HCO_3

Solution:

Dissolved $CO_2 = 0.03 \times 56$ = 1.68 mM/liter
Total $CO_2 = 1.68 \times [1 + \text{antilog } (7.24\text{-}6.1)]$
$= 1.68 \times [1 + \text{antilog } (1.14)]$
$= 1.68 \times 14.8$ = 24.9 mM/liter
$HCO_3 = 24.9 - 1.68$ = 23.2 mM/liter

3. *Given:* Arterial pH = 7.58, and total arterial CO_2 content = 19.2 mM/liter

   Calculate: P_{CO_2}

Solution:

$$P_{CO_2} = \frac{19.2}{0.03 \times [1 + \text{antilog } (7.58\text{-}6.1)]}$$

$$= \frac{19.2}{0.03 \times [1 + \text{antilog } (1.48)]}$$

$$= \frac{19.2}{0.03 \times 31.2}$$

$$= 20.3 \text{ mm Hg}$$

The answers to such calculations can be checked by fitting them into the H-H equation to see whether the equation balances.

Exercise 4-2

	Given		*Calculate*
(a)	P_{CO_2} = 32 mm Hg	Total CO_2 = 55 vol%	pH
(b)	P_{CO_2} = 56 mm Hg	Total CO_2 = 66 vol%	pH
(c)	P_{CO_2} = 72 mm Hg	Total CO_2 = 30 vol%	pH
(d)	Total CO_2 = 55 vol%	pH = 7.26	P_{CO_2}
(e)	Total CO_2 = 44 vol%	pH = 7.55	P_{CO_2}
(f)	Total CO_2 = 30 vol%	pH = 7.35	P_{CO_2}
(g)	P_{CO_2} = 55 mm Hg	pH = 7.41	Total CO_2; HCO_3
(h)	P_{CO_2} = 38 mm Hg	pH = 7.52	Total CO_2; HCO_3
(i)	P_{CO_2} = 26 mm Hg	pH = 7.30	Total CO_2; HCO_3

CLINICAL ACID-BASE STATES

Table 4-6 tabulates the nine fundamental acid-base conditions, illustrating the chemical characteristics of each and introducing the term *compensated.*

When several factors work together to maintain a physiologic balance and one of the factors behaves abnormally to threaten the equilibrium, the other factors readjust their levels of function in an attempt to make up for the deficiency and maintain stability of the system. This is called *physiologic compensation.* Thus, each of the four types of acid-base upsets can exist as uncompensated or compensated. The differentiation is not as clear-cut as indicated in the table, which is exaggerated for emphasis. In fact, compensation actually starts as soon as the balance is upset, and although we have shown the disturbances in equilibrium and their compensation as isolated stages purely for demonstration purposes, it should be appreciated that these processes occur simultaneously. Finally, compensation is often incomplete, becoming less effective as the imbalance increases until it eventually breaks

Table 4-6. *Table of acid-base states*

Normal balance	*24 mM/1 / 1.2 mM/1 (40 mm Hg)*	*20/1*	*7.40*
Respiratory acidosis	24 mM/l / 2.4 mM/l (80 mm Hg)	10/1	7.10
Respiratory acidosis (compensated)	48 mM/l / 2.4 mM/l (80 mm Hg)	20/1	7.40
Respiratory alkalosis	24 mM/l / 0.6 mM/l (20 mm Hg)	40/1	7.70
Respiratory alkalosis (compensated)	12 mM/l / 0.6 mM/l (20 mm Hg)	20/1	7.40
Metabolic acidosis	12 mM/l / 1.2 mM/l (40 mm Hg)	10/1	7.10
Metabolic acidosis (compensated)	12 mM/l / 0.6 mM/l (20 mm Hg)	20/1	7.40
Metabolic alkalosis	48 mM/l / 1.2 mM/l (40 mm Hg)	40/1	7.70
Metabolic alkalosis (compensated)	48 mM/l / 2.4 mM/l (80 mm Hg)	20/1	7.40

down. For the severe levels of decompensation shown, full physiologic compensation would be impossible, and all degrees of partial compensation could be found in a real clinical situation.

The following general rule will help to keep acid-base disturbances in a reasonable mental order: *respiratory* disorders upset the *denominator* of the acid-base ratio because ventilation regulates the blood CO_2 and compensation attempts to adjust the numerator to restore a 20:1 ratio; *metabolic* disorders upset the *numerator* of the ratio as bicarbonate is either increased or decreased and compensation attempts to adjust the denominator. The dissolved CO_2 can be changed, either primarily or as a secondary compensation, only by modifying the ventilatory pattern with hypoventilation or hyperventilation. The HCO_3 compensates by an increase in production or by varying the amounts excreted in the urine.

Respiratory acidosis

Respiratory acidosis is *always* the result of *alveolar hypoventilation* with its retention of CO_2 in the arterial blood. The hypoventilation may be due to (a) chronic cardiopulmonary disease with failure of the ventilatory control system, (b) neuromuscular or skeletal disease with inadequate ventilatory muscular action, or (c) the action of drugs such as narcotics and sedatives which depress respiratory center action. Regardless of cause, there is an increase in the partial pressure of arterial CO_2 and, depending upon the state of compensation, a drop in arterial pH.

Compensation begins as soon as the CO_2 starts to accumulate and is a major function of the kidney. The body attempts to increase the amount of bicarbonate, keeping pace with the rising dissolved carbon dioxide, to maintain the necessary 20:1 ratio for a pH of 7.40. Reference to Fig. 4-6 will recall the mechanism of the chloride shift, whereby, as the amount of CO_2 increases in the blood, chloride moves out of the plasma into the erythrocyte in exchange for bicarbonate. As a result, during the compensation for respiratory acidosis, the level of plasma chloride drops and the bicarbonate increases. It is here that the action of the kidney is of extreme importance, for the kidney uses two mechanisms to regulate the essential electrolyte levels. First, it selectively rejects the excretion of the bicarbonate ion in the urine, conserving it in the plasma for its use as a blood buffer. At the same time it also reduces the excretion of sodium, retaining it to combine with the increased amounts of bicarbonate. The additional amounts of sodium bicarbonate thus made available to counter the increasing retained carbon dioxide are referred to as the *alkaline reserve.* Second, in place of sodium, the kidney removes from the blood increasing amounts of hydrogen ion, as HCl and NH_4Cl. This serves the dual purpose of maintaining electrolyte balance, by substituting one positive ion for another in the urine; but most important, for the health of the body, it reduces the overall acidity of the blood. In a sense, the perceptive kidney, recognizing that retained carbon dioxide represents increasing amounts of carbonic acid, removes as many hydrogen ions as it can from the blood to "compensate" for the respiratory-induced acidity. If the onset of respiratory acidosis is rapid and acute, renal compensation may not be able to keep up with the rising carbon dioxide on a minute by minute basis, and the compensatory exchange of hydrogen for bicarbonate may not reach its maximum efficiency for 3 or 4 days. In slowly developing acidosis, as is often seen with chronic pulmonary disease when repeated infections and the progressive lung destruction span months or years, the compensatory process may adjust proportionately to the acidosis. In such instances, pH levels may be maintained stable, within the normal range, not less than 7.35. It should be emphasized that, because kidney action is able to prevent a serious drop in pH, this does not mean that acidosis is not present. Examination of arterial blood would reveal an elevated P_{CO_2}, and this is conclusive evidence of respiratory acidosis in a patient with ventilatory failure, but an acidosis compensated by renal action. As should be anticipated, there is a limit to which the body can compensate an acid-base upset, beyond which there is a "break" in compensation. With chronic respiratory disease, in the absence of complications, the kidney is able to maintain a normal pH until the P_{CO_2} exceeds 60 mm Hg, but there is invariable decompensation when the P_{CO_2} reaches 70 mm Hg.[32] This does not mean that every patient with chronic lung disease and an arterial carbon dioxide tension under 70 mm Hg will have a normal pH. It means that under no circumstance can the unaided kidney effect complete compensation beyond this level. The therapist will see many patients with varying degrees of hypercapnia and accompanying acidosis, and frequently they will have associated conditions that influence acid-base balance, especially metabolic disorders and cardiac failure.

When alveolar hypoventilation is a manifestation of the inability of the respiratory center to respond to the amount of CO_2 perfusing it, the inactivity of the center may be the result of depressing drugs, as mentioned above, or may represent a sort of fatigue of the center after prolonged subjection to gradually increasing CO_2 tensions accompanying chronic ventilatory failure, as is found in pulmonary emphysema. In any instance, central innervation of the ventilatory muscles diminishes, tidal air exchange is reduced, and arterial P_{CO_2} rises. During progressive ventilatory failure, as tidal airflow drops, in addition to *hypercapnia* (increased CO_2 in the blood), there is also a fall in alveolar P_{O_2} and consequently in arterial P_{O_2}. This reduced blood oxygen state is called *hypoxemia,* and the subsequent deprivation of tissue oxygen, *hypoxia.* With a reduced oxygen content, arterial blood has an increased amount of unsaturated hemoglobin, which, in sufficient quantities, can darken the color of the blood and impart to the skin a bluish tinge called *cyanosis.* Mechanisms of hypoxia and cyanosis will be discussed in detail in Chapter 6, but these brief descriptions will permit us to use the terms in the meantime. Thus, in severe failure of the respiratory center, the major stimulus to breathing may be the so-called *hypoxic drive* of the carotid and aortic bodies, described in Chapter 3, as the presence of arterial hypoxia stimulates the chemoreceptors to innervate the muscles of ventilation to prevent a further drop in oxygen content. It is important to note that hypoxia must be present for the chemoreceptor drive to function and that this function ceases when hypoxia is corrected. Here is a circumstance in which **indiscriminate use of oxygen can be fatal.** In ventilatory failure, respiratory exchange is inadequate for prolonged survival, but *some* ventilation is better than *none,* even though it maintains a state of hypercapnia and hypoxia. Should the patient be given oxygen to relieve his hypoxia, the chemoreceptors will cease to function, and with an already inactive respiratory center *breathing will stop.* In this state of apnea, acidosis will rapidly increase to a fatal level and the patient will expire, often with a paradoxically healthy-appearing pink complexion. This is a very real risk in the treatment of patients in failure and must be guarded against by all those involved in the patient's management. Safe and effective techniques will be discussed elsewhere.

The patient in respiratory acidosis will manifest hypoventilation in one of two ways. His tidal volume will be small, sometimes with barely perceptible chest and epigastric motion, or he will be tachypneic, with rapid shallow movements that accomplish little more than ventilation of the dead space. Laboratory examinations will show a low pH, an elevated P_{CO_2} and HCO_3, a low serum Cl, and an acid urine. If acid-base compensation is poor, the patient's mental state will be obtunded or he may be in a coma and, almost always, the ventilation is enough impaired that hypoxia produces visible cyanosis. Although much of the management is directed toward the underlying disease, the most critical treatment is the correction of hypoventilation, usually best accomplished by assisting the patient with mechanical ventilators or controlling his breathing completely. *While being adequately ventilated,* the patient can be given oxygen as needed to correct his hypoxia, blood gas and pH determinations being used frequently to monitor the effectiveness of therapy. Other details of management will be considered later.

Respiratory alkalosis

Alveolar hyperventilation removes CO_2 from the blood, dropping the P_{CO_2} to low levels and elevating the pH. The respiratory center can be stimulated to excessive activity by brain injury or a tumor's increasing pressure on the center, by excessive salicylate ingestion, by fever, by inflammation of the brain, or by emotional stimuli. Of immediate concern to the inhalation therapist, however, is the hyperventilation that *he* can induce by the use of mechanical ventilators. Artificial ventilation of a patient with a normal respiratory tract can very easily be overdone and the patient hyperventilated into respiratory alkalosis. The therapist must watch very carefully to prevent this development.

Compensation is accomplished by an increased renal excretion of bicarbonate, retention of chloride, and reduction in the formation of ammonia and excretion of acid salts. This lowers the blood bicarbonate level, bringing the acid-base ratio back toward 20:1 and reducing the pH.

Alkalosis is as hazardous to the patient as is acidosis. He is seen to be breathing deeply and his blood shows an elevated pH, a depressed P_{CO_2}, and, depending upon the degree of compensation, low bicarbonate and total CO_2. Serum chloride may be slightly elevated, and the urine alkaline. The patient may complain of *paresthesias* of the extremities, a sensation of "pins and needles" or of the extremities "being asleep." Reflexes are hyperactive, true tetanic contractions may occur, and somnolence increasing to coma may develop. One of the major complications of alkalosis is its impairment of cerebral circulation, as a rapid decrease in P_{CO_2} produces a contraction of cerebral arterioles, with a reduction in blood flow to the brain. This can be severe enough to cause speech difficulty and muscular paralysis, which may be permanent. Hypocapnia also predisposes the patient to serious disturbance in cardiac rhythm (arrhythmia), which may lead to arrest. Treatment is usually directed toward the underlying cause, but symptomatic relief can often be obtained by the use of sedation to suppress the respiratory center and by the inhalation of carbon dioxide to build up the blood P_{CO_2}.

Metabolic acidosis

In metabolic disorders, acid-base balance is dependent upon the electrolytic balance in the body, or the relation between the positively charged ions (cations) and the negatively charged ions (anions).[33,34] The former consist of Na, Ca, K, Mg; the latter, HCO_3, protein (serum protein and hemoglobin), HPO_4, Cl, SO_4, and organic acids. The HCO_3, protein, and HPO_4 ions we already know comprise the buffer systems of the body and are appropriately named *buffer anions.* The remaining anions are designated as *fixed anions.* The cations are combined with a variety of anions, and those that are in combination with the buffer anions (mostly sodium as $NaHCO_3$, but small amounts of the other cations as well) are termed *buffer cations,* and sometimes *buffer base* or *total body buffer.* The remaining cations, combined with other than buffer anions, may be considered as *fixed cations.* The sum of the anions must equal the sum of the cations, and they are measured in meq/liter or mM/liter, depending upon the ion.

The total ionic content of plasma in concentration per liter is depicted schematically in Fig. 4-7. Here, two columns contain the cations and anions, and their average normal values are indicated. H_2CO_3 dissociates so little that it is indicated in both columns as mM/liter of CO_2. The buffer anions are clearly delineated from the fixed anions; the buffer cations are not different cations from the fixed cations but rather are portions of the latter that are combined with buffer anions. It can be seen, for example, that if chloride should decrease in amount the buffer anions would increase in order to keep the total unchanged. Also, it is easy to visualize a loss of sodium, with an accompanying loss of bicarbonate, and chloride expanding to replace the bicarbonate.

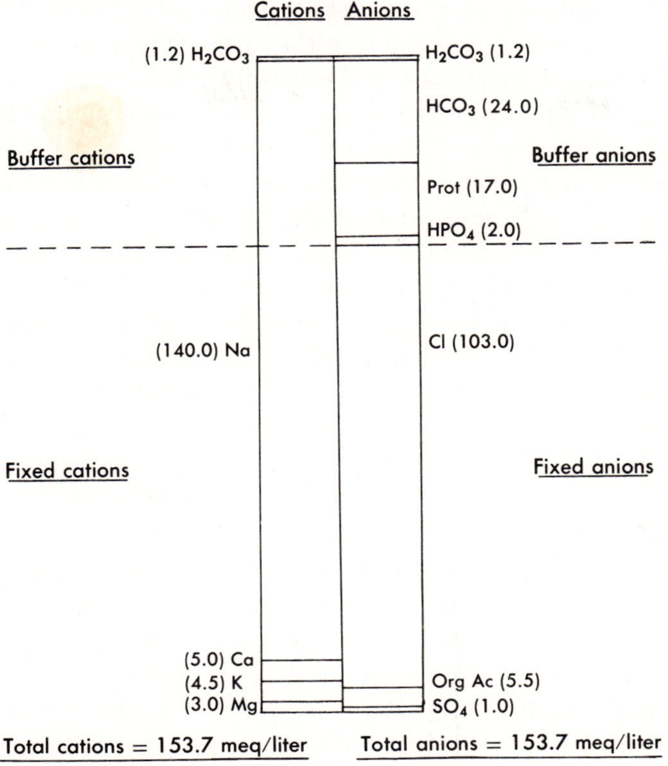

Fig. 4-7. Balance between fixed and buffer electrolytes of plasma.

Thus, the interchanges between the electrolytes due to metabolic reactions modify the buffer anions and through changes, especially in the HCO_3, regulate pH. Although the metabolic relation to acid-base balance is not of primary concern to the inhalation therapist, a general understanding of the basic principles should be of interest to him since many of his patients will have systemic diseases associated with respiratory.

Any systemic disease that causes a depletion of the fixed cations (or buffer base), or an increase in the fixed anions, can produce metabolic acidosis. The production of abnormal acids in the blood, or the retention of acids through failure of the kidney to excrete them, will replace buffer anions. This may be viewed as the depletion of the buffer ions while neutralizing the acids. Again, in the plasma, HCO_3 is the major anion involved since the most prevalent protein, Hb, is found only in the erythrocyte and phosphate is present in but small amounts. Keeping in mind the H-H equation, we can conveniently visualize an abnormal buildup of acids in the body (especially organic) with which the plasma HCO_3 reacts to neutralize the acidity. This effort depletes the available HCO_3, lowering the numerator of the H-H equation and reducing blood pH. Retention of chloride, incident to an excessive intake of this ion, will replace some of the bicarbonate in the anion column, lowering the blood pH. Surprisingly, and somewhat paradoxically, loss of potassium, which might be expected to produce acidosis, raises the pH. This is the result of a complex chain of electrolytic exchanges by which there is, in the presence of potassium loss, a disproportionately larger renal loss of chloride so that the net result is an increase in bicarbonate.

Compensation for metabolic acidosis is by an increase in the respiratory removal of CO_2 proportionately to the bicarbonate through the mechanism of hyperventilation. It should be noted in Table 4-6 that, from the blood findings alone, it is not possible to distinguish between *compensated* respiratory alkalosis and *compensated* metabolic acidosis. In this case, the clinical picture of the patient's condition will be the deciding factor. The treatment of metabolic acidosis is obviously that of the underlying disease, since the respiratory abnormality is a conpensatory act and not a reflection of respiratory disease.

Metabolic alkalosis

It is apparent that metabolic alkalosis is the product of any systemic disease that causes an excess of buffer through a relative increase of fixed cations over fixed anions. This can be the result of the loss of chloride of gastric HCl in protracted vomiting, the retention of large amounts of sodium by the ingestion of alkalis (the sodium thus combining with additional bicarbonate), the disproportionate loss of chloride over sodium common to mercurial diuretics, or the effect of potassium loss just mentioned. (This is often found in potassium loss that occurs with intubation and drainage of the bowel, long-term use of corticosteroids, or a reduced potassium intake.) Compensation is attempted by a conservation of H_2CO_3 through hypoventilation to raise the acid denominator of the H-H equation and to restore a 20:1 ratio. Again note that *compensated* metabolic alkalosis is undistinguishable chemically from *compensated* respiratory acidosis, which emphasizes the fact that diagnostic reliance cannot be placed completely upon the laboratory.

Mixed acid-base states

By now it may be obvious to the student that combinations of disorders may occur in the same patient.[35,36] Any of the four respiratory states may coexist with any of the four metabolic states, and patients with simultaneous respiratory and metabolic diseases often present complicated pictures. Referred to earlier, and emphasized again, is the patient with respiratory acidosis who swings rapidly into respiratory alkalosis because of too vigorous therapy and thus demonstrates not simultaneous, but alternating acid-base disorders. It is theoretically possible for a respiratory imbalance in one direction to be offset by a metabolic imbalance in the other, with a resulting normal pH. Differentiation between these possibilities is a medical problem requiring the finest diagnostic acumen and intelligent use of the laboratory, and the difficulties encountered should be appreciated by the inhalation therapist.

Chapter 5

Cardiovascular system

In view of the great volume of texts written on the structure, function, and pathology of the heart, it is unnecessary for us to undertake a comprehensive review of cardiology. However, because the functions of the heart and lungs are so interrelated, it is felt that a brief explanation of some selected features of the cardiovascular system is pertinent, with emphasis on those aspects relating most directly to principles and practice of inhalation therapy. From references already made, it should be apparent to the therapist that he will frequently be called upon to treat patients with both pulmonary and cardiac diseases, and in his approach to his work he should always be aware of *cardiopulmonary* function. With this as a start, it is hoped that he will be encouraged to pursue the topic further as his interest and experience develop.

THE CARDIAC CYCLE

In the performance of its function as a pump, the heart works through a ceaseless series of cycles, from a prenatal period to the moment of death. Each cardiac cycle is composed of a contraction of the myocardial fibers, followed by a period of rest. Contraction of the involuntary muscle is achieved by a forceful shortening of each fiber so that, as the total muscle mass contracts, it builds up a pressure in the cavities it encloses, reduces their volumes, and expresses their contents into the cardiac outflow tracts. Nerve impulses from the higher centers of the central nervous system are carried to the heart by the vagus nerve, which contains parasympathetic fibers, and by sympathetic nerves arising from the upper thoracic segments of the spinal cord. The former inhibit heart action, the latter stimulate it, and the net sum of the constant barrage of impulses through these channels determines the final controlling influence.

Within the heart itself, a highly specialized system of conducting tissue is responsible for the precisely timed distribution of impulses to all parts of the myocardium. Under suitable conditions, the intact heart removed from all nerve connections can continue to beat for a period of time, which fact demonstrates that, despite its control over cardiac contraction, the central nervous innervation is not essential for heart action. There must be, therefore, an automatic stimulus in the heart capable of maintaining contraction but, in the

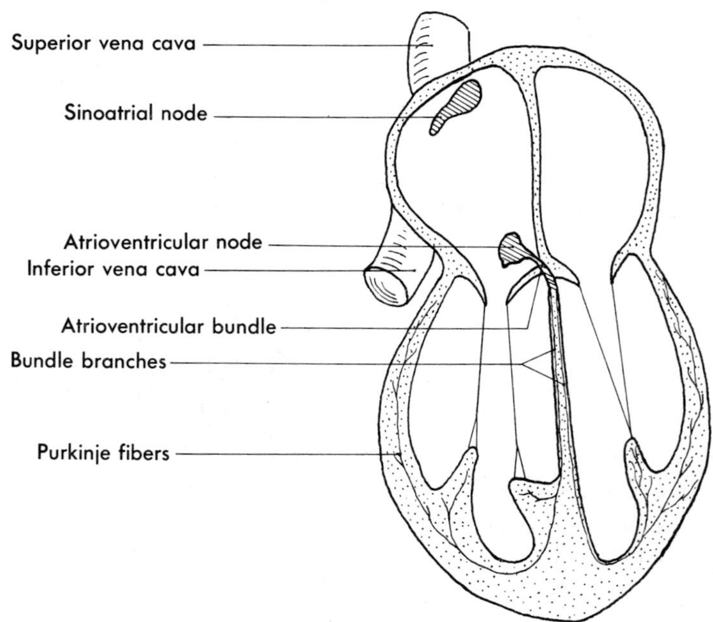

Fig. 5-1. Conduction system of the heart. See text for description.

intact subject, greatly influenced by the central nervous system. This is labeled the *conduction system* of the heart. Fig. 5-1 schematically illustrates the major portions of this system: the sinoatrial node (sinus node), the atrioventricular node (A-V node), the atrioventricular bundle (bundle of His), and the bundle branches and Purkinje fibers. The histology of the conduction system is that of highly specialized muscle fibers rather than nerve fibers but capable of conducting muscle-stimulating impulses.

Sinoatrial node (sinus node). This structure is called the *pacemaker* of the heart and is a small nodule of conducting tissue, about 0.75 inch long, located in the muscle of the right atrium just in front of the opening of the superior vena cava. The sinus node initiates electrical impulses (to be described later) which radiate from it in the fashion of circular ripples from a stone dropped into water. Traveling at a rate of 1000 mm per second, these impulses are discharged at variable rates, from 50 to 90 per minute, but average about 70 per minute at rest. They excite the atrial myocardium to contract, both atria functioning simultaneously. The discharge rate of the sinus node is modified by nervous control, increased by the sympathetic nerves and inhibited by the parasympathetic through vagal innervation. Cardiac rate can be increased by excessive stimulation of sympathetic nerves or by drugs simulating sympathetic action, and the heart can be slowed or stopped by parasympathetic action, especially through the action of certain reflexes carried by the vagus nerve. Both effects are of considerable clinical importance.

Atrioventricular (A-V) node. Similar in structure to the sinus node, the

A-V node is located in the right atrium on the lower part of the interatrial septum just above the septal leaf of the tricuspid valve. It functions as a pickup and relay station for sinus impulses. With no structural connection to the sinus node, the A-V node is stimulated by the radiating sinus impulses, and it relays these onward into the ventricles. Should the sinus node fail to function because of disease, the A-V node then assumes the duties of pacemaker, but it is less effective than the sinus node.

Atrioventricular bundle (bundle of His). A well-defined bundle of muscular tissue originates at the A-V node and runs horizontally forward over the septal tricuspid valve leaf to the upper part of the interventricular septum. The sinus impulse received by the A-V node is transmitted through the bundle and is thus carried to the myocardium of the ventricular chambers. This is the only conduction link between atria and ventricles, and when it is damaged or destroyed by disease, a condition of *block* is said to exist, a cardiac condition commonly encountered in clinical medicine.

Bundle branches and Purkinje fibers. On the upper part of the interventricular septum the A-V bundle terminates by dividing into two *bundle branches,* the right and left, each going to its respective ventricle. The bundles pass down the septum, beneath the endocardium, giving off branches to the papillary muscles, and then continue into the ventricles, where they divide into innumerable fine filaments and form a network (Purkinje fibers) interlacing the depths of the ventricular muscle. The impulse, originating in the sinus node, is carried at a rate of some 5000 mm per second to every portion of the ventricles, in effect stimulating all myocardial fibers simultaneously, for uniform contraction of both ventricles.

The sequence of the cardiac cycle is contraction of both atria, driving blood into the ventricles, followed by contraction of both ventricles, which expels the blood into the cardiac outflow tracts. These phases of muscular contraction are respectively called atrial and ventricular *systole.* Following systole, both sets of chambers enter a period of rest and muscular relaxation called *diastole.* Because systole and diastole of the two sets of chambers are not of uniform duration, there is some overlapping, schematically illustrated in Fig. 5-2, which shows the start of a cardiac cycle with ventricular systole, as a matter of convenience. Note that the atria spend most of their time in diastole, during which time blood flows into these chambers from the venae cavae and pulmonary veins and, with the tricuspid and mitral valves closed, the atria distend with blood. After about 0.3 second of atrial diastole, a point corresponding to the end of ventricular systole, the atrioventricular valves open and atrial blood flows into the ventricles. Then, at 0.7 second, atrial systole occurs for a brief 0.1 second, forcibly ejecting the last of the auricular blood into the ventricles. During atrial diastole, ventricular systole takes place, for about 0.3 second; then as the A-V valves open, the semilunar valves close and the ventricles enter their diastolic phase. For approximately 0.4 second, atrial and ventricular diastoles coincide and the entire heart is quiet, as blood

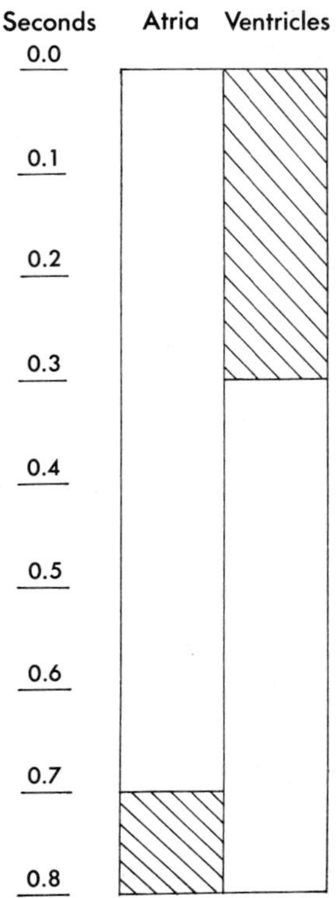

Fig. 5-2. The duration and relationships of the systolic (shaded) and diastolic (clear) components of the cardiac cycle are shown for a rate of 75 per minute.

is flowing by gravity from atria into ventricles. It is important to note that myocardium has a peculiar quality that assures the heart of maximum contractile effort. Once systolic contraction begins, the fibers are *refractory,* or resistant to further stimulation, until they have had time to recover and regain their energy. This means that repeated stimuli cannot maintain them in a state of continued contraction, which would eventually lead to serious fatigue. The refractory period of the myocardium is maintained through systole and for an additional period of time approximately equal to the duration of systole, when it once again is responsive to stimuli.

The heartbeat, as palpated through the chest wall and at the peripheral arterial pulses, reflects the force of ventricular systole only, since the contraction of the atria is not sufficiently strong to be transmitted. The pause between beats consists of ventricular diastole, the last part of atrial diastole, and the unnoticed atrial systole. It is apparent that as the heart rate varies the duration of the cycle segments will vary inversely. Thus, rapid rates (tachycardia) often associated with disease not only reduce the rest periods of the myocardium but also, by shortening filling time, can reduce the cardiac output per beat (stroke volume).

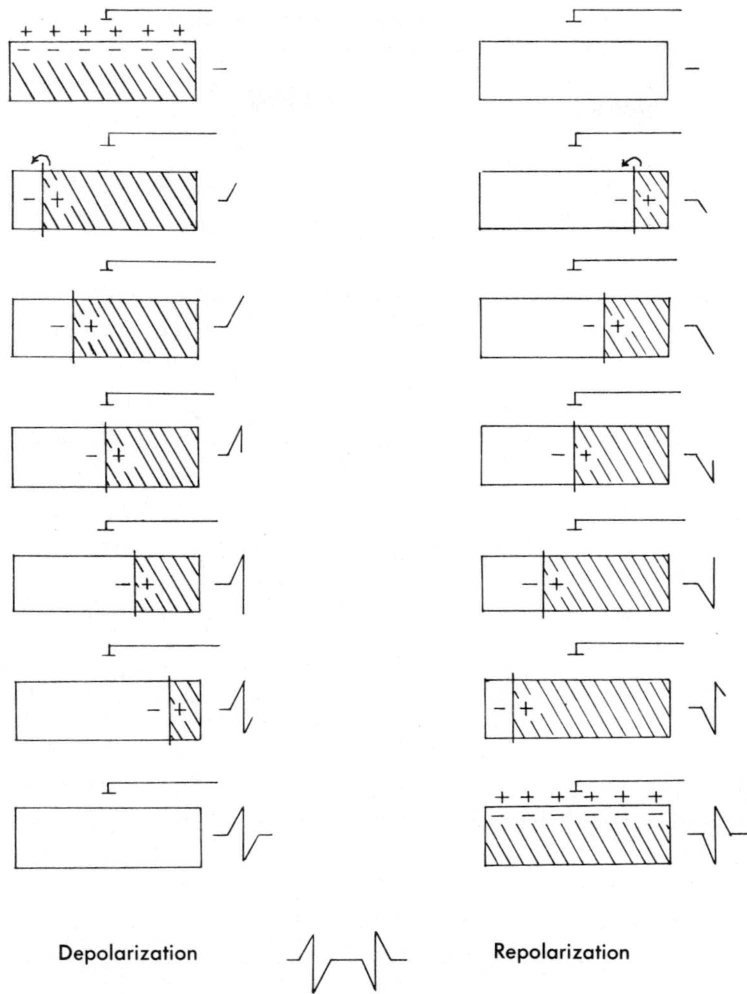

Fig. 5-3. Schematic representation of depolarization and repolarization of heart muscle. See text for description. (Adapted from Barker, J. M.: The unipolar electrocardiogram, New York, 1952, Appleton-Century-Crofts.)

ELECTROPHYSIOLOGY OF THE HEART

As with other muscles, contraction of myocardial fibers is an electrical phenomenon consisting of the buildup and discharge of a minute electrical current. A strip of muscle fiber may be visualized as covered with positive and negative charges, these charges being equally distributed throughout the strip so that in the resting state the net electrical charge is neutral. With an electrical potential present, the muscle strip is polarized and is neither predominately positive nor negative. Should a portion of a muscle strip become excited or activated, or suffer injury, the area so affected becomes electronegative in relation to the rest of the muscle, as the zinc electrode of a battery is electronegative to the copper electrode. Wtih this disruption in the even distribution of the electric charges, zones of opposite polarity are formed and a current flows from the positive zone to the negative. The muscle strip undergoes a process of *depolarization*, whereby all of the charges are used up in the current flow, until the strip is completely depolarized, or without electric potential. Functionally, this is the stage of muscle contraction, or cardiac systole. During diastole the muscle strip undergoes *repolarization*, with reestablishment of the original polarity. This process proceeds in the reverse direction from depolarization, starting with the end of the strip most recently depolarized, and since it involves zones of opposite polarity, a current is also produced during repolarization. Fig. 5-3 schematically demonstrates those two important phenomena. The rectangles represent muscle strips; those fully shaded at the top of the left column and the bottom of the right column are in the resting, polarized state, with equal numbers of positive and negative charges. Over the center of each strip is an electrode to pick up current flow and lead it to a recording device that will translate the flow into a curve. The recorder is so designed that when the electrode is opposite positively charged tissue an upright curve is written, and when opposite negative a downslope. Representative curves are illustrated adjacent to each rectangle.

Because the polarized strip in the left column has a net neutral charge evenly distributed about it, no current flows and the electrode records a straight, or *isoelectric* line. After a suitable stimulus, depolarization begins as a zone of negativity at the left end of the strip, and this depolarized area is delineated in the illustrations from the remainder of the still polarized muscle by a vertical boundary line. The opposite side of the boundary is positively charged, and the direction of current flow is depicted by arrows. As depolarization progresses, the electrode is faced with the approaching positive charge and records an upstroke. When the boundary is directly beneath the electrode, because it is neither positive nor negative, the curve drops to the isoelectric line. Almost at once, very strong negative charges are recorded, the curve drops sharply below the baseline, and, as the negativity moves gradually away from the electrode, its influence wanes, the curve returning up to the baseline. At this point the strip is completely depolarized and charges are absent. The right column shows the repolarization proceeding in the opposite direction, recording curves that are the reverse of those of depolarization.

The above principles are widely used in diagnostic electrocardiography and in monitoring devices for the continued observation of cardiac action in acutely ill patients. The electrical characteristics of the intact heart are more complex than those of the isolated muscle strip, and the currents recorded by the electrodes are the net sums of many currents in the areas being explored. It is not intended to present a course in electrocardiographic interpretation, but only to describe the basic major features of this important diagnostic tool.[37] Fig. 5-4 represents a typical "average" electrocardiographic segment,

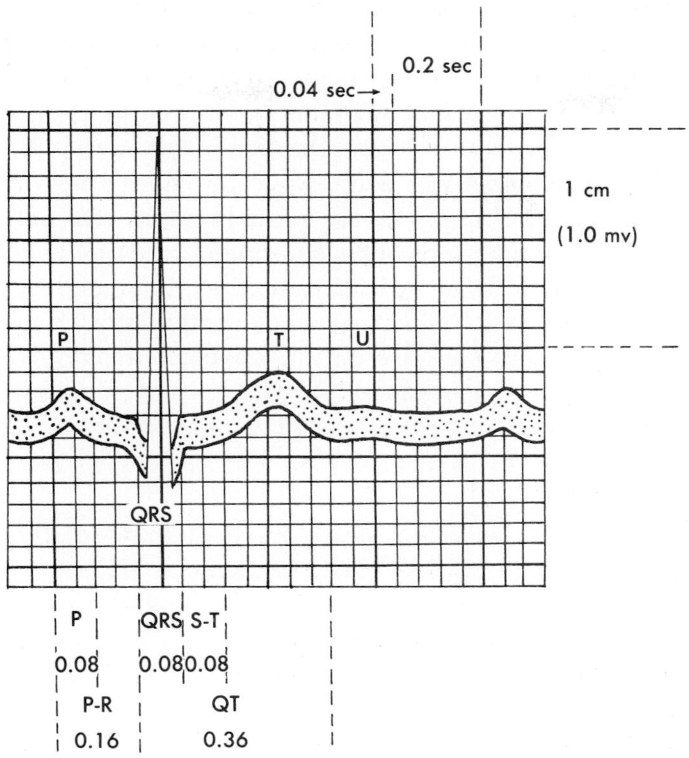

Fig. 5-4. Sketch of a normal electrocardiographic pattern. See text for description.

showing the characteristic curves recorded from a normal heart. The electrocardiographic machine amplifies the small electric currents brought to it by the electrode leads and passes them through a *galvanometer,* in which is located a pivoted writing arm called a *stylus.* Depending upon the polarity of the current passing through the galvanometer, the stylus is attracted to one or the other pole of the galvanometer magnet. By convention, positive deflections move the stylus upward, and negative downward. The movements are recorded on specially calibrated graph paper, which moves at a fixed speed, and the curves thus written can be measured in terms of voltage (vertical amplitude), and time (horizontal distance). Many different leads are used to give various electric "views" of the heart. For monitoring purposes, one lead is employed and the current projected through a cathode tube onto a fluorescent screen, where the record of each heartbeat can be seen as it is formed. Such an instrument is called an *oscilloscope.*

Although the contour of each lead differs from the others, the major components of an electrocardiographic tracing are illustrated in Fig. 5-4. The bold vertical lines represent time intervals of 0.2 second, subdivided into increments of 0.04 second. Bold horizontal lines are 1 cm apart, measuring an amplitude of 1.0 millivolt (mv), and each interval between represents 0.1 mv. Some normal values of amplitude and duration are indicated in the illustration. The P wave records the electrical activity of atrial systole, whereas the QRS complex represents ventricular depolarization. The P-R interval (actually, the P-QRS interval) is the length of time taken by the atrial impulse to reach the ventricles. The QT time is referred to as electrical ventricular systole (not mechanical systole). Diastole extends from the end of T to the next P and often contains a small U wave, the significance of which is not well understood. The S-T interval is the pause between ventricular depolarization and repolarization and represents a period of *absolute* ventricular refractoriness, during which the ventricles cannot be stimulated since they have not yet become polarized. Ventricular repolarization records the T wave, during which time the ventricles are only relatively refractory, since they can respond to stimuli in proportion to the degree that repolarization has been completed. After the T, of course, ventricular myocardium is fully responsive.

SYSTEMIC BLOOD FLOW

With each ventricular systole, approximately 60 to 70 ml of blood leave each ventricle, so the stroke volume of the heart is 120 to 140 ml. Obviously, the minute volume, or cardiac output, will depend upon the stroke volume and the cardiac rate, a situation analogous to the relation between the ventilatory tidal volume, rate, and minute volume. The speed and power with which systemic arterial blood will disseminate to all parts of the body depend upon a balance between two forces—that of left ventricular contraction and that of the resistance of the arterial tree. The latter is referred to as the *peripheral vascular resistance*, an important factor in determining systemic blood flow. Peripheral vascular resistance may be defined as the resistive force against which the left ventricle has to pump; it is produced by the "tone" of the arterial tree. We recall that arteries contain both elastic and muscle fibers in their structure and the arterial system as a whole is a continuously branching and narrowing arborization of channels. The elastic recoil of the larger arteries provides the initial resistance to the bolus of blood expelled from the left ventricle, whereas the tone of the muscle fibers of the smaller vessels maintains resistance distally. The apposition of the forces of ventricular contraction and peripheral resistance makes for a relatively smooth flow of blood with a minimal surge effect, which would result if a strong jet of blood were propelled into a rigid conducting system. If the system were flaccid, the ejection force would be dissipated before the stream reached the distal vessels, and again the flow would be uneven. Under the impact of the left ventricular blood, the proximal aorta stretches across its diameter to accommodate the blood volume; then as the aortic valve closes, the elastic aorta recoils. The recoil force is exerted against the column of blood in the arterial system and, since the valve does not yield, forces the blood distally. A wave of expansion and contraction, gradually diminishing, thus carries the blood through the major arteries, with no significant loss of velocity. The smaller arteries and arterioles maintain resistance and also determine the quantity of distal blood flow by appropriate contraction and relaxation of their muscle fibers. The function of these fibers, which is under reflex nervous control, assures adequate blood supply to those areas of the body in greatest need.

Each left ventricular contraction must be of sufficient force to impel the systemic column of blood in a continuous circuit, carrying the venous blood back to the right heart, much of it against gravity. This force is called the left ventricular systolic pressure. Direct measurement of this pressure can be made only by the technique of threading a catheter into the chamber, attaching the proximal end to a pressure recording device. However, an excellent approximation of this ejection force can be reached by measuring the pulsatile force transmitted to the column of blood in the brachial artery. This is the measurement of the familiar *blood pressure.* An inflatable cuff is secured about the upper arm and is connected by a rubber tube to a mercury manometer. By means of a hand bulb, the cuff is inflated until the brachial arterial flow is occluded, the inflating pressure being transmitted to the manometer. The cuff pressure is gradually released until blood just starts to flow again in the artery, and at this precise moment the manometer pressure is noted. At this point, the force of left ventricular contraction is enough to overcome (or is equal to) the pressure in the cuff as recorded by the manometer. It is reported as so many millimeters of mercury. In practice, the escape of blood past the occlusion of the cuff is determined by listening with a stethoscope over the artery in the antecubital fossa, at which time a characteristic sound is heard. This is the *systolic* blood pressure, with a wide range of normal from about *90 to 150 mm Hg* and an average in the adult of approximately *120 mm Hg.* After noting the systolic pressure, if one continues to listen while still slowly releasing the cuff pressure, he can detect another point manifested either by a definite change in the character of the arterial sound or, occasionally, by its disappearance. This event coincides with the elastic recoil of the artery on the blood column, and the closure of the aortic valve. The pressure noted at this time is called the *diastolic* blood pressure and has a normal range of *70 to 90 mm Hg* with an average of 80 mm Hg. The complete blood pressure reading thus has two components, systolic and diastolic, and is recorded as, for example, 120/80.

The physiologic significance of blood pressure values can be summarized in a simplified manner as follows:

Elevated systolic pressure implies an increase in the resistance of the arterial tree such as occurs with pathologic thickening of arterial or arteriolar walls, and/or reduction in their elasticity.

Reduced systolic pressure indicates a drop in conducting system resistance, as may result from peripheral vascular collapse, a state of shock, or weakness of the left ventricular myocardium.

Elevated diastolic pressure is consistent with an increase in peripheral resistance, often accompanying systolic pressure increase, but usually implies more advanced resistance than does a systolic increase alone.

Reduced diastolic pressure is found with a loss of resistance or myocardial weakness, as described above, but also occurs with an incompetent aortic valve, which allows retrograde flow of blood back into the left ventricle during diastolic recoil.

Although much of the systolic thrust of the left ventricle has been dissipated by the time capillary blood has perfused tissue cells, the return venous circulation is under a significant head of pressure. Venous return is dependent upon the impetus of the arterial flow, aided by the "milking" effect exerted upon the veins by surrounding muscles (especially of the lower extremity), the tone of the abdominal musculature, and the negative inspiratory intrathoracic pressure. Thus, venous return from the lower limbs is more effective when leg muscles are active than when at rest, a matter of some practical importance, whereas return flow from the head and neck is dependent upon gravity and the intrathoracic negative pressure. The effect of intrathoracic pressure on venous return to the heart is of considerable importance to the inhalation therapist, as it relates directly to his work. Spontaneous natural breathing is characterized by a relatively long inhalation followed by a short exhalation, so that the time interval of falling intrathoracic pressure is greater than the time of rising pressure; and we know that except under conditions of forced exhalation thoracic pressure never exceeds ambient. The thorax thus acts like a large suction pump, aiding the venous blood in its return to the heart, and by virtue of the ventilatory pattern, maximum return occurs during inhalation. It can be properly inferred, then, that any condition which raises the mean intrathoracic pressure will impede the venous return; and it readily follows that if the volume of blood returning to the heart is reduced the cardiac output will drop. We can easily demonstrate the effect on venous flow of increased intrathoracic pressure by holding the breath, straining, and then observing the color changes in the face from stasis of blood in the veins. Under some conditions we can note marked distention of the superficial veins of the neck. If such a buildup of thoracic pressure is significant and prolonged, venous blood unable to return to the heart will pool in venous reservoirs of the liver and abdominal circulation. It is pertinent to observe here that one of the major tools of inhalation therapy, the positive-pressure ventilator, is a potential prime offender in this regard, a matter that will be discussed in detail later. Because the venous pressure varies markedly in different parts of the body and with position of the body, its measurement is made under standard conditions. A vein in the antecubital fossa is chosen as the site, and the patient is placed in a flat supine position with the arm arranged so that the antecubital fossa is at the same level as the right atrium of the heart. A needle is inserted into the vein and is attached to a special manometer so that the pressure of the column of blood in the vein is balanced against a column of *saline* in the manometer. The normal range of venous pressure is very wide, from 50 to 110 mm of *water*. Of more limited value than the arterial pressure, venous pressure is especially useful in quantitating the retarding effect upon venous return of weakness of the right ventricle. In certain pathologic conditions elevated venous pressure is readily apparent by visible distention of cervical veins and constitutes an important clinical sign.

PULMONARY BLOOD FLOW

The pulmonary circulation, when compared with the systemic, is a low-pressure system. The total circuit distance from right ventricle to left atrium is short, and the pulmonary capillary bed is extensive, so that relatively low pressures suffice for blood flow. As an average, the pulmonary artery pressure is about 25/8 mm Hg. It should be apparent that recording pulmonary pressure is not as simple as measuring the systemic and can only be accomplished by means of intracardiac catheterization. By this technique, it is possible to measure pressures in the right atrium, the right ventricle, and for a considerable distance into the pulmonary arteries. Such serial readings make it possible to differentiate between lesions, e.g., stenotic heart valves, which lead to increased pressures within the heart in the presence of a normal pulmonary system, and an actual increase in the peripheral resistance of the pulmonary arterial tree. Many of the diseases with which the inhalation therapist will have contact produce thickening and/or narrowing of the pulmonary vessels, the resulting increased resistance requiring added ejection force of the right ventricle. Also, destruction of a sufficient portion of the pulmonary capillary bed by disease of the lung, even in the presence of normal remaining vessels, may produce resistance to right heart output, since the same output is forced through a smaller cross-sectional capillary bed. Whenever resistance to pulmonary flow is present, the right ventricle is put under strain and, if persistent, will lead to weakening of the right ventricle. If this is due to pulmonary disease, the effect upon the heart is called *cor pulmonale*, or "pulmonary heart," to be described shortly.

Despite the vital importance of the pulmonary arterial blood supply, we cannot overlook the systemic component of the total pulmonary blood flow.[38] The student is encouraged to review the anatomic relationships of the bronchial arteries and note that, whereas the pulmonary arteries give off no visceral branches before the level of the alveoli, the bronchial vessels supply the entire length of the bronchial tree to the bronchioles with oxygenated blood. The returning bronchial venous blood follows an interesting variety of routes, which have some clinical significance. The accompanying bronchial veins are imperfect and irregular and can probably accommodate no more than a third of the bronchial venous blood as they empty into the azygos vein. From the distal portions of the airways, bronchial venous blood drains into the *pulmonary veins* (arterialized blood) and thus contributes to the normal small degree of unsaturation of the systemic arterial blood. At the capillary level there are microscopic communications between bronchial and pulmonary capillaries. Here, there is a mixture of arterialized systemic blood (bronchial capillaries) with venous blood (pulmonary capillaries). This relationship is unimportant under normal circumstances, but in certain disease states in which there is interruption of pulmonary arterial flow, these communications may become grossly enlarged and provide a significant volume of blood perfusing alveoli, even though it is arterial. This so-called *bronchial collateral flow* can reach tremendous proportions in destructive pulmonary diseases, best exemplified by bronchiectasis.

At this point the essentials of *acute pulmonary edema* will be described because, although not necessarily the product of intrinsic lung or heart disease, edema of the lung involves a serious disruption of the pulmonary circulation and marked interference with pulmonary gas exchange. It can provoke an acute, life-threatening clinical situation frequently encountered not only in the hospital emergency room but also on inpatient divisions, and the inhalation therapist plays an important role in its treatment. Theoretically, edema of the lung can be of three types: intracellular, interstitial, and alveolar, but our present interest will be centered about the alveolar edema.[39]

Acute pulmonary edema is a condition in which there is a rapid movement of some or all of the blood components across the pulmonary capillary wall into the minute pericapillary space, from which they flow into the alveoli, alveolar ducts, and bronchial tree. Among the many factors that determine the degree of edema are (a) the net osmotic pressure across the capillary wall, between the blood and interstitial lung fluid, (b) the permeability (ease of penetration) of both capillary and alveolar walls, and (c) the capacity of the pulmonary lymphatic drainage, or the ease with which the lymphatics can remove excess interstitial fluid. An upset of the physiologic balance between these factors, whatever the cause, can produce an often massive outpouring of fluid (transudation) into the lungs in a matter of minutes. Despite the frequency with which acute pulmonary edema occurs, little is known about the exact mechanism responsible for it. Presumably, a precipitating underlying disease stimulates some autonomic nervous system reflexes that enhance alveolar-capillary permeability. Afferent autonomic nerve endings are found in many organs (heart, vessels, lungs, hollow viscera of the abdomen) that communicate through brain centers with efferent nerves supplying peripheral and pulmonary blood vessels. Abnormal reflexes can be initiated that upset the usual balanced vasomotor tone responsible for smoothly related pulmonary flow and hydrostatic pressure.[40]

Acute pulmonary edema is more a clinical syndrome than a disease entity and accompanies a variety of specific diseases. Among the latter, in which acute edema may play a significant role, are cardiovascular disease, especially coronary heart disease, heart failure, valvular disease, lung diseases, severe infections, brain injury, metabolic disorders, extensive surface burns, and severe body trauma. The acute edema, itself, may be responsible for the loss of a great enough volume of circulating fluid to precipitate a serious state of shock (acute circulatory failure, see below), but the outstanding signs and symptoms are the result of the extensive obstruction of airways and alveoli, with resulting hypoxia and impaired ventilation. Often, the onset of acute pulmonary edema may be preceded by a sense of anxiety and then openly manifest itself by sudden dyspnea. The fluid permeating the respiratory tract is churned into a froth by the rapidly moving tidal air exchange, is often pink or frankly blood tinged, and may be of such quantity as to bubble from the mouth under the stress of the patient's strenuous breathing. The neck veins may be markedly distended, and frequently the blood pressure is elevated, unless shock is present. Air passing through the edema fluid produces a bubbling sound known as *rales,* which often can be heard by the unaided ear as well as by the stethoscope, and not rarely the wheezing sounds of air moving through narrow passages are also present. The patient labors hard to breath and is usually markedly cyanotic from his severe obstructive hypoxia. The treatment of acute pulmonary edema will be discussed later, but the student can certainly perceive that thereapy will be of a dual nature—that of the underlying disease, and of the edema itself.

CORONARY BLOOD FLOW

Although we are not concerned with specific diseases at this point, because of the great prevalence of coronary heart disease—especially in the age group comprising the bulk of patients receiving inhalation therapy—a few observations should be made of this important segment of the cardiovascular system. If the student reviews the anatomy of the heart, he will recall that the myocardium receives its blood supply through the coronary arteries and that these vessels are the first branches of the aorta, thus assuring that perfusion of the myocardial cells will be supported by the maximum delivery pressure of the left ventricle. Not only is the contractility of the heart muscle dependent upon an adequate blood flow, but the conducting system of the heart is very sensitive to circulatory interference. Because the work demand of the heart is so variable and the organ's response to demand must be prompt, the circulatory system of the heart must be flexible and able to adjust blood flow from moment to moment. As long as the coronary vessels are normal in structure, this presents no problem; but when diseased, they subject the function of the entire body to a serious hazard.

From the middle years on, the incidence of impaired coronary circulation increases, yet despite the prevalence of coronary artery disease, relatively little is known about its specific causes. It is believed that the vessels may respond to unknown stimuli, neurogenic or humoral, by a spastic contraction of their muscle fibers. Such episodes reduce the blood flow to the myocardium, often with drastic but usually transient effects, most frequently manifest by acute chest pain. A recurring condition, it is clinically referred to as *angina pectoris* (literally, "pain in the chest"). The coronary vessels are also subject to the same sclerosis, or hardening process, that so often affects the general arterial tree. Attributed to such factors as the degeneration of aging, toxic effects of nicotine directly or indirectly, cholesterol ingestion, neurogenic stimuli, and many others, thickening of the coronary arterial walls effectively and permanently reduces their caliber and elasticity. Such vessels are unable to respond to myocardial need for a rapid increase in cellular perfusion and seriously handicap the cardiac function. Further, the arteries, whether already damaged or not, are subject to the formation of thromboses (blood clots) from causes that again are not clear, with acute or gradual occlusion of their lumens. The inhalation therapist will have frequent occasion to see patients suffering from acute coronary occlusion, many of whom are ill enough to require the services of specialized care units in the hospital.

Interference with myocardial perfusion damages the muscle cells, and when such damage is severe enough to be permanent, the affected myocardium is replaced with fibrosis. Over a period of time the accumulation of fibrosis can reach a point at which there is not enough normal-functioning myocardium for adequate cardiac function, and heart failure develops. Also, should myocardial circulatory insufficiency involve a segment of the conducting system of the heart, rate and rhythm disturbances will be an important part of the clinical picture. The term *infarction* is given to a localized area of the heart where myocardial cells have been replaced by scarring, and *diffuse myocardial fibrosis* to a more generalized distribution of fibrous replacement.

It should be emphasized that the myocardium is very susceptible to hypoxia, and the coronary vessels to a sudden drop in arterial carbon dioxide tension. These facts must be kept in mind by the inhalation therapist, and although he may be treating a patient primarily for a respiratory ailment, he should try to acquaint himself with the general state of the patient's myocardial health.

CARDIOVASCULAR FAILURE

The inhalation therapist will have constant contact with patients in heart failure, and he must be aware of the basic physiologic defects involved. A heart is considered to be in failure when it can no longer fulfill its function of ensuring adequate cellular perfusion to all parts of the body without assistance. Such a state is called *cardiac decompensation.* With its underlying disease still present but its function restored by supportive therapy (i.e., digitalis, bed rest, etc.), the heart is said to be in a state of "compensation," full or partial. A heart may decompensate because of an increase in the work load imposed upon it (increased resistance in the circulation, defective function of the cardiac valves), a decrease in the ventricular contractile power (myocardial damage from fibrosis, infection, toxins), or a combination of both. There are a host of classifications of cardiac and vascular functional derangements, based on physiologic and clinical criteria, but it would be inappropriate to attempt to summarize briefly, with any degree of clarity in these few pages, that which is not done with much uniformity in large texts. Because our purpose is to provide the inhalation therapist with a basic orientation to those forms of disease relative to his work, we will describe but two types of cardiovascular incompetence that are of great importance to him: *congestive heart failure* and *acute circulatory failure.*

Congestive heart failure

The term *congestive* implies an overcrowding and refers to a packing of vessels with blood as a result of a backup of circulation. In this type of failure, since the forward flow of blood is reduced, the blood backlogs in the return vessels, which become distended, and there is pooling in venous and capillary reservoirs. Velocity is reduced, and there is interference with cellular gas exchange. There are two types of congestive failure, which need differentiation, *left ventricular congestive failure* and *right ventricular congestive failure.*

Left ventricular failure. Strong though it is, the left ventricle can fail if it is opposed by increasing resistance in the systemic circulation or if the myocardium is weakened by disease. Blood returning to the left heart from the lung cannot be ejected rapidly enough, and it backs up in the pulmonary circulation. Vessels in the lung, especially the arterioles, capillaries, and veins, become "passively" congested. Often pressure in these channels increases to the point that blood water is forced from them into the pulmonary pericapillary and interstitial spaces and the alveoli. Although this state justifies the title of pulmonary edema, there are some important differential points that separate it clinically from the acute pulmonary edema discussed above. The edema produced by left ventricular failure is of a passive nature, due to the increased hydrostatic pressure of blood stasis in the pulmonary circulation. This is entirely different from the "active" acute edema, which is the result of dynamic changes in the A-C membrane and its environment, mediated through nerve reflexes in response to disease that may be remote from the lung. In addition to etiologic and physiologic differences, the functional impairments of these two types of edema vary. However, it should be emphasized that a patient with passive pulmonary congestion and edema may also be subject to a superimposed acute edema, a not infrequent occurrence. We have already noted that acute pulmonary edema generally has an abrupt onset, runs a stormy course, and is of relatively short duration. Passive edema, on the other hand, is always due to heart disease and is chronic in nature. The extravasation of fluid into the lung is of much smaller volume than that of acute edema, and its clinical and physiologic effects upon ventilation are of different quality.

Whereas the functional impairment in respiration of acute pulmonary edema is generally obstructive in nature, that of passive congestion and edema is less easily categorized. The congested pulmonary vessels and edema fluid are space-occupying and encroach upon alveolar air space, with reduction especially noted in the vital capacity. With engorgement of the vessels and perivascular and interstitial fluid increased, the lung becomes less flexible, and loss of pulmonary compliance is an important sequella to left heart failure. The congested vessels also offer increased resistance to the work of the right ventricle, putting it under strain. Of great significance is the combined effect of pulmonary congestion and edema to disrupt normal ventilation-perfusion relationships, interfere with alveolar gas exchange, and produce hypoxia. It is reasonable to suppose that if sufficient edema fluid should accumulate in alveoli and perhaps terminal bronchioles it would obstruct airflow to the alveoli. In this respect, chronic passive edema may simulate, but to a lesser degree, the effect of acute edema. However, much of the edema of passive congestion may be interstitial, exerting its influence by increasing the thickness of the A-C membrane, creating a "diffusion defect" for oxygen rather than an obstruction to ventilation. It is very probable that both obstruction and diffusion interference play simultaneous or reciprocating roles, depending upon the exact dynamics of the congestion at any given time. Because the quantity of pulmonary blood flow can be variable in left heart failure, depending upon the degree of compensation or decompensation, its relation to ventilation will also be an important determinant in effective gas exchange. Thus, obstruction, diffusion defect, and disturbed ventilation-perfusion relationships may all be important effects of chronic passive edema. These conditions will be described more generally, individually, in the next chapter. Finally, the hydrostatic pressure in the congested lung vessels and in the lymphatics of the thorax may reach such heights that fluid will escape into the pleural space, producing a hydrothorax (literally, "water in the chest"). Up to several liters may accumulate here, and because of the obvious effect of lung compression by the fluid, we see that restriction of lung expansion is also a potential risk of left heart failure.

Right ventricular failure. The most frequent cause of failure of the right ventricle is preexisting failure of the left ventricle, and we have already noted that increased back pressure in the pulmonary circulation can produce a pulmonary hypertension, the resistance of which can strain the capacity of the right ventricle beyond its normal compensation. In addition, other intrinsic cardiac diseases, valvular and congenital, can overburden the right heart, but we are interested in a specific type of right failure, that due to pulmonary disease. *Cor pulmonale* implies compromise of the right ventricle, by the effects of intrapulmonary pathology, and is characterized by right ventricular enlargement (hypertrophy, a thickening of the myocardial wall; or dilatation, an enlargement of the chamber due to stretching of the myocardial fibers; or both) associated with pulmonary disease known to interfere with right ventricular function.[41] The disease so affecting the right heart usually produces an elevated pressure in the pulmonary circulation, but pulmonary hypertension, itself, does not constitute cor pulmonale.

Cor pulmonale is most commonly seen, and has been best documented, in the disease complex of which we will learn more later, obstructive bronchitis–pulmonary emphysema. Studies of this condition, along with others characterized by ventilatory failure, indicate that the most important elements in the genesis of cor pulmonale are probably bronchiolar obstruction, alveolar hypoventilation, and hypoxia.[42] The exact interrelation of these factors is not entirely clear, but it has been suggested that hypoxia may exert its influence directly on the myocardium. On the other hand, the effect of chronic hypoxia may be more indirect, perhaps initiating a rise in cardiac output and a subsequent elevation of pulmonary arterial pressure. Others place more emphasis on the prerequisite of chronic airway obstruction as a prime mover in the development of right heart strain but with hypoxia and hypercapnia as necessary factors.[43] Whatever the mechanism, the right ventricle is subjected to increasing resistance in providing pulmonary perfusion, and it responds by increasing its mass of myocardial tissue for greater contractile force (hypertrophy) or by elongating its myocardial fibers for greater contractile leverage, enlarging the ventricular cavity (dilatation); or the two may exist together. The right side of the heart becomes prominent by x-ray examination and shows certain electrocardiographic patterns suggesting enlargement.

When the right ventricle fails, it no longer is able to maintain an adequate output (although the early signs of impending failure may be an increased output) and stasis or congestion occurs in the systemic circulation that supplies it. There is pooling of blood in the veins of the lower extremities and in the venous and capillary beds of the abdominal viscera, especially in the liver. Again, with the weakened right ventricle unable to accommodate the returning venous blood, hydrostatic pressure in the veins promotes the escape of fluid into surrounding tissues, with the production of edema of the feet and legs, demonstrable swelling of the liver (hepatomegaly), and the outpouring of fluid into the abdominal cavity (ascites). With pure right failure there may be no signs of circulatory embarrassment of the lung, only evidence of its underlying disease. Prominent distention of the superficial neck veins, especially in the supine position, may be a prominent feature of right heart failure, and there will be an expected elevation of peripheral venous pressure. In summary, then, because the heart is a mated pair of pumps, each with its own circuit but with each circuit interacting with the other, it is easy to see that each pump is subject to individual failure. Because of the relationship of the two pumps, we can see how the right can fail without materially affecting the left but that failure of the left will eventually strain the right to the point of decompensation. The therapist will see many patients with diseases of the systematic cardiovascular system who will have both left and right congestive heart failure and who will demonstrate to varying degrees any or all of the signs and symptoms characteristic of each.

Acute circulatory failure

This term embodies a large number of different diseases and conditions with a variety of etiologies, but they all have one thing in common—a serious drop in cardiac output due to either cardiac or noncardiac causes, with subsequent tissue hypoxia. In contrast to the reduction in cardiac output found in the congestive heart failures discussed above, that which characterizes acute circulatory failure occurs rapidly, allowing the body little time to adjust to the acute change. The student will encounter this condition frequently, will often be part of the therapeutic team involved in its management, and will soon get accustomed to hearing it referred to as "shock." The name *shock* is not a precise one, for it may have different connotations to different people, and although some have recommended its discontinuance, a name once established is difficult to change.[44] Shock involves many interacting physiologic phenomena of great complexity, and there is no unanimity on classification, either clinical or physiologic. Since we do not wish to get embroiled in controversial theories but rather wish to develop a practical clinical appreciation of this significant condition, we will describe the cardinal features of shock as a composite of those characteristics most frequently accepted.[45-47]

We will avoid the complex classifications of shock that involve the many specific etiologies and describe it as an abnormal physiologic state with a disproportion between the circulating blood volume and the size of the vascular bed, which leads to circulatory failure (the inability to maintain an adequate minute volume of blood flow for tissue needs) and cellular hypoxia. The three important factors in its genesis are the blood volume, the effectiveness of the cardiac pump, and the "tone" of the peripheral vasculature. Should one or more of these fail, shock will develop if the remainder cannot compensate for the deficiency. With the major component of the shock syndrome a reduced cardiac output, we can rightfully expect there to be an accompanying drop in arterial blood pressure. It is these two factors that subject the body tissues to the risk of hypoxia, since adequate cellular gas exchange requires both a minimum blood volume and a perfusing pressure. In the presence of this threat, the body must protect its most hypoxia-sensitive vital organs, the brain and heart, from oxygen want. Compensation consists of redistributing the arterial circulation to assure adequate cerebral and cardiac perfusion, even at the expense of other tissues, especially the abdominal organs and peripheral areas (skin). This is accomplished by widespread vascoconstriction to shift the available blood flow to the two vital structures and also to maintain suitable blood pressure through an increase in peripheral resistance. The blood pressure may continue to fall, a characteristic of shock, but cerebral and cardiac perfusion can remain ample for a long time. Should the shock state progress into what is termed *irreversible shock*, compensation will fail and vascoconstriction may give way to vasodilatation at the capillary and venular level, with the pooling of large volumes of blood in the capillary beds. This further reduces the circulating blood volume (hypovolemia) and initiates a vicious cycle that may continue to death. There are some types of acute circulatory failure that initially show vasodilatation rather than vasoconstriction, and in these the underlying disease prevents the constrictor compensation just described. It is perhaps evident to the student that there can be a period of imminent or potential shock before the classical symptoms of hypotension warn of falling cardiac output. Patients suspected of having conditions predisposing to shock are carefully observed for its signs.

We can summarize in a brief outline the major causes of reduction in cardiac output as follows:

(1) *Reduction in blood volume*
   (a) Loss of blood by hemorrhage
   (b) Extravasation of blood or plasma from vessels into intercellular spaces, as result of damage to capillaries and larger vessels by trauma and surgery
   (c) Dehydration, with loss of fluid through skin, kidney, gastrointestinal tract

(2) *Reduced venous return from capillary and venular pooling*
   (a) Vasodilatation, due to loss of vasomotor stimuli from toxins (bacterial sepsis)
   (b) Vasodilatation, due to loss of vasoconstrictor action, as from spinal anesthesia

(3) *Failure of cardiac pump action*
   (a) Cardiac filling defect, as from tamponade (compression of heart from pericardial fluid) and tachycardia (insufficient diastolic filling time due to rapid rate)
   (b) Cardiac emptying defect, as from an obstructing intracardiac thrombus, large pulmonary embolus
   (c) Impaired cardiac function, especially from myocardial infarct

From a very practical point of view, the inhalation therapist will see patients go into shock mostly as the result of severe trauma (automobile or industrial accidents, gunshot wounds), extensive surgery (manipulation of viscera, loss of blood and plasma), massive acute blood loss, and overwhelming sepsis (blood invasion by bacteria). Of special interest to the therapist, and the prime reason why he should understand the basic principles of shock, is the circulatory failure that can follow a disturbance in intrathoracic pressure dynamics. Any disorder that can produce a significant elevation in intrapleural pressure, elevating the mean pressure from the negative to the positive range, by virtue of interfering with venous return through the thoracic vessels and by restricting diastolic filling of the heart, can generate shock. It cannot be emphasized too frequently or too strongly that this is an inherent risk in the use of positive pressure ventilating equipment.

The clinical picture of shock will be a familiar one to the therapist in a general hospital. The patient may be restless or apathetic and lethargic, but he will show marked physical weakness. His skin will be pale, cold, and moist or will show a grayish cyanosis. The superficial veins will be collapsed and difficult to find, a point of considerable therapeutic concern. The blood pressure will be low, at least less than 80 mm Hg, systolic, and in severe states may be so weak as to be unobtainable, and the peripheral pulse will be faint or "thready" and rapid. Urinary output falls off as kidney perfusion is seriously compromised. Body temperature is often below normal. It is beyond the scope of this text to detail the particulars of therapy, which frequently taxes the ingenuity of the medical attendents, but among all the necessary supportive measures it should be evident that the administration of oxygen is of prime importance. The alert therapist will observe the other techniques employed to maintain maximum tissue perfusion, including the "shock position," fluid and blood replacement and cardiovascular stimulants.

CARDIAC ARRHYTHMIAS

The importance of the cardiac arrhythmias lies not so much in their relation to inhalation directly as in the frequency with which they occur in the hospital population most apt to be serviced by inhalation therapy. In the performance of his duties, the inhalation therapist will see and hear much attention directed to this class of cardiac disorders, and especially in critical care units he will see visual evidence of them on oscilloscope monitor screens. As with the preceding examples of heart disease, we will outline the minimal features of arrhythmias most commonly encountered in hospital practice, ignoring the more bizarre, and leave it to the individual therapist to supplement this material with independent reading, according to his interest.

Although *dysrhythmia* (a malfunctioning rhythm) is probably more accurate, *arrhythmia* has become the standard expression for a cardiac rhythm that deviates from the usual and natural pattern, interrupting the automatic rhythmic heart action which was initiated before birth. Many of the rhythm disturbances can be diagnosed with certainty only by the electrocardiogram. others can be readily detected clinically, and the presence of yet others may be highly suspected. The presence of an abnormal heart rhythm is not necessarily a bad omen, for many of them are innocuous and occur in normal hearts; but others may indicate serious underlying pathology, and a few signify imminent death. A simple physiologic concept must be understood if one is to appreciate the great variety of abnormal rhythms to which the heart is subject. We have already established that the sinus node (sinoatrial node) is the normal focus for the start of cardiac contraction, but any site in the myocardium or the conducting system is capable of initiating excitation. It is as though an almost infinite number of trigger points are kept subdued by the normal action of the dominant sinus node but express themselves when some factor causes the latter to lose its tight control. We will briefly describe the following, all of which the therapist may expect to see in the general hospital: sinus arrhythmia, premature contractions, paroxysmal tachycardia, atrial flutter, atrial fibrillation, ventricular fibrillation, atrioventricular block, and sinus arrest.[48,49]

Sinus arrhythmia

The most frequent and least harmful of all the arrhythmias, sinus arrhythmia, is a normal variant in the young but can often be found at almost any age.

It is characterized by a change in cardiac rate synchronous with the respiratory cycle, as the heart rate increases during inspiration and decreases with expiration. It can be exaggerated by inspiratory breath holding and eliminated by exercise. The mechanism for its presence is an alteration in the strength of vagal (parasympathetic) influence on the normal pacemaker. Presumably, during inspiration the increased vagal impulses brought into play by the Hering-Breuer reflex quantitatively detract from the vagal impulses serving the sinus node. With lessened parasympathetic inhibition during this phase of respiration, the excitation rate of the node increases with a similar response by the ventricles. This condition has no pathologic implications, and no treatment is indicated.

Premature contractions

Localized areas of the atria, atrioventricular (A-V) node, and ventricular myocardium may initiate an excitation impulse independently of the sinus node. Because they occur away from the normal focus of stimulation, they are referred to as *ectopic foci.* Premature contractions may be prognostically benign or serious, as they can occur in both normal and diseased hearts. They result from the irritation of some spot in the myocardium or conducting system by a variety of stimulants, among which the following are frequent offenders: excitement, anxiety, smoking, alcoholic ingestion, fatigue, gastrointestinal disturbances, and procedures such as thoracic surgery, cardiac catheterization, and digitalis (a vital drug used in the treatment of heart failure but which can irritate the myocardium).

The premature contraction is a sort of "extra" beat and is so named because it is activated before a normal beat would be expected, inserting itself between two normal contractions. If the stimulus is great enough or there is more than one stimulus, there may be a short string of premature contractions. Also, in pathologic states, different stimuli may generate impulses from more than one ectopic focus. There are three general types of premature contractions: atrial, nodal, and ventricular. In the first, an ectopic atrial impulse follows the usual path, and the extra beat cannot be distinguished from a normal. A nodal premature contraction starts in the A-V node (not the sinus node) and also follows the usual path into the ventricles, but because it travels a shorter distance than a sinus impulse, characteristic time measurements on the electrocardiogram identify it. Since a ventricular premature contraction starts at the opposite end of the excitation chain, its path through the ventricular muscle is grossly abnormal, and the electrocardiographic configuration is often quite bizarre. Ventricular extra systoles may occur with regularity, alternating with normal sinus beats, producing a coupled rhythm referred to as "bigeminy."

An interesting characteristic of premature contractions, which can sometimes be noted clinically, and usually by the electrocardiograph, is the slightly longer than normal refractory period of myocardial fibers. Because the extra ectopic stimulus occurs out of phase, it interferes with the usual sequence of excitability and refractoriness and causes a lag before the next following contraction. This is called a *compensatory pause.* In an atrial premature contraction, the ectopic impulse encompasses the sinus node, which must wait until it recovers before it can initiate its own normal beat. Thus, the interval between the premature beat and the next normal one is longer than the interval between two normal beats. After ventricular extra contractions, and usually nodal ones as well, the ventricles are refractory to the next normal sinus impulse, leading to a longer pause that is designated as "fully compensated." In this instance, the time interval between the normal beats preceding and following the ectopic is exactly twice the time interval between any two other normal beats.

The clinical significance of premature contractions usually depends upon the patient's tolerance of them, their frequency, and the presence or absence of underlying disease. Symptoms may be absent, or the patient may complain of "palpitations" or a "thumping" in the chest. The patient is actually aware of the *absence* of heart action during the compensatory pause as well as the difference in contractile force between normal and some abnormal beats. Sometimes dizziness and a sense of fullness in the chest or neck are bothersome.

Paroxysmal tachycardia

Chains or bursts of atrial, nodal, or ventricular premature contractions constitute paroxysmal tachycardia, which may last for prolonged periods of time. During an attack, the cardiac rate may range from 160 to 240 per minute. The rhythm is usually regular, is not affected by breathing or exercise, and may terminate abruptly. Atrial and nodal paroxysms can often be stopped by strong vagal stimuli, accomplished by exerting pressure on the eyeballs or carotid sinus, or by gagging. Ventricular ectopic foci will not respond to these maneuvers, since the ventricular myocardium is less influenced by vagal innervation than is the atrial.

From a clinical point of view, this abnormality may be functional (not due to organic disease) or due to cardiac disease. It often produces weakness and dizziness, and if prolonged, there will be a drop in cardiac output due to the sharp reduction in diastolic filling time from the rapid rate. A diseased heart may be thrown into congestive failure, and shock is a real threat. There is also the risk that paroxysmal tachycardia will progress to the very grave ventricular fibrillation, to be described below. Its presence is always an indication for careful observation, and drug therapy of the arrhythmia is a usual precaution.

Atrial flutter

In atrial flutter there is either a rapid circular movement of a stimulus or a repetitive single ectopic focus exciting the atria at rates of 200 to 350 per minute, with a clocklike regularity. It is named from the flutterlike contraction imparted to the atria. The refractoriness of the A-V node does not permit it to transmit usually more than 180 impulses per minute, so many of the atrial signals are blocked. The ratio of blocked to transmitted impulses may be quite constant in a given instance, such as 2:1, 3:1, 4:1, etc.

Flutter is usually due to disease, and even with a partial block, the ventricular rate is still high enough to compromise cardiac filling and output. Because of the fixed atrioventricular ratio, the cardiac rate does not increase with exercise, even in those instances in which the block may permit a near normal rate. This interferes with the normal cardiac reserve and its response to exercise.

Atrial fibrillation

Atrial fibrillation is the most common of the significant abnormal rhythm disturbances and is the usual end point of a preexisting flutter, although a flutter is not a prerequisite. Fibrillation always means cardiac pathology. The atria are subjected to a completely uncontrolled, randomly irregular barrage of impulses at rates of 350 to 500 per minute. The A-V node transmits as many of these as it can, and the result is a chaotic ventricular response of grossly irregular contractions of varying intensities. Some of the contractions are too weak to be palpated in the peripheral pulses, and this leads to a *pulse deficit*, a discrepancy between the cardiac rate as counted over the chest and the rate of arterial pulsations.

The therapist will see many patients with this defect, for its causes span the extremes of life. It is a common sequella to such childhood diseases as rheumatic fever and is often seen with degenerative cardiac diseases of later years. It is not incompatible with fairly normal activity, and many people carry it for years. However, the fibrillation (weak, shaky, ineffectual contraction) of the atria promotes poor atrial emptying, with the retention of blood in these chambers and the subsequent risk of intra-atrial thrombus formation, often a source of future emboli. For this reason attempts are usually made to convert such hearts to a normal rhythm. Atrial fibrillation is readily detected by physical examination, but its electrocardiographic picture is characteristic, with the absence of definitive P waves and their replacement by an irregularly wavy baseline.

Ventricular fibrillation

So grave as to be imminently fatal if not quickly corrected, ventricular fibrillation consists of a rapid tremulous shaking of the ventricular myocardium completely incompatible with any useful cardiac output. Frequently preceded by persistent or recurring ventricular paroxysmal tachycardia, fibrillation can be caused by many conditions, among which are electric shock, anesthesia, mechanical irritation of the heart, severe hypoxia, myocardial infarction, and large doses of digitalis or epinephrine. The rapid drop in cardiac output produces an acute cerebral hypoxia, often manifested by convulsions, and death ensues within a few minutes. From a functional viewpoint, ventricular fibrillation may be considered a form of "cardiac arrest," for although there is some ventricular activity, it is of no value. This abnormality, like sinus arrest to be described below, constitutes a true emergency situation, with survival dependent upon the immediate application of the techniques of emergency resuscitation.

Atrioventricular block

Disorders of the myocardium such as inflammations, infarction or arteriosclerotic ischemia, and digitalis toxicity can reduce or destroy the ability of the A-V node or the bundle of His to transmit the sinus impulse to the ventricles. If every impulse is conducted but with a prolonged time (prolonged P-R interval on the electrocardiogram), the block is considered as *first degree.* If some impulses are conducted but others dropped, the block is *second degree.* If no atrial impulses are conducted to the ventricles, the block is *third degree* or "complete." The last is the most important, for with no sinus impulse the ventricles must develop their own pacemaker and are able to do so only at very slow rates of between 25 and 45 per minute. Under conditions of stress, or in the presence of other arrhythmias, the bradycardia may be inadequate for cerebral blood flow, and the heart may even stop for several seconds. Acute unconsciousness may occur without warning, the so-called *Stokes-Adams syncope* (fainting). Convulsions and death may accompany such episodes. The disability of complete heart block is obvious and the need for treatment urgent. Whereas some patients respond to medical therapy, others have realized new leases on life with the use of newly developed electric pacemakers implanted in their bodies.

Sinus arrest

Like ventricular fibrillation, sinus arrest is a second cause of sudden cardiac standstill. The basic defect is failure of the sinus node to initiate an impulse and may be considered a suppression of the node by overwhelming vagal impulses. An ectopic pacemaker may compensate, but often the entire stimulus production of the heart is adversely affected, and no contraction occurs. Death is obvious unless excitation can be resumed. Sinus arrest is apt to accompany the early stages of anesthesia or certain bodily manipulations that are able to set up a strong vagal reflex. These include instrumentation during such examination of body cavities as cystoscopy, bronchoscopy, or pharyngeal probing and occasionally traction on thoracic organs during surgery. Many hearts so affected are perfectly normal and need only a stimulus such as massage or a sharp blow to the sternum to set them back into rhythmic activity.

• • •

Of special interest to the inhalation therapist, we can briefly summarize three factors related to cardiac arrhythmias. Prolonged deep hypoxia can stimulate the production of ectopic foci of excitation and precipitate conduction block in a myocardium already partially ischemic. Physical manipulation of the body can trigger vagal reflexes that are able to arrest heart action by inhibiting the sinus node. Although such incidents are not common, presumably moving the head or neck of some patients or initiating pharyngeal vagal stimuli by instrumentation are among maneuvers with this potential risk. Finally, high blood levels of carbon dioxide in themselves, or because of the accompanying reduced blood pH, can activate ectopic focal activity. It is also felt that a sudden reduction in a previously elevated carbon dioxide tension can stimulate ventricular arrhythmias.[50,51] These points must be kept in mind in the treatment of patients in ventilatory failure.

CONGENITAL HEART DISEASE

No attempt will be made to classify and describe this large and important group of cardiac abnormalities, for the number of texts and articles in the literature on the subject are so vast that the student can find material to any desired depth of sophistication for his own self-study. A few principles will be discussed that should make further pursuit of the subject more meaningful.

Congenitally deformed hearts are the victims of incomplete or erroneous prenatal development, occasionally the result of maternal disease, but most often are due to some unknown cause. The scope of defects ranges from the very slight, compatible with normal life, to the very severe, incompatible with no more than a few minutes of survival. Most defects are detected during childhood or adolescence, and because many are increasingly benefited by surgery, every attempt is made to establish an accurate diagnosis and prognosis. The inhalation therapist, in a hospital actively engaged in cardiac surgery, will have occasion to see many patients with congenital heart disease, since many of them have associated respiratory problems, and postoperative care often uses inhalation therapy services.

The two broad classifications of congenital disease that concern us here are *acyanotic* (absence of cyanosis) and *cyanotic* congenital defects. The differentiation between the two depends upon whether significant amounts of unsaturated blood mix with arterialized blood to produce cyanosis. Many congenital defects consist of communications between the two sides of the heart through septal defects, or openings in the interatrial and interventricular septa. These are called *intracardiac shunts*, since blood can pass from one side of the heart to the other without following the usual channels. Because the pressure in the left heart is greater than in the right, an uncomplicated septal defect will shunt blood from the left to the right. In other words, variable amounts of left heart blood, depending upon the size of the imperfection, will pass directly into the right heart, mixing arterialized blood with venous. This, of course, does not produce cyanosis. However, the increased load of blood perfusing the lung, some of which is coming back for a second round, increases the pressure in the pulmonary circulation. Physical exercise may further raise the pulmonary pressure temporarily to a level that exceeds the systemic pressure, reversing the pressure gradient across the septum and converting the shunt from a left-to-right to a right-to-left. During this interval, venous blood will mix with arterial and may produce cyanosis. Also, progressive pulmonary hypertension may strain the right ventricle to the point of failure, and an interatrial shunt may be reversed to cause cyanosis. If narrowing of the pulmonary valve or the pulmonary artery is part of the cardiac defect complex, then cyanosis will be present from the early stages in the presence of associated septal openings because of initial pulmonary hypertension. There are conditions that permit cyanosis even in the absence of pulmonary hypertension—e.g., septal defects so large that venous blood mixes with arterial even without a reverse gradient, or an aorta that arises from the right ventricle. Generally speaking, however, the presence or absence of cyanosis in septal cardiac defects depends upon the presence or absence of high pressure in the pulmonary circulation.

Chapter 6

Clinical cardiopulmonary pathology

The purpose of this chapter is to consider some of the disturbances in cardiopulmonary physiology with which the inhalation therapist can be expected to come into frequent contact. The topics to be discussed will not constitute specific disease entities but rather will consist of some of the major physiologic changes that underlie the common respiratory disorders. This might be a good point to mention a basic philosophy of inhalation therapy. Generally speaking inhalation therapy is not directed toward the cure of disease in the sense of removing a specific etiology. A surgeon removes an inflamed appendix and cures the clinical condition of acute appendicitis; a physician administers an antibiotic and cures a disease by destroying the causative organism. In contrast, inhalation therapy is fundamentally supportive or symptomatic in nature. In the former instance, therapy helps to maintain respiratory and cardiac integrity until more etiologically specific treatment can be effective, and in the latter, it attempts to counter the effects of disease and to help restore maximum function. In a broad sense, then, and with some obvious exceptions, the technology of inhalation therapy is concerned not so much with what the disease under treatment is as with what the disease has done to cardiopulmonary physiology. Although it is important that an effective therapist have a practical working knowledge of relevant clinical diseases, it is far more important that he understand the malfunction of respiration brought about by these diseases. With this in mind, we will discuss major features of five pathologic conditions, some or all of which are common to cardiopulmonary disease in general—hypoxia, airway obstruction, pulmonary distention, pulmonary restriction, and ventilation-perfusion imbalance.

HYPOXIA

Hypoxia is a general term that implies an inadequate availability of oxygen for cell function, whereas *hypoxemia* refers to a diminution in the actual content of oxygen in arterial blood.[52-54] Although there is an obvious difference in their meanings, the two are frequently used interchangeably, and as a matter of convenience, the shorter term, hypoxia, will be used in the following text. It will be assumed that the reader can make his own mental differentiation according to usage of the terms. It is even more important that the student clearly understand the difference between two quantitative expressions of blood oxygen content, *arterial oxygen saturation* and *arterial oxygen tension.*

Since a major step in the process of oxygen transport is the union of oxygen with hemoglobin, the degree to which hemoglobin is saturated with oxygen is a valuable indication of the efficiency of the hemoglobin carriage. Thus, hypoxia can be said to exist if the arterial oxygen saturation, breathing room air at 1 atm, is less than 97%. It should be carefully noted, however, that saturation reflects only the relationship between oxygen and hemoglobin. Partial pressure, on the other hand, is a measure of the kinetic activity of the gas, the force permitting it to overcome diffusion barriers and make it available to the body cells. Because both saturation and tension are interrelated and both influenced by the acid-base balance, neither gives us really different information, just different views of the same phenomenon—like inspecting a house from various angles. Although the same structure is seen, one view may show it off to better advantage than another and give the viewer a clearer perspective to judge its features. In our kinetic approach to pulmonary physiology we were concerned with partial pressures of gas in the atmosphere and in the alveoli, and it is logical that we follow through in our evaluation of gas in the blood. Historically, the clinical use of saturation as a measure of blood oxygen content antedates partial pressure, for it is only within relatively recent times that equipment has been available for the rapid and accurate determination of oxygen tension. Generally, then, arterial oxygen partial pressure more readily indicates abnormalities in the oxygen transport route than does hemoglobin saturation.

For example, inspection of the oxygen dissociation curve reveals that approximately identical saturation values around 97% can be found on the pH curves of 7.20, 7.40, and 7.60, at P_{O_2} values of 120, 100, and 80 mm Hg, respectively. Thus, the same saturation can accompany hyperoxic, normal oxygen, and hypoxic gas tensions. Although the saturation implies a normal state, two of the oxygen tensions are significantly abnormal. Also, at the upper end of any pH curve, a slight drop in saturation of 3% or 4%, which might not seem a cause for alarm, can mean a tension drop of 20 mm Hg or more, certainly an indication of a respiratory abnormality. Obviously, for best evaluation, tension, saturation, and pH adjusted for temperature deviation should be determined, but serial oxygen tensions will best reflect the progress or regress of hypoxia and the disease responsible for it.

Classification of hypoxia

There are many classifications of types of hypoxia, but the following includes the principal causative factors.

Reduced alveolar oxygen. This can result from either of the following.

LOW AMBIENT P_{O_2}. Breathing a mixture with a low concentration of oxygen at atmosphere, or oxygen at subatmosphere, provides an inadequate alveolar oxygen tension for normal diffusion into pulmonary blood. A common example of this problem is encountered during travel to high altitudes, where the unaccustomed visitor often suffers ill effects of hypoxia for several days, the so-called "mountain sickness," or hypobarism.

HYPOVENTILATION. Always associated with hypercapnea, hypoventilation reduces the amount of air ventilating the alveoli so that there is not enough oxygen available for normal arterial saturation.

Impaired alveolar-capillary diffusion. Faced with pathologic changes in any of the structures of the A-C membrane, such as fibrosis, granuloma, proliferation of connective tissue, or interstitial edema, fewer oxygen molecules will be able to penetrate the barrier even with normal alveolar gas tension, and the arterial tension will be considerably less than the alveolar. The student may see this condition referred to in the literature as *alveolar-capillary block*, but in current terminology it is more properly called a *diffusion defect*. A pure diffusion defect is relatively uncommon, and because it is often absent in some conditions in which the pathology would seem to make it probable, much is not known about its exact mechanism. The diagnosis of impaired diffusion is basically a laboratory procedure, and further reference will be made to it during the discussion on ventilation-perfusion imbalance.

Anatomic shunts. A shunt is a bypass, or a short circuit, and in a cardiopulmonary sense it consists of a direct communication between the arterial and venous circulations. The result of congenital defects, disease, or trauma, a shunt may consist of a local communication between a peripheral artery and a nearby vein, or a large defect in the septa separating the left and right chambers of the heart. The latter type is the most clinically important; it is common in congenital heart disease and is described in Chapter 5.

Hemoglobin deficiency. This defect may be of two varieties.

ABSOLUTE. Anemia, with a quantitative lack of circulating hemoglobin, can seriously impair the oxygen-carrying capacity of the blood, even in the presence of normal supply and adequate diffusion.

RELATIVE. For adequate oxygenation, not only must there be enough hemoglobin, but it must be capable of transporting oxygen because abnormal hemoglobin can produce clinically significant hypoxia. For example, carbon monoxide in a breathing mixture will combine with hemoglobin much faster than will the oxygen present, and it forms carboxyhemoglobin, which is incapable of carrying oxygen. It is this mechanism that makes carbon monoxide such a lethal agent. Another abnormal form of hemoglobin is methemoglobin, an oxidized (not oxygenated) form in which the iron is in the ferric instead of the normal ferrous state. The result of hereditary defects or the ingestion of certain drugs in toxic doses, methemoglobin, like carboxyhemoglobin, is unable to transport oxygen and is an important cause of hypoxia.

Circulatory failure. Should the systemic circulation lose its thrust, there will be reduced tissue cell perfusion with resulting hypoxia. This may also be of two types.

GENERALIZED. In the presence of generalized circulatory failure, as in shock or with a failing heart, oxygen deprivation will be widespread.

LOCAL. Venous or arterial obstruction can interfere with local circulation, causing tissue hypoxia of the affected area.

Histotoxins. Chemical substances that interfere with the enzyme systems of body cells responsible for oxygen utilization can produce lethal cellular hypoxia, in the presence of adequate oxygen supply. Cyanide poisoning is one of the best known clinical examples of this category.

Ventilation/Perfusion ratio imbalance. Because of the clinical importance of this cause of hypoxia, its principles and the consequences of its disturbance will be discussed in considerable detail later in this chapter, under its own heading.

Acute hypoxia

Acute hypoxia is caused by a rapid reduction of available oxygen as from asphyxia, airway obstruction, blockage of alveoli by the fluid of edema or infectious exudate, abrupt cardiorespiratory failure, and acute hemorrhage. Some patients, depending upon the cause, may exhibit hypoventilation, and others hyperventilation to the point of "air hunger," a seemingly insatiable attempt to breath more and more air. In the latter, hyperpnea is usually present, and the increased ventilatory volume blows off excess carbon dioxide, dropping the blood level significantly and elevating blood pH. Arterial oxygen tensions and saturation are both low. If the degree of hypoxia is less than critical, the mental state it produces has been likened to that of alcoholic intoxication.[55] Headache is a frequent complaint, and there is often mental confusion. However, in the early stages of oxygen deprivation, mental stimulation may be strikingly evident, the subject reacting in a euphoric and sometimes hilarious manner. This is followed by a state of depression and drowsiness. Muscle weakness ensues, accompanied by lack of coordination, and as the hypoxia progresses, there is serious loss of discrimination and judgment.[56] With a more sudden hypoxia, there may be an acute abrupt loss of consciousness; this is not common except in those instances when the subject finds himself suddenly in an airless environment, such as a gas-filled compartment.

The most critical target organ of hypoxia is the central nervous system, and, with a few exceptions, survival of acute hypoxia is dependent upon its effect on the brain. One of the early responses of the brain is vasodilatation and an increased cerebral blood flow. However, because nerve tissue is so vulnerable to oxygen lack, a few minutes of severe hypoxia may produce irreversible damage to brain cells, and prolongation of lesser degrees can lead to death or permanent damage. Comas of days' or weeks' duration are not uncommon; and the half-living vegetative existence of the not-quite-dead brain may be the most tragic consequence of hypoxia.

Other organs are affected by hypoxia. Although the healthy heart can tolerate hypoxia to a considerable degree, one slightly compromised by disease may suffer seriously. This is especially evident in the patient with subclinical cardiac disorders (not quite to the symptom-producing stage), such as early or mild coronary artery narrowing or early heart failure. Functioning with a minimum reserve, such hearts, when perfused with hypoxic blood, will be adversely effected. Myocardial fibers, with a high oxygen demand, may weaken or die, or the cardiac rhythm may be seriously disturbed. Patients with known or suspected heart disease, especially those in the middle and older age groups, must be watched very closely, from the cardiac point of view; electrocardiographic changes are frequent indications of impending or actual myocardial hypoxia. Kidney cells also require constant and adequate oxygenation, and hypoxia can precipitate renal failure, interfering with the ability of the kidney to maintain normal electrolyte and water balance and to eliminate waste products efficiently. Finally, the carbon dioxide transport mechanism is less effective with hypoxia, since oxyhemoglobin is needed to displace carbon dioxide in the lung.

The depth of hypoxia that the body can tolerate and still survive is a matter of considerable interest. There are so many obvious modifying variables, such as the state of the circulation (especially the cerebral), the general body cellular health, the total metabolism, and the intensity of therapy, that there is no clear-cut lower limit of oxygenation. A guiding rule of thumb for some time has held that an arterial P_{O_2} below 20 mm Hg is probably incompatible with life;[57] yet values as low as 9 mm Hg followed by recovery are known.[58] It is most likely that the modern therapy of respiratory failure has reduced the hypoxic threshold of viability.

Special mention will be made of a common sign of hypoxia, *cyanosis*, present in both acute and chronic hypoxia although not invariably in either. Cyanosis is a blue or gray-blue color imparted to skin, mucous membranes, and nail beds in the presence of hypoxia. Evaluation of the degree of cyanosis, or even its presence, depends upon the perception of the examiner, modified by such factors as the ambient lighting, the color of the environment, and especially the skin color of the subject. In dark-skinned patients cyanosis may be detected only in nail beds or mucous membranes. Thus, although failure to see cyanosis does not rule out hypoxia, its presence is a strong positive sign of hypoxia.

Cyanosis is related to the degree of oxygen *unsaturation* of *capillary* blood perfusing body surfaces, and generally it requires the presence of about *5 gm%* of unsaturated hemoglobin to be detected. Obviously, the greater the concentration of unsaturated hemoglobin, the deeper will be the cyanosis, since it is the reduced hemoglobin that gives to blood its bluish red "venous" appearance. Normally, capillary blood contains about *2.5 gm of reduced hemoglobin per 100 ml of blood,* a value derived as follows: Since capillary blood represents blood continuously giving up oxygen as it passes from the arterial to the venous end of the capillary, its unsaturated Hb content may be considered the *average* of the unsaturation of the arterial blood entering the capillary and the venous blood leaving. At a normal O_2 saturation of 97%, 15 gm% of arterial Hb have 3% unsaturated Hb, or 0.45 gm%. Venous blood 70% saturated has 30% unsaturated Hb, or 4.5 gm%. The average capillary unsaturation would thus equal:

$$\frac{0.45 + 4.5}{2} = 2.5\% \text{ of unsaturated hemoglobin}$$[59]

Assuming a hemoglobin concentration of 15 gm% and an a-v oxygen saturation difference of 24% (corresponding to an a-v oxygen content difference of 5 vol%, as described earlier), we can calculate that an arterial oxygen saturation of 79% will produce a mean capillary unsaturation of 5 gm% (Appendix 11). Hypoxia below this level, which the oxygen dissociation curve shows to be the equivalent of about 45 mm Hg partial pressure of oxygen, will probably produce visible cyanosis. However, since cyanosis depends upon a specific concentration of unsaturated capillary hemoglobin, in anemia, with its reduced quantity of available hemoglobin, there may not be enough unsaturated hemoglobin to produce cyanosis until the arterial saturation drops well below 80%. Conversely, polycythemia, with its increased supply of hemoglobin, may show cyanosis even though there is adequate circulating oxygen.

Chronic hypoxia

If the onset of hypoxia is slowly progressive, the body may adjust to it without any acute reactions. Diseases most apt to cause chronic hypoxia include gradually destructive or fibrotic lung diseases, congenital or acquired heart diseases, and chronic blood loss. In general, a persistent state of chronic hypoxia simulates a condition of persistent mental and physical fatigue. Mental responses may become sluggish and acuity diminished, and patients frequently complain of inability to perform physical tasks with the same ease as formerly. As a rule, however, chronic hypoxia itself is not a common cause of disability; rather it is the underlying diseases responsible for the hypoxia. Often, relief of the hypoxia only, with oxygen breathing, will have little effect on disability. In many of the patients with whom the inhalation therapist will have contact it is the physical effort to maintain normal oxygen and carbon dioxide levels that is the real cause of disability. Just as in acute hypoxia, if the oxygen lack is severe enough chronically, cyanosis will be present.

People who are born at high altitudes and who continue to live for several years at those altitudes must physiologically adjust from the prenatal period to an environment with a lower oxygen tension than that which exists at sea level. Inhabitants of mountainous areas, especially those of the South American Andes and our own Rocky Mountains, have been extensively studied over many years, up to and including the present, to determine how the body adjusts to hypobaric conditions. Many people live normal and active lives at partial pressures of oxygen in the same range as that found in patients at atmosphere who are suffering from hypoxia due to disease. It is obvious that altitude residents must be endowed with some type of adaptation to their "hypoxic" environment; and although many of the details of their physiologic responses, cardiac as well as pulmonary, are still under investigation, a few pertinent facts have been established. These people have a larger "red cell mass" than do natives of lowlands. This means that the total mass (or volume) of all their circulating erythrocytes is greater than that of the average human population, generally accomplished by an increased number of such cells. In addition, altitude dwellers have significantly larger lung volumes. In a general way, it may be safe to assume that mountain life has certain rigors not found at sea level, if for no other reason than the nature of the terrain itself and the fact that the economy of such areas has often been agrarian. The survival of generations in such an environment attests to the efficiency of natural adaptation. Indeed, extensive studies have failed to show any ill effects in the indigenous populations, as long as they remain at altitude. Apparently, however, if high-altitude dwellers leave their original environment for the lowlands for a certain period of time, they often lose their natural adaptation; and a return to low ambient oxygen tensions puts them at the same disadvantage as is experienced by any other transient from sea level. For the individual with a normal cardiorespiratory system, a period of several days may be required to acclimatize to the reduced oxygen partial pressure, during which time he may experience weakness and lassitude, headaches, and a marked impairment of his usual physical performance.

In a sense, the pulmonary hypoxic patient, with his low arterial oxygen tension, is in a situation much like that of the altitude dweller or visitor, with the important difference that he has a defective respiratory mechanism. Nevertheless, chronic hypoxia is accompanied by an attempt on the part of the body to accommodate to the limited amount of oxygen that is able to reach the arterial blood. Hypoxia stimulates the bone marrow to increase its production of erythrocytes (an action called *hematopoiesis*) so that, as in the altitude dweller, there is an increase in the number of circulating red cells or, more specifically, an increase in the red cell mass. This state is referred to as *secondary polycythemia,* meaning a more than normal number of red cells secondary to the underlying pulmonary disease. As may be expected, there is also a condition called primary polycythemia, or polycythemia vera, entirely unrelated to cardiopulmonary dysfunction. In secondary polycythemia there is no increase in the other cellular blood components. The presence of polycythemia is always suspected in a chronically hypoxic patient, but its actual identification may not be apparent. In many patients it may be readily detected by examination of the blood and by noting an increase in the *hematocrit,* which is the ratio between the volume of cells (mostly red cells, of course) and plasma, in a centrifuged sample of blood that has been treated with an anticoagulant.

Normally, this does not exceed about 45%, but in polycythemia it may be nearly double. The hemoglobin content is similarly elevated from its usual upper limit of 15 gm% to perhaps 20 gm%, and measurement of the circulating erythrocytes will often show an excess above the normal high of around 5 million per cubic millimeter of blood.

It has been demonstrated, however, that such simple measures do not always reflect the hypoxic hematopoiesis responsible for polycythemia.[60] There is usually an associated increase in plasma volume; and if this if of sufficient degree, those measurements that relate red cell numbers or hemoglobin content to blood volume may appear erroneously normal. The most definitive diagnostic technique is an actual measurement of circulating red cell mass, using procedures that employ the dilution of dye by the blood, or the "tagging" of red cells by radioactive substances, which permits evaluation of both the total circulating blood volume and the erythrocyte mass. It is felt that polycythemia is common in patients with chronic lung disease and, if such tests are performed, many who would not otherwise be detected will be revealed.

Enough patients show elevated hematocrits and hemoglobin contents to warrant a few remarks about the clinical significance of such findings. With a sufficient increase in the ratio of red cells to blood fluid, viscosity of the blood can be expected to rise, constituting a matter of concern in the management of this condition.[61] At least in principle, the retarding effect upon blood velocity and ease of flow of increasing viscosity may outweigh the advantages of the additional oxygen-carrying capacity of the enlarged red cell mass, and cellular distribution of oxygen may be impaired by a slowing of or interference with perfusion of body cells. It has been suggested that viscosity is not physiologically significant until the hematrocrit reaches 55% to 60%.[62] Still, there is justified fear that the sluggish circulation of polycythemia may cause intravascular thromboses, especially in vessels that may already be damaged by sclerosis or narrowing from other causes, because slowly moving blood clots more readily than does swiftly moving blood.

The patient with overt polycythemia is usually cyanotic, despite an actual increase in the volume of oxygen carried by the blood. This is because the cyanosis depends upon the amount of circulating unsaturated hemoglobin, not saturated, and the patient with a greater than normal number of red cells can have a corresponding increase in the amount of hemoglobin that is unsaturated as well as saturated. There are often complaints of headache, fullness in the head, nasal stuffiness, lethargy, difficulty in taking a deep breath, and epistaxis (nosebleed). The small vessels of the sclera (the white of the eye) may be seen as grossly congested from an increased blood volume. Finally, the increased volume of circulating blood, especially if associated with significant viscosity, places an abnormal work load on the heart to overcome the resistance to flow. The less muscular right ventricle is especially affected; it becomes strained, enlarges in an attempt to sustain its increased load, and eventually fails. This produces the so-called *cor pulmonale,* or "pulmonary heart," right-sided heart disease secondary to pulmonary disease

The inhalation therapist will commonly encounter a physical sign in his patients called *clubbing.* Although this condition is not exclusively associated with hypoxia, because of its frequency in this state, it is felt to be pertinent to the discussion here. Clubbing is one state of a more generalized process that affects bones and joints known as hypertrophic osteoarthropathy.[64,65] The essential lesion of osteoarthropathy is a chronic inflammatory process with thickening of periosteum, especially of the long bones, accompanied by the deposition of new bone. By x-ray examination the bones are seen to be thickened, giving rise to the term *hypertrophic.* Joints may also be affected with swelling and inflammation. In a well-developed case, many bones and joints may be affected with pain and disabling limitation of motion. Since the changes in the joints and long bones may frequently be detected by x-ray examination only and since lesser degrees are more frequently encountered in patients seen by the inhalation therapist, we will describe in greater detail that aspect of the process known as clubbing.

Clubbing may occur as an early stage of hypertrophic osteoarthropathy, or it may be found without subsequent long bone changes. It is manifested by a bulbous swelling of the terminal phalanges of the fingers and toes, which become enlarged and rounded, often but not always cyanotic. There is an increase in all diameters of the tips of the extremities, giving them a "drumstick" appearance. In contrast to the process found in long bones, pain is not usually a symptom of clubbing, although the soft tissue swelling at the ends of the digits may be considerable. A characteristic feature of clubbing is the contour of the nail, which becomes rounded both longitudinally and transversely. Curvature of the nail is not in itself necessarily a sign of disease and often is only a variation of the normal. In clubbing, however, the distortion of the nail is accompanied by a loss of the cuticular angle, the angle at the junction of the skin and nail as viewed from the side of the finger. This is shown in Fig. 6-1, illustrating a normal flat nail, a normal curved nail, and early and late clubbing. The marked cuticular angle in both normal nails is evident but is

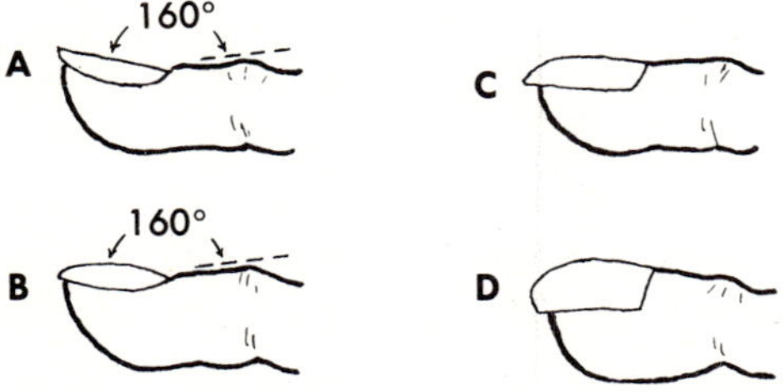

Fig. 6-1. Clubbing is characterized by marked curvature of the nail, a loss of the cuticular angle, an increase in the angle the surface of the nail makes with the terminal phalanx above the normal of 160 degrees, and a bulbous soft tissue swelling of the terminal phalanx. Sketches **A** and **B** show the contours of normal straight and curved nails; **C** and **D** represent increasing degrees of clubbing.

absent in clubbing. As the clubbing progresses from mild to severe, the degrees of curvature gradually increase. The first indication of imminent clubbing, before significant rounding is evident, is loss of the cuticular angle, associated with a "floating" nail base. This latter is characterized by a sponginess palpated under the base of the nail which allows the nail to be moved up and down with compression.

Despite the frequency with which clubbing is seen, the specific etiology of clubbing, or the full osteoarthropathy, is not known. It has been speculated that some or many of the following are responsible: chronic infection, unspecified toxins, capillary stasis from increased venous back pressure, arterial hypoxia, and local hypoxia. There is some disturbance in the circulation of the terminal portions of the digits, manifested by an increased blood flow. This has been demonstrated, through microphotography of a nail bed, as an increase in the width of the capillaries.[66] Nonetheless, this sign is an extremely important clinical one, even though it does not always indicate hypoxia, or even pulmonary disease. In adults approximately 75% to 85% of clubbing is due to pulmonary disease (lung tumors, bronchiectasis, fibrosis, empyema); 10% to 15% to cardiac disease (congenital right-to-left shunt, subacute bacterial endocarditis); 10% to liver or gastrointestinal disease (cirrhosis, chronic diarrhea conditions); 5% to miscellaneous causes (heredity, tumors of the thyroid or pharynx, aneurysms of large branches of the aorta). In children, clubbing is predominantly found in cystic fibrosis, bronchiectasis, empyema, and congenital heart disease.[67] In summary, it can be said that clubbing suggests disease, first, of the respiratory tract, second, of the heart, and third, of the liver or gastrointestinal tract. It is of interest to note that the appearance of clubbing may antedate the x-ray signs of carcinoma of the lung by as many as 48 months. Finally, in many instances successful treatment of the underlying disease results in the resolution of the clubbing and a return of the digits to normal.

Treatment of hypoxia

The obvious need in hypoxia is oxygen to preserve the life of body cells, but the details of its administration will be dealt with elsewhere. It should be emphasized, however, that the objective of therapy is to restore arterial oxygen tension to normal, not to overload the blood with high pressures, except in very specific and limited circumstances. While hypoxia is being relieved, every effort must be made to correct the underlying pathology responsible for the hypoxia, for only when the latter is accomplished, can we feel that the patient is improved. The therapist will see many patients in whom disease has left permanent lung damage of such a degree that sustained normal oxygenation is impossible to achieve, and the management of such patients will strain the ingenuity of physician and therapist alike. Again, to emphasize a point that cannot be overstressed, when hypoxia is associated with hypercapnia in the presence of an unresponsive respiratory center and the chemoreceptor hypoxic drive is active, ventilation must be supported mechanically during the administration of oxygen to prevent fatal apnea.

Where polycythemia is clinically significant, *phlebotomy* is often a useful procedure. Literally meaning "opening of a vein," phlebotomy entails the venous withdrawal of blood, in increments of about 300 ml, at intervals of 3 to 4 days. The objective of therapy is to lower the hematocrit to a maximum of about 50%, removing a segment of the red cell mass. Since blood water is restored by a shifting of the body fluids, the result is a reduction of blood viscosity. Some feel that the beneficial effects of phlebotomy are attributed to relief of the enlarged blood volume, not just to lowered viscosity. The clinical results are often very rewarding, as patients feel better both physically and mentally and the progress of cor pulmonale is retarded.[62] During an acute hospitalization, a patient may have several phlebotomies and then return as an outpatient for follow-up treatment as needed, usually with gradually decreasing frequency.

AIRWAY OBSTRUCTION

Obstruction of the airways is one of the most common causes of cardiopulmonary disability and is almost always an important factor in the disease of patients treated by the inhalation therapist except for those with nonpulmonary ventilatory problems. Obstruction may be transient and reversible, or it may be permanent. We considered the effects of airway resistance on the mechanics of ventilation earlier and will now concern ourselves with a description of the physiologic and pathologic changes brought about by obstruction. For our purposes, we will not include gross obstruction, as from an inhaled foreign body or a large tumor, but rather will classify the causes of obstruction as *mucosal edema, bronchial spasm, increased secretions,* and *bronchiolar collapse.*

Mucosal edema

Edema is an increase in the amount of interstitial fluid that bathes the body cells; pathologic changes cause a shift of body water from the plasma to the intercellular spaces, with resulting swelling of the affected area, which may be localized or extensive over larger areas of the body. The most common example of edema of the respiratory tract is the nasal swelling and inflammation (rhinitis) of the common cold, with the accompanying obstruction to breathing. This same reaction can be visualized in the lower portions of the respiratory passages. Severe edema of the larynx is well known as *croup,* and the same relative degree of airway narrowing can occur in the small bronchi and bronchioles.

Mucosal edema can be caused by:

(1) Mechanical irritation or trauma to the respiratory mucosa, as from instrumentation, the presence of a foreign body, or the inhalation of caustic liquids or irritant fumes

(2) Infection, bacterial or viral, in which the reaction represents a body defense against the invading organisms

(3) Allergy to inhaled liquids or particulate matter, exemplified by the common allergic bronchial asthma

Respiratory mucosa becomes boggy in acute edema, soft, spongy, and waterlogged. There is usually an accompanying arteriolar and capillary congestion, which adds to the swelling. If of short duration, acute edema may be easily reversible following removal of its cause. However, if the edema is long lasting or frequently recurring, it may become *indurated*, giving to the tissue a permanent thickening and a firm, rather than soft, consistency. Such changes markedly interfere with mucosal function, especially through destruction of cilia, and the removal of the normal mucus blanket. Chronic respiratory infection aids in the perpetuation of such induration.

Bronchial spasm

Spasm may be defined as an involuntary excessive contraction of a muscle. Common examples are found in extremity muscle cramps, spasm of neck muscles following injury, and intestinal cramps. Bronchial spasm is produced by excessive and prolonged contraction of the involuntary muscle fibers in the walls of the bronchi and bronchioles. Such contraction can seriously reduce airway lumens and may be localized or general. The causes of bronchial spasm are the same as those of edema listed above, but especially bronchial asthma, of which spasm is the major physiologic derangement.

Increased secretions

By *increased bronchial secretions* we mean an actual increase in volume of secretions produced, an increase in their viscosity, or both. Although such reactions may follow exposure of the respiratory mucosa to many irritants, infection is the most frequent offender, and the common cold is again a familiar example with its abundance of sputum.

Bronchial secretions are composed of many ingredients[68]: *mucus*, secreted by the goblet cells and mucous glands of the bronchial mucosa; *DNA* (deoxyribonucleic acid, as a protein salt) and *RNA* (ribonucleic acid, as a protein salt), released from nuclei and cytoplasm of disintegrating cells; *plasma fluid* and *proteins*, including fibrinogen, escaping from pulmonary capillaries. The differentiation between normal and pathologic secretions depends upon the relative concentrations of their components.

For purposes of discussion we can make a distinction between two broad types of sputum—mucoid and purulent. *Mucoid* secretions may be considered as a response by the airways to foreign matter invasion, infective or noninfective, in an attempt to remove the offending agent. One of the characteristics of a well-established chronic bronchitis is an actual increase in the number of mucous glands in the bronchial walls. The secretions so produced will consist of a high concentration of mucus, in respect to the other constituents. Mucus contains mucoproteins, a combination of any of several proteins with substances known as mucopolysaccharides, and long-chain carbohydrate-containing compounds, and it is these mucoproteins that are responsible for the viscosity of the secretions. Thus, when stimulated to overproduction of sputum by some irritative or pathologic process, the airways will contain larger amounts of fluid of a greater than normal viscosity. It should be added, because it is so important, that viscosity of normal secretions (normal relative concentrations of its components) can be raised to dangerous degrees simply by dehydration. This will be considered again later with the subject of humidification. *Purulent* secretions, on the other hand, are the result of invasion of the respiratory tract by pathogenic bacteria and the effect of such infection on the sputum. The natural inflammatory response to bacterial infection brings many leukocytes to the area, and they engage the organisms in destructive battle. The mucoid secretions, which are the first response, become grossly infiltrated with intact and fragmented bacteria, leukocytes, and tissue cells damaged by the process. Disruption of the cytoplasm and nuclei of the cells releases into the secretions a large amount of nucleoproteins, the DNA and RNA noted above. It is principally the deoxyribonucleic acid protein that gives to the secretions their purulent characteristics of viscosity to the point of tenacious stringiness and a yellow to green discoloration, in contrast to the colorless, clear or frothy, mucoid type. If the bronchial inflammation is acute, the sputum may have streaks of dark red or brown from extravasated blood. Finally, depending upon the offending bacteria or the presence of secondary or mixed infection, putrefactive organisms will often distinguish purulent sputum with a disagreeable odor.

The usually effective mucus blanket with its escalator cleansing action becomes less effective as its viscosity and volume increase, and these factors interfere with ciliary action. Often much of the cilia is destroyed, removing a valuable protective mechanism from the respiratory tract. As viscosity increases, the ordinary cough mechanism is less able to remove the secretions, and these plug airways, seriously interfering with ventilation. Parts of the lung may become airless, a condition referred to as *atelectasis,* with potentially grave consequences.

Bronchiolar collapse

Usually associated with advanced bronchopulmonary disease, bronchiolar collapse is a clinically important form of small airway obstruction that, in many patients, becomes the most critical factor in ventilatory disability. The mechanism of its action is based upon two components. First, there must be damage to the integrity of the bronchiolar walls so that they are unable to maintain patency in the face of the second factor, a pressure gradient across the bronchiolar walls. The conditions predisposing to bronchiolar collapse are most frequently found in the destructive lung diseases such as emphy-

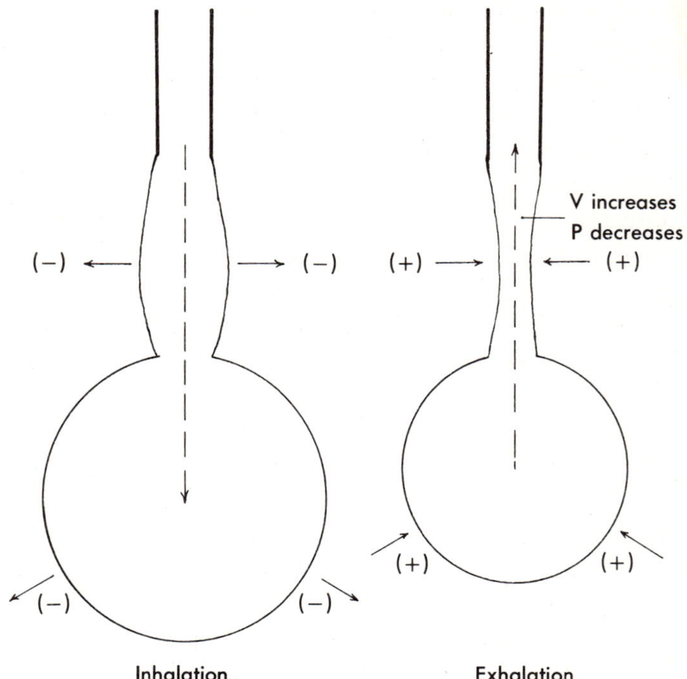

Fig. 6-2. A disease-weakened bronchiole is shown as thin walled and flaccid. Negative intrathoracic pressure inflates the alveolus with little difficulty. During exhalation, however, rising intrathoracic pressure compresses the diseased bronchiole as well as the alveolus, impeding airflow. In addition, the velocity of air through the bronchiolar restriction reduces intralumenal pressure, encouraging further collapse and worsening the obstruction.

sema, bronchiectasis, and cystic disease; and, by far, emphysema is the predominant influence.

The bronchioles, devoid of cartilaginous support, are essentially highly pliable soft-walled tubes that depend for their patency upon surrounding structures. Encompassed by masses of alveoli whose septa are arranged in a radial fashion apparently attached to their walls, the lumens of the bronchioles are kept from collapsing by the weblike support of these air sacs. During normal exhalation the rising intrathoracic pressure is exerted upon the bronchiolar walls, as on all other thoracic structures, and does slightly narrow them; but the intact surrounding alveoli prevent further collapse. Fig. 6-2 illustrates diagrammatically what happens in the presence of bronchopulmonary disease. With destruction of alveoli and the loss of their supportive septa, the bronchiolar walls are responsive to pressure changes between the intrabronchiolar lumens and the pleural space. During inhalation the increasingly negative intrathoracic pressure and the inflow of air are sufficient to dilate the bronchioles to full patency. During exhalation, however, the rising thoracic pressure, unopposed by alveolar septal countertraction, compresses the resilient bronchioles and narrows them to the point of interference with airflow. At the same time, as the exhaled air is being forced through the narrowing bronchioles, its velocity progressively increases. In keeping with the Bernoulli principle, with the increase in intralumenal velocity, there is a drop in intralumenal pressure and the negative pressure gradient thus established across the bronchiole wall between the lumen and pleural space favors further narrowing. A vicious cycle is thereby set in motion which perpetuates the continuing airway collapse.[69]

The patients in whom this condition is clinically significant are usually those who already have expiratory difficulty from their underlying disease and must exert exceptionally great effort during exhalation. It is thus evident to what degree the element of bronchiolar collapse can contribute to a steadily worsening disability. In addition to its chronic influence on exhalation, bronchiolar collapse can produce an acute state referred to as *acute air trapping.* Frequently, without warning, a patient may suddenly find he is unable to complete a phase of exhalation he has already started. His chest is immobilized in a position of partial exhalation and he is unable either to inhale or to further empty his lungs. He may struggle to move his chest and become severely cyanotic, especially in the face and neck. Such an episode may be triggered by an unnoticed early expiratory effort of greater force than usual; and as the sequence of events described above comes into play after the movement of part of his exhaled air, a number of his bronchioles completely collapse, trapping the remainder of his tidal volume. Although frightening to the point of panic, to the patient and observers alike, these attacks are usually self-limiting. A series of sharp forceful lateral squeezes applied to both sides of the thorax will often supply spurts of air of sufficient pressure to overcome the collapse and empty the lungs. This is a technique learned by many patients and especially by members of their families. To prevent acute trapping and to accomplish the maximum exhalation with the minimum of effort, patients either learn spontaneously or are taught the technique of "pursed-lip breathing." In the maneuver, the patient slightly purses his lips as he exhales, deliberately prolonging exhalation and trying to maintain an even flow of air. The moderate obstruction he effects at the mouth builds up a back pressure in his airways, not enough to make exhalation difficult but enough to retard air velocity and reduce the transbronchiolar pressure gradient to prevent collapse.

Effect of obstruction on ventilation

Obstruction markedly increases the work of breathing because of the elevated resistance of smaller air passages and the retarding effect of air turbulence. Resistance to breathing may be more pronounced in one phase or the other of ventilation. For example, the laryngeal obstruction of childhood croup may necessitate such a strong inspiratory effort that there will be noticeable retraction of the sternum and epigastrium during inspiration, and the flow of air past the obstruction may produce a harsh sound known as a *stridor.* Most often, however, obstruction is a major problem in chronic bronchopulmonary diseases, and then exhalation is impeded. To a considerable degree, the ventilatory muscles can overcome obstruction to inhalation, but the passive nature of normal exhalation is unable to deflate the lung to its resting position and exhalation must employ muscular effort, at times very strenuous. The tremendous work involved in moving air against obstruction utilizes so much physical energy that it constitutes one of the major factors in the disability of chronic pulmonary diseases. Indeed, muscular fatigue may lead to ventilatory failure, hypercapnia, and respiratory acidosis.

Expiration time is usually prolonged beyond that of inhalation, and often contraction of the upper abdomen is evident during the latter part of exhalation. If bronchospasm is extensive or mobile secretions are present, characteristic breath sounds can be heard by the unaided ear or by the use of the stethoscope (auscultation) during exhalation. *Wheezes* are high-pitched squeaky noises produced by air passing with some velocity through passages narrowed by spasm or thick secretions. *Rhonchi* are coarser, lower-pitched sounds caused by vibration of bronchial secretions in the airflow. *Rales* are fine bubbling or crackling sounds, usually noted during inhalation as air passes through fluid in the alveoli, and are not necessarily reflections of obstruction.

Treatment of obstruction

Details of treatment will be considered elsewhere, but the general procedures will include the following.

Aspiration. This is the removal of secretions through the use of suctioning. It may be accomplished by means of *bronchoscopy,* the passage of a long, lighted tube, under direct vision, into the lobar bronchi, allowing examination of these structures as well as extensive aspiration. Frequently employed is the insertion of a catheter into the main-stem bronchi in patients in whom a *tracheostomy* tube has been placed just below the larynx, or in whom an *endotracheal* tube has been passed through the mouth and larynx into the upper trachea. Small catheters, passed through hollow needles inserted between the tracheal rings just below the larynx, are occasionally used for aspiration of thin secretions.

Aerosols. The inhalation of very fine particles of liquids, in the form of a mist, is extensively used and includes the following:

(a) Water—to thin secretions by increasing their water content
(b) Bronchodilators—agents that reduce bronchial spasm
(c) Decongestants—agents that reduce vascular congestion
(d) Liquefacients—agents that liquify secretions by altering their physical or chemical characteristics

Systemic liquefacients. Some medications, taken by mouth or vein, make bronchial secretions more liquid and easier to raise.

Postural drainage. Physical therapeutic techniques that utilize gravity in mobilizing secretions, by positioning the patient, are an important part of both short-term and long-term therapy.

PULMONARY DISTENTION

Pulmonary distention is a state of hyperinflation of the lung characterized by an increase in the functional residual capacity (FRC), and its two major causes are *airway obstruction* and *loss of lung elasticity.* As a rule, distention due to obstructed airways is generally of a temporary and reversible nature, exemplified by an attack of acute bronchial asthma. In this condition, diffuse bronchial spasm is the outstanding feature, and during such an episode the FRC may be markedly increased. On subsidence and in the absence of complications (especially bronchial infection), the resting thoracic level returns to normal and the FRC is reduced. It is also probable that some distention may accompany acute episodes of obstructive bronchitis, but this is apt to be variable and evanescent.

From a practical, inhalation therapy point of view, *pulmonary distention* usually refers to the hyperinflation of pulmonary emphysema. Although we have not considered the clinical and pathologic nature of this disease in a specific discussion, we have mentioned it so many times that the student may already be forming a mental picture of its characteristics. There are many excellent descriptions of emphysema (often called obstructive emphysema, bronchitis-emphysema, and chronic obstructive lung disease, among its many names) in any number of texts, and the student is encouraged to familiarize himself well with it, for it will probably be the most prevalent disease he will encounter. We will note only a few of its details here, as they pertain to distention. Basically, emphysema is a destructive disease characterized by disruption of variable numbers of alveolar walls; the more disruption, the more severe is the disease. This destructive process converts the lung from an organ with a large number of uniform-sized air spaces into one with a smaller number of variable-sized spaces and fewer gas diffusion surfaces. A consequence of the resulting architectural change in the lung is a marked uneveness of airflow and air distribution and, most serious, a great loss of elastic fibers.

Until fairly recently, it was generally felt that destructive distention was a sequella of progressive or persistent airway obstruction. It was postulated that because of any of the common causes of bronchial and bronchiolar obstruction, the resistance to expiratory airflow developed an intra-alveolar back pressure that eventually destroyed the alveolar walls. Somewhat oversimplified, it was like the rupture of a hyperinflated balloon. The continued expiratory resistance was then supposed to have trapped air in the enlarged air sacs. However, studies on normal individuals whose lungs are subjected to very high intrapulmonary pressures from back pressure for long periods of time (e.g., wind instrument musicians) have failed to show any adverse effects upon lung function and no signs of distention.[70] Refined pathologic techniques that permit better correlation between pathology and function have demonstrated that in many if not most instances the distention precedes and causes the airway obstruction so frequently seen with it. It is speculated that some factors not yet clearly defined (sometimes infectious?) destroy the alveolar walls, with loss of diffusing surface and elasticity. Bronchiolar collapse, described above, causes obstruction, which is worsened by an ensuing chronic bronchitis subsequent to failure of cough-clearance of the airways.[69,71] By this mechanism, following alveolar disruption, the actual pulmonary distention is the result of loss of elasticity, rather than of obstruction, since the thoracic expansile forces are now relatively unopposed.

Less well defined as a pathologic entity is the degenerative change that accompanies the aging process and that diminishes the tone of elastic tissue throughout the body. The loss of skin elasticity in the elderly is a common observation, and apparently a similar phenomenon takes place in the lung. The increase in FRC often seen with advancing age is sometimes unwisely referred to as *senile emphysema*, although there is no concrete evidence that this constitutes a true disease.

Effect of distention on ventilation

The adverse effects of distention upon ventilation can be described in the following three categories: reduced inspiratory capacity, low position of the diaphragm, and enlarged FRC.

Reduced inspiratory capacity. The elevated end-expiratory resting level of the thorax and the low, flat diaphragm (to be described next) produce the inspiratory position of the thorax. Thus, at the resting level, the lungs are already in a position of partial inspiration, since the lung-thorax relationship is unbalanced in the direction of the thoracic forces. The inspiratory capacity is encroached upon, and increase in tidal volume in response to exertional needs is limited (Fig. 3-20).

Low position of diaphragm. Increase in the FRC forces the chest into the inspiratory position as the lung-thorax resting level rises, and the overdistention of the lung depresses and flattens the contour of the diaphragmatic domes. In a low position, contraction of the diaphragm, even though feeble, instead of lowering itself, pulls in the costal margin and reduces the volume of the thorax during inhalation, rather than enlarging it. With loss of effective use of the diaphragm, reduction in intrathoracic pressure is dependent upon contraction of the intercostals and the accessory ventilatory muscles. The pull of the accessory muscles causes an upward and outward displacement of the sternum, an increase in the sternal angle (the junction of the manubrium and body of the sternum, at the level of the second rib), and eventually an increase in the anteroposterior diameter of the chest. This produces the *barrel-chest* deformity common to long-standing distention. The thoracic negative pressure, generated at a tremendous energy cost to the patient, also acts upon the ineffective diaphragm, pulling it *upward* during inhalation, the so-called "paradoxical ventilation." Thus, while the intercostals and accessories are working hard to enlarge the thorax, the rising diaphragm, sucked upward by their action, partially negates their efforts, and the net gain in intrathoracic volume is small in proportion to the physical effort expended. When inspiratory efforts are strenuous enough, not only is the diaphragm elevated during inhalation, but the abdominal wall is also retracted in a contrary manner. Exhalation, lacking the effective use of the abdominals, is a slow process, depending upon inadequate passive recoil and expiratory action of the intercostals; and during exhalation, rising intrathoracic pressure drives down the diaphragm as the abdominal wall balloons outward. The clinical picture is one of a short, gasping inhalation, with extensive use of accessory muscles of ventilation and epigastric retraction, followed by a prolonged exhalation accompanied by varying degrees of epigastric protrusion. The presence of a barrel-chest defect, with or without paradoxical ventilation, signifies serious disruption of the normal lung-thoracic architecture, and the attentive therapist should always be on the watch for it.

Large functional residual capacity. The physiologic significance of an enlarged FRC can be appreciated only if the part it plays in ventilation is visualized clearly. Since the FRC is a substantial volume of air remaining in the lung at the end of a quiet exhalation, the next tidal volume of inhaled air must mix with it in order to reach the alveoli. In other words, air that is ventilating the alveoli with each breath is a mixture of air already in the lung and new air entering. The larger the residual air volume, the greater is the dilution of incoming tidal air. Since enlarged FRC is usually accompanied by airway obstruction, large and variable-sized air spaces, or both, an even distribution of tidal air to all alveoli is impossible. Thus, *uneven distribution of inspired air* is a characteristic of severe pulmonary distention and results in nonuniform alveolar ventilation, a hazard to gas exchange since it interferes with the normal ventilation-perfusion balance to be described below. An estimate of the evenness with which inspired air is distributed among the alveoli can be made in the cardiopulmonary laboratory. One technique involves the breathing of pure oxygen for a number of minutes, gradually washing out nitrogen remaining in the lung from previous air breathing. The exhaled air is monitored by an analyzer that measures the gradually decreasing concentration of nitrogen removed, and the time-concentration relationship is noted. In a lung disrupted by severe obstruction or especially in which variable-sized air spaces empty in an irregular fashion, the relationship will be markedly abnormal. Another technique utilizes the inhalation of a known concentration of inert helium; by measurement of the time it takes for the lung air to reach equilibrium with the inhaled gas the distribution characteristic of the lung can be determined.

Treatment of distention

The treatment of distention is nonspecific and is aimed to achieve the following.

Reduce obstruction. The methods employed to reduce obstruction are those described above, with emphasis upon the use of aerosols and postural drainage.

Improve pulmonary air distribution. Closely related to the management of obstruction, treatment of distention employs the intermittent use of mechanical ventilators to assist air distribution by providing air under pressure. Aerosols to reduce obstruction, frequently delivered at the same time, help to maintain the integrity of the airways while ventilating alveoli that are otherwise poorly supplied with air.

Improve mechanics of ventilation. To help consolidate gains realized from the above two therapies, patients are retrained in the proper use of their ventilatory muscles through breathing exercises. Emphasis is placed upon restoration of effective use of the diaphragm and upon aiding the patient to limit his reliance on his accessory muscles. This approach is incorporated into the long-term management of the patient, and its techniques become part of his daily activities.

PULMONARY RESTRICTION

Pulmonary restriction is defined as an interference with easy or adequate lung expansion and is often associated with a decrease in lung and/or thoracic compliance. There are many pathologic states that can restrict expansion of the lung, some of which will be briefly described in the following four groups: thoracic, intrathoracic (nonpulmonary), pulmonary, and abdominal.

Thoracic. Some of the thoracic causes of restriction are the result of structural changes in the chest, others of reduced flexibility:

a. Kyphoscoliosis is an abnormal curvature of the spine that, when it affects the dorsal segment, distorts the thoracic cage by compressing one side or the other. In general, it is produced by an imbalance between the bilateral skeletal muscle groups, weakness of one group allowing unopposed traction by the other, with eventual tilting and rotation of the spine and chest cage. Poliomyelitis is a frequent offender, as are developmental defects of childhood and adolescence from causes as yet unknown. The disfigured thorax may imprison portions of the lung, preventing normal expansion.
b. Destructive bone diseases of the spine and thorax, such as tuberculosis and osteoporosis, may produce restrictive distortion not classified as kyphoscoliosis.
c. Trauma, such as sternal and costal fractures, will cause severe although usually temporary restriction.
d. Reduced thoracic flexibility can result from such diseases as arthritis, scleroderma, and fibromyositis.
e. Paralysis of ventilatory muscles, as in poliomyelitis and myasthenia gravis, although not reflecting a decrease in compliance, markedly interferes with lung expansion.

Intrathoracic (Nonpulmonary). Diseases within the chest often impede lung expansion because of the following:

a. Pleurisy limits ventilation by restrictive pain or by subsequent restrictive pleural thickening.
b. Fluid in the pleural cavity restricts pulmonary expansion by direct compression of the lung. Such fluid may be *serous* in character, from pleural inflammation or heart failure; *purulent*, from pleural infection or extension of a lung infection into the pleural space or from infected chest trauma; or *hemorrhagic*, from trauma or destructive lung disease.

Pulmonary. Most of the pulmonary causes of lung restriction can be put into one of two categories:

a. Fibrosis or scarring of the lung accounts for most of the restrictive problems. It is a sequella of recurrent respiratory infections, often accompanying chronic bronchopulmonary disease such as emphysema, and follows such destructive diseases as tuberculosis, bronchiectasis, and many industrial or occupational diseases.
b. Intrapulmonary vascular congestion can significantly impair the compliance of the lung. Due to a failing heart, blood in the pulmonary circuit may back up, distending the vaculature of the lung with an increased blood volume. Since the total compliance of the lung is dependent upon all structures in it, as the flexibility of the pulmonary vessels lessens with their congestion, the overall flexibility of the lung will be reduced. Mobility of the lung will be further impaired if the congestion is accompanied by pulmonary edema, with its increased fluid in the pulmonary intercellular spaces, and fluid in the alveoli.

Abdominal. Through immobilization of the diaphragm, abdominal pathology is a frequent cause of pulmonary restriction:

a. Abdominal splinting, a rigid contraction of the musculature of the abdominal wall, is usually an unconscious reaction to pain from intra-abdominal disease or postoperative discomfort. Ventilation can be seriously impeded, and the combination of restriction and hypoventilation comprises a common respiratory complication of abdominal disease.
b. Abdominal distention results from excessive accumulation of gas or air in the stomach or intestinal tract. This may be of such a degree that the abdominal wall is pushed outward into a rounded dome under great tension.
c. Abdominal fluid, referred to as *ascites*, usually the result of liver disease, heart failure, or some pathology causing widespread peritoneal irritation, increases intra-abdominal pressure to interfere with diaphragmatic descent.

Effect of restriction on ventilation

Restriction reduces the vital capacity, and in severe instances may limit it nearly to the resting tidal volume. In this case, as with distention, there may be little or no inspiratory reserve volume to accommodate the needs of exertion. The FRC may be normal in the absence of associated distention, but despite this, the measured residual volume is often enlarged since the rigidity of the lung, or the lack of muscular effort, reduces the size of the forced expiratory reserve volume. More often than not, other ventilatory disturbances accompany restriction, especially in patients with chronic bronchopulmonary disease.

Treatment of restriction

Some specific objectives of treatment are obvious, such as the removal of pleural or abdominal fluid, the removal of pleural adhesions, the repair of structural defects of the thorax, and the improvement of circulation. In many patients, however, such corrective causes are not present, and relief of the restrictive agent is not possible. In general, the treatment is that outlined for pulmonary distention. The more specific techniques of maintaining controlled mechanical ventilation of the restricted patient in ventilatory failure will be discussed separately.

VENTILATION-PERFUSION IMBALANCE

A disturbance in the ratio between ventilation and pulmonary perfusion is always secondary to some other disorder and is a condition that may be found with many types of diseases. In addition, this imbalance may also be the result of some of the disturbances already discussed in this chapter, but its clinical effects are so widespread and important that it deserves detailed consideration in any discussion of pathophysiology.

In terms of the body as a whole, with its myriad of individual cellular demands, the total exchange of oxygen for carbon dioxide is called the body *respiratory quotient* (RQ) and is expressed as the ratio of the quantity of carbon dioxide produced to oxygen consumed per unit of time, $\dot{V}_{CO_2}/\dot{V}_{O_2}$. Depending upon the net metabolic needs of all parts of the body at a given moment, this ratio ranges from 0.7 to 1.0, with an average of 0.8. Because of biochemically limiting factors of metabolism, the RQ cannot exceed 1.0. Thus, less carbon dioxide is produced by the body than oxygen is utilized, and to maintain necessary tissue gas exchange, there must be a comparable exchange in the lung between alveoli and blood. For this, the tidal flow of air into and out of the alveoli constitutes the pulmonary ventilation, and the pulmonary capillary blood flow, in direct contact with the alveolar walls, provides the perfusion of the lung. The relationship between the ventilation and perfusion is referred to as the *ventilation/perfusion ratio,* or the *respiratory/exchange ratio* (R), symbolically designated as $\dot{V}_A/\dot{Q}_c$. It is the ratio between the minute flow of air into the alveoli and the minute flow of blood through the pulmonary capillaries. The respiratory exchange ratio of the whole lung is the same as the respiratory quotient, averaging 4:5, or 0.8.[72] This means that for every 4 liters of alveolar ventilation, there are 5 liters of pulmonary capillary blood flow.

A normal R in itself, however, is not adequate insurance of effective gas exchange since it does not tell us how the ventilation and perfusion are distributed throughout the lung. Consider the hypothetical example of all the ventilation going to one lung and all the perfusion to the other. In this situation, although the total amount of ventilation and perfusion may be normal, and R equal to 0.8, it is obvious that gas exchange will be absent and survival impossible. It is important to grasp the concept of a whole host of respiratory exchange ratios scattered throughout the lungs, the so-called "regional distribution of R's." Each lobule of the lung might well have its own ratio, depending upon the local balance between ventilation and perfusion, but the overall lung R will be the same as the respiratory quotient. One can imagine generalized or localized disease or injury modifying both ventilation and perfusion so that the final functional effect upon ventilation would depend on which was the more disturbed. Thus, when we attempt to classify the physiologic effects of disease as either ventilatory or circulatory imbalance of the ratio, we must recognize that either or both elements may be at fault.

Measurement of regional ventilation/perfusion ratios is difficult, but useful data have been obtained by using inhaled radioactive oxygen or intravenous radioactive xenon, recording the relative distribution of ventilation and perfusion by counters placed regionally over the chest. The speed and

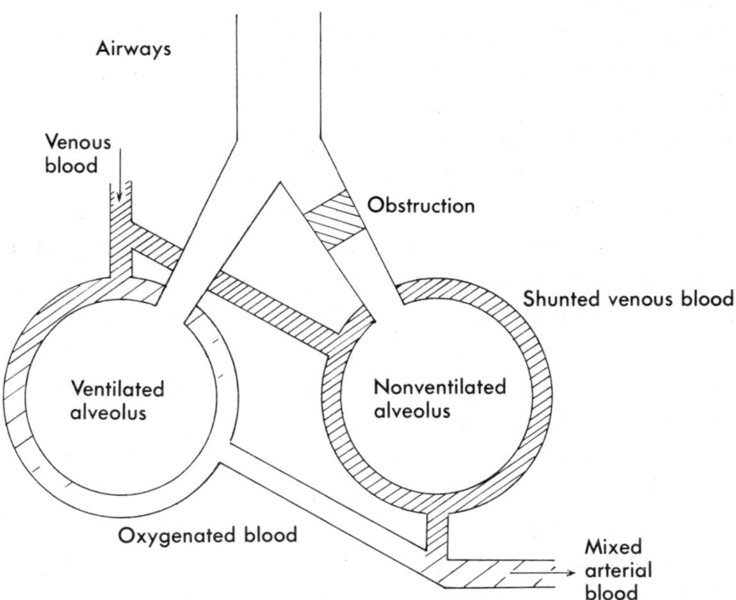

Fig. 6-3. *Venous admixture* is a term given to mixed arterial blood leaving the lung when it contains both fully oxygenated blood from normally ventilated alveoli and incompletely oxygenated "shunted venous blood" from poorly ventilated alveoli. In the sketch, ventilation to one alveolus is normal but is blocked to the other, and capillary shading represents a quantitative index of unsaturation. In the normal subject quietly breathing ambient air at 1 atm pressure, mixed arterial blood is approximately 97% saturated with oxygen.

extent of distribution of radioactivity reflects ventilation, and its clearance from the lungs perfusion.[73]

Let us now consider some of the implications of decreased and increased regional respiratory exchange ratios.

Low $\dot{V}/\dot{Q}$**.** A ratio less than the normal average body RQ of 0.8 results from a decrease in regional alveolar ventilation, physiologically producing what is known as a *venous admixture,* or from the introduction into the arterial system of unsaturated blood, with an attendant drop in arterial oxygen content. Through some pathologic process, variable numbers of alveoli are subjected to differing degrees of underventilation. If they remain fully perfused, the blood leaving them will not be normally saturated with oxygen and will be at least partially venous in nature as it combines with the mixed arterial blood leaving areas of normal R. Fig. 6-3 schematically illustrates this mechanism with the complete obstructure of one alveolar unit.

The venous admixture is actually a *physiologic venous-arterial shunt,* although the term *admixture* is preferred in current terminology. It is a shunt because the effect, on mixed arterial oxygenation, of perfused blood denied its normal quota of oxygen is the same as that of blood bypassing the lung physically. It is termed physiologic because it is caused by a functional derangement of an organ that may have basically normal structure. The natural human environment of ambient air at 1 atm pressure produces a small normal venous admixture, at least during quiet breathing, because the distribution of ventilation throughout the lung is not even and with any given breath some alveoli are incompletely ventilated. Thus, the normal arterial oxygen saturation is about 97%, although it can often be raised to 100% with hyperventilation. Fig. 6-4 diagrams the normal physiologic shunt, or venous admixture, showing the shunted blood as if it bypassed the lung.

We shall take some time to discuss the effect of a venous admixture on blood oxygenation. This will serve the double purpose of acquainting the

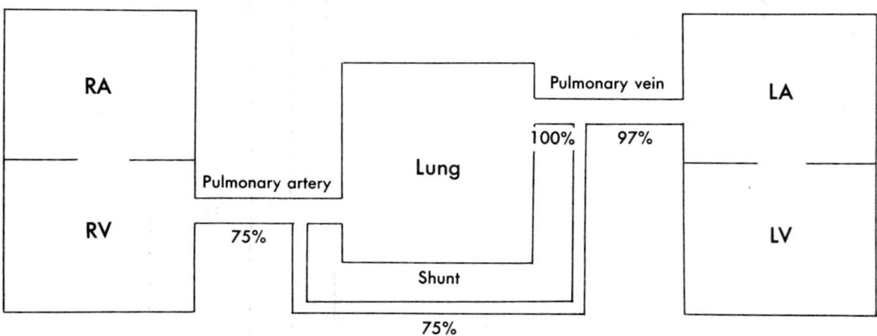

Fig. 6-4. This diagrams the normal physiologic shunt, or venous admixture, during tidal ventilation of air at 1 atm pressure. It shows some venous blood, with an O_2 saturation of 75%, as if it bypassed the lung as a result of perfusing scattered, nonventilated alveoli. The mixture of the shunted with the fully oxygenated blood gives arterial blood its usual saturation of about 97%.

student with a useful technique of evaluating cardiopulmonary function and at the same time enabling him to call upon some of the concepts of physiology that he has studied in an unavoidably isolated fashion so that he can put them to practical use. The important fact is not overlooked that our purpose is to educate the inhalation therapist, not a professional postgraduate student; and although the detailed concepts of ventilation-perfusion relationships often tax the minds of the experienced physiologist, there is no reason why the therapist should not be stimulated to learn as much as he can about the patient he will be treating. We will use two hypothetical situations, with a graphic illustration of each, to show the clinical effect of a significant venous admixture. In the interest of simplicity, we will take some liberties with reality. First, the situations we will create will be exaggerated for emphasis, and, as shown in Figs. 6-5 and 6-6, the lung in question will consist of but two alveoli, each with its own perfusing capillary. One alveolus will be completely nonventilated and will resemble a closed space; the other will ventilate under differing conditions. Second, in considering blood oxygen content, we will concern ourselves only with oxygen combined with hemoglobin, at 15 gm%, ignoring the dissolved fraction. This facilitates calculations and, because of the minute quantities of dissolved gas at atmosphere, introduces very little error. We will further assume that, as the venous blood enters our simple systems, its flow divides so that equal volumes perfuse each al-

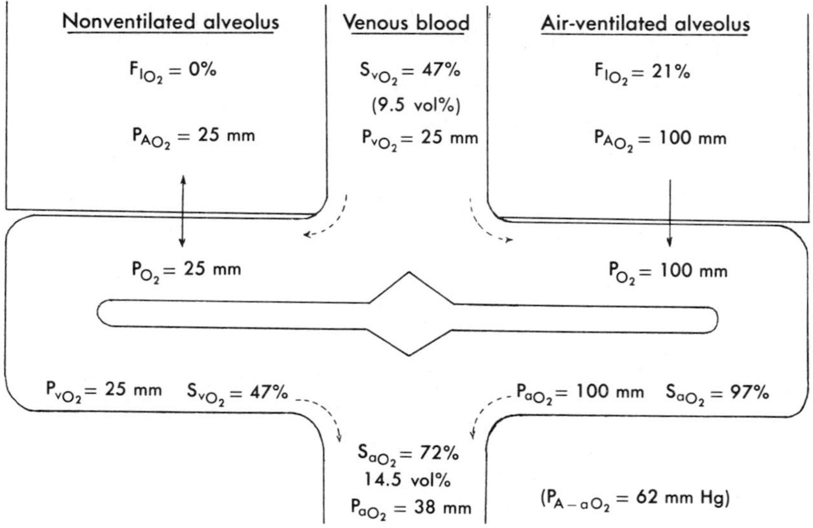

Fig. 6-5. The sketch represents an alveolus with no ventilation and one with normal air ventilation, each being perfused by one half the venous blood entering the system. The data are based on a hemoglobin content of 15 gm% and an a-v oxygen difference of 5 vol%. Arterialized blood leaving the ventilated alveolus combines with shunted (venous) blood leaving the nonventilated alveolus, giving the mixed arterial blood a saturation of 72% and a P_{O_2} of 38 mm Hg. There is thus an oxygen tension difference, or gradient, between the alveolar air and the mixed arterial blood, of 62 mm Hg. This is called an A-a_{O_2} gradient, symbolized as $P_{A\text{-}a_{O_2}}$.

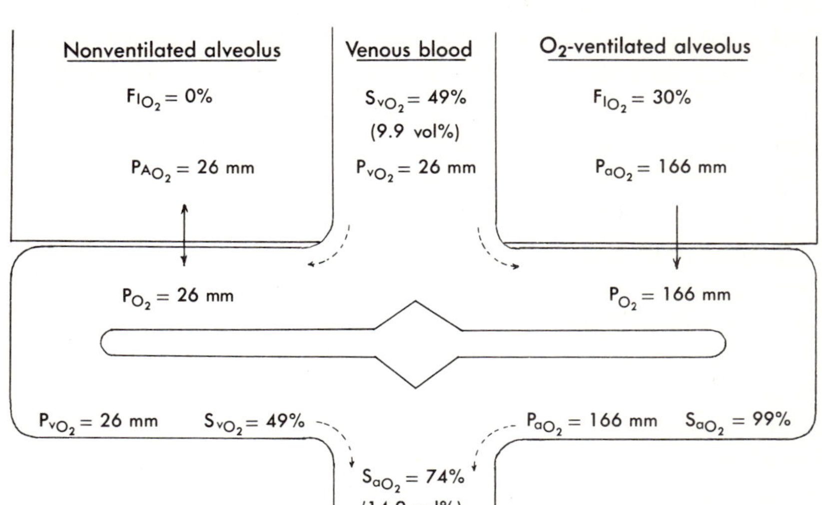

Fig. 6-6. This system is the same as that of Fig. 6-5, except that the functioning alveolus is ventilated with an inspired gas mixture containing 30% oxygen, resulting in a calculated $P_{A_{O_2}}$ of 166 mm Hg, and an A-a_{O_2} gradient of 126 mm Hg. Thus, as long as blood is being shunted, an increase in $F_{I_{O_2}}$ will lead to a disproportionately smaller increase in $P_{a_{O_2}}$ and a widened A-a_{O_2} gradient.

veolus and the arterial blood leaving is thus a mixture of equal parts from each alveolus. Finally, we will assume that in each instance the a-v oxygen difference (representing oxygen given up to body cells) will remain steady at 5 vol%. To accomplish this, we have calculated values that allow the fully arterialized blood from the ventilated alveolus, when diluted with the shunted blood of the nonventilated alveolus, to have an oxygen content 5 vol% greater than it has when it returns to the lung as venous blood after perfusing body cells. The student will notice that all values are exceedingly lower than the normals to which he has been exposed, but he must observe that these conditions represent what can be called a 50% shunt, in which half the circulating blood is denied oxygenation. Although they are grossly abnormal, there are clinical states that closely match them.

In Fig. 6-5 blood perfusing the air-ventilated alveolus, with its oxygen tension of 100 mm Hg, is fully oxygenated and approaches the outflow tract with a P_{O_2} of 100 mm Hg and a saturation of 97%. On the other hand, blood perfusing the nonventilated alveolus picks up no oxygen. In fact, theoretically, there could be a diffusion of oxygen from the venous blood into the closed and oxygen-poor alveolus, maintaining a $P_{A_{O_2}}$ equal to the 25 mm Hg tension of the perfusing blood. This half of the blood volume thus reaches the outflow still as venous blood, with its P_{O_2} of 25 mm Hg and a saturation of 47%, and here the two streams unite and thoroughly mix. The oxygen content of the *mixed* arterial blood is dependent upon the degree of saturation of each of its two components, since saturation is volumetrically related to hemoglobin content. In this instance the final saturation is the average of the values of the two halves, or 72%, and by the normal oxygen dissociation curve this represents a partial pressure of 38 mm Hg. Note that a saturation of 72%, in this very hypoxic arterial blood, is the equivalent of a combined oxygen content of 14.5 vol% (72% of 20.1 = 14.5). On this basis, the oxygen content of the venous blood was established as 9.5 vol%, at a partial pressure of 25 mm Hg.

If this were a subject under study and we were to get a sample of exhaled alveolar air to measure its oxygen content, or if we calculated it according to the alveolar air equation, we would find a $P_{A_{O_2}}$ of about 100 mm Hg.* The nonventilating alveolus, of course, contributes nothing to alveolar sampling. The difference between the oxygen tensions in the alveoli and in sampled arterial blood constitutes a gradient, called an *alveolar-arterial oxygen tension gradient,* or more simply an A-a_{O_2} gradient, symbolized as $P_{A\text{-}a_{O_2}}$. Under normal conditions, with the small physiologic shunt usually present, the A-a gradient does not exceed 10 mm Hg. The gradient in our example is 62 mm Hg (100 − 38). A large gradient usually identifies a state of hypoxia as due to some cause other than an inadequate alveolar supply of oxygen and generally resolves the diagnosis to a differential between a venous admixture and a diffusion defect. Although we have illustrated the manner in which a gradient can be caused by shunting, a block to diffusion of oxygen across the A-C membrane theoretically could just as well have been responsible. Let us now describe a procedure that will help us differentiate between an A-a_{O_2} gradient resulting from a shunt and one from a diffusion defect.

Fig. 6-6 represents the same general arrangement as described above, but now the ventilating alveolus carries a 30% oxygen mixture instead of the 21% of air. An a-v oxygen difference of 5 vol% is still assumed for uniformity. With this breathing mixture the alveolar oxygen tension is calculated to be approximately 166 mm Hg, and the perfusing blood leaving the ventilated alveolus equilibrates at this tension. The arterial oxygen saturation corresponding to a partial pressure of 166 mm Hg is difficult to read with accuracy from the flat upper portion of the dissociation curve, but according to a table designed to overcome this problem, it is approximately 99%.[74] Employing the same technique as above in determining the characteristics of the mixed arterial blood leaving the lung, we find a final arterial oxygen saturation of 75% and an oxygen tension of 40 mm Hg. If we now compare the alveolar and arterial oxygen partial pressures, we find an A-a_{O_2} gradient of 126 mm Hg (166 − 40). These two examples make it evident that, as we increase the oxygen concentration in the breathing mixture and as long as some of the blood is consistently bypassing ventilated alveoli, we will get a decreasing proportionate increase in the oxygen content of the mixed arterial blood. This should be expected, and if the student will examine the data carefully,

*See Appendix 12 for an explanation of the alveolar air equation.

he will see how the characteristics of the oxygen dissociation curve limit the value of increasing the oxygenation of the ventilated alveolus. We can thereby make the following generalization: If an alveolar-arterial oxygen tension gradient exists when room air is breathed and it is primarily due to a shunt, the gradient will widen, with increasing concentrations of oxygen in the breathing mixture. It should be pointed out that this holds true for the normal subject since his negligible gradient will also increase as he breathes oxygen-enriched air. Finally, whereas an A-a oxygen gradient is characteristically present with a lowered $\dot{V}/\dot{Q}$, an arterial-alveolar P_{CO_2} gradient or difference is not. The greater diffusibility of carbon dioxide permits its easy escape through ventilated alveoli, aided by the often present hyperventilation accompanying hypoxia.

In contrast to venous admixture, the hypoxia due to an impairment of oxygen diffusion is generally felt to be overcome by an elevation of the inspired oxygen concentration. With increasing alveolar oxygen partial pressure, enough additional oxygen molecules are diffused into the blood to bring the latter above the hypoxemic level, although at times breathing concentrations close to 100% may be necessary. Because of this, a subject with an A-a oxygen gradient from a diffusion defect will show a reduction in his gradient as he breathes an increased oxygen mixture since the rise in his blood gas tension will be proportionately higher than that of his alveoli (although, of course, the former can never exceed the latter). It might be

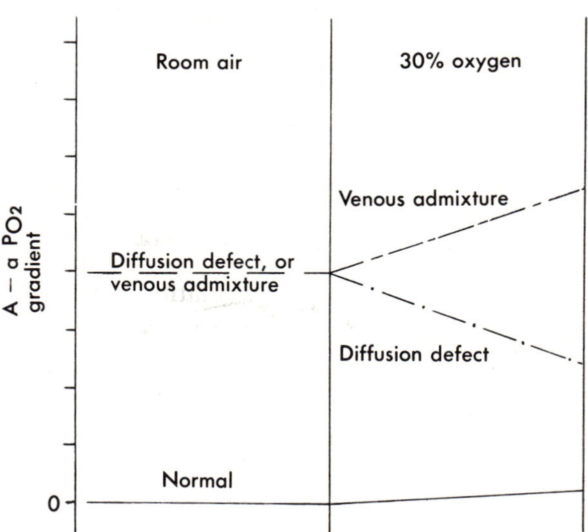

Fig. 6-7. Simplified schematic of differentiation between normal and abnormal A-a P_{O_2} gradients, the latter shown in nonspecific arbitrary units, using the double gradient technique. Normal lungs show no significant gradient with air breathing, but a slight one with 30% oxygen. Both diffusion defects and venous admixture produce gradients with air, but the gradient (*not* the absolute alveolar and arterial tensions) with 30% oxygen decreases with diffusion defects and worsens with shunting.

added that in both shunt and diffusion defect the hypoxia will worsen with exercise and gradients will widen as the increased tissue use of oxygen lowers the venous gas content in the shunt and as the increased blood flow of exercise further reduces pulmonary gas exchange time of a diffusion defect.

The technique of subjecting a patient to two breathing mixtures with differing oxygen concentrations (often room air, and 30% to 40% oxygen) and calculating the two A-a gradients is termed a *double-gradient study.* It is a valuable diagnostic tool and, though by no means foolproof, gives a dynamic perspective to cardiopulmonary function hampered by hypoxia. Fig. 6-7 is a nonquantitative sketch showing the double oxygen–gradient characteristics of the normal state, shunt, and diffusion defect.

High $\dot{V}/\dot{Q}$. Regional elevations of the respiratory exchange ratio (R), which may reach 3.0 or more, result from the loss of adequate perfusion of ventilated alveoli; and when capillary flow to alveoli is reduced or absent, there is reduced or absent gas exchange even in the presence of normal or increased tidal alveolar airflow. As illustrated in Fig. 3-1, this constitutes *dead space ventilation.* The basic effects of a highly localized elevated R are schematically illustrated in Fig. 6-8, which shows two normally ventilated

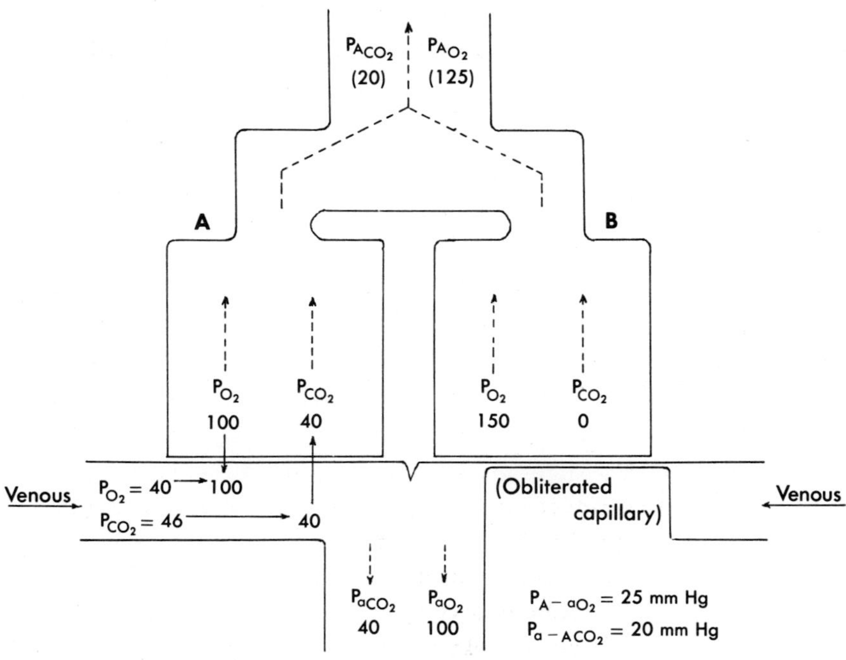

Fig. 6-8. Two normally air-ventilated alveoli are shown, one with full perfusion, **A,** the other without perfusion because of obstruction to (or destruction of) its capillary, **B.** Mixed arterial blood leaving the system has normal gas tensions, but sampled mixed alveolar air is high in O_2 and low in CO_2. This produces an A-a_{O_2} gradient of 25 mm Hg and an a-A_{CO_2} difference of 20 mm Hg. The latter normally does not exceed 5 mm Hg, and higher values indicate ventilation of non-perfused alveoli, or dead space breathing.

alveoli, one (A) with normal perfusion and the other (B) unperfused because of a block in its perfusing capillary. Because alveolus B is not perfused, it receives no carbon dioxide and its P_{CO_2} is zero. In the absence of carbon dioxide the gas of the alveolus consists of oxygen, nitrogen, and water vapor, and its oxygen partial pressure is approximately 150 mm Hg. With no component from the obstructed capillary, mixed arterial blood from the area has normal tensions of carbon dioxide and oxygen. The gas values of a mixed alveolar sample, however, are the averages of those of each alveolus, with a $P_{A_{CO_2}}$ of 20 mm Hg, and a $P_{A_{O_2}}$ of 125 mm Hg. Because of the perfusion defect, then, there are gas tension gradients present between the alveoli and arterial blood: an A-a oxygen gradient of 25 mm Hg and an a-A carbon dioxide gradient of 20 mm Hg. Again, this example is quite exaggerated, since one might expect to find a normal carbon dioxide gradient not in excess of 5 mm Hg and a value of twice this would be considered highly significant. The only specific information that an elevated carbon dioxide gradient gives us is to indicate that there is a general increase in pulmonary ventilation over pulmonary perfusion. This is dead space ventilation, but physiologically it means that there is a certain amount of work being invested in ventilation from which there is not a proportionate return in profitable blood gas exchange. The term *wasted ventilation* has been given to this uneconomical state.[75]

Clinically, this concept has a practical diagnostic application. Pulmonary embolism is a relatively common phenomenon and may express itself as a massive obstruction of a large branch of the pulmonary artery or as frequently recurring blockage of small arteries or arterioles. Within a few hours after the onset of such an episode, evidence of a high $\dot{V}/\dot{Q}$ may be noted. The terminal portion of the patient's tidal air, considered to be alveolar in quality, is analyzed for its carbon dioxide concentration and tension, while a sample of arterial blood is drawn for the same purpose. A significant difference between the carbon dioxide tensions of the two samples, indicating an elevated $\dot{V}/\dot{Q}$, is often helpful in complementing other data to support a diagnosis of embolism, although it obviously is not pathognomonic. The nature of the test has given it the familiar title of an *end-tidal CO_2 determination.*

In summary, two statements can be made:

1. A low $\dot{V}/\dot{Q}$ produces a venous admixture, with hypoxia and an A-a oxygen tension gradient resulting from a drop in arterial oxygen tension but with little effect on the carbon dioxide.
2. A high $\dot{V}/\dot{Q}$ produces alveolar dead space ventilation, with little hypoxia but with an A-a oxygen gradient due to an elevation of alevolar oxygen tension and an A-a carbon dioxide pressure difference.

It is important to remember that these concepts are to be used to explain *local* events in the lung, not necessarily the lung as a whole. Also, in disease, all degress of both ratio imbalances may be present, with the final state of lung function dependent upon the net resulting mixed pathophysiology.

Chapter 7

Aerosol and humidity therapy

We will introduce the subject of clinical inhalation therapy with a discussion of aerosols and humidity. This deliberate pairing was chosen because the use of water in the treatment of bronchopulmonary disease requires an understanding of the principles of aerosols, and we will learn that of all the pharmacologically and physically active aerosols, water is the most important. From this point on, our attention will be directed primarily toward the patient—his needs, and how we can best serve these needs. This does not mean that we will not frequently pause to consider some basic principle, but our thinking will be patient oriented, and we will lean heavily upon the physical and chemical fundamentals covered in the preceding pages.

PHYSICAL PROPERTIES OF AEROSOLS

The therapist will better understand the clinical use of medical aerosols, as well as the important health effects of atmospheric contaminants, if he has a background knowledge of the nature of aerosols in general. An aerosol is defined as a suspension of very fine particles (particulate matter) of liquid or solid in a gas. In general, aerosol particles are considered to fall within the size range of 0.005μ to 50.0μ in diameter, but from a practical point of view only those are important that are less than 3μ in diameter, for it is at this mass size that gravity begins to lose its influence, a point of some importance, as we shall soon see. Atmospheric aerosols can be considered to be either *natural* or *man made* and may consist of windblown dusts, bacteria, yeast, molds, water, dusts from explosions or earth-moving equipment, smoke, industrial wastes, and products of incomplete combustion of a large variety of commercial fuels, to list but a few of the more prevalent. Another classification of atmospheric particulate matter, which is especially revealing in its relationship to disease production, is that which describes *neutral particles,* commonly referred to as dusts and "condensation nuclei." These are made up of hygroscopic substances (substances able to absorb water).[76] The neutral, dustlike particles range in size from 10^{-5} to 10^{-3} cm in diameter, have mostly a nuisance value, and are generally less harmful than the condensation nuclei. The latter are smaller, from 10^{-7} to 10^{-5} cm in diameter, and are composed mostly of chloride salts, sulfuric acid, phosphorous compounds, nitrogen oxides, and nitric acid. In the air, such nuclei grow rapidly in size by the acquisition of water, as the relative humidity exceeds 70%, and easily produce haze and fog. It should be apparent also that any hygroscopic aerosol might undergo the same change during inhalation into the moist environment of the respiratory tract. Finally, although we are not studying the atmosphere as such, it is relevant to note that condensation nuclei, often consisting of toxic or irritant trace gases, tend to form on the most minute speck of matter, giving stability to these otherwise vaporous substances so that they are able to enter the respiratory tract, with harmful effects.[77] Their participation in the damaging action of contaminated urban air and smothering smogs is a matter of record.

To communicate clearly in a discussion of aerosol technology, we must learn some basic terms that are descriptive of the physical activity of particles. *Stability* of an aerosol refers to its ability to remain in suspension for significant periods of time or, in fact, to maintain its integrity as an aerosol. Such stability depends upon a number of characteristics, including size and nature of the particulate matter, concentration of particles, ambient humidity, and the degree of mobility of the carrier gas. *Instability* is the reverse of the above, the propensity of a suspended particle to remove itself, or be removed, from suspension. From a therapeutic point of view it is apparent that the stability or instability of a given aerosol will bear directly upon the aerosol's effectiveness and be a matter of considerable concern to the manufacturer. It is not surprising that, among the many regulating mechanisms of nature and through a process almost like that of natural selection, a measure of stability is achieved among the atmospheric aerosols. Although the size range of particulate matter is great, as the myriad particles intermingle, some will condense on others, some will coalesce to from larger masses (agglomerate), and others will vanish through instability. A large population of aerosols thus undergoes a process of "aging," whereby there is a gradual increase in the number of particles of optimum size and concentration for maximum stability, with a reduction in the range of sizes. This *ideal* state consists of particles from 0.2μ to 0.7μ in diameter, in concentrations of from 100 to 1,000 particles per cubic centimeter of gas.[77] Fig. 7-1 is a graphic illustration of this phenomenon, showing the relationship between population, distribution of particulate diameters, and time.

Related to the characteristics of stability and instability, but especially pertinent to the therapeutic use of aerosols, are *penetration, deposition* or *retention,* and *clearance,* terms that are descriptive of the fate of particles once they have come into contact with the respiratory tract. "Penetration" refers to the maximum depth that suspended particles can be carried into the tract by the inhaled tidal air. "Deposition" is the result of an aerosol's eventual instability, permitting it to "fall out" on a nearby surface, whereas "retention" implies the depositon of a particle within the confines of a structure, such as the respiratory tract. Aerosol "clearance" is the opposite of re-

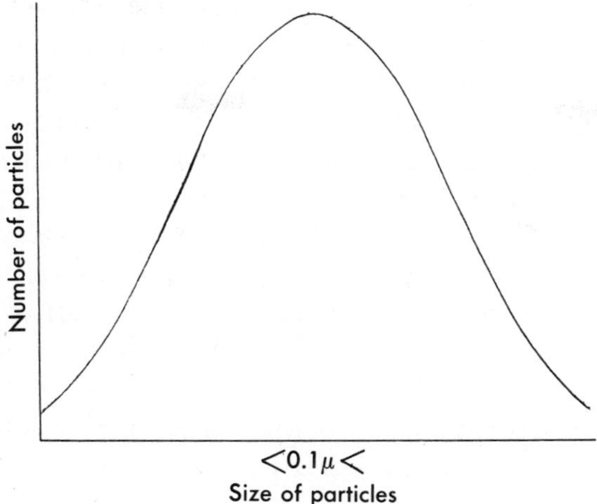

Fig. 7-1. This graph is a distribution curve of aerosol particle sizes. If a population of particles of many sizes is allowed to settle, the largest number will have diameters somewhere around 0.1μ, with decreasing frequency of sizes larger and smaller. (Adapted from Lovejoy, F. W., and Morrow, P. E.: Aerosols, bronchodilators and mucolytic agents, Anesthesiology **23**:460, 1962.)

tention and, depending upon its specific use, may have two meanings. Most authors refer to aerosol clearance as the process of removal of particles once deposited in the respiratory tissues by one of several biologic mechanisms that will be considered later. Occasionally the term implies the excretion of still-suspended particles in the exhaled air. Let us describe these activities in more detail.

Penetration and deposition of aerosols

Because of their interrelation, penetration and deposition will be discussed tgether. Of significance is the location of the deposition of inhaled particles, for there is a considerable physiologic difference between particle contact with the relatively rugged and exposed nasal tissue and particle contact with the more secluded and reactive bronchial and alveolar cells. The latter areas are of more interest to us in the therapeutic use of aerosols. The depth of penetration of the respiratory tract increases as the particle size decreases. In fact, unless a particle is considerably less than 100μ in diameter, it will not even gain entrance. The nasal filtering process (deposition in the nose) is so effective that it will remove completely particles down to 5μ in diameter, whereas sizes below 1μ are able to pass the upper tract and are retained in pulmonary tissue. We can make the generalization that the overall retention of particulate matter in the total respiratory tract is 100% for particles down to 5μ in diameter, which are trapped in the nose, and about 25% for particles down to 0.25μ, which are deposited and retained along the rest of the tract. Deposition in the upper respiratory tract (conducting airways to the respiratory bronchioles) varies from 100% for large particles to 0% for particles of 1μ, whereas deposition in the alveoli is 90%

to 100% for sizes down to 1μ.[78] There are five major factors that influence aerosol penetration and deposition—*gravity, kinetic activity of gas molecules, inertial impaction, physical nature of the particle,* and the *ventilatory pattern.*

Gravity. The speed with which a particle will "settle" is a measure of its ease of deposition. The settling rate is related to the force exerted by gravity on the particle mass or the combination of its density and size. The greater the mass of any body, the greater will be the influence of gravity upon it. Suspended particles between 0.1μ and 70μ generally follow the prediction of Stoke's law of sedimentation.[79] In its entirety, Stoke's law relates the velocity at which a small particle falls toward the earth with such physical factors as particle volume, density, acceleration of gravity, and viscous resistance of air. For our purposes, however, we can use it in a simplified proportionality and state that, within the above size range, the settling velocity of a particle is proportional to the product of its density and the square of its diameter. Thus:

$$\text{Settling rate} \cong \text{Density} \times \text{Diameter}^2$$

In Table 7-1, compare the relative velocities with which the three hypothetical particles will deposit under the influence of gravity. Particle x, with a density of 1 unit and a diameter of 2 units, will settle with a velocity of 4 units. Particle y, of the same density but with twice the diameter, will settle four times as fast; whereas particle z, with the same diameter but twice the density, will settle twice as fast.

Kinetic activity of gas molecules. This interesting force of particle deposition is effective on sizes 0.1μ or smaller. Because of their minute size, such aerosols are almost molecular in character and, as such, are subject to some of the physical activities attributed to molecules. They present the phenomenon of *Brownian movement* under the influence of the kinetic activity of the molecules of their carrier gas. The suspended particles are under constant bombardment from the gas molecules and are thus impelled into high-speed random movements for very short distances. The smaller the particles, the greater will be their velocities. This transferred activity and mobility causes many of the particles to come into contact with nearby surfaces, and it is referred to as *diffusion* of the aerosol. The resulting surface impaction is called *diffusion deposition.* How much of the suspended material will deposit is a function of its "diffusion coefficient," defined as the volume of particles that can diffuse

Table 7-1. *Gravity deposition*

Particle	*Density*	*Diameter*	*Velocity*
x	1	2	4
y	1	4	16
z	2	2	8

a distance of 1μ over an area of 1 cm^2 at a pressure of 1 atm, and is inversely proportional to particle size. Whether a given particle will deposit or what fraction of a given volume of suspended particles will fall out is determined by the distance of the particles from the nearest suitable surface. The probability of deposition is related to time as well as to diffusibility and distance, and the average distance that the force of diffusion will move a minute particle is expressed by the following proportionality:

$$\text{Average distance traveled} \cong \sqrt{\text{Diffusion coefficient} \times \text{Time}}$$

We are not interested in quantitative values for such physical phenomena, but we should be aware that they play an important role in the efficiency of aerosol therapy, and we should recognize that consideration of these many factors in the design of aerosol generators can mean the difference between good and indifferent equipment.

Inertial impaction. A particle being carried in an airstream tends to continue on a straight course when the stream undergoes a sudden change in direction.[80] This divergence of the particle's path from that of the airstream is referred to as a "sideways slip." Because it occurs at angulations in the conducting channel, such a slip can precipitate a particle on a nearby surface. Whether a particle will deposit in such a manner depends in part upon its location within the airstream, the probability increasing with the particle's proximity to the periphery of the stream. Whether it will deposit depends also upon the force of inertia, which opposes any change in direction of a moving particle, being great enough to free the particle from its fellows in the stream. To do this, inertia must overcome the resistance of air friction, so another probability of deposition depends upon the net effect of the two forces of inertia and friction. In summary, then, it can be said that inertial precipitation of aerosol particles of uniform density is related to particle velocity and size.

Physical nature of particles. Of the many physical and chemical characteristics of minute matter, probably the most important in terms of deposition and retention is its hygroscopic nature, noted above. Initially small, a particle may absorb relatively large amounts of water from ambient air, especially in transit through the respiratory tract, and increase many times its diameter. This, of course, will alter its original probable point of impact. The solubility and chemical nature of particles, especially those in a heterogeneous atmospheric mixture, may play an important role. Very small particles may dissolve in or chemically react with aerosolized water or other solvents of a larger size and thus eventually deposit at levels different from those dictated by their original sizes. Finally, particle contour can influence deposition. Although we speak of aerosol particles as though they all had regular diameters like the spheroids of liquid particulates, some hard and brittle substances produce particles with many angulations and irregular plane surfaces. Such particles may follow transit and deposition paths considerably different from those predicted on the basis of physical laws we have been discussing. We might note here that our application of aerosol principles in the treatment of disease is somewhat simplified in that most therapeutic aerosols currently in use are liquids, and the aberrations that might be attributed to solid particles need not concern us.

Ventilatory pattern. In general, deposition and retention of aerosol particles is directly related to inhaled volume and inversely related to respiratory rate. This generalization, however, is not applicable to sizes less than 1μ in diameter. The character of air movement on particle behavior is significant down to the level of the terminal bronchiole, but air in the alveolar sacs is almost stagnant. Thus, depth and frequency of ventilation have little influence on the deposition of particles once they have reached the alveolar level.[81,82] The nature of ventilation higher in the tract does help to determine the volume of particles reaching alveoli and thus exerts an indirect influence. Deposition of particles is increased with both increasing tidal volume and decreasing frequency, and the effects of both are additive. Shallow breathing carries a reduced volume of aerosols per tidal volume, and a rapid breathing rate reduces the time available to the particles to settle. If penetration and deposition are the objectives as in aerosol therapy, the ideal ventilatory pattern consists of slow, moderately deep breathing, with breath holding at end-inspiration. This facilitates the introduction into the respiratory tract of a significant volume of particles and allows adequate time for the smallest to enter the alveoli by diffusion, and to settle by diffusion. This is a practical point that the therapist will have to keep in mind as he supervises and teaches patients the techniques of effective aerosol therapy.

Clearance of aerosols

We will concern ourselves with the removal of particles from the respiratory tract by means other than the exhaled air and will discuss clearance of the upper and lower segments of the tract separately. The mechanism for cleansing the upper tract is referred to as the *ciliary mucus transport*; and there are several mechanisms to service the pulmonary areas.

Ciliary mucus clearance. It is assumed that the student already knows the anatomic structure of the airways and the pulmonary lobules. Of critical importance to the subject under discussion is the nature of the mucosal lining of the respiratory tract. We will recall that the mucosa is characterized by the presence of microscopic hairlike structures called cilia that extend from the beginning of the trachea through all the ramifications of the airways to the level of the terminal bronchioles. Approximately 3μ to 4μ long, the cilia are in constant wavelike motion called "beating," which goes on at a rate of some 1300 strokes per minute. The unique function of the cilia is made possible by more rapid upward strokes than downward recovery strokes. As the cilia wave cephalad (in the direction of the head), they propel an overlying thin layer of fluid called mucus. Respiratory mucus is a thin clear substance, produced by specialized cells (*goblet* cells) throughout the tract to the respiratory bronchioles, and is on the average 5μ thick.[83,84] Its function is to entrap foreign particles and, with the aid of the cilia, to remove them from the tract. Lying like a blanket over the cilia, the mucus layer is carried cephalad in an escalator fashion by the ciliary action at rates up to 13.5 mm per minute. The mucus, with its captive particles, is brought into the trachea and then into the lower pharynx by a normal and almost imperceptible "throat clearing" action to be either expectorated or swallowed, depending upon its volume. The system is extremely efficient as long as both cilia and mucus are in a healthy state. Should a pathologic process increase the depth of the mucus layer, its upward propulsion will gradually slow, becoming ineffective when the thickness of the fluid approaches four to five times the height of the cilia. Similarly, function will be impaired following damage to or destruction of the cilia. It is evident that airway obstruction from the prolific thick secretions accompanying bronchial irritation or infection can be self-perpetuating, as the increase in the secretory load retards its own removal.

Pulmonary tissue clearance. Particles in the lobular lung units can be removed by several routes. Some may be considered "functionally" removed in situ through encapsulation and immobilization by a deposit of fibrous tissue, remaining for the duration of the subject's life. It is not surprising that enough such reactions throughout wide areas of the lung might, in themselves eventually present a problem. Other solid aerosols are picked up by wandering scavenger cells called *phagocytes,* whose mobility permits them to gather at sites of foreign matter deposition. After engulfing the particles within their own protoplasm, the phagocytes can transport them into the cilliary-mucus escalator for removal as described or into the interstitial lymphatics for incarceration in regional lymph nodes. Depending upon solubility, some particles may dissolve in tissue fluid and diffuse into the general circulation to be disposed of by the body's metabolic processes.

Let us summarize the relation between particle size and deposition in the respiratory tract and point out that although much of the research done on inhaled particulate matter has used nontherapeutic solid particles the results give us a practical insight into the expected behavior of the liquid aerosols we will have occasion to use. It is generally agreed that there is a particle size of *minimum* deposition, around 0.4μ in diameter, and that above and below this size the incidence of deposition somewhere in the tract increases. The observed maximum particle diameter found in alveolar air never exceeds 1.2μ.[82] Thus, the highest probability for pulmonary deposition is attributed to particles in the 1μ to 2μ range (gravity settling) and below 0.2μ (diffusion precipitation); the lowest probability is found with particles 0.25μ to 0.50μ, for which the effects of both gravity and diffusion are minimal.[85,86] These data are summarized in Table 7-2.

The student should understand that in the above discussion of the properties of aerosols there are included many generalizations and assumptions that may or may not be valid. The current great interest in aerosols has produced

Table 7-2. *Particle size and site of deposition*

Particle size (μ)	*Deposition in respiratory tract*
100	Do not enter tract
100-5	Trapped in nose
5-2	Deposite somewhere proximal to alveoli
2-1	Can enter alveoli, with 95% to 100% retention of those down to 1μ
1-0.25	Stable, with minimal settling
0.25	Increasing alveolar deposition

many changes in investigative techniques, making it difficult to correlate data from one source to another. These differences in technique account for much of the variance found in the literature, especially pertaining to effective particle sizes[87] and to the degree of alveolar penetration by aerosols.[88] Nevertheless, we have reviewed the most widely accepted behavioral characteristics of aerosols as they apply to clinical medicine, and we can only be alert to new developments in this interesting field.

CLINICAL USE OF AEROSOLS AND HUMIDITY

Aerosols and humidity are used to achieve the following four general objectives: *relief of bronchospasm and respiratory mucosal edema, mobilization of bronchial secretions for easier removal, administration of antibiotics,* and *humidification of the respiratory tract.* Without attempting to penetrate the field of pharmacology to any depth, we will describe some of the more commonly used medications, for although the inhalation therapist does not prescribe, he must be aware of the major effects of all therapy he administers. Only with such knowledge can he give safe and effective care to his patients, always on the alert for adverse reactions to treatment.

Relief of bronchospasm and mucosal edema

These two conditions are paired, for not only are they frequently associated, but many of the medications employed in therapy are effective against both. Those agents designed to reduce bronchospasm and edema are called, respectively, *bronchodilators* and *decongestants.* It should be emphasized that we are here referring only to those that are used as aerosols, for there are many bronchodilators and a few decongestants that can be administered parenterally (by injection) or orally. Bronchodilators increase the lumen of the airways by relaxing the spasm of the bronchial muscle, which was triggered by disease or irritation. Decongestants (agents that relieve "congestion") function in one of two ways. Most cause a contraction of the muscle fibers of the arterioles and small arteries, thereby reducing blood flow to the affected area and lowering the hydrostatic pressure that permits fluid to move into the tissues. Others interfere with the natural defense mechanism that stimulates increased blood flow to an injured area and are called "anti-inflammatory" in action. For purposes of discussion, a bronchodilator and decongestant can be classified as *sympathomimetic, parasympatholytic, xanthine,* and *adrenocorticosteriod.* Awkward as they appear at first glance, these names have meanings that indicate either their origins or modes of action, features that are common to the terminology of many drugs with which the therapist will come into contact.

Sympathomimetic. This type of drug "mimics" the physiologic action of the sympathetic nervous system, and because both it and the sympathetic system are so important to medicine generally, a brief review of the latter at this point should be of value. In addition to the extensive system of nerves that govern actions of the voluntary muscles and carry the various bodily sensations to the brain, there is an important segment of the overall nervous system called the "autonomic nervous system." This functions beyond the level of our conscious control, does not respond to our voluntary demands, and is under the control of various centers of the brain. In short, the autonomic system performs its many duties, minute by minute, whether we are awake or asleep, according to impulses received by the higher centers that are transmitted to them automatically. The autonomic nerves, among other things, govern the activities of the cardiac muscle, the smooth or involuntary muscle of all bodily systems, the digestive and genitourinary systems, the sweat glands, and certain endocrine glands. In a general way it may be said that autonomic control maintains stability among the many interacting systems of the body, combatting any factor that would change the so-called "internal environment" much as our voluntary actions help us to adjust to the external environment. This internal balance is referred to as *homeostasis.*

The autonomic nervous system is itself divided into two subsystems—the *sympathetic* and the *parasympathic* divisions—and most of the structures listed above are innervated (supplied with nerves) by both. Broadly speaking, we say the effects of each subdivision on a given receptor organ are antagonistic to the other; inactivity of one allows the action of the other to dominate the organ response. Each thus exerts a constant action against the other, like two forces maintaining a steady pull on each end of a rope. This action is called *tone,* and it establishes a balance of influence on receptor function, assuring fine control over function and rapid response. Generally, the sympathetic division is designed to protect the integrity and maintain the safety of the organism, which involves the expenditure of energy. The parasympathetic, on the other hand, is less kinetic in its objectives and is more concerned with conservation and restoration of function. A few examples of these opposing actions are listed in Table 7-3.

To relate this to the field of aerosol therapy, the student is encouraged to consult a standard text on physiology and review the autonomic innervation of the cardiovascular and respiratory systems. He will then see clearly how a "sympathomimetic" drug will elict such responses as bronchial dilatation, arterial and arteriolar constriction, elevation of cardiac rate and blood pres-

Table 7-3. *Sympathetic and parasympathetic action*

Organ	*Sympathetic*	*Parasympathetic*
Ocular pupil	Dilatation	Constriction
Bronchi	Dilatation	Constriction
Heart	Stimulation	Inhibition
Intestine	Inhibition	Stimulation

sure, and stimulation of the central nervous system with wakefulness and jitteriness. It should be added here, that the action of a drug which elevates the blood pressure by increasing the peripheral arterial resistance through vasoconstriction is referred to as a *vasopressor effect.* It is evident that most of the sympathetic responses do not contribute to the objectives we are now discussing but constitute what we term "side effects." Thus, the ideal drug would be one that gives the maximum bronchial dilatation and local vasoconstriction and a minimum of other reactions. The search for such a drug is responsible for the large number of commercial preparations and combinations available on the market.

EPINEPHRINE (Adrenaline, Suprarenin). The "parent" therapeutic sympathomimetic from which most others are derived or to which they are related, epinephrine is a biologic produced in the *medulla,* or central portion, of the adrenal glands. It performs important functions in regulating the body's metabolism and maintaining a state of alertness to cope with the environment. The therapist will see this drug used frequently in the hospital for its effect on the circulation and to combat allergic reactions, for which purposes it will be administered by injection under the skin, into muscle, or into superficial veins. It is practically completely inactivated in the stomach; thus oral use is not feasable, but it has been used parenterally for many years for the relief of acute bronchial asthma.

Epinephrine is one of the most powerful bronchodilators and decongestants, whether given by injection or by aerosol. Indeed, its action by aerosol is both *topical* (local, by application to a surface) and *systemic* (distributed to many parts of the body), since the small particles act by direct contact with the bronchial mucosa and are also absorbed into the circulation by way of the pulmonary flow. Thus, inhalation generally affords quicker response than does subcutaneous or intramuscular injection, although not exceeding the intravenous route. There are two major hazards to aerosolized epinephrine. First, the unwanted side effects may be a danger as well as a nuisance, and the effect upon the cardiovascular system may outweigh its benefits. This is especially true in elderly patients or those with known heart or vascular disease. Second, repeated use of epinephrine often leads to a condition of "fastness," in which there is a progressive decreasing response to the drug and dangerously larger doses are required for therapeutic effect. A patient exhibiting this phenomenon is considered to be epinephrine-fast. Less commonly seen but worthy of note is a third complication apparently attributable to any of the sympathomimetic compounds by which the symptoms of acute bronchial asthma are made worse by these aerosols. It is felt that this adverse effect is due to the development of an allergy to some of the metabolic end products of the drugs.[89]

If epinephrine is to be used as a bronchodilator-decongestant aerosol, nothing stronger than a 1% aqueous solution (1:100) should be considered safe, and this must not be mistaken for the 1:1000 solution used parenterally. Two effective inhalations from 30 to 60 seconds apart should suffice, and treatments should be spaced at least 4 hours apart. Because of the development of safer preparations, some of which are described below, the use of epinephrine aerosol has rapidly declined in recent years.

RACEMIC EPINEPHRINE (Vaponefrin, Asthmanefrin). A synthetic form of epinephrine but with one half its vasopressor effect, racemic epinephrine has actions similar to those of regular epinephrine. As an aerosol it is used in a 2.25% solution, with the same precautions kept in mind as with epinephrine. The inhalation therapist will soon learn that the response to any given medication varies markedly from patient to patient and what is well tolerated by one patient may elicit severe undesirable reactions in another. Because of this, no matter what degree of safety is claimed for a particular product, the therapist must ever be aware of potential side effects.

ISOPROTERENOL (Isuprel and Aludrine as the hydrochloride, Norisodrine as the sulfate). A major advantage of this aerosol is its somewhat better bronchodilating effect than that of epinephrine, with nearly complete absence of vasopressor action. In contrast to epinephrine, isoproterenol produces vasodilatation and thus has negligible decongestant value. It tends to lower diastolic and not systolic blood pressure but may encourage a sinus tachycardia. Its symptomatic side effects are infrequent, tend to be mild, and include nausea, excitement, tremors, and rapid heart action.[90]

Although available in aqueous concentrations of 1:100 and 1:200, for routine aerosol use the *1:200 strength is recommended.* For intermittent short-term therapy, as in self-administration, two to four well-spaced inhalations at 4-hour intervals is a conservative program although the general safety of the drug allows for considerable flexibility according to clinical need. It can be noted here that, since all aerosols are, in a sense, foreign bodies, overuse of them often causes severe pharyngeal and laryngeal irritation, further aggravating the very condition being treated. Warning of this possibility should be included in instructions given to all patients who are to treat themselves. For prolonged bronchodilatation, especially as administered with mechanical ventilators, the isoproterenol should be further diluted to concentrations of 1:400 or 1:600.

CYCLOPENTAMINE (Clopane hydrochloride). Used alone in a 0.5% to 1.0% aqueous solution, cyclopentamine is a powerful vasoconstrictor administered by fine spray (atomization) or direct application to the nose for control of nasal mucosal congestion and nasal bleeding. For pulmonary aerosol therapy, it is an ingredient in a compound trade-named Aerolone. Cyclopentamine, 0.5%, is combined with isoproterenol, 0.25%, in water and propylene glycol to afford the dual actions of bronchodilatation and decongestion. The usual precautions must be observed as with any potent sympathomimetic, and occasionally such side effects as insomnia, nervousness, and tachycardia may be expected.

The inhalation therapist may have occasion to note the presence of propylene glycol in many liquid preparations, and its function might well be explained at this time. Propylene glycol is a fairly simple organic compound, related to glycerin but less irritating, that is frequently used as a vehicle or solvent for active substances to be administered by intramuscular injection and is itself completely inert physiologically. In liquids designed for aerosol use, advantage is taken of another characteristic of propylene glycol: it is hygroscopic, and through its ability to absorb water it supposedly will minimize shrinkage of aerosol particles by evaporation as the particles enter the warmth of the respiratory tract. However, the probability is just as great that aerosol size may so increase through hygroscopic growth that penetration will be hampered; and it is sometimes suspected that aerosol particles may become so stable that they exert no therapeutic effect in the respiratory tract and are exhaled intact.

PHENYLEPHRINE (Neo-Synephrine as the hydrochloride). This is a vasopressor and as such is a potent decongestant, frequently used in nasal preparations. Phenylephrine is less a bronchodilator than is isoproterenol, but the two compounds are combined as a solid-particle aerosol (one of the few in common use) in a pressurized capsule for simultaneous relief of constriction and congestion. It has been claimed that decrease in airway resistance (an objective sign of bronchodilatation) is longer lasting following the administration of both phenylephrine and isoproterenol than following the administration of isoproterenol alone, regardless of the method of aerosolization.[91]

ISOETHARINE (Dilabron). With a bronchodilating effect less than that of isoproterenol, isoetharine is more potent than epinephrine. It can be given orally and for this purpose is often combined with an antihistamine and a decongestant. The cardiovascular effects of isoetharine are similar to those of isoproterenol but are less intense.[92] It is reported to be more effective in conditions characterized predominantly by bronchospasm, such as bronchial asthma, than by increased secretions, as in chronic bronchitis.[93]

This by no means exhausts the list of available sympathomimetics used as aerosols, and there are a great variety of combinations. The therapist will develop a habit of reading the descriptive literature of all new medications with which he comes in contact and will at least note those products pertaining to his work that are advertized in the medical journals.

Parasympatholytic: In contrast to the sympathomimetic type of drug just described, the parasympatholytic does not imitate the parasympathetic system but rather *inactivates* the system's function. The suffix *lytic* derives from the verb to lyse, or destroy. Thus we can expect, in a general way, that a parasympatholytic will produce a response similar to that of an administered sympathomimetic by allowing sympathetic system effect on the target organ free of parasympathetic restraint. The only drug of this type applicable to aerosol therapy is *atropine,* and even though it is but slightly used in current techniques, it is of sufficient potential interest to deserve description. The systemic and topical administration of atropine, its derivatives, and synthetic preparations has wide application in many other medical fields.

ATROPINE. This is an alkaloid derived from the plant *Atropa belladonna.* As is characteristic of all alkaloids, plant or animal, atropine is a complex nitrogenous organic compound with potent physiologic and toxic properties. In its pharmacologic action it depresses the reactions of structures supplied by the parasympathetic nervous system. The most extensive of the cranial nerves are the paired vagus nerves, large conveyors of parasympathetic fibers. Coursing from the brain, the vagi pass through the neck, supplying all the organs in the thorax, and continue into the abdomen, where they innervate the digestive system and other abdominal viscera. Thus, in our area of interest the action of atropine inhibits vagal stimulation of the heart and respiratory tract, elevating blood pressure and cardiac rate and dilating bronchi by paralyzing the terminals of the vagal parasympathetic nerve endings. In addition, atropine is felt to have action in the central nervous system, stimulating the cerebral respiratory center to generate rapid, deep breathing.[94]

The beneficial effect of atropine on bronchoconstriction has been well demonstrated in airways that were subjected to dust inhalation and protected by the drug parenterally administered.[95] Aerosol studies have employed 1.0% and 0.2% concentrations of atropine in equal parts of propylene glycol and water.[96] It has been emphasized that the medication must be microaerosolized, with mean particle diameters from 0.03μ to 0.05μ. This avoids potential toxic effects from the powerful drug by assuring maximal deposition in the alveoli and minimizing absorption from the upper tract. Through the use of very small particle size, total dosage of the alkaloid is kept within safe limits, but microaerosolization to such a controlled degree can be achieved only with specialized equipment, to be described later. With the proper administration of atropine aerosol, airway resistance can be significantly reduced in normal subjects as well as in obstructed patients. Bronchi are also protected against the induced bronchospasm of inhaled irritants such as carbachol and aluminum dust. It was also found that results were equally satisfactory with the 0.2% as the 1.0% solution. It has been suggested that atropine in small amounts be added to sympathomimetic mixtures, if microaerosol generators can be used.

Xanthine (aminophylline). There is a group of vegetable organic compounds called the xanthines, of which the three most important are *caffeine,* *theophylline*, and *theobromine*. We are all familiar with caffeine as the important ingredient of coffee, tea, and cocoa, but the xanthine group as a whole has some specific physiologic actions that make them valuable as pharmacologics. Although the degree to which these three react varies, in general, their activity includes the following: central nervous system stimulation, respiratory stimulation, smooth muscle relaxation, diuresis (increased production of urine), coronary artery dilatation, cardiac stimulation, and skeletal muscle stimulation. It is evident that there is a great potential for the medical use of these substances. Frequently used in the past for cardiac stimulation (caffeine) and diuresis (theobromine), for the most part, they have been replaced by more effective agents, with the exception of theophylline. This agent, compounded as theophylline ethylenediamine is known as aminophylline and still plays an important role in therapeutics. It is useful in certain types and stages of congestive heart failure and is especially valuable in correcting Cheyne-Stokes ventilation, but we will confine our discussion to its use as a bronchodilator.

The therapist will see aminophylline frequently used for patients with diffuse bronchospasm, and in cases of intractable bronchial asthma, especially when there is refractoriness to the sympathomimetics. The usual mode of administration is intravenous, adding to a saline infusion the contents of a 20 ml ampule of the drug, containing 0.5 gm. Intramuscular and rectal routes are sometimes used, but these are less effective, and aminophylline is extremely irritating to the gastric mucosa unless given as a specially coated tablet. Rapid administration may produce such side effects as headache, rapid heart action, dizziness, hyperventilation, nausea, and hypotension; but with care, these are usually not a significant problem.

As an aerosol, aminophylline has not enjoyed as widespread usage as the sympathomimetics, although the effectiveness of this technique has been recognized for many years.[97] The intravenous preparation is used for aerosolization, by any convenient method available. Continuous nebulization has been used, until relief is obtained, often requiring as much as 0.5 to 0.7 gm of aminophylline. Intermittent therapy, with positive pressure or an aerosol mask, alone or in conjunction with sympathomimetics, is also effective in bronchial asthma. Because of the relatively small amounts of the drug absorbed, side effects of aerosol administration are very rare.[98,99] It seems practical to consider aerosolized aminophylline in those patients with diffuse bronchospasm who no longer respond to safe doses of sympathomimetics, for the speed of action and economy of the latter still justify their consideration as first-line drugs.

Adrenocorticosteroid. The drugs in this group have assumed a position of great importance in the therapy of almost all branches of medicine. Again, although we are interested in a relatively limited aspect of their use at present, some general background knowledge of them is essential because the therapist will encounter them throughout his patient care experience. For the sake of convenience, we will use the commonly employed abbreviated expression "steroid," with the understanding that we mean adrenocorticosteroid. We must understand also that, like many familiar terms, it is not really correct; for steroids comprise a large group of organic compounds, many of which have other physiologic properties than those in which we are interested. The steroids that will concern us are potent hormones secreted by the *cortex* (outer layer) of the adrenal glands, as opposed to the sympathomimetic products of the adrenal medulla, already described. There are some five general groups of complex organic compounds produced in the adrenal cortex, of which the only one of importance to our present needs is the *glucocorticoids.* The name of this group derives from its involvement in carbohydrate metabolism, and its two most clinically useful members are *cortisol* and *cortisone.* There are available many commercial preparations and modifications of these two, with variable potencies and supposed specific responses.

The adrenal steroids exert a tremendous influence upon the body physiology, touching all organ systems. They have been referred to as "stress hormones" because they are excreted in excessive amounts when the body is put under stress, and severe trauma or prolonged grave illness may cause a depletion of their supply. In a complex way, the steroids give support to the body to aid it through a crisis, and if they are acutely depleted or if their production is interrupted by abrupt destruction of the adrenals, the body functions deteriorate rapidly. On the other hand, a slow, chronic increase of cortical function does not produce a catastrophic picture but rather a multiplicity of signs and symptoms described as *Cushing's syndrome.* A patient beginning to show evidence of excessive steroid action is often referred to as "Cushinoid." We will describe some of the more common and important effects of hyperadrenalism, to illustrate the wide range of steroid action. The glucocorticoids have the following effects.[100-102]

FORMATION OF GLUCOSE FROM BODY PROTEIN. When excessive, this can raise the blood sugar level high enough to produce "steroid diabetes" or to activate a latent, subclinical true diabetes. There can be associated protein loss with muscle wasting and weakness.

DEPLETION OF BONE CALCIUM. Through a process of resorption, calcium is removed from bone, so thinning its consistency that fractures are frequent. This state of the bone is called *osteoporosis.*

INCREASE IN FAT PRODUCTION. Excessive amounts of fat are produced, also from body protein, and are characteristically deposited in the subcutaneous tissues of the head and trunk. This results in a marked rounding of the facial contour, referred to as *moon face,* and an accumulation of fat at the base of the neck and upper back, called *buffalo hump.* These are two of the most prominent visible signs of a Cushinoid state.

IMPAIRMENT OF IMMUNOLOGIC RESPONSE. Steroids inactivate circulating antibodies and thus can protect the body against the harmful effects of severe allergies. By the same token, however, this function lowers the body's resistance to infection, a point of significance in the therapeutic use of steroids.

REDUCTION OF INFLAMMATORY RESPONSE. There is a decrease in the local vascular congestion and cellular infiltration that is the natural response to injury or infection. In addition, the deposition of fibrous tissue as part of the reparative process is inhibited. Of use in controlling the adverse effects of inflammation, this function also facilitates the spread of infection, since it interferes with the usual process of localization. This is a serious threat to the patient with quiescent tuberculosis.

INCREASE OF GASTRIC ACIDITY. This predisposes to the development of stomach ulcer, or the worsening of one already present. Bleeding and rupture are ever-present risks.

ELEVATION OF BLOOD PRESSURE. Steroids, through the mediation of certain electrolytes and other hormones, elevate the blood pressure. Of therapeutic significance, in state of shock, when the cardiovascular system no longer responds to sympathomimetics, steroids often aid the vasoconstrictors to regain their pressor effects on the arterioles.

To complete the review of steroid action, mention should be made of the pituitary gland. The adrenal cortex is directly controlled by the anterior division of the pituitary gland, through a pituitary hormone called *adrenocorticotropic hormone.* The name itself describes a substance that stimulates *(-tropic)* the adrenal cortex and, not surprisingly, is almost always referred to as ACTH. Administration of ACTH can be expected to elicit the same response as cortisol and cortisone, by stimulating the adrenal production of these substances. This presupposes that the adrenal cortex is in a functioning state, able to respond. Because, during the therapeutic administration of steroids, the adrenals are apt to slacken in their activity (the body is receiving adequate hormone from its outside source), there is risk of adrenal atrophy with prolonged loss of function. Under such circumstances, ACTH may be given for periods of time to stimulate the adrenals to function and to prevent their atrophy.

For the most part, in the treatment of respiratory diseases, steroids are administered orally and parenterally. They are used for their potent anti-inflammatory and antifibrogenic effects in acute and chronic obstructive diseases and in resistant allergies of the respiratory tract. The therapist will have occasion to witness dramatic responses to steroid therapy, especially in the patient acutely obstructed by intractable bronchospasm and mucosal edema. However, because of the almost inevitable development of some side effects or because so many patients have conditions that contraindicate these drugs, it has been hoped that aerosol administration might offer a safer route for prolonged therapy. It was felt that such topical application directly to the target organ might give enhanced action with a smaller total dose. So far, no unanimity of opinion has brought this hope to reality, and although steroid aerosol enjoys moderate acceptance, it has not yet become a major agent.

Many steroids have been tried, but the one most generally used, potent and of small molecular size, is *dexamethasone,* which we will describe.

Dexamethazone sodium phosphate. Commercially available in a gas-propelled pressurized capsule, dexamethasone can be used alone or mixed with isoproterenol. It is the general concensus of its users that this steroid is therapeutically active and effective throughout the entire respiratory tract from the nose to the bronchioles in the treatment of nasal allergies, allergic asthma, and some chronic obstructive states.[103,104] However, with no doubt concerning its local effects, dexamethasone has been found to have very definite systemic effects, readily detected by special urinary excretion tests. Some investigators feel that the local responses in the respiratory tract are significantly greater than the systemic and thus justify its use.[105] Others have found a safe dosage difficult to control by aerosol administration, with Cushinoid symptoms of prior oral administration unrelieved by the change to aerosol, and believe that it has no place in therapy at this time.[106] Still other users have found therapeutic results with aerosol application as effective as the oral route, but they warn of the risk of complications of self-administered medication.[107] This is always a hazard inherent in any procedure when the patient is responsible for his own therapy on a home-treatment program. The risk is increased with use of a drug whose unfavorable side effects may develop insidiously rather than acutely.

Other steroids have been investigated for their therapeutic potential as aerosols. *Prednisone* (as the acetate), a popular oral form of this group, has been found to have satisfactory physiologic effects, but it apparently tends to produce bronchospasm.[108] Although the addition of bronchodilators to the program aleviates the spasm, the irritant effects of the steroid are not completely eliminated and dexamethasone remains the aerosol drug of choice.

Determination of the actual dose of steroid aerosol to be administered is a matter of professional judgment and is the responsibility of the attending physician. By and large, since steroid aerosols are usually packaged in self-administered gas-propelled units, the physician gives directions for the use directly to his patient. However, should the therapist be assigned to oversee the patient's treatment program, he should make certain that the physician is specific in his orders. Whereas this should be the practice for any treatment, there are many instances in which established routines can be used, allowing the therapist some flexibility to adjust techniques to individual needs. The great potency of the steroids and the possibility of adverse reactions mitigate against their administration by anything less than specific instructions for each patient. The many variables that influence the efficiency of aerosol treatment, such as function of the nebulizer, depth of ventilation, and ventilatory rate, make it impossible to predict the systemic absorption of the drug. The physician must "play it by ear," judging total dosage necessary by clinical response.

Mobilization of bronchial secretions

Of all the agents used to modify the character of respiratory tract secretions, rendering them more fluid for easier removal, none is more important than water; but the very importance of water justifies a separate discussion, which will be undertaken below. Our concern here will be with those physical and chemical substances that are used with water for sputum mobilization. We are already well aware of the great hazard to health and life from airway obstruction, and the relief of bronchospasm and mucosal edema corrects only a part of this serious defect. In a large percentage of patients suffering from chronic bronchopulmonary disease, the presence of increased amounts of sputum, or increased viscosity of the sputum, is a major cause of ventilatory disability. We will describe the aerosols most frequently used for removal of bronchial secretions, arbitrarily dividing them into the two groups of *mucolytics* and *proteolytics*. The former are most effective against sputum that is predominantly mucoid, and the latter against purulent sputum with its high protein content. Some products are claimed to be of equal value against both.

Mucolytics. Although *mucolysis* means the disruption of the long chains of organic compounds that constitute mucoid sputum, fragmenting them into smaller more mobile molecules, we will include here, for convenience, *wetting agents*. These substances do not break molecular bonds, but through their surface-active effects they lessen the integrity of secretions and aid in their separation from airway walls.

WETTING AGENTS (detergents). Tyloxapol and sodium ethasulfate are two such agents in clinical use, the former prepared commercially as Alevaire and the latter as Tergemist. Because of the greater general experience with tyloxapol, it will be discussed as the prototype of wetting agents. Tyloxapol actually has two active ingredients: it is an aqueous solution of 0.125% tyloxapol (also known as Superione) and 2% sodium bicarbonate (along with 5% glycerin for stability, as described above for propylene glycol). Sodium bicarbonate in this concentration has, itself, mucolytic properties, for some of the polysaccharides will separate in a sufficiently alkaline medium. In vitro studies of the action of tyloxapol on homogenized specimens of sputum demonstrated its surfactant action. The sputum, with a measured surface tension of 52 dynes/cm, was not altered in the addition of water; but when subjected to the action of tyloxapol, the surface tension dropped 20%.[109] It was concluded that a second major function of the wetting agent took place at the wet surface interface between the respiratory mucosa and the mucoid layer, breaking the adherence of the mucus to the bronchial wall. This allowed the mucoid layer to be separated and then removed by cough.

Tyloxapol has been used for several years, and although the mechanical effect of its detergent on mucoid specimens in the laboratory is unquestioned, there is still not a uniform opinion as to its value in clinical application. Many feel that it is effective in removing secretions from both sinuses and bronchi and can be used continuously for long periods of time for its humidifying effects as well as its mucolysis.[110,111] In the treatment of acute infections of the respiratory tract, tyloxapol has been found to increase the effectiveness of simultaneously administered antibiotics.[112] Other users feel strongly that the value of tyloxapol lies in the humidifying effects of its water-glycerin solvent and that the wetting agent does not influence viscosity or amount of sputum or clinical improvement.[113] It has been suggested that subjecting the bronchioles and alveoli to detergent action may produce such histologic changes in the lung as membrane damage and interstitial infiltration, sometimes seen in postmortem examination of patients succumbing to ventilatory failure. Such diverse opinions are not unusual on any type of treatment. When a new therapy is proposed, there is typically great enthusiasm for its hoped-for success, much of which is generated by its promoter, and it is only after considerable practical experience that exaggerated claims are disproved, more specific indications for its use are recognized, and effective techniques for its application are developed. Then its proper role in clinical medicine can be evaluated. It might be opportune to note here that the anticipated results of any treatment are usually in direct proportion to the skill with which the treatment is administered. This is especially pertinent to inhalation therapy, in which, because of its rapid growth and extensive use, we can never be certain that uniformly efficient techniques are employed in a given circumstance. This point must be kept in mind when we try to reconcile conflicting clinical data. The therapeutic use of wetting agents might be summarized by saying that they do have a limited effect on bronchial secretions and, by rendering these secretions less viscid, will supplement the efforts of an existing effective cough mechanism. They are physiologically nontoxic and, when employed as a vehicle for other active substances, enhance the latter's probability of contact with respiratory tissue. It should be emphasized, however, that detergents have little value against frankly purulent sputum.

ACETYLCYSTEINE (*N*-acetyl-L-cysteine, Mucomyst). In the search for agents other than detergents effective in breaking the mucoproteins responsible for the viscosity of sputum in chronic respiratory diseases, the action of the naturally occurring amino acid, L-cysteine, was studied. Although it was found to be a potent mucolytic, it had irritating properties that could be eliminated by modifying the acid into an acetyl form, as it is now employed. The chemical reaction between acetylcysteine and bronchial mucus has been extensively studied,[114] and basically it consists of a disruption of chemical bonds holding together segments of the long-chain mucoproteins by the direct action of specific groups of the amino acid. It is thus a true mucolytic and reduces the viscosity of mucoid sputum in direct proportion to its concentration. Some claim is made for a liquefying action on purulent sputum, but since acetylcysteine has no specificity for the ribonucleic acids characteristic of purulency, such action is probably indirect and mediated through associated mucoid components.

Some studies have indicated that, when acetylcysteine is used as a 20%

solution, mucolysis is as effective with a 10% concentration and, whereas the stronger preparation tends to induce bronchospasm in some patients, the lesser strength is a neglibile hazard.[115] Other studies have found both 10% and 20% to be harmless, neither producing significant bronchospasm.[116] The possibility of damage to alveolar surfactant has been of concern with the inhalation of microaerosols of any kind, and especially with one of potent lytic qualities. Examination of both human and animal lung tissue after use of 10% acetylcysteine aerosol showed no change in surface activity.[117] Serious complications are rare. A burning sensation in the upper passages is occasionally reported, and nausea may be experienced. Some patients complain of the rotten-egg odor, but most become adjusted to it quickly and appear to ignore it.

In general, the clinical response to this aerosol for the removal of mucoid secretions has been favorable, with indications for its use covering a wide range, from the cystic fibrosis of childhood (in which it seems to have scored considerable success), through the suppurative lung diseases, to the chronic bronchitis-emphysema of late adulthood.[118,119] Nevertheless, a small minority have felt that acetylcysteine, though effective in vitro, has not shown any benefit in patients and is of no clinical value.[120] Of interest, in reference to comments made above, one source felt that the aerosol was effective in cleansing the upper airways but did not aid the lower regions, and expressed the opinion that this is probably the fault of inadequate equipment or techniques currently available.[121] We shall see shortly that there are aerosol generators able to supply particles of a tremendous size range for the deposition of medication to any level of the respiratory tract. Failure of particles to reach the target area should not be a reason for lack of anticipated response.

A very practical point to note is the chemical reactivity between acetylcysteine and certain component parts of nebulization equipment, especially iron, copper, and rubber. To avoid the loss of potency of such reactions, parts coming in contact with the amino acid (liquid or aerosol) should be made of glass, plastic, aluminum, chromed metal, silver, or stainless steel.

There is no critical dosage schedule for administering acetylcysteine aerosol; it is used according to individual needs. It can be administered by hand nebulizer, pump, or aerosol mask, and in positive-pressure breathing devices, but the drug itself should not be put in a heated nebulizer. In addition to the aerosol route, acetylcysteine is often effectively used by direct instillation, especially to facilitate bronchial aspiration through tracheostomy or endotracheal tubes.

ETHYL ALCOHOL (ethanol). With an indication, real or optional, in almost all aspects of man's activities, we should not be surprised to find alcohol included among the therapeutic aerosols. In contrast to most of its uses, however, its virtue as an aerosol depends upon its local action in the respiratory tract. As a matter of convenience, alcohol is included with the mucolytics, although not without some justification, for it is used to reduce surface tension of pulmonary fluids. Its action is not directed primarily to abnormal mucoid substances but rather to the thinner but equally hazardous edema fluid that frequently obstructs bronchioles and alveoli. Aerosolized alcohol performs a valuable service in the treatment of acute pulmonary edema and can often be helpful in cases of low-grade edema. Before positive-pressure ventilators had reached their present sophisticated state of efficiency, recognition of the potential of aerosolized alcohol added an important new weapon against pulmonary edema.[122]

From whatever cause, acute pulmonary edema is characterized by the accumulation in the alveoli and bronchioles of a thin watery fluid, often containing some blood. There is enough protein in edema fluid to produce froth as air passes through it with tidal ventilation. A relatively small volume of fluid can thus be increased to a much larger volume of massed bubbles that severly obstruct the small airways and alveoli. It is this frothy edema fluid that so seriously compromises the alveolar ventilation/perfusion ratio and in a sense drowns the patient in his own water.

The function of aerosolized alcohol is to mix with the edema fluid and lower its surface tension so that the bubbles will lose their stability, rupture, and return to the liquid state. Liquid not only occupies less alveolar space, but its removal is made easier by way of the cough mechanism and the perfusing circulation. Considering the surface tensions of both tissue fluid and blood plasma, if for the sake of illustration we assume edema fluid to be composed of equal parts of each, we can give to the alveolar and bronchiolar froth a surface tension of somewhere around 60 dynes per centimeter. In contrast, four concentrations of alcohol are shown with their approximate surface tensions in dynes per centimeter: 25% = 34; 30% = 32; 50% = 28; 100% = 22. Mixing any of these with edema fluid will lower the surface tension of the resulting solution, and froth will be converted to liquid. At times, this phenomenon produces dramatic clinical results, with relief of acute hypoxia evident in a few minutes.

Concentrations between 25% and 50% are suitable for therapeutic effect, without undue risk of local airway irritation. Although absorption does occur in the alveoli, the actual amounts of alcohol in the bloodstream at any one time are well within the limits of sobriety. Alcohol can be given by any standard aerosol generator by way of oropharyngeal catheter, mask, or positive pressure. The latter two applications are preferred for the treatment of acute episodes. More will be said of therapy in the discussion of mechanical ventilation, for an inhalation therapist on night duty in an active general hospital will have many opportunities to treat acute pulmonary edema in his emergency room.

SODIUM BICARBONATE (baking soda). Reference was made to the mucolytic effect of this common household commodity in the above discussion of the action of tyloxapol. Large mucoid molecular chains tend to break as the pH of their environment rises, and local bronchial alkalinity can reach a pH of 8.3

without untoward irritation or damage.[109] Indeed, the treatment of acutely obstructive episodes of cystic fibrosis often includes, along with other modalities, the deliberate production of systemic alkalosis by the intravenous and oral administration of bicarbonate, to make full use of its mucolytic properties. Although this regimen is less necessary with the availability of more potent mucolytics, such as acetylcysteine and proteolytics (to be discussed next), sodium bicarbonate aerosol still has a place not only in this disease but also in chronic states of the adult. It is not uncommon to encounter patients in whom mucolysis from the usually effective agents lessens, and for such patients it is occasionally beneficial to switch to aerosolized 2% sodium bicarbonate to see whether mucus flow can be stimulated. For home use, a teaspoonful of the soda in a cup of water makes a readily available solution.

Proteolytics. As the name indicates, members of this group lyse the protein material found in purulent sputum, and although there is only one commercial preparation for all practical purposes, enjoying widespread use, a brief description of the development of this therapy is felt to be pertinent here. Because the effectiveness of mucolytics decreases with increasing purulency of bronchial secretions, the early efforts to find an adjuvant agent centered on *trypsin,* a proteinase (enzyme active against protein) of the pancreas. Trypsin plays an important role in the natural digestion of ingested protein, but it is most effective on protein that is already partially digested. It also acts on respiratory and intestinal mucin and on fibrin. The use of trypsin as an aerosol demonstrated its effectiveness in cleansing the upper airways of proteinacious accumulations, apparently without damage to living cells or impairment of ciliary function. Some early investigators were disappointed with its results, feeling that it sometimes worsened the obstruction. Hoarseness was a frequent and troublesome complication, attributed to too high concentrations of the drug or too rapid administration.[123-125] Aerosolized trypsin was used for several years, and in my opinion produced fairly satisfactory results, superior to other products then available. There were a few febrile reactions noted, and because of the real or imagined risk of an allergic reaction, it was common to include an antihistamine in the treatment program. The effectiveness of a proteolytic aerosol was enough to prompt further search for better products, and trypsin has now been replaced by dornase.

DORNASE (pancreatic dornase, pancreatic deoxyribonuclease, Dornavac). Dornase is not a digestant in the same manner as trypsin although it, too, is an important natural proteolytic. It is more specific in its action than is trypsin, since it depolymerizes (breaks long chains into smaller ones) deoxyribonucleic acid (DNA).[126] Therapeutically, this is most important, since it has been determined that from 30% to 70% of the solid matter of purulent secretions is composed of DNA.[127] The principle source of dornase is beef pancreas, but dornase is also produced by the pathogenic bacterium hemolytic streptococcus. Indeed, the filtrate of a culture of hemolytic streptococcus contains two active enzymes, streptococcal fibrinolysin (streptokinase) and streptococcal deoxyribonuclease (streptodornase). We might infer from its name that streptokinase acts mostly on fibrous tissue and as such is not particularly relevant to our present needs. A combination of these two enzymes is commercially prepared as Varidase, and although it is rather widely used for local application and intracavitary instillation, it has had limited use as an aerosol.[128,129]

Clinically, dornase is indicated in any bronchopulmonary condition in which the accumulation of purulent sputum interferes with ventilation or with the resolution of an infection. It is thus of use in pneumonia, pulmonary abscess, bronchiectasis, cystic fibrosis, and especially in an acute respiratory infection superimposed on chronic lung disease.[130] As might be expected, there are some who feel that enzyme aerosols have no useful role in clinical medicine.[131] However, after using pancreatic dornase for many years, I believe it to be one of the most valuable of available aerosols, for *specific* use. It is effective only against infected sputum, and indications for its use can be determined by visual examination of the sputum for color and consistency. For predominantly mucoid secretions it is of little value. No significant side reactions have been noted, and the only common patient complaint is post-treatment burning of the mouth, easily prevented by a vigorous mouthwash immediately following therapy. Inhalation of 100,000 units two to three times daily for 2 to 4 days is generally sufficient, but such a course can be repeated as frequently as necessary. Dornase is also useful for intralumenal instillation, as an adjunct to aerosol therapy, when gross airway obstruction is present. During dornase therapy, the attending therapist must always be ready to aspirate the liquefied secretions if the patient's cough is inadequate, a precaution of great importance in the unresponsive patient being supported by mechanical ventilation.

Administration of antibiotics

When it became apparent that a new effective route was available for the administration of drugs, interest soon developed in the use of this new route in treating respiratory tract infections, especially such localized bronchopulmonary diseases as lung abscess, necrotizing pneumonia, and bronchiectasis, which were especially resistent to conventional therapy. In the mid-1940's sulfonamides were aerosolized, but the advent of penicillin and subsequent antibiotics stimulated extensive use of aerosols and the accumulation of a significant background of experience.[132-137]

The rationale for aerosol therapy was based on the speculation that, even with adequate blood levels of systemically administered antibiotics, the diffusion of the drug from blood into infected tissue for its direct antibacterial action was blocked by tissue reaction to the infection. In localized lesions, especially, it was felt that the presence of thick bronchial and alveolar exudates comprised a formidable diffusion barrier. Also, it was felt probable that interstitial edema and fibrosis of the diseased area were additional factors in preventing therapeutic antibiotic tissue levels. These observations were borne out by the frequent observation of active microbial growth in sputum while intensive systemic therapy was being administered.

At one time or other, most of the standard antibiotic drugs have been tried in aerosol form. The list includes, at least, penicillin, streptomycin, neomycin, polymixin B, novobiocin, tetracycline, oxytetracycline, chloramphenicol, kanamycin, gentimicin, and colistin. The reported results make it apparent that there is no magic cure in the technique of aerosolization and that although some patients respond dramatically others show little or no benefit.[138,139] In view of the modifying factors listed above and with the variability of bacterial susceptibility encountered in systemic therapy, this is not surprising. However, the efficacy of aerosolized antibiotics can be significantly increased by using a technique that deserves special mention.[140] The same exudates and secretions that impair drug diffusion from blood to tissue are able to interfere with the action of aerosolized particles, and they are probably responsible for many instances of therapeutic failure. The prior or concommitant use of bronchodilators will aid penetration of antibiotic particles but will not bring them into bacterial contact in the presence of thick secretions. The most promising procedure entails combining antibiotics with pancreatic dornase. The latter reduces viscosity of purulent sputum and, while so doing, exposes the infecting organism to the action of the inhaled antibiotic. Assuming that the antibiotic has significant potency against the organism, therapeutic bactericidal levels of the drug can be delivered directly to the diseased tissue. The choice of antibiotic is a matter of professional medical judgment, not in the province of the inhalation therapist, and is based upon clinical experience, identification of the offending bacteria, and sensitivity tests of several antibiotics against bacterial cultures. Since most patients with these resistant infections are seriously ill, they are usually treated with a combination of systemic and aerosol antibiotics of the same or different type. In all probability, the effectiveness of the systemically administered drug is enhanced by liquefication of the intrapulmonary diffusion barrier through the action of the proteolytic alone, but in several reported instances clinical and bacteriologic improvement was delayed until aerosol antibiotic was added. Soluble or intravenous preparations of the drugs are used, and their dose-calibrated solutions can be conveniently mixed with the dissolved dornase for joint administration or, if desired, the two may be used sequentially.

In summary, we can say that, for the most part, aerosolized antibiotics are not intended to supplant the systemic but rather to supplement them in treating diseases characterized by copious purulent sputum. The inhalation therapy reduces the amount of secretions and clears it of bacterial growth, but we must remember that the risk of distant spread of infection to other parts of the body can best be controlled by maintaining therapeutic blood levels by systemic antibiotics. Of special interest to the therapist is the frequent appearance of *Pseudomonas aeruginosa* (*Bacillus pyocyaneus*) in the respiratory tract of patients suffering from chronic respiratory disease, or who have been receiving treatment from poorly maintained inhalation therapy equipment, especially patients who have been tracheotomized and require frequent tracheobronchial suctioning. A potentially serious infection, it is notoriously resistant to systemic therapy, even by those drugs which sensitivity tests would indicate to be effective. The most encouraging results appear to follow the combined therapy of pancreatic dornase and either polymixin B or kanamycin. Although these drugs, as well as other useful antibiotics, have considerable toxicity in their own right, because systemic absorption from the aerosol is so slight, they can be used safely.

Humidification of the respiratory tract

Water is a major therapeutic agent in the treatment of bronchopulmonary disease and the most important of all the aerosols. In an earlier chapter we considered some of the physical properties of water in the atmosphere, but we will now discuss water and its relation to respiratory hygiene, defining some terms and general principles with which the inhalation therapist should be very familiar.[141] Unfortunately, the inhalational use of water is associated with a variety of terms and expressions, and it is helpful to have an understanding of some precise definitions to avoid confusion of meaning. Inhaled water fits into two categories, and we must differentiate between humidity and vapor, on the one hand, and mist, aerosol, "cold steam," and fog, on the other. We will use *vapor* to refer to the first classification and *aerosol* for the second. Recall that water vapor is water in a gaseous form, sometimes referred to as "molecular water," and as such is invisible. By definition, on the other hand, aerosolized water is water in a very fine particulate form, suspended in the air. Thus water aerosol is "liquid water" and exerts no partial pressure as does the vapor. Depending upon the size of its particles, water aerosol is visible or reveals its presence by light diffraction, giving rise to the terms "mist," "fog," and the descriptive but inaccurate "cold steam" used in water aerosol therapy.

The amount of water vapor in a given volume of gas is measured according to the principles of absolute and relative humidity, with which we are acquainted. For evaluation of respiratory humidity the convenient term "percent body humidity"[142] is sometimes used. It refers to the amount of water vapor in a volume of gas as the percent of the water in gas saturated at body temperature. For example, air at 20° C, saturated with vapor, contains 18.5 mg of water per liter, whereas saturated air at body temperature contains 43.8 mg/liter. The room air could be said to have 42% body humidity.

Liquid water particles can be measured, as any aerosol, by particle size. Less frequently they are measured as the number of particles per cubic millimeter of gas. Finally, aerosolized water production is calibrated in the number of milliliters of water aerosolized per minute, especially useful in comparing the performances of large-volume aerosol generators.

The therapist will recognize that there is considerable overlapping in the therapeutic use of water vapor and water aerosol, but it is still convenient to describe their indications separately for clarity and to emphasize their basic differences.

Water vapor. Water vapor is used specificially to prevent or correct a "humidity deficit" in the respiratory tract. Normally, the tracheobronchial tree is able to maintain saturation of inspired gas at body temperature by evaporation from the respiratory mucosa, most of which probably occurs proximal to the carina. Gas thus reaching the pulmonary tissue contains 44 mg of water vapor per liter of gas. If the inspired gas contains less than this amount of water, its vapor pressure will be less than the 47 mm Hg of body humidity, and a vapor pressure gradient will be established between the inspired gas and the respiratory mucosa. Evaporation of body water from the mucosa into the gas brings the latter to full humidification. When the respiratory tract and the general body hydration are in good health, this humidifying mechanism works efficiently, but a humidity deficit of pathologic degree, which the body may have difficulty in compensating, can be produced under two circumstances.

BREATHING DRY GAS. The administration of therapeutic gases from a tank or central supply subjects the respiratory tract to large volumes of vapor-free gas. The normal humidification process may be inadequate to cope with this load and may have to draw on the water content of the entire mucosal surface. Such failure will be hastened or aggravated by an associated dehydration incident to systemic disease. Depletion of mucosal moisture increases the viscosity of the mucus blanket of the tract and a slowing of its escalator movement. At the same time ciliary action is adversely affected. The increased or abnormal secretions, so often present in patients requiring gas therapy, become dehydrated and less mobile, contributing significantly to airway resistance.

MUCOSAL CRUSTING. The same secretions noted above, resulting from bronchopulmonary infection and irritation or systemic disease, can cover the mucosal surface with a dry and crusted coat. Impervious to the diffusion of moisture, it blocks the normal humidification process from the underlying mucosa, and its own desiccation may be perpetrated by the inhalation of therapeutic gases that are inadequately humidified.

Water aerosol. Water aerosol serves a double function. Its principle duty is to deliver liquid water, in minute particle form, to the mucosal surface. The site of its maximum deposition is determined by factors that we already know, particle size and ventilatory pattern. The water which "rains out" in the airways is intended to dilute thick secretions or moisten dry crusts for easier removal by cough or aspiration. In addition to this local effect of physical water particles contacting the airway surfaces, aerosols provide an important source of moisture for humidifying the inspired carrier gas. As the gas enters the warmth of the body and its vapor *capacity* increases, suspended water particles evaporate into the gas, raising its vapor tension to that of body humidity. Humidification can be increased by heating the water to be aerosolized so that it reaches the respiratory tract with no humidity deficit, not only increasing the inhaled water content but also sparing the respiratory tract its duty of humidifying the air. Reference will be made again to this maneuver when equipment is discussed.

The clinical indications for water therapy are many, and the therapist is responsible for seeing that it is properly administered. It is an old therapy, going back through many generations, as man has often used inhaled steam to relieve his respiratory distress. Our current techniques are more efficient, but the objectives are the same. The therapist will use aerosolized water to treat laryngeal croup of childhood, the thick secretions of cystic fibrosis, and chronic bronchial infections, and he will routinely include it with the administration of all therapeutic gases. Unless otherwise specified, distilled water is preferred to tap water because its cleanliness and freedom from solutes are a protection for both the patient and the equipment.

There is one special use of water aerosol therapy that deserves individual attention because of its widespread use and importance—the induction of sputum specimens for laboratory examinations. Such examinations are done for two general reasons. First, specimens are prepared by skilled technicians called cytotechnologists and are carefully examined under the microscope for the presence of malignant cells, in suspected cases of cancer of the respiratory tract. Often, if such disease is in communication with the airway, cells from the surface of the tumor will desquamate, mix with bronchial secretions, and be expectorated. Although the absence of malignant cells in this test, called a *cytologic* sputum examination, does not eliminate the possibility of cancer, their presence is strong evidence of the existence of cancer somewhere in the bronchi or lungs and necessitates a careful search for its location or for some other explanation for the abnormal cells. Second, a *bacteriologic* sputum examination attempts to determine the presence or absence of bacteria in the secretions, and to identify those present. Initially the specimen is smeared on a glass slide, stained with a dye, and microscopically examined for organisms. This often gives a good idea of the general type of microbe present and permits the start of therapy. The rest of the specimen is mixed with several kinds of culture media (nutrients that promote bacterial growth) and incubated from a few hours to several days or weeks to allow maximum growth. Examination of the culture allows specific identification of the bacteria.

Most of the patients treated by the inhalation therapist will have little trouble providing sputum specimens for analysis, and no special procedures will be required. On the other hand, patients with suspected malignancy or nonacute tuberculosis may have very scanty sputum or none at all, and to obtain specimens from them may be critical. For these patients, techniques are available to procure an *induced sputum* specimen, so-called because agents are used by inhalation to promote an increased flow of bronchial secretion and to stimulate a cough. It has been indicated earlier that bronchial secretions will respond to almost any inhaled irritant and for induction many have been tried, including 10% sodium chloride, dornase, acetylcysteine, sterile or distilled water aerosols, and sulfur dioxide gas.[143] The last, although effective, has been found too irritating and is not generally recommended, and the mucolytics and proteolytics have little value in the absence of secretions. The salt-and-water aerosols, when delivered by standard aerosolization, are preheated to 140° to 185° F by any suitable means, but usually by an immersion heating unit in the aerosol generator.[144] This "superheated" aerosol is well saturated with humidity as the patient inhales it, and it also contains large numbers of particles for deposition throughout the bronchial tree.

The distilled water particles condense on the bronchial mucosa and mix with and increase the volume of the normal thin layer of mucus present. The abundance of fine particles also has an irritant effect, stimulating a cough that expectorates the diluted secretions. Sodium chloride aerosols have the same effect, and one additional: because a 10% concentration is more saline than the average body fluids (approximately 0.9%), this aerosol is hypertonic, and as it contacts the bronchial wall, its osmolarity draws fluid from the mucosal layer into the bronchial lumen, increasing the volume of secretions available for expectoration. With both fluid aerosols, the stimulated cough causes the secretions thus moved to carry with them loose or superficial cells from the mucosal surface as well as any available bacteria close to the bronchial lumen. Cells and bacteria, which the subject would be unable to produce by voluntary cough, can thereby be examined.

When the technique of sputum induction became accepted, it was customary to use a 20% solution of propylene glycol as the saline solvent because of the stabilizing properties attributed to this agent. It was felt that the inclusion of propylene in the mixture assured the penetration and deposition of a maximum number of particles in the respiratory tract. However, further experience demonstrated that propylene glycol itself had an inhibiting effect on the causative organism of tuberculosis *(Mycobacterium tuberculosis)*, destroying it or preventing its growth in culture.[143] This was a serious handicap, for the recovery of tubercle bacilli is an important function of sputum induction. From a practical point of view of the overall use of this technique, since the technique is diagnostic and the condition of the subject to be examined is therefore not known, it is advisable to omit propylene glycol from induced sputum mixtures and to use simply 10% sodium chloride in water. The units especially available for administration of heated aerosol are compact and easily portable, lending themselves well to private office and outpatient use as well as to general hospital use. However, some hospitals that have ultrasonic aerosol generators (to be described below) have found them to be most effective in inducing cough. Using distilled water at room temperature, these generators produce finely uniform particles that stimulate a heavy cough, usually after but a few breaths. As yet there are no available data comparing the relative amounts of secretions produced by ultrasonic aerosols as against the standard heated hypertonic saline aerosols. Precautions should be taken to protect medical personnel from possible contamination, especially when they are obtaining specimens suspected of containing tubercle bacilli. The use of a specially ventilated hooded table has been suggested and appears to be as practical a method as any.[145]

The usefulness of this procedure is widely recognized. For many years it was a common practice to aspirate the stomach through a long tube swallowed by the patient and to examine the gastric secretions for tubercle bacilli that the patient had inadvertently swallowed after unnoticed small coughs. Although not a difficult procedure, it was a nuisance that has been replaced by the much more convenient induced cough, which most investigators find to have a far greater bacterial yield.[146,147] It has proved to be a great boon to cancer detection, at times eliminating diagnostic procedures much more hazardous.[148,149] In addition to its diagnostic value, sputum induction often affords excellent symptomatic relief of airway obstruction by removing inspissated mucus, and not infrequently the technique of heated supersaturated aerosolization is used for its therapeutic benefit. The duration of exposure to the aerosol, for diagnosis or therapy, can be varied to suit each individual. The patient is instructed to inhale the aerosol through his mouth in an easy and comfortable manner, resting as often as necessary, and at most the session should not exceed 15 minutes. Samples of sputum should be collected over the ensuing 30 minutes, and care should be taken not to collect saliva but only secretions that obviously arise from the depths of the airways. Sterile containers should be available for all specimens. If sputum is to be examined for malignant cells, it *must* be free of foreign particles. This is best accomplished by having hospitalized patients wash their teeth and thoroughly rinse their mouths prior to collection, and outpatients to at least rinse. As a maximum precaution against contamination, it is helpful to collect as many cytology specimens as possible before breakfast; sputum yields are usually most abundant at that time.

The pharmaceutical and physical agents described in this section are by no means an all-inclusive list of available or potential aerosols, and there is every indication that increasing numbers of substances will be found to lend themselves well to this form of administration. Interest has been shown in treating diseases characterized by surfactant deficiency by an aerosol substitution of this important agent. Synthetic dipalmitoyl-lecithin, a manufactured form of one of the active ingredients of surfactant, has been given a limited trial and apparently promises to be more effective than other detergents so far used. It has been used as a 0.25% solution, microaerosolized to a particle size of 0.25μ for deep alveolar penetration, but further experience must tell whether it will develop into a safe and useful drug.[150] For an entirely different area of medicine, experimental work has tested the feasibility of the aerosol administration of heparin. An anticoagulant, widely used in the treatment and prevention of vascular thromboses and emboli, heparin is usually given according to an inconvenient parenteral schedule. There would be obvious advantages of a simply administered aerosol dosage, and although work on this project is much too early to be conclusive, it is interesting that aerosols are being considered for diseases other than pulmonary.[151] Such apparently unlikely substances as dyes have a limited aerosol use. The inhalation therapist will have occasion to note the concern caused by finding heavy sputum cultures of a yeastlike fungus called *Candida albicans,* and he will learn of the dispute centered about the question of whether or not this organism is a true pathogen. A frequent normal inhabitant of the mouth, throat, and upper respiratory tract, *C. albicans* is usually considered to be pathogenic in its own right if it is accompanied by a sufficient overgrowth. A clinical infection with it is often called "moniliasis." Moniliasis frequently accompanies chronic or debilitating diseases and can be very resistant to treatment. Some of the coal-tar dyes, especially *brilliant green* and *methylene blue,* have been found to be effective by aerosol. Treatment is carried out for several weeks, with either a 0.2% solution of brilliant green or a 0.1% solution of methylene blue, in 50% propylene glycol, aerosolizing 2 ml five times daily. Repeated courses of 10 days each until clinical improvement is evident have proved satisfactory.[152,153] Staining of skin and linens poses nonmedical complications, but the effectiveness and freedom from toxicity of these drugs justifies their consideration whenever clinical moniliasis is a threat.

With the improved aerosol equipment and techniques of the past few years, and especially with the development of skilled technical personnel to administer them, it is hoped that increasing advantage will be taken of this relatively easy and painless method of treating disease.

AEROSOL AND HUMIDITY GENERATORS

This section is not intended to be a technical manual, describing the details of specific equipment or comparing the characteristics of competitive products, for such information is available through the commercial brochures and specification tables provided by all manufacturers. We will discuss principles involved in the design and operation of aerosol and humidity generators so that the therapist will recognize and understand the features of any piece of equipment with which he will have to work. He will develop his own criteria for judging equipment, based on his experience, and will soon learn that he must thoroughly read all descriptive literature provided with each item before he attempts to put that item to clinical use. He will make it a point to disassemble the parts, familiarizing himself with the location and function of each component, with an eye to the ever-present problems of maintenance and repair. Although most ethical manufacturers of quality medical equipment are straightforward in their advertising, their objective is to sell, whereas the main interest of the therapist is the welfare of patients under his care. Thus, the therapist will try to determine for himself such features of his equipment as safety, probable patient acceptance, quality of performance, ease of cleaning, durability, and economy. This type of critical appraisal is the mark of a safe and effective therapist.

Instruments used to generate aerosols are called *nebulizers* (from "nebula," meaning a cloud or mist), and those that increase water vapor content, *humidifiers*, although there is a considerable overlap between them both in function and in application and they sometimes differ only in degree or in the use to which they are put. It may be generalized, however, that nebulizers are designed to deliver a maximum number of particles of desired size, of pharmaceutics or water, for penetration and deposition in the respiratory tract, and that humidifiers are designed to deliver a maximum amount of water vapor with a minimum of particulate water. Some humidifiers produce varying amounts of aerosolized water, but the prime difference between them and nebulizers is the tremendous volume of particles of the latter. Nebulizers and humidifiers are both available for use with water at room temperature or, by the inclusion of heating devices, with water at elevated temperatures. By raising the water temperature far above that of the body (up to 60° C), some humidifiers can add enough vapor to the inspired gas so that, despite the drop in temperature in transit from instrument to patient, when gas inters the body it will be at or near body humidity. Some nebulizers, when used to deliver liquid water to the respiratory tract, employ the same principle so the carrier gas will have its quota of vapor and will not "steal" it from the suspended particles intended for deposition.[154] To help us keep in mind that there is a basic therapeutic difference between humidification and nebulization, let us employ the following rough classification of the types of equipment used for each: *humidifiers*—jet (aerosol), pass-over, and bubble-diffusion; *nebulizers*—jet impeller and ultrasonic. We will describe some of the characteristics of each of the five different types.

Jet aerosol-humidifier

Although the jet instruments can be used for both aerosol generation and humidification, for the sake of simplicity we will refer to them as nebulizers and differentiate between their specific uses when indicated. The jet nebulizer is the most versatile of all this group of instruments and enjoys the most widespread usage. It is simple, can function without moving parts, and is based on the Bernoulli effect as illustrated in the simplified sketch of Fig. 7-2. Although jet nebulizers assume many shapes and sizes, they all have the fundamental features shown in the illustration. A source of gas pressure must be provided that may be a simple hand-operated rubber bulb, a motorized compressor, or tanked gas. The gas enters the nebulizer chamber through a restricted orifice, providing a jet stream of high velocity (A). The jet is directed across the end of a fine capillary tube (B), the other end of which is immersed

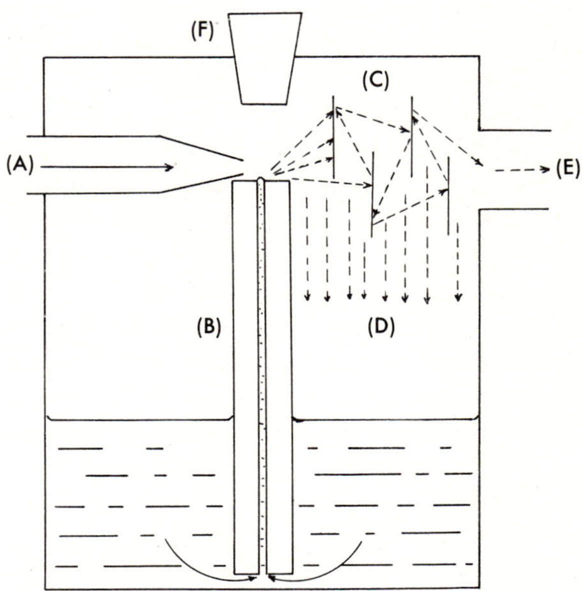

Fig. 7-2. Principle of jet nebulization. See text for explanation. (Adapted from Egan, D. F.: Humidity and water aerosol therapy, Conn Med **31**:353, 1967).

in the solution to be nebulized. The high velocity of the gas produces a local drop in pressure immediately adjacent to the capillary ostium (Bernoulli effect), and because the reservoir surface is subjected to atmospheric pressure, liquid is forced up the capillary (solid arrows). As it reaches the top of the tube, the liquid is continuously blown off by the gas jet as small particles, and thrown against one or more barriers called baffles (C). Again, these baffles can be of many shapes such as small spheres, rods, or plates, or the configuration of the nebulizer chamber may function as a baffle. Here, the particles are further fragmented, and many coalesce into masses too large to transport; these return to the reservoir as a condensate (D). The outflow gas to the patient (E) contains aerosol particles of the desired therapeutic size. Many chambers provide an optional opening for the introduction of air into the gas-particle mixture (F). When opened, a venturi is created as the jet gas draws room air into the chamber (termed *air entrainment*), providing an increased flow rate through the nebulizer to the patient, increasing the rate of nebulization of the reservoir, and thus administering more liquid per unit of time. The need for such an additional source of gas varies with the instrument and its specific use, a matter to which we will have occasion to refer later. However, it must be remembered that changing the physical environment of a nebulization chamber may alter the character of the aerosol output, especially in terms of the effect of the turbulence of higher flow rates on particle stability. These are influences that the interested therapist can determine for himself by carefully controlled measurements of equipment performance under various conditions.

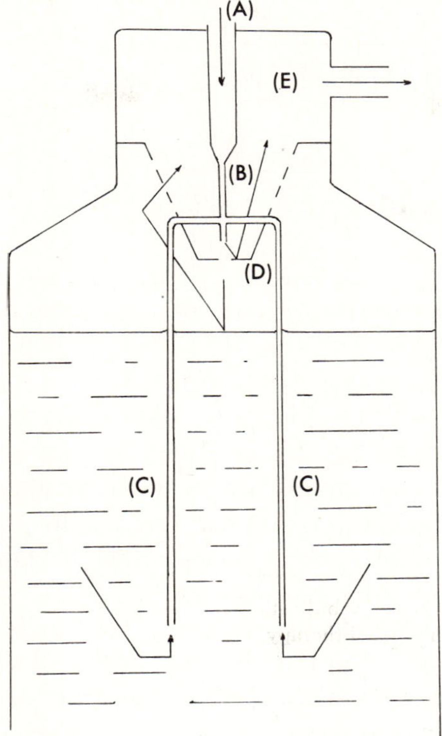

Fig. 7-3. Components of a jet humidifier. See text for description.

Essentially, the structure of the baffle system of a jet instrument determines whether it is to function as a nebulizer or as a jet humidifier. Fig. 7-3 depicts the jet principle employed in humidification. The power gas enters at A, passing through a restriction (B) into which twin capillary tubes (C) open. The venturi at B produces a foaming mixture of liquid and gas that meets a baffle (D) as it emerges from the jet orifice. The baffle may be a perforated plate against which some liquid particles impinge, fracture, and are reflected into the vapor chamber (E). Other particles penetrate the plate and are further baffled by the reservoir surface, which retains the larger ones; the remainder are screened once more as they enter the vapor chamber through the plate baffle. Baffled particles condense and return to the reservoir. The minute water particles that continue into the chamber evaporate into the gas to raise its vapor content, supplemented by water of evaporation from the reservoir surface. Gas issuing from the unit will thus have a maximum amount of water vapor and a minimum of liquid water particles, and it is with this type of humidifier that electric immersion heaters are most frequently used. The amount of humidity can be easily increased, but the output temperature must be monitored to avoid overheating in case of malfunction of the thermostatic control of the unit, and special attention must be paid to prevent the reservoir of water from being depleted.

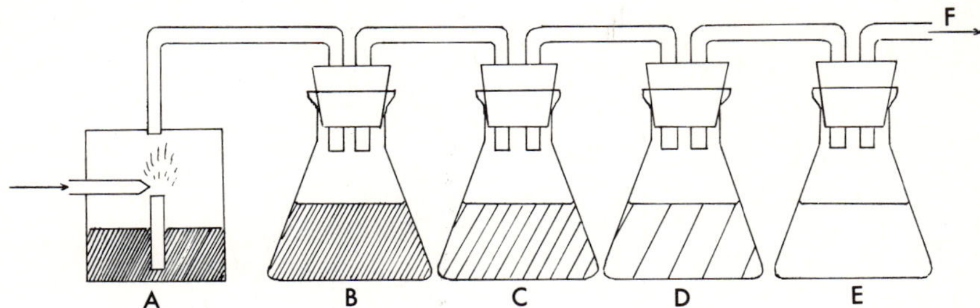

Fig. 7-4. Demonstration of the principle of liquid filtration in the production of microaerosols. Shading of the liquid represents the concentration of dye. See text for further explanation.

There are two interesting variations of the jet nebulization principle that deserve comment—liquid filtration and self-propulsion.

Liquid filtration.[155] Nebulizers of this type are reportedly able to produce aerosol particles consistently less than 0.5μ in diameter, the so-called "microaerosols," or submicronic particles. Technically, they are classified according to a "D" series, such as D.10, etc., up to D.37, depending upon size, particular structure, and other specifications. The basic feature of these nebulizers is the use of the nebulized solution as the baffling system of the units. The principle depends upon the observation that, if a mass of aerosolized liquid particles of heterogeneous sizes is brought into contact with successive volumes of the liquid, particles of increasingly smaller size will be removed from the aerosol until only completely stable particles of a very small size remain in suspension. Fig. 7-4 demonstrates this in the simplest fashion. Container A represents a typical air jet, nebulizing a dye-colored solution, whereas B to E are a variable number of glass flasks containing, initially, volumes of the uncolored solvent used to prepare the nebulizing solution. The flasks are connected in series so that the total output of the nebulizer will pass through each one in succession. In operation, it will be noted that the solvent in each flask becomes decreasingly colored, until one flask will show none. Thus, relatively large numbers of large particles are trapped by the solvent in flask A, deeply staining the fluid, but by the time the aerosol issues from the last flask (at F), the particles are of such a uniformly small and stable size that none are baffled.

The use of this "scrubbing" process for the removal of unwanted large liquid particles in commercial nebulizers is modified according to the need of space economy and is illustrated in Fig. 7-5. A heterogeneous aerosol is generated by an air jet immersed in solution at A and passes upward through a series of constrictions (B). Turbulent flow removes from the stream all but the smallest and most stable particles, condensing them so that they return to the reservoir. Those particles leaving the ports (C), in order to have escaped the scrubbing turbulence, are submicronic in size.

Self-propulsion. Popular because of their compactness and ease of operation, nebulizers with a self-contained power supply are in widespread use.

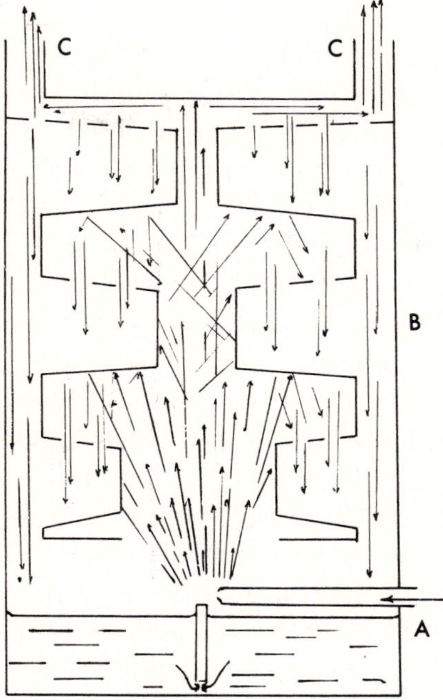

Fig. 7-5. Utilization of liquid filtration in an aerosol generator. Turbulent flow through the constrictions removes all but the smallest particles. See text.

They are made of a small vial containing the solution (or powder) to be nebulized and a physiologically inert gas under pressure as a propellant. With the supplied mouthpiece in place, a slight squeeze releases a small valve allowing the gas to nebulize the medication and deliver it in self-limited premeasured doses.

For the purpose of discussing the clinical use of jet nebulizers, we can arbitrarily divide them into two classes—intermittent nebulizers and reservoir nebulizers—although it will be obvious that there is no clear-cut line of demarcation between the two.

INTERMITTENT NEBULIZERS. This group comprises the relatively small instruments with a capacity of about 5 ml used for limited periods of time on an intermittent basis, mostly for the administration of pharmaceutical aerosols rather than water or humidity. The prototype is the so-called "hand nebulizer," which combines a simple glass or plastic air jet powered by a hand-operated rubber squeeze bulb and is especially suited to the short-term administration of sympathomimetic bronchodilators, for which it was originally designed. The therapist should acquaint himself with the energy required to operate a hand bulb so that he will appreciate the difficulty experienced by a patient attempting to use such a nebulizer for a long period of time. Most units of this type have air ports that permit two velocities of airflow and nebulization. In general, the slower rate without air entrainment is satisfactory, but the option permits adjusting therapy to individual needs. Simple though the instrument is, proper technique in its usage is essential for good results. All patients should be instructed in the nebulizer's use, with a demonstration by the therapist, and should not be permitted to rely only on the manufacturer's directions. Two major points should be emphasized. First, the patient should be instructed to open his mouth widely so that the lips and teeth will not obstruct the aerosol flow, then hold the nebulizer so that its delivery port is directed toward the mouth but is about 1 inch away from the lips. This allows the aerosol to be entrained in the inspiratory airflow, but if the nebulizer tube is inserted into the mouth and the lips tightly pursed about it, much of the aerosol will be deposited in the mouth. Second, the patient should be taught to inhale as slowly and deeply as possible and to deliver the first charge of aerosol just after he starts his inhalation. The therapist will observe that many patients release the aerosol at, or even before, the start of inhalation, depositing much of it outside the respiratory tract. Depending upon the length of inhalation, two or three aerosol doses may be delivered in one breath. At end-inspiration, the breath should be held for 2 or 3 seconds to allow maximum aerosol distribution and deposition.

Usually two to four good inhalations of a sympathomimetic at one time, repeated in 2 to 4 hours, are adequate. The therapist will see many patients for whom this schedule is not completely satisfactory, and he will be asked how often the patient can use the nebulizer. In cases of severe bronchospasm it may be necessary to allow more frequent treatments, but it must always be kept in mind that bronchodilator drugs are potent, with possible serious side effects. Sympathomimetics are locally irritating to the respiratory tract, and too frequent use can actually aggravate the very condition for which they are being used. If relief cannot be obtained with a safe conservative schedule, some other or additional therapy may be indicated, but unrestrained use of the bronchodilator is not. In this regard, the very convenience of the self-propelled gas-operated nebulizer, described above, is a hazard. In principle, such units are both effective and safe as they deliver measured doses well within limits of tolerance. However, their ready availability and the ease with which they can be used leads to frequent patient abuse and disregard for advised schedules. It is not unusual to see patients using these nebulizers every 5 or 10 minutes, and one can imagine the chemical irritation of the respiratory mucosa added to the disability of the underlying disease. Overuse of the hand bulb nebulizer is apt to be less harmful because of the work involved in its operation, which may be considerable for the patient with respiratory distress. It is often prudent to prescribe this type of instrument for the patient suspected of a tendency to self-medication.

For the administration of mucolytic, proteolytic, or antibiotic aerosols, or for longer therapy with dilute bronchodilators, the small-volume hand nebulizers can be adapted to a power source. A small compressor is most practical, since it does not need the pressure regulator or flowmeter of tanked gas and is safe for home use. For treatments that may last up to 30 or 60 minutes, the use of an aerosol mask is advisable. Not only is the patient spared the nuisance and fatigue of holding a nebulizer to his face, but the design of such a mask holds a mass of aerosol particles about the mouth as a reservoir from which the patient can inhale. Since nebulization during the exhalation is wasteful of medication, a simple Y-connector can be inserted in the tubing from the pump to the nebulizer, with the stem of the Y connected to the pump, and one of the arms to the nebulizer. The other arm, left free, can be obstructed by the finger during inhalation to permit nebulization and can be released during exhalation to shunt the airflow away from the nebulizer. Although the same general pattern of slow deep breathing is advised for prolonged therapy as was described earlier, the patient should be warned about overbreathing to the point of discomfort from either the effort involved or possible hypocapnia. In addition to directions included in the original medication prescription, specific dose measurements should be given to the patient, in drops or milliliters, depending upon the technique used in filling the nebulizer, and he should be taught not to flood the capillary tube by overfilling. Finally, the patient should be instructed to rinse his nebulizer after use by nebulizing a small amount of water to prevent clogging of the capillary or jet with dried medication.

RESERVOIR NEBULIZERS. As the name applies, these nebulizers have a large capacity for the solution to be nebulized and are intended for prolonged intermittent or continuous use. Thus, they are predominantly used for aerosolized water or humidity therapy although occasionally for more active agents such as mucolytic detergents. For purposes of discussion we can consider the use of reservoir jet nebulizers in the two categories of prolonged intermittent and continuous.

Prolonged intermittent. Prolonged intermittent use refers to the administration of water (usually) aerosol for periods longer than would be practical with a small-volume nebulizer, to avoid the inconvenience of repeated replenishment of the latter. The use of heated aerosol of hypertonic saline, with or without propylene glycol, for sputum induction or for the removal of thick bronchial plugs is a common example. This technique was discussed in the previous section of this chapter and needs no further amplification except to stress its therapeutic as well as its diagnostic value. Intermittent water aerosol is not new in the treatment of acute laryngitis, for several generations have taken advantage of the relief afforded by the inhalation of steam. Aerosol generators, however, are more efficient than the heated tea kettle, providing a steady volume of particles of more uniform size than can be found in steam. Water aerosol can be generated for prolonged periods of time at room temperature ("cold steam") or warmed by an immersion heater or by setting the reservoir in a container of water on a hot plate. Jet humidifiers (or aerosol generators) are effective in the daily management of patients with permanent tracheostomies, for whom high humidity should be added to the inspired air at regular intervals to maintain the integrity of the respiratory tract mucosa. This procedure can easily be carried out at home with a tracheostomy mask to direct the maximum amount of humid air directly into the trachea.

Continuous. Continuous use implies an uninterrupted administration of humidity or water particles for long periods of time. Probably the most common and important example is the humidification of therapeutic oxygen, for, except during short-term emergency use, oxygen (or any other compressed gas) should never be given without adequate humidification. Inhalation of the bone-dry gas not only is uncomfortable to the patient after a few minutes, but its desiccating effect on the respiratory mucosa can be critically harmful. For most patients receiving oxygen, unless bronchial secretions are a major problem, a simple jet humidifier is effective and easy to set up. The patient with an "acute trach" must have continuous humidification until his underlying disease has become stabilized. This is the patient whose acute respiratory problem required a tracheotomy operation and whose resultant tracheostomy is used either to ease his spontaneous breathing or to assist him with mechanical ventilation. Details of the management of the tracheotomized patient will be discussed later, and at this point we will only emphasize that the life of the patient may be in jeopardy if adequate water is not provided for his respiratory tract. Aerosolized water is a standard part of therapy for childhood croup, or acute laryngotracheobronchitis. The laryngeal edema, characteristic of this condition, can rapidly and fatally obstruct the airways of small children but often is dramatically relieved by water-saturated inspired air or oxygen. As noted above in reference to the treatment of laryngitis, steam has long been used for croup, but because the benefit of mist therapy is directly proportional to the concentration of water particles and the length of patient exposure, boiling water as a source of aerosol has limitations. Many hospitals have special "croup rooms" equipped with jets that fill the temperature-controlled room with a dense fog or use a more elaborate combination of air and live steam to create "natural fog."[156] Although effective, these units waste valuable hospital space when not in use. Large-volume jet nebulizers have had extensive use in the past few years, for when combined with a bed or crib canopy, they constitute a personal croup room about the individual patient. They are most effective when used with a temperature-controlled oxygen tent, which we will describe in another section; such a unit is then called a mist tent. Instruments designed for just this type of therapy are available, the most recent innovation being the ultrasonic nebulizer, which will also be described, later in this chapter. The ultrasonic nebulizer produces a large volume of water aerosol and has thus gained great popularity over the jet nebulizer for prolonged high-humidity therapy. However, some of the most recent jet models have nearly the same mist production as the ultrasonic, and the simplicity, lower initial cost, and minimal maintainance of the jet nebulizers make them still the front-line instruments for humidity and mist. Finally, patients hospitalized with chronic bronchopulmonary disease frequently have serious problems with obstructive secretions, and the aerosol deposition of water in the respiratory tract is an important part of their therapy. It should be repeated here for emphasis that, for this type of patient, the most important of all the aerosol medications is water, a point we will have occasion to note more than once when we consider other therapeutic techniques.

One of the virtues of a skilled inhalation therapist is his versatility. With his knowledge of equipment and the objectives of therapy, he is able to choose the right instrument, or combination of instruments, to accomplish these objectives. He will frequently be called upon to use imagination and ingenuity in setting up equipment to suit the needs of patients with special problems. Because of the great variety and numbers of jet aerosol-humidifiiers, it would be impractical as well as needless to attempt to describe the idiosyncrasies of each, but we will mention a few operational principles common to all, which the therapist should bear in mind. To begin with, the relationship between the output of the jet nebulizer and the main flow of gas being humidified is important, and it may be described in one of two ways, *sidestream* nebuliza-

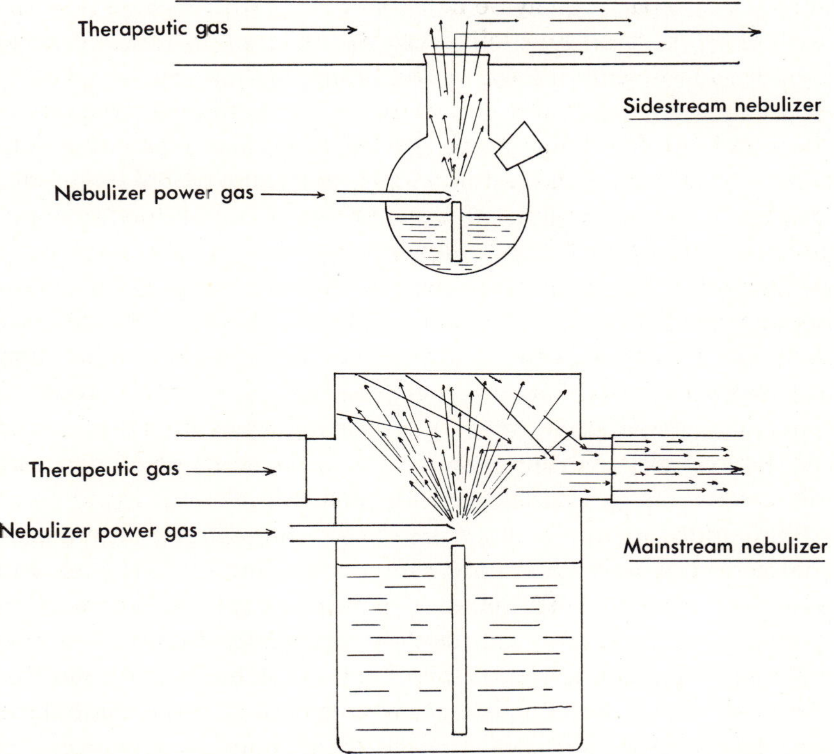

Fig. 7-6. Diagrammatic comparison of sidestream and mainstream nebulizers. The aerosol of the sidestream unit is considerably diluted by the large volume of dry therapeutic gas and provides limited humidity. It is used primarily to administer medication. The entire therapeutic gas flow passes through the mainstream nebulizer chamber and is able to pick up significant moisture. The effectiveness of this nebulizer can be increased by heating the fluid reservoir.

tion and *mainstream* nebulization.[157] In sidestream nebulization, the aerosol is discharged into the therapeutic gas flow between the delivery instrument and the patient, as shown in Fig. 7-6. The nebulizer has its own separate gas power supply, which is smaller than the therapeutic gas flow, and when the aerosol mixes with the greater volume of dry gas in the patient delivery tube, it is too diluted to raise the humidity of the gas to maximum. The sidestream method is mostly used with mechanical ventilators of the intermittent positive-pressure type, and although it is limited in the humidity it contributes, the moisture is usually sufficient for short-term therapy; but for prolonged ventilator therapy the humidity is not adequate, and frequent refilling is necessary. Primarily, it is an effective way of administering medication during a treatment, and all the pharmaceutical agents described in the last section of this chapter can be given by this route. In mainstream nebulization, the entire gas flow to the patient passes through the chamber of the nebulizer. These units are reservior nebulizers, and with the high aerosol production, the outflow gas to the patient can be supplied with a therapeutic level of humidity, up to 100% if a heating element is included. The importance of a heated water reservoir cannot be overstated, if the goal is 100% humidification. It has been demonstrated that, in unheated nebulizers, either jet or bubble (to be described shortly), as oxygen flows through the unit the water temperature drops significantly.[158] At flow rates up to 12 liters per minute the temperature of the reservoir water may drop as much as 13° C below its starting ambient temperature within 1 hour. Even the small-volume sidestream nebulizer will show a temperature drop of up to 5° C in 10 minutes. The temperature of the water thus becomes the limiting factor in the final humidity of the delivered gas. Even if the gas in the nebulizer chamber is saturated at its temperature, at the end of the gas delivery tube the humidity may fall to 50%, at the temperature of that point. The use of a heating device in the nebulizer to raise the water temperature to 53° C (125° F), in conjunction with a delivery tube of 1.9 cm internal diameter to prevent water clogging, will permit vapor saturation at body temperature. The jet oxygen humidifiers, as illustrated in Fig. 7-3, are theoretically mainstream units when the oxygen supply powers the jet; but oxygen concentrations can be varied by diluting the oxygen with air either in the nebulizing unit or at the patient end of the delivery tube, and the added volume of inspired gas at room temperature and humidity can lower the net humidity of the total inhaled gas. Combinations of sidestream and mainstream nebulization are often used together, especially during mechanical ventilation. The ventilator output is directed through the larger reservoir nebulizer, and a small sidestream nebulizer is added to the flow just before it reaches the patient. Such a combination allows a continuous humidification of the main gas flow and the continuous or intermittent addition of medication. However, if the reservoir nebulizer is heated for maximum humidity, there will be a drop in temperature as the gas traverses the delivery tube, with precipitation of excess water in the tube. In addition, the considerable volume of gas powering the sidestream nebulizer, which is not heated, will further lower the final delivery temperature; and although theoretically the inhaled gas might be saturated at its given temperature, the volume of vapor it contains may be lower then 100% body humidity. If the therapist thoroughly understands his equipment, he may be able to modify it to deliver heated gas to the medication nebulizer and increase the delivered humidity.

Attention should be given to the effect of the air jet on flow in the reservoir nebulizers, especially when they are used as mainstream humidifiers. Most units are designed to operate at power gas pressures of 50 pounds per square inch (50 psi) delivered through a flowmenter that regulates the number of liters per minute (lpm) available to the nebulizer. Because the jet through which the gas must pass is a restricted orifice, a considerable back pressure develops at the jet, according to the principles of pressure, resistance, and flow rate discussed in earlier chapters. There will thus be a limit to the amount of gas per unit of time that can go through a given nebulizer under operating conditions. This is information that every therapist should know about his equipment, either through information supplied by the manufacturer or by the process of testing the equipment himself, measuring and recording the data. Jet nebulizers are frequently used with canopy tents or other enclosures for high-humidity or mist therapy, and care must be taken to see that there is adequate airflow for the patient's needs. Some jet nebulizers may not be able to exceed an output of more than 8 lpm and, if used with tent oxygen therapy requiring a minute turnover of 12 liters, will be inadequate. Separate oxygen supply lines will be needed for nebulization and ventilation. If an air compressor is used to power a nebulizer, the flow output of the pump must be known, not when functioning unrestricted but when attached to the nebulizer. Thus, a pump may be rated at 20 lmp but when attached to an instrument may deliver only 10 lpm, and if this is the sole ventilatory supply to a mist tent, additional sources of air must be made available either through air-entrainment ports in the nebulizer or through the canopy itself. Many of the large nebulizers have provisions for diluting the oxygen they deliver. These consist of a port with variable openings to draw in room air, calibrated for concentrations of oxygen at various settings. This added air increases the total flow rate output from the nebulizer. The lower the concentration of oxygen in the delivered mixture, the greater will be the volume of ambient air added, and the greater the total flow. Some manufacturers provide data that relate the flowmeter reading with the oxygen concentration and the total output, but if these are not available, the therapist must determine them himself. The air-dilution ports are closed when heated nebulization is used, because the inflow of diluting air cools the air-mist mixture and negates the purpose of the instrument. With the output of the nebulizer functioning at its lowest level, there are many times when the flow rate will not be adequate for the patient's need, and full advantage cannot be taken of the 100% humidity potential of the nebulizer.

Safety pressure release valves are necessary in the large jet nebulizers, and they should be periodically checked. There is always the risk of compression or kinking of the output line, and the buildup of pressure in the unit is potentially dangerous. Also, because such an event would stop the therapy, relief valves usually have audible signals to warn of the shutoff of gas supply to the patient.

Pass-over humidifier

The pass-over humidifier is the simplest of all and depends upon evaporation to supply humidity to air directed across its surface. Although its efficiency can be increased by heating either the water or the air, this type of humidifier has been replaced, for the most part, by the other humidifiers and nebulizers under discussion.

Bubble-diffusion humidifier

One of the oldest methods of humidifying oxygen consists of bubbling it through a reservoir of water, thus providing a large number of gas-liquid surfaces to enhance evaporation. Fig. 7-7 illustrates two commonly employed techniques. Gas enters the unit at A and passes through a tube immersed

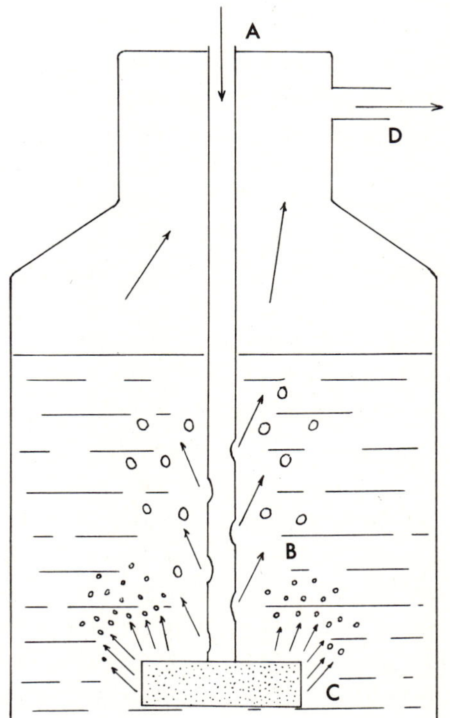

Fig. 7-7. The bubble-diffusion humidifier bubbles therapeutic gas, *A*, through a perforated tube, *B*, or a porous diffusion head, *C*. The larger the number of small bubbles, the greater will be the evaporation area to humidify the gas leaving outflow port, *D*.

nearly to the bottom of a jar containing water. Sometimes the tube contains multiple perforations (B) through which the gas escapes as bubbles of a size determined by the size of the openings. The relatively small amount of gas in each bubble, surrounded by a large amount of water, picks up water of evaporation to varying degrees of humidity and leaves the outflow port (D). Instead of the holes, the immersed oxygen tube may be fitted with a porous stonelike *diffusion head* (C) at its lower tip. This breaks the gas into much smaller bubbles than the perforated tube, thus increasing the total gas surface for evaporation of water among the much larger number of small bubbles. At best, humidity of between 40% to 50% is all that can be expected at the outflow, and this probably drops to less than 20% in the warm respiratory tract. Although the old "bubble bottles" have been replaced by more effective humidifiers, the bubble-diffusion principle has not been altogether discarded, and there are some new designs of this instrument that have proved to be very effective. Made especially for adaptation to mechanical ventilators, one such unit, known as a "cascade" humidifier, effectively breaks the inspired gas into minute bubbles and passes them through water heated by an adjustable immersion heater. The temperature of the humidifier can be raised to such a level that the moist gas will still be humid when it reaches the patient and 100% saturation can be achieved.

Impeller nebulizer

Physical force of a rapidly rotating disc is used to break up water into fine particles and to emit it as a heavy mist. The disc, driven by an electric motor, sucks water from a reservoir and literally throws it through a meshed or slotted baffle. Of less uniform size than the particles from a well-constructed jet nebulizer, the aerosol does produce a grossly visible fog and affords the inspired air a good supply of water particles for evaporation, although, with the heterogeneous particle sizes, there tends to be more "rain out" about a patient enclosed in a tent. Because there is no need for a compressed gas source and the units are compact and easy to operate, the impeller nebulizer is popular for home use. It is available in a number of sizes and output capacities, some decorator styled for room size humidification.

Ultrasonic nebulizer

It was noted earlier that the most recent addition to therapeutic nebulizers is the ultrasonic, based on a totally different principle from that employed by the others we have discussed. It is a complex electronic instrument that has been adequately described in much detail elsewhere, but we will review its major features and applications briefly.[159,160] The nebulizer has two components—a power unit and a nebulizing unit. The power unit, utilizing standard alternating house current, converts the current to an ultrahigh frequency of 1.35 megacycles per second, in one commercial instrument, and 1.4 megacycles per second, in another. This is conveyed to the nebulizing unit, where the great vibrational energy is focused on a piezoelectric transducer, in the form of a small cupped ceramic disc. With water on its concave surface, the ceramic disc responds to the energy applied to it, vibrating in sympathy, and transmits the vibrations to the enclosed water, which is referred to as a *couplant.* Set in the couplant fluid is a container into which is placed the water to be nebulized. The high-frequency vibrations of the ceramic transducer, picked up by the couplant, are transmitted into the nebulizer, where their intense energy physically breaks the water into a large volume of small particles. The transfer of energy is accompanied by the production of a small amount of heat, varying from 3° to 10° C above ambient. The aerosol particles can be carried to the patient by a small blower, provided with the instrument, or by oxygen as a carrier gas, or the patient can draw the aerosol with his own ventilation. Depending upon the make and model, there are adjustments for variable aerosol concentrations, and up to 6 ml of water can be nebulized per minute. Because of the high aerosol output, heating is not necessary, and the therapy can be administered at room temperature.

Clinical response testifies to the efficacy of ultrasonic nebulization and its ability to deposit water in the respiratory tract, but there is little specific information regarding mean particle size produced. On the one hand, it is asserted that measured mean values varied from 1μ to 10μ in diameter but with a narrow distribution range[161] and, on the other, it is claimed that the mass of particles falls within the 0.8μ to 1.0μ range with probable 80% deposition within the lung.[162] The lack of condensation of moisture on a piece of glass held in the aerosol stream indicates an effective stability of particle size. In the process of determining the degree of humidity actually delivered to the respiratory tract, a revealing experiment was conducted on dogs.[162] Very small humidity transducers were introduced into the primary division of the bronchi and were attached to recorders responsive to the amount of water vapor with which the transducers were in contact. Calibrations were in arbitrary "humidity units," depending upon the deflection of the recorder with known humidity. This permitted the comparison of the amount of moisture delivered to the airway with air-activated and ultrasonic nebulizers. Standard nebulizers increased bronchial vapor content an average of 0.18 units, whereas the ultrasonic achieved 0.71 and 4.03 units, on two volume settings. In addition, the duration of maintained humidity was longer with the ultrasonic than with the air-generated instruments.

With the large aerosol production of which the ultrasonic nebulizer is capable and the obvious penetration of water into the respiratory tract, the question of possible harm to the lung arose. Washing the lung with water or saline is known to disrupt its surface tension stability, presumably by the removal of pulmonary surfactant; and because it was important to know whether ultrasonic aerosolization posed the same risk, animal experimentations were carried out.[163,164] The lungs of dogs subjected to nebulization of isotonic saline and distilled water were examined, and no evidence of interference with surface tension stability was detected, even after 72 hours of aerosols. It was speculated that the small particle size and the total low fluid volume were not harmful, in this respect. On the other hand, it was noted that after prolonged aerosol exposure all animals receiving saline mist, and a few of those on distilled water, showed microscopic pulmonary changes consistent with bronchopneumonia. The deposition of hypertonic saline, the result of water evaporating from normal saline, was felt to be responsible. It was concluded that continuous wetting of the lung with ultrasonic mist for long periods of time might be deleterious, although no time-limit safety guides were suggested.

In addition to its large aerosol volume, the ultrasonic nebulizer has other physical virtues. Of importance is the independence of the aerosol production from the flow rate of the breathing gas. Whereas the output of the jet nebulizer is dependent upon the flow of its power gas, the ultrasonic nebulizer can dispense a steady particle volume regardless of the flow. This is an advantage when the nebulizer is incorporated into an oxygen therapy or mechanical ventilation procedure, for it will not materially disturb the therapeutic gas flow pattern. Because the only grossly moving part of the instrument is the small blower, operation is quiet and inoffensive. Parts are easily cleaned and sterilized, and the inflow can be filtered.

The clinical use of the ultrasonic nebulizer is extensive, but it is of prime value when the actual deposition of water in the respiratory tract is desired. The basic indication, therefore, is the liquefaction by dilution of bronchial secretions, and a secondary use is the maximum humidification of inhaled air. It is effective in stimulating cough for both therapeutic and diagnostic purposes, when its full output volume is held close to the mouth and slowly inhaled. Water aerosol is usually more irritating than saline for this purpose and is valuable in inducing a sputum specimen for laboratory examination, but it is equally useful in wetting thick bronchial secretions and stimulating expectoration. In general, the ability of the adult patient to cooperate with the techniques employing simpler aerosol generators and humidifiers obviates the need for the ultrasonic instrument except for unusual circumstances. However, it has reached its greatest potential in treating respiratory conditions in children.

Ultrasonic nebulization has been used in all the usual pediatric diseases characterized by obstructive secretions, but its most outstanding success has been in the treatment of cystic fibrosis (cystic fibrosis of the pancreas,mucoviscidosis). Of unknown etiology, cystic fibrosis is a complex hereditary disease involving several organ systems, characterized by a malfunction of mucus-secreting glands with the production of markedly viscid mucus. Early descriptions of the disease emphasized cystic destruction of the pancreas secondary to plugging of its excretory ducts by thick secretions and gave the disease its not quite accurate name. Because this disease is not uncommon, the student is encouraged to familiarize himself with its many clinical features.

but we will concern ourselves here with its pulmonary complications. Fatalities are usually due to respiratory failure from pulmonary mucoviscidosis. Along with secretions elsewhere in the body, bronchial mucus is remarkably thick and tenacious, severely obstructing airways and leading to secondary bronchitis, bronchiectasis, emphysema, and repeated pulmonary infections. Although the total treatment program involves many aspects, none is more important than the constant effort to maintain airway patency. To this end, the prolonged inhalation of aerosolized water has long been standard therapy, either on an intermittent basis when secretions develop acutely or on a regular regimen of a prescribed number of daily hours in a mist tent. In these situations ultrasonic nebulization has become a valuable tool.

The deposition of water in the respiratory tract is able to thin secretions by dilution and to facilitate their removal by the natural cough mechanism, by vigorous postural drainage, and occasionally by aspiration. This requires subjecting the small patient to an atmosphere filled to as near capacity as possible with water particles able to penetrate the depths of the respiratory tract, assuring not only 100% humidity but also a significant excess of particulate water for intrabronchial deposition. Such a "supersaturated" state of therapeutic effectiveness is difficult to attain with jet or impeller nebulizers, without using two or three at a time, but it is possible with the high aerosol output of the ultrasonic. With a minimum of appliances and noise, the smallest child can rest undisturbed in a mist tent served by this unit, and the particle stability prevents any significant external wetting from fallout. The small infant in a dense water aerosol atmosphere must be watched carefully for overhydration since relatively large amounts of water can be absorbed from the lung into the circulation. Infants are weighed frequently to assess water uptake, and the amount supplied by nebulization is deducted from the daily total dietary source. For prolonged nebulization, there is no universal agreement as to the relative values of water (preferably sterile) or isotonic saline. Some feel that water is safer, because the immature kidney of infants and small children has difficulty in excreting the added sodium load of saline, retention of which might seriously disturb water and electrolyte balance.[165] Others prefer normal saline because of the irritating effects of such a large volume of water particles.[166] For safety's sake, even during an acute obstructive exacerbation, patients are removed from the mist tent at intervals. During "normal" or nonacute phases of cystic fibrosis, as a prophylactic measure, many patients are placed in a mist tent during the sleeping hours, a technique employed as part of home care that often reduces the number of hospitalizations for acute obstruction.

It should be evident that, in addition to cystic fibrosis, ultrasonic nebulization is valuable in the treatment of the acute obstruction of croup, as described earlier. Although water and saline are the two most frequently used media in the ultrasonic nebulizer, there is increasing interest in the use of other substances, with pharmacologic action. There has been some concern that the vibrational energy of ultrasonic nebulization might degrade or disrupt the structure of chemical substances and either destroy their specific action or produce harmful by-products. Although there is evidence that this concern is unwarranted, until more precise information is available, water and saline remain the medications of choice.[165]

In summary, with the widespread indications for aerosol therapy and the increasing variety of equipment appearing on the market, the inhalation therapist who has supervisory responsibility is faced with a difficult test of judgment. The medical director of a department of inhalation therapy and the hospital administrator will often rely on his recommendations as to type and quality of equipment to be purchased, and he must weigh the therapeutic value of each proposed addition to his inventory against its expected use and cost. His objective will be to provide the maximum service to a heterogeneous hospital patient population, within the limits of his budget, and he will have to consider the initial cost of new equipment, the service required to maintain it in workable condition, and the probability that all members of his department will use it with the same degree of efficiency and uniformity. The decision may be a compromise between what the therapist would like to have and what is practical. He will find from experience that it is generally unwise to disburse a large fraction of his budget for the purchase of a few expensive items which, although desirable, may be essential for only a few patients when the same expenditure could provide more less sophisticated items that would be satisfactory for many. Again, this underscores the need for a competent therapist to understand fully the merits of his equipment and the general therapeutic needs of his hospital's patients.

Chapter 8

Gas therapy

MEDICAL GASES

The administration of therapeutic gases is the most important function of the inhalation therapist. Indeed, it is from the humble beginning of the so-called "oxygen service" of the average general hospital that the present skilled technology of inhalation therapy evolved, and even though the therapist has now assumed a host of duties and responsibilities, gas therapy is the foundation of his work. We have covered many aspects of gases—something of their behavior and characteristics, the mechanics of introducing them into the body through ventilation, and the activities of some of them as they participate in bodily functions. In this chapter we will consider the packaging and distribution of compressed therapy gases and the clinical equipment and techniques for using them to treat patients. We will call upon some previously discussed principles as we describe both the gaseous and liquid forms of gases. Much of the data in this section of the chapter are drawn from two sources with which all inhalation therapists should be familiar, the codes of the National Fire Protection Association[147] and pamphlets of the Compressed Gas Association, Inc., especially those that describe the common medical gases and the many important safety measures for which the therapist must be held responsible.[168] In addition, the student will find useful information in the many good brochures and other publications of the manufacturers of gases and gas equipment.

As noted in Chapter 1, the commercial gas industry and the various fields of related engineering use the English system of measurement almost exclusively, and the student must familiarize himself with the necessary units when considering the packaging of gases; but he will find himself back in the metric system when discussing their application to the patient. Before we attempt to discuss the matter at hand, there is one variation of measurement we have not had occasion to use in the past but which is essential in considering gas therapy. Pressure in the English system is expressed as pounds per square inch and, in the parlance of commercial gases, is abbreviated *psi*. However, it is often necessary to be more specific and to denote whether a given pressure includes that of the atmosphere or is in excess of atmospheric. This need arises because of the use of calibrated gauges to measure and record pressures. A pressure gauge, which usually consists of a numbered circular dial with a centrally pivoted needle indicator, registers zero pressure under atmospheric conditions. In other words, at zero gauge pressure, there is already 1 atmosphere of pressure (14.7 psi) active, and any deviation above zero by the gauge indicates pressure above atmospheric. Therefore, the recorded pressure is referred to as *pounds per square inch, gauge* (psig). Less commonly used in ordinary gas therapy, but widely used in hyperbaric medicine, is the concept of "absolute pressure." This means the actual total pressure of a gas, including that exerted by the atmosphere, and is called *pounds per square inch, absolute* (psia). To orient his thinking, the student can remember that psia is always 1 atm, or 14.7 lb/in^2, greater than psig. Thus 14.7 psig = 29.4 psia; 371.2 psig = 385.9 psia. For completeness, it should be noted that hyperbaric terminology frequently employs units of atmospheres and refers to so many atmospheres, gauge (atg), or atmospheres, absolute (ata), with the same relationship described for pounds per square inch. By common usage, in compressed gas data, gauge pressure is implied unless otherwise specified, and psi and psig are used interchangeably, although the latter is more correct.

Cylinder gases

Of all the many gases that are compressed into cylinders for distribution, we will be interested in the few that are called medical gases. Even of these, we will discuss in detail only some, because a few are used mainly in the laboratory and others are anesthetics, which are not in the province of the inhalation therapist. Initially, we will include in our discussion the groups of gases listed in Table 8-1. These, prepared and packaged for medical use, will give us a wide scope to discuss techniques involved and characteristics of compressed gases; then our clinical discussions will be limited to the therapy gases.

From a safety point of view, compressed gases are classified as nonflammable (will not burn), nonflammable but will support combustion, and flammable (will burn readily). The above gases can be grouped according to their flammability as indicated in Table 8-2.

Table 8-1. *Therapy and anesthetic gases*

Limited therapy, Laboratory gases	*Therapy gases*	*Anesthetics*
Nitrogen (N_2)	Air	Cyclopropane $(CH_2)_3$
Carbon dioxide (CO_2)	Oxygen (O_2)	Nitrous oxide (N_2O)
Helium (He)	Oxygen-nitrogen (O_2/N_2)	Ethylene (C_2H_4)
	Oxygen-carbon dioxide (O_2/CO_2)	
	Helium-oxygen (He/O_2)	

Table 8-2. *Flammability of gases*

Nonflammable: N_2, CO_2, He
Support combustion: O_2, N_2O, air, O_2/N_2, O_2/CO_2, He/O_2
Flammable: $(CH_2)_3$, C_2H_4

Gas cylinders. The containers used to hold and ship compressed or liquid medical gases are high pressure units, carefully controlled in their specifications by regulations, both federal and industrial. They are made of seamless steel, finely tempered and nonreactive with their gaseous or liquid contents, and are classified as type "3A" or "3AA" cylinders. We will compare various pressures used in medical gas cylinders; but regardless of the cylinder pressure, all tanks used for therapy have valves that, in clinical use, are fitted with devices to reduce the pressure going to the patient to a "working pressure" of 50 psig. The valves also have safety releases that will give way before the cylinders burst should exposure to sudden heat dangerously elevate the gas pressure.

Cylinders are given a letter designation according to size. Following is a list of most of the common sizes, in inches of diameter and height including valve, with an asterisk indicating the relatively few with which the inhalation therapist can expect to have frequent contact:

A	B	D*	E*	F	M	G*	H&K*
3 × 10	3½ × 16	4¼ × 20	4¼ × 30	5½ × 55	7⅛ × 46	8½ × 55	9 × 55

Sizes A through E are referred to as small cylinders and are used most often for anesthetic gases and portable emergency oxygen supply. These small tanks differ from the larger ones in the mechanism by which they attach to the appliances they serve. They employ a connector called a *yoke,* whereas the large cylinders (F to H&K) have a threaded outlet from their valves to which a nut attaches a pressure reducer. Fig. 8-1 illustrates the general structure of the cylinder valves and the yoke used with small cylinders. *A* represents a small cylinder valve, but the principle of the large valves is similar. 1 is the stem on which a handgrip is placed when in use; 2 is the valve plunger with its threaded lower end; 3 is the outlet of the valve, a recess in the small valves but a projecting threaded nipple in the large ones; 4 is the valve seat; 5 is an emergency pressure release; 6 is one of a pair of borings in the valve body of the small cylinders only, part of the Pin-Index Safety System, to be described later; 7 is the gas channel into the valve; 8 is the threaded connection between the valve and the cylinder. *B* is an illustration of a yoke connector for the A to E cylinders that fits about the cylinder valve, showing the aperture that is slipped about the valve; a screw that holds the yoke firmly onto the valve; the small receiving nipple that fits snugly into the gas outlet (3, in *A*); and the pins of the Index System noted above.

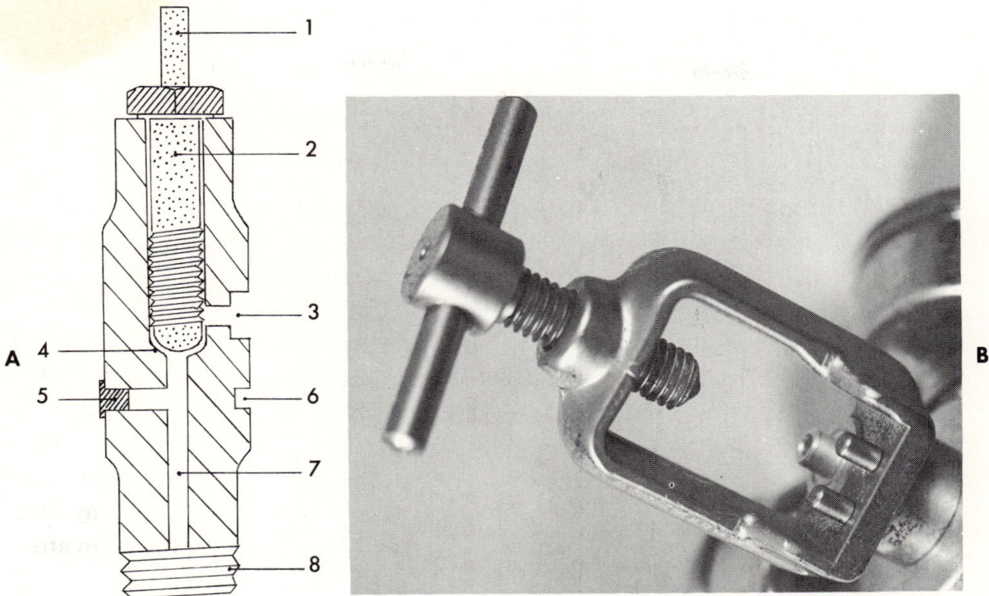

Fig. 8-1. A, Diagrammatic sectional sketch of a small cylinder valve. **B,** Photograph of the yoke connector used with small cylinders. See text for description.

Medical gas cylinders are marked by metal stampings on their shoulders that are supposed to supply specific information. The letters ICC, standing for the Interstate Commerce Commission, are followed by the designation of the cylinder as a 3A or 3AA type and then by the maximum working pressure of the cylinder in psi. This is the filling pressure of the tank, which can usually be exceeded by 10%. For example, a frequently encountered cylinder has a marked pressure of 2015 psi but is usually filled to about 2200 psi. Below these data the letter size of the cylinder is marked (E, G, etc.) followed by the serial number of the cylinder. A third line of stampings includes the initials of the company that owns the cylinder, and as a fourth line there is a mark identifying the inspecting authority. On the opposite surface of the tank there is another set of stampings the first line of which indicates the method by which the cylinder was manufactured, often noted as "Spun Cr-Mo," indicating the use of chrome-molybdenum. Below are a series of symbols that include the identification of the manufacturer of the cylinder, the data of its original safety test, dates of all subsequent tests as prescribed by regulation, and frequently the notation "E.E." followed by a number that indicates the cubic centimeter elastic expansion of the cylinder under test conditions. In addition to these permanent marks, all tanks should have securely attached to them labels clearly identifying the contents and their concentrations, and some will tell the cubic feet or gallon measurement of the gas.

As an aid to the easy identification of medical gases, Table 8-3 lists the

Table 8-3. *Color code for size E gas cylinders*

Gas	*Color*
Oxygen	Green
Carbon dioxide	Gray
Nitrous oxide	Light blue
Cyclopropane	Orange
Helium	Brown
Ethylene	Red
Carbon dioxide and oxygen	Gray and green
Helium and oxygen	Brown and green

Table 8-4. *Gas volumes conversion factors*

Cubic feet	*Liters*	*Gallons*
1.0	28.316	7.481
0.03531	1.0	0.2642
0.1337	3.785	1.0

color code for the size E cylinders, specifically those intended for use on anesthesia machines, that has been adopted by the Bureau of Standards of the United States Department of Commerce.

It is strongly emphasized that the color of a cylinder is to be used only as a rough guide and the therapist *must always check* the cylinder contents by *carefully reading its label.* Many of the larger cylinders employ essentially the same color scale, but there is enough variation among the many tanks the therapist may have occasion to handle to make the color identification unreliable. It is hoped that soon there will be a fully uniform international color marking system.

Every 5 years compressed gas cylinders must be subjected to a safety inspection and testing. Under compression, such factors as leaks, cylinder expansion, and wall stress are determined, and the cylinders are inspected internally and cleaned. The date of each such testing is stamped on the cylinder shoulder.

Because of the many ways of expressing gas volume measurements, it is helpful to be able to convert from one to the other by the use of the factors in Table 8-4.

It should be kept in mind that, because of the different filling pressures of gases, volumes of different gases in the same size cylinder will vary. For example, a G-cylinder contains about 187 cubic feet of oxygen but only about 147 cubic feet of helium. Table 8-5 gives an idea of the approximate filling pressure ranges of medical gases, depending upon the types of cylinders used, calibrated at 70° F.

Table 8-5. *Pressure ranges of medical gases*

Gas	*Physical state*	*psig*	*Gas*	*Physical state*	*psig*
Air	G	1800	CO_2	L	825
O_2	G	1800-2400	He	G	1650-2000
O_2/N_2	G	1800-2200	$(CH_2)_3$	L	75
O_2/CO_2	G	1500-2200	N_2O	L	745
He/O_2	G	1650-2000	C_2H_4	G	1250
N_2	G	1800-2200			

Filling (charging) cylinders. We will differentiate between gases and liquid gases.

GASES. The general rule is that gas cylinders will be filled at a temperature of 70° F to the pressure specified for a given cylinder, as stamped on its shoulder. However, certain gases, including oxygen, helium, helium-oxygen, and oxygen-carbon dioxide, may be filled to 10% in excess of the stated pressure. Thus a cylinder certified for 2015 psi may be filled to a pressure of 2217 psi and is generally referred to as a 2200 lb tank.

LIQUID GASES. For those gases that are packaged in liquid form, there is a limiting "filling density" that determines how much may be put in each cylinder. The filling density is the ratio between the weight of liquid gas put in a cylinder and the weight of water that the cylinder is able to contain. Thus, the carbon dioxide filling density of 68% means that the weight of the liquid gas allowable to charge a cylinder is equal to 68% of the weight of water that the cylinder has the capacity to hold. The filling densities of cyclopropane and nitrous oxide are 55% and 68%, respectively.

It should be noted that cylinder pressures for liquid gases are considerably lower than those for vaporous gases and the critical temperatures of the three liquid gases under consideration are all above average room temperature (CO_2 = 88° F; $[CH_2]_3$ = 256° F; N_2O = 98° F). Because liquid gas does not fill the entire volume of a given cylinder, the space above the liquid surface contains vapor of the gas in equilibrium with the liquid, and the measured pressure in the cylinder is the pressure of the *vapor* at any given temperature. Thus, although the pressure of a tank of carbon dioxide at its critical temperature of 88° F would be 1071 psig (critical pressure) and would rise with continued elevation of temperature, at room temperature of 70° F it is only about 825 psig. Similarly, the pressure of cyclopropane at its critical temperature of 256° F is 797 psig but is only 75 psig at room temperature. To compare vapor gas cylinders with liquid gas, we can say that the pressure in the former represents the force required to squeeze into a cylinder a given volume of gas; whereas in the latter it is the vapor pressure of the gas over the surface of a given weight of liquid poured into the closed container. The liquid gas pressure is dependent upon the temperature and is the result of the filling of the cylinder, not the cause.

Measuring cylinder contents

GAS CYLINDERS. The volume of gas in a cylinder is directly related to the cylinder pressure at a constant temperature. If a tank is full at 2200 psig, it will be but half full as usage drops the pressure to 1100 psig. The usual method of monitoring the depletion of cylinder contents is by the use of gauges. If greater accuracy is needed, weighing the cylinder when the weight of the empty cylinder and the density of the gas are known is more precise.

LIQUID GAS CYLINDERS. Since the pressure in a liquid gas cylinder is that of the gas vapor in balance with the liquid at a given temperature, it gives no indication of how much liquid remains in the cylinder at any one time. As long as there is liquid in the cylinder the vapor pressure, and thus the recorded gauge pressure, will remain unchanged even though gas is being drawn off. When the liquid is finally gone and the cylinder contains only vapor, then the pressure will fall in proportion to the reduction in the remaining gas volume until the tank is empty. Thus, gauge pressure is of use in monitoring cylinder contents only terminally; if contents must be determined, the cylinder must be weighed. Fig. 8-2 compares the pressure behavior of gas and liquid gas cylinders. Of course, the vapor pressure of liquid gas cylinders will

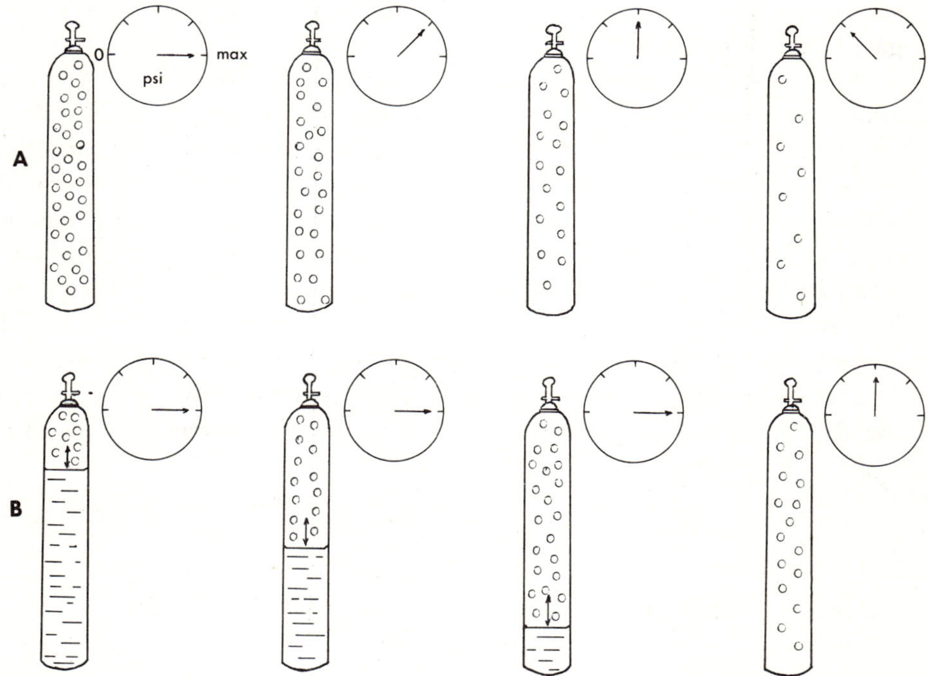

Fig. 8-2. The content of a gas-filled cylinder, **A**, is directly proportional to the gas pressure. As gas is withdrawn, for example, a pressure drop of 50% indicates a loss of 50% of the contained gas. In a liquid-gas cylinder, **B**, gauge pressure measures only the vapor pressure of gas in equilibrium with the liquid phase, and this remains constant at a given temperature as long as liquid is present. Only when all the liquid phase has vaporized, as the cylinder nears depletion, does the gauge pressure drop proportionately to the terminal volume of remaining gas.

vary with the temperature of their contents. Whereas carbon dioxide has a cylinder pressure of 838 psig at 70° F, at 60° F it has a cylinder pressure of only 733 psig. Then, as the temperature rises and approaches the critical point, more liquid will vaporize in the cylinder with an accompanying rise in pressure. Should a tank of carbon dioxide warm up to 88° F, the entire liquid contents will convert to gas; and if the temperature does not drop, as the gas is withdrawn, the cylinder gauge pressure will fall proportionately. Ethylene, on the other hand, is a gas at room temperature but with a relatively high critical temperature of 49° F; should it cool below this value, it will liquefy and its gauge pressure will stabilize as long as liquid remains in the cylinder.

Estimating duration of cylinder flow. When we set up a therapeutic procedure that utilizes cylinder vapor gas and that is expected to cover an extended period of time, it is a matter of both safety and convenience to be able to predict the approximate time to prepare for the replacement of the cylinder. Although this cannot be done with unerring accuracy because of the possibility of irregular flow rates, a practical rough estimate can be made on the basis of the average anticipated gas flows, the cylinder size, and the cylinder pressure at the start of therapy. Factors that can be used to convert these data into a time estimate can be calculated from the information on commonly used gases and cylinder sizes in Table 8-6.

Here is an example of the cumbersome combination of both the English and metric systems of measurement. Commercial gas cylinder calibrations and values are usually recorded in the English system; but once a therapeutic gas leaves the cylinder pressure reducing gauge, it is subject to the medical custom of using metric measurements. In essence, we wish to determine the length of time a given number of liters of gas per minute (lpm) will flow from a source of a given cubic footage of gas under a measurable pressure in psig. We now know that at a given temperature, the cylinder gas volume will decrease in proportion to the drop in gauge pressure; therefore each reduction in pounds per square inch of pressure represents a specific volume of gas loss from the cylinder. This factor, relating pressure drop to gas volume, is calculated as follows:

$$\frac{\text{Cubic feet of gas in full cylinder} \times \text{Factor to convert from cubic feet to liters}}{\text{Pressure of full cylinder in psig}}$$

Table 8-6. *Pressures and volumes of commonly used cylinders*

		Cubic feet of gas			
Gas	*Full cylinder pressure*	*D*	*E*	*G*	*H & K*
O_2	2200	12.7	22	187	244
O_2/CO_2	1800	12.7	22	187	244
He/O_2	2200	10.8	17.7	150	194
O_2/N_2	2200			187	244
Air	2200			187	244

Table 8-7. *Factors to calculate duration of cylinder flow in minutes*

Gas	*Cylinder size*			
	D	*E*	*G*	*H & K*
O_2, O_2/N_2, Air	0.16	0.28	2.41	3.14
O_2/CO_2	0.20	0.35	2.94	3.84
He/O_2	0.14	0.23	1.93	2.50

For example, an oxygen G-cylinder contains about 187 cubic feet of gas under a filling pressure of 2200 psig. Therefore, the volume of gas leaving the cylinder for every psig drop in pressure would be $(187 \times 28.3) \div 2200 = 2.41$ liters per psig.

Factors, so calculated for the gases and cylinders listed above, are shown in Table 8-7.

The principle employing the use of these factors is based on the relationship that tells us: liter loss in cylinder volume per drop in each pound per square inch of cylinder pressure, multiplied by the observed cylinder gauge pressure and divided by the liter per minute gas flow rate delivered to the patient, equals the number of minutes the gas will flow until the cylinder is empty. Thus:

$$\text{Duration of flow in minutes} = \frac{\text{Gauge pressure in psi} \times \text{Factor}}{\text{Liter flow}}$$

As an example, let us estimate the duration of a G-cylinder of oxygen with a gauge pressure of 800 psi, if we use a flow rate of 8 lpm. Referring to Table 8-7, we find the oxygen G-cylinder factor of 2.41 and set up the simple fraction:

$$\frac{800 \times 2.41}{8} = 241 \text{ minutes, or approximately 4 hours}$$

Bulk oxygen

Because of the tremendous volume of oxygen used in the average general hospital, a separate discussion of special large bulk storage systems is warranted. Bulk oxygen storage consists of any system capable of accommodating more than 12,000 cubic feet of the gas ready for use or more than 25,000 cubic feet including unconnected reserves. Such systems may be located out of doors or in a special building set aside for the purpose. Strict regulations for locating and maintaining bulk oxygen systems have been established by the National Fire Protection Association, subject to further control by local community fire and building codes. The supervision and maintenance of bulk oxygen units are not always functions of the inhalation therapist but often are responsibilities of oxygen service companies and hospital departments of engineering and maintenance. Nevertheless, the therapist should be acquainted with the systems since they concern his most important therapeutic tool and because he should be knowledgeable enough to be able to participate in dealing with emergency interruption of gas supply.

Bulk oxygen systems may provide either gaseous or liquid oxygen, and these will be discussed separately below. Bulk oxygen is used as a "central supply," or "piped-in system," in which the gas is carried from its station to the hospital divisions by a system of pipes built into the walls of new construction or often added to the wall surfaces of older buildings. It is thus possible to have an oxygen outlet conveniently located by each patient's bed and any other area desired. The great values of such a centrally located oxygen supply should be obvious. There is practically no risk of a depletion of oxygen during therapy, and the inconvenience and hazard of transporting and storing individual tanks are obviated. Finally, pressure reduction of oxygen is accomplished at the central station, and the gas is piped to the clinical areas already reduced to the standard working pressure of 50 psig. This eliminates the need for pressure-reducing valves at the patient outlets and requires the use of only flowmeters. As opposed to cylinder gas supply, a central system is referred to as a low-pressure system.

Gaseous bulk oxygen. There are three general systems that employ large central supplies of the gas form of oxygen.

STANDARD CYLINDERS. Large-sized standard cylinders can be banked together, usually pressurized at 2400 psig. Numbers of them can be tied together by a *manifold,* which, essentially, converts the individual units into one continuous supply. The manifold mechanism contains pressure-reduction valving and flow-control and alarm systems that warn of impending depletion or malfunction. As tanks empty, they are replaced by others. Sometimes packages of six or more tanks are manifolded together, each package replaced as needed.

FIXED CYLINDERS. In contrast to the cylinders just described, this system consists of large banks of up to 75 cylinders permanently fixed at a stationary site. When empty, they are refilled on location from a truck that contains liquid oxygen and converts the liquid to gas for pumping into the cylinders.

TRAILER UNITS. Mounted on trailers, tanks of a variety of sizes can be towed to the central area and connected to the distribution circuit. For heavy oxygen consumption, there are available large trailers with up to 30 permanently attached long horizontal tubes. Replacement is a simple matter of switching trailers. Like the other tank systems, trailer gas is also at 2400 psig pressure.

Liquid bulk oxygen. An extremely economical method of transporting and storing oxygen, liquid gas systems are widely used where the demand justifies their installation. Although we have already discussed the liquid form of some medical gases packaged in standard cylinders, because of its physical characteristics, liquid oxygen deserves special consideration. The major physical difference between oxygen and those liquid gases noted above is its very low critical temperature (−181.1° F) and boiling point (−297.3° F). The mechanisms for producing and maintaining the liquid state of oxygen are much more complex than are those for other medical liquid gases, but the practical returns justify the effort. Of prime importance is the fact that, at its boiling point, 1 cubic foot of liquid oxygen is the equivalent of 860.6 cubic feet of gaseous oxygen at ambient temperature and pressure.

Brief reference has been made earlier to the method of producing liquid oxygen from the compression and cooling of air. To prevent the liquid from reverting to gas, the liquid must be kept below −297° F, both in transportation and in storage. This is accomplished by keeping it in special containers, under a pressure not to exceed 250 psig. All such containers for liquid oxygen, whether trucks for transporting the substance or hospital supply stations, are constructed on the principle of a large thermos bottle, with which we are all acquainted. They consist of inner and outer steel shells, separated by a vacuum, which effectively blocks the transfer of heat into the liquid. This evacuated space is filled with a noncombustible insulation, and the inner shell is silvered to aid in repelling heat. The containers are vented so that vaporized liquid oxygen can escape if warming occurs. It should be apparent that when liquid oxygen is kept below its boiling point it can be exposed to atmospheric pressure, at least for short periods of time, without immediately vaporizing. Otherwise, transferring the material from supply truck to bulk container, for example, would be difficult. There are two types of containers for hospital use of liquid oxygen—the liquid oxygen cylinder and the permanent station.

LIQUID OXYGEN CYLINDER. This unit is not necessarily classified as part of a bulk system because individual tanks of liquid gas can be used. These cylinders measure 58 inches high and 20 inches in diameter and hold the equivalent of 3000 cubic feet of gas at ambient temperature and pressure, matching the contents of more than 12 large gas cylinders. As with the gas tanks, the liquid cylinders can be banked by manifold to provide a space-saving supply of oxygen.

FIXED STATION. These units are cylindrical or spherical containers with capacities up to a gaseous equivalent of 130,000 cubic feet. The liquid is con-

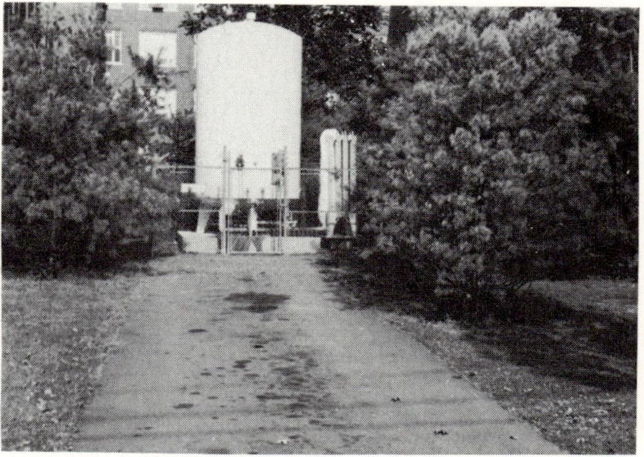

Fig. 8-3. Typical liquid oxygen storage facility in a hospital setting.

verted to usable gas by a heating unit called a *vaporizer,* which may be heated by steam, hot air, electricity, or hot water. Elaborately controlled to assure a steady even conversion of liquid to gas according to need, these systems assure an unlimited gas supply no matter what the peak demand load may be. They are refilled from service tank trucks according to schedules suited to each hospital. All liquid gas sources reduce their already low pressure to the 50 psig hospital line pressure. Fig. 8-3 illustrates a typical unit.

Regulation of gas flow

Whatever the source of medical gas, a device is needed to regulate its flow as it is administered to a patient. This ensures that the gas will be given at a safe pressure and allows adjustment of the volume of gas to suit the patient's needs. Such a device is called a *regulator* and it performs two functions: it reduces the high pressure of the gas in the cylinder to a safe working pressure, about 50 psig, and it allows the controlled release of gas over a narrow range of flow rates, usually from 1 to 15 liters per minute. The student may wonder why this would be necessary for central oxygen supply, when the outlet pressure already has been reduced to 50 psig. In such instances the entire regulator mechanism is not needed and only the flow rate control is used. We will discuss separately the following four topics: regulation of high-pressure cylinder gas, regulation of low-pressure centrally supplied systems, pressure compensation and safety indexed connector systems.

High-pressure cylinder gas regulators. There are three types of cylinder regulators, and though they function on the same basic principle, they deserve individual description. They may be designated as preset, adjustable, and multiple-stage regulators.

PRESET REGULATOR. Fig. 8-4 shows a schematic illustration of this instrument. Attached to the cylinder outlet, high-pressure gas enters the regulator through A, with cylinder pressure (and thus contents) recorded on the pressure gauge (B). The body of the regulator is divided into a pressure chamber (C) and an ambient pressure chamber (D) by a flexible diaphragm (E). Attached to the diaphragm, in the atmospheric chamber, is a spring (F) fixed to the other side of the chamber. Also attached to the diaphragm, but in the pressure chamber, is a valve stem (G) the other end of which controls the flow of gas through a valve (H). Gas goes to the patient through the outflow (I), passing through a Thorpe-tube flowmeter (J). The amount of gas released to the patient is regulated by the needle valve (K) and is read on a calibrated scale as liters per minute according to the height at which the ball is elevated in the Thorpe-tube flowmeter. The pressure chamber is supplied with a safety vent (L) that prevents an accidental buildup of pressure beyond 200 psig in the event of malfunction. This regulator is called *preset* because it is so constructed that the spring (F) will give if pressure on the diaphragm (E) exceeds 50 psig. When this happens, the valve stem (G) will be pulled back and the valve (H) will close, preventing further entry of gas into the regulator. As long

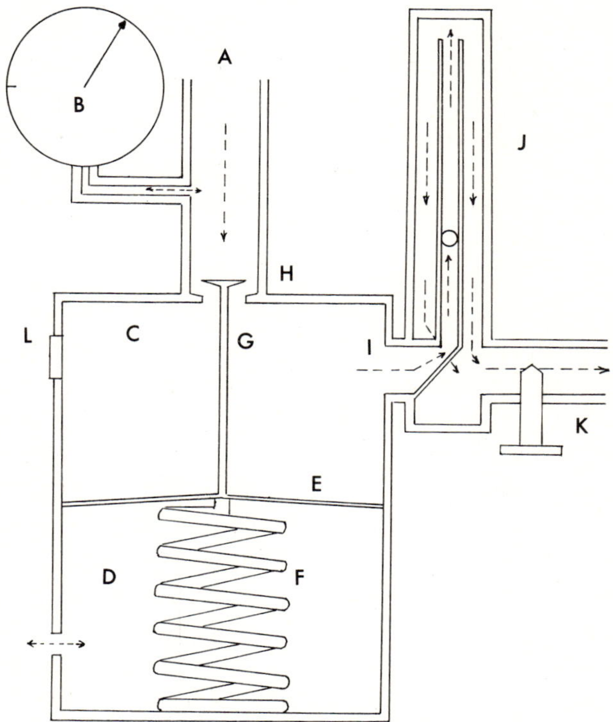

Fig. 8-4. Diagram of preset, high-pressure gas regulator. See text for details.

as the needle valve (K) is open, allowing the escape of gas from the pressure chamber, the valve at H will remain open and permit gas flow. Thus a balance will be established so that the valve at H is open just enough to meet the demand of valve K and the automatic adjustment of the diaphragm-spring combination will prevent excessive pressures from building up in chamber C.

ADJUSTABLE REGULATOR. This is one of the most commonly encountered regulators, differing from the preset type in two aspects, as shown in Fig. 8-5. The identifying feature of this regulator is the threaded hand control on its face (K). This is attached to the end of the spring and allows displacement of the diaphragm. Whereas the valve (H) in the preset regulator is open until gas enters the pressure chamber and closes it by pressure against the diaphragm, in the adjustable regulator the valve (H) is closed until the hand screw advances the whole mechanism and opens it to allow gas flow. The valve can thus be opened to permit a wide range of flows, and the pressures in chamber C will vary according to the relation between the amount of high-pressure gas entering and the amount leaving the regulator, but the spring will prevent the pressure from exceeding 50 psig. In the preset regulator, pressure in the chamber is always 50 psig; but in the adjustable one, it can be anything up to 50 psig. A second characteristic of the adjustable regulator is the use of a

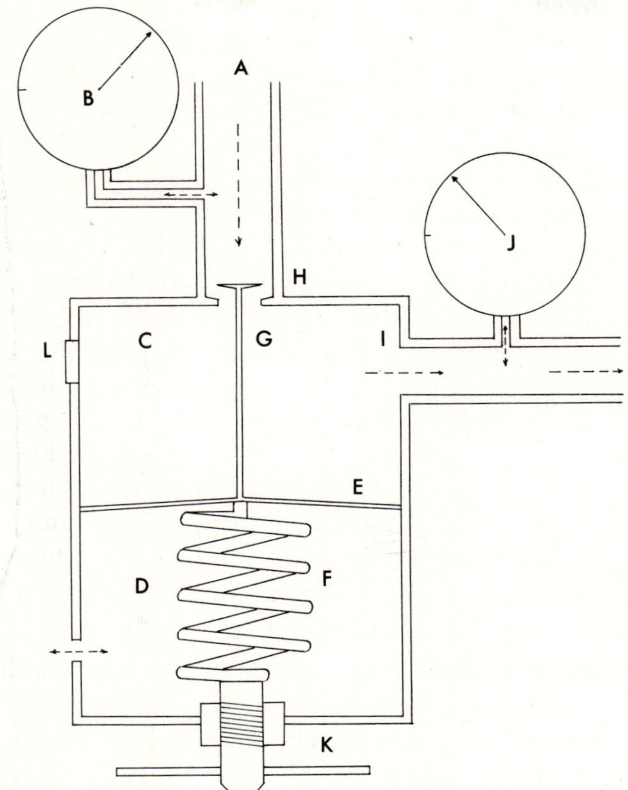

Fig. 8-5. Diagram of an adjustable, high-pressure gas regulator. See text for details.

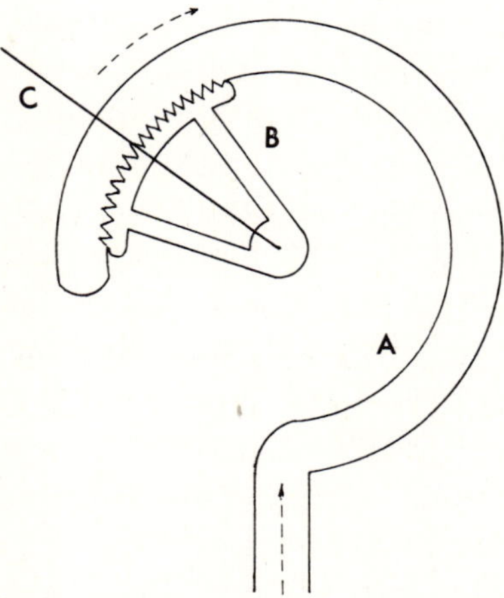

Fig. 8-6. Crude diagram of the principle of a gas-pressure gauge. See text for description.

Bourdon flowmeter (J) instead of a Thorpe. In reality, the Bourdon meter is a pressure gauge, like that at the regulator inflow (B), and functions on the principle crudely schematicized in Fig. 8-6. The heart of the gauge is a curved flexible closed tube (A) that responds to the pressure of gas entering it by changing shape. The force of the gas tends to straighten the tube, causing its distal end to move as indicated by the arrow; and through a gear mechanism (B) this motion is transmitted to an indicating needle (C). A numbered scale is calibrated by its manufacturer to read the needle movement either as pressure or liter flow, and gauges are constructed to varying degrees of sensitivity according to the ranges of pressure to which they are to be subjected. The Bourdon gauge is a low-pressure device (less than 50 psig) that meters the gas leaving the regulator, with a scale that converts pressure to flow rate in liters per minute.

MULTIPLE-STAGE REGULATOR. As the name implies, this instrument accomplishes pressure reduction in two or three steps instead of one and is essentially one or two valves in one. Therapists may have occasion to use two-stage reducing valves, but rarely three. The first stage of high-pressure reduction is preset at the factory and lowers cylinder pressure to an intermediate level, somewhere around 700 psig; in three-stage units the second stage lowers it to about half the first. The final stages, second or third as the case may be, therefore work off a lower pressure than does a single-stage valve and presumably are able to effect somewhat more precision and smoothness in flow control. A multiple-stage reducing valve may be provided with either a Bourdon or a Thorpe-tube metering device. It is larger and more costly than a single-stage and is indicated where minimal fluctuations in pressure and flow rates are critical factors. For routine hospital work the simpler single-stage regulators are satisfactory. The number of stages in a reducing valve can be easily determined by noting the number of safety vents present; there will be one for each pressure chamber.

Low-pressure gas regulators. It was emphasized earlier that one of the assets of a central gas supply system is the reduction of pressure at the central location so that the gas is at its working pressure when it reaches the outlets. This eliminates the need for pressure-reducing devices for patient administration and requires only a simple flowmeter. The Thorpe-tube flowmeter is used for this purpose, since it is calibrated to work off a pressure of 50 psig, as shown in Fig. 8-4. With outlets of a low pressure–oxygen or compressed-air system located by the patient's bed, therapy can be instituted in moments merely by plugging in a flowmeter and adjusting its flow as desired.

Pressure compensation. The term *pressure compensation* refers to a design in the Thorpe-tube flowmeter to prevent changes in gas pressure flowing through it from affecting its liter flow calibration. Although all standard manufacturers of these devices now supply them pressure compensated, the therapist should understand the importance of this and be on the alert for old equipment still in use that might not conform to present standards.

The problem of pressure compensation is the result of the effect of back pressure on a flowmeter, when the gas outlet of the meter is connected with a therapeutic instrument. Practically all gas-administering equipment contains some restrictions in its circuits; and in some, such as jet aerosol generators, these restrictions are acute. When gas flow encounters a restriction, a back pressure is generated. At this point we might define back pressure as a pressure drop across a restriction, according to concepts we considered in some detail earlier, when we learned of Bernoulli's principle, and the relation between pressure, flow, and resistance. Therapeutically, we are interested in the delivered pressure distal to an obstruction, and if this is lower than the line pressure entering the restriction, we have a back pressure proximal to the restriction. Let us now compare three flow-measuring devices, a Bourdon flow (pressure) gauge, an uncompensated flowmeter (Thorpe-tube), and a compensated flowmeter.

BOURDON GAUGE. As just described and illustrated in Figs. 8-5 and 8-6, the Bourdon gauge measures pressure and is thus not a flowmeter. It measures the pressure of gas flowing from the pressure chamber of an adjustable reducing valve, and at the factory it is calibrated to indicate given flow volumes of gas at different pressures with its outflow *open to the atmosphere.* Thus the face of the valve shows supposed flow rates. In clinical use, however, the gauge output is faced with the back pressure resistance of therapeutic appliances, and it responds to this pressure, indicating a flow higher than the patient actually receives. At low flow rates, the pressure drop across an obstruction may be slight, but if the patient needs higher flows, the reducing valve must be opened further to supply gas at a higher pressure. At these increased rates, there will be more of a pressure drop across the obstruction, and the gauge-indicated flow may be considerably greater than that which actually reaches the patient. Indeed, because the gauge records reducing valve chamber pressure, it will register pressure (flow rate on its printed face) with the valve open and the output completely blocked.

UNCOMPENSATED FLOWMETER. This type is also calibrated in liters per minute against the atmosphere, without restriction. Gas flow at 50 psig into the meter is controlled by a needle valve *proximal* to the meter, as shown in Fig. 8-7, *A*. The heart of the meter consists of a tapered transparent tube with a float, as shown much exaggerated in Fig. 8-8, with its diameter increasing from below upward. The float is suspended in the tube by the flow of gas past it, and its position is noted against an adjacent scale, which indicates the flow rate. Because the tube is part of the gas conduction system, the float cannot occlude it and must depend for its support on the Bernoulli effect. The space between the float and the inner surface of the tube constitutes a restriction, and the increased velocity of gas through this restriction produces a pressure drop immediately above the float. In Fig. 8-8, pressure above the float (P_2) is less than that below it (P_1), and the float rises in the tube until its own weight equals the lifting force. When therapy equipment is attached distal to the

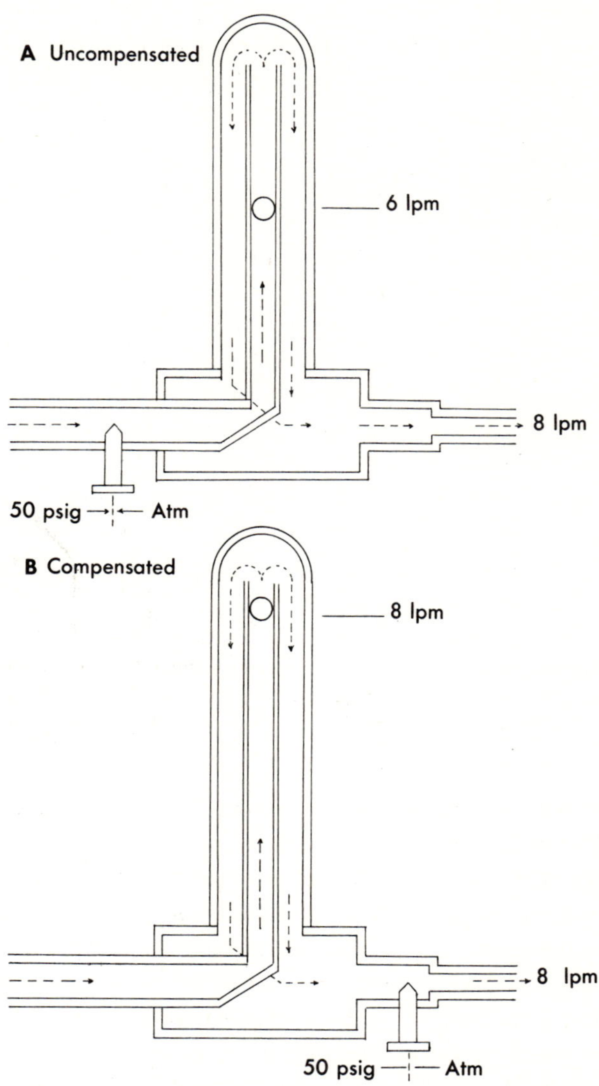

Fig. 8-7. Comparison of, **A**, pressure-uncompensated, and **B**, pressure-compensated flowmeters. In the former, the flow-control valve is proximal to the meter, and the gauge records less than the actual output. In the latter, location of the valve distal to the meter correlates the gauge reading with the output. See text for detailed explanation.

meter, back pressure is generated in the atmosphere-equilibrated circuit, from the point of restriction in the equipment back through the flow tube to the needle valve, Fig. 8-7, A. As long as the back pressure does not exceed the source pressure of 50 psig, gas will continue to flow into the tube, but the back pressure does increase the pressure distal to the float (P_2 in Fig. 8-8). This reduces the pressure differential from P_1 to P_2, lessens the lift effect, and lets the float drop to a lower position. Therefore, a flowmeter that does not

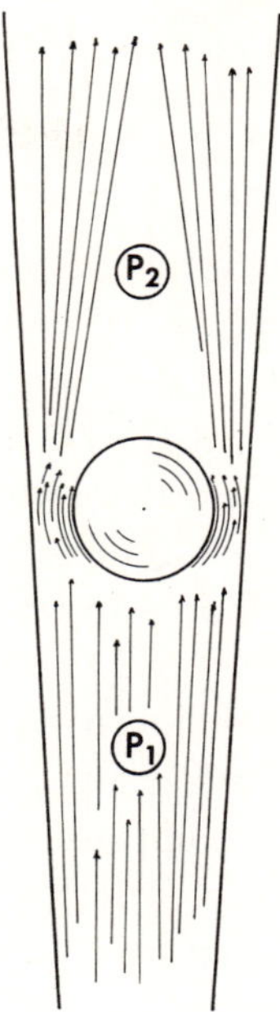

Fig. 8-8. The position of a flowmeter float depends upon a Bernoulli-generated pressure differential across it so that $P_1 > P_2$. Back pressure on the float increases P_2, reducing the differential and permitting the float to drop even though actual flow rate may be maintained.

compensate for back pressure, when faced with a restriction, records less gas flow than the patient actually receives.

COMPENSATED FLOWMETER. In contrast to the above two instruments, the scale of the compensated flowmeter is calibrated against a constant pressure of 50 psig instead of the atmosphere, and its major structural feature, shown in Fig. 8-7, *B*, is a flow control needle valve *distal* to the flow tube. Thus, the entire meter, including the tube, to the needle valve is at a constant pressure of 50 psig, whereas in an uncompensated meter the 50 psig inlet pressure stops at the needle valve proximal to the tube. With a restriction distal to the meter, back pressure will develop in the atmosphere-equilibrated portion of the circuit, from the restriction back to the needle valve. However, as long as the back pressure does not exceed 50 psig, it can have no effect in the tube and will not alter the flow kinetics, which are responsible for the lifting force on the float. Such a pressure-compensated flowmeter, regardless of restrictions, will accurately record the flow to the patient and is the preferred instrument for clinical use.

Safety indexed connector systems. With the tremendous number of compressed gases in current commercial, medical, and scientific use, one of the greatest risks in medical gas therapy is the inadvertant administration of a wrong gas to a patient. Certainly, care on the part of the medical attendant in reading labels or other identifying marks is the most important deterrent to such an accident. The human error, however, must always be considered a potential risk, and to compensate for this there have been developed specially designed connectors for compressed gas tanks and their accessories. The purpose of an indexed connector system is to make impossible certain connections between cylinders and delivery systems. When properly used, for example, a cylinder of any gas other than oxygen could not be functionally attached to any system for which only oxygen is specified. The importance of such a precaution for anesthetic gases is obvious. The systems commonly in use will be briefly described, but the therapist is encouraged to familiarize himself with their details as set forth in publications of the Compressed Gas Association. There are three basic indexed connector systems: the American Standard Compressed Gas Cylinder Outlet and Inlet Connections, the Diameter-Index Safety System (DISS), and the Pin-Index Safety System.

AMERICAN STANDARD COMPRESSED GAS CYLINDER VALVE OUTLET AND INLET CONNECTIONS. In the United States and Canada the specifications for threaded connections between compressed gas cylinders and their attached tubing have been standardized according to the type of gas concerned and are explained in detail in one of the publications of the Compressed Gas Association, Inc.[169] This system is confined to cylinders with threaded outlets from their valves and includes specifications for the mating nipples and hexagonal nuts by which an appliance (usually a pressure regulator) is attached to the valve. Fig. 8-9 illustrates a cutaway of a joined threaded outlet and nipple. The gas channel through the nipple of the regulator is aligned with the channel through the threaded outlet, and the two parts are secured by a wrench-tightened hexagonal nut that is held loosely on the nipple by a shoulder and flange mechanism.

The Standard system is based on varying dimensions of the cylinder out-

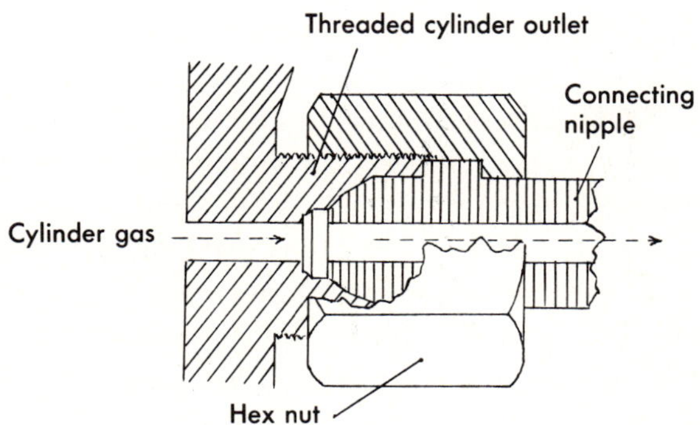

Fig. 8-9. This sketch illustrates the structure of a typical American Standard connection, such as might be used to attach a reducing valve to a large high-pressure cylinder. The hexagonal nut is held onto the nipple of the reducing valve by a circular collar, seen as a cross-sectional projection on the nipple. As the hex nut is tightened on the threaded cylinder outlet, the end of the nipple is snugly seated into the conical outlet. (Adapted from CGA Pamphlet V-1, p 28, connection no. 540, Compressed Gas Association, Inc., New York.)

let and nipple, to limit the introduction of cylinders into a gas circuit specific to certain groups of gases. There are four fundamental divisions of the calibrated system—internal and external threads and right-handed and left-handed threads. Each division is further segmented by varying the number, pitch, and diameter of the threads. In general, left-handed threads are used for fuel gases, and right-handed threads are used for nonfuel. Most of the valve outlets have external threads, and their corresponding nipples internal threads. The threads of the Standard system are usually classified as NGO (National Gas Outlet), but a few are NGT (National Gas Taper). Each gas does not have its own specific connection, but 1 to 13 gases may share the same one since there are some 26 different connections for about 62 listed gases. The Standard system of classification is not binding on manufacturers, and the inhalation therapist must certainly read the specifications of cylinders supplied to his hospital so that he will be completely familiar with any deviations from standard design.

In catalogues of cylinder gas dealers, the therapist will see the connection specifications listed for each type of cylinder and gas. A typical description is as follows, for a large cylinder of oxygen:

CGA-540 0.903-14NGO-RH-Ext

This tells us that the connection for the threaded outlet of this cylinder is listed by the Compressed Gas Association as connection no. 540, that the outlet has a thread diameter of 0.903 inch, that there are 14 threads per inch of the National Gas Outlet type, and that the threads are right-handed and external.

Generally, the inhalation therapist will use but one or two outlet connections, since most of the relatively small number of different gases he employs are grouped within a few connector sizes. He should be familiar with the classifications, however, since expanding instrumentation and scope of services may bring him into increasing contact with gases and tubing systems in the future.

DIAMETER-INDEX SAFETY SYSTEM (DISS). As a sequential companion to the American Standard system described above, the DISS was established to prevent accidental interchanging among the removable threaded connectors used for medical gas–administering equipment at pressures of *200 psig or less.* Specifically, DISS in inhalation therapy is utilized in effecting safe union between pressure regulators or flowmeters and any threaded connectors that are frequently engaged or disengaged in routine use. Such connections will also be used with therapy equipment and anesthesia apparatus. It should be noted that the standard removable threaded oxygen connector that has been in long use, 0.5625 inch in diameter, 18 threads per inch, has been retained and is not a part of the Diameter-Index System.

The system is designed as follows: Each connection consists of an externally threaded body (like the threaded outlet of a cylinder but smaller) and a mated nipple with hex nut, illustrated in Fig. 8-10. The body of the connector has two concentric borings, a primary bore, noted as Bore 1, and a counterbore, Bore 2. The accompanying nipple has two shoulders, identified as 1 and 2, and a loose hex nut secured by a flange behind Shoulder 2. It can be seen that, as the two parts are joined, the corresponding shoulders and bores mate and the union is held by the tightened hex nut. Indexing is achieved by varying the dimensions of the borings and shoulders; starting with a basic set of dimensions, bore 1 is increased and bore 2 decreased in increments of 0.012 inch. The nipple shoulders are changed accordingly. The final connection is a smooth-bored body and a nipple of regular diameter. There are 11 indexed connections, which accommodate 11 gases or gas mixtures, and Table 8-8 lists the DISS connection numbers with the gases assigned to each from data of the Compressed Gas Association.[170]

To illustrate the use of the DISS, let us imagine an equipment catalogue listing the specifications of a pressure regulator to be used on a cylinder of 100% carbon dioxide. The *inlet* (inlet of regulator, which mates with the threaded outlet of the cylinder) will require an American Standard connection designated as CGA-320. According to CGA data this will be a 0.825 inch

Table 8-8. *DISS connection numbers and assigned gases*

Connection number	*Gas*	*Connection number*	*Gas*
1020	Unassigned	1140	C_2H_4
1040	N_2O	1160	Air
1060	He	1180	He/O_2 (He 80% or less)
	He/O_2 ($O_2 < 20\%$)	1200	O_2/CO_2 (CO_2 7% or less)
1080	CO_2	1220	Suction
	O_2/CO_2 ($CO_2 > 7\%$)	1240	O_2 (standard)
1100	$(CH_2)_3$		
1120	Unassigned		

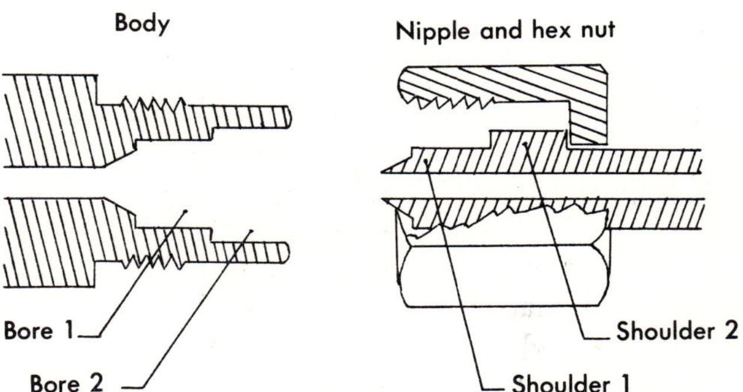

Fig. 8-10. Schematic illustration of components of a representative DISS connection. The two shoulders of the nipple allow the nipple to unite only with a body having corresponding borings. If the match is incorrect, the hex nut will not engage the body threads. (Adapted from CGA Pamphlet V-5, p 9, DISS connection no. 1100, Compressed Gas Association, Inc., New York.)

14NGO-RH-Ext cylinder outlet for which there is a specific regulator nipple.[169] The *outlet* (of the regulator, to which a low-pressure line is attached to supply an appliance) will require a DISS connection CGA-1080.

Most of the time the therapist will use oxygen from a regulator, utilizing the standard removable connection designated as CGA-1240, which is not a DISS unit; but he will frequently have occasion to administer helium-oxygen mixtures and oxygen–carbon dioxide mixtures, both of which have DISS connections. To avoid the cumbersome stocking of a large variety of pressure regulators and to make economical use of those on hand, he can use adapters to convert the outlets of the common oxygen regulators to suitable DISS dimensions for special gas use.

PIN-INDEX SAFETY SYSTEM. Pin-Indexing is incorporated in the specifications of the American Standard listing just described but as a special section applicable only to the flush valve outlets of the small cylinders, up to and including size E, which use a yoke connection. These valves do not have a threaded outlet but rather a recess in a flat face of the valve into which fits a nipple on the yoke to receive the gas (Fig. 8-1). The Pin-Index is intended for use on anesthesia machines or similar equipment, where fixed yokes are attached to internal gas circuitry, and is designed to prevent the wrong cylinder from being attached to a given yoke.

Two holes are drilled in the face of the valve, their exact position varying with the gas in the cylinder. There are two pins in corresponding positions on the yoke, and unless the pins and holes align perfectly, the yoke nipple will not seat in the recess of the valve. Six hole-pin combinations comprise

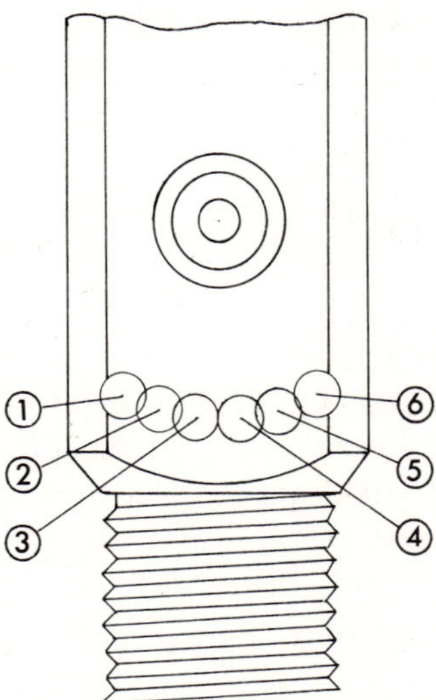

Fig. 8-11. Location of the Pin-Index Safety System holes in the cylinder valve face, various pairs of which constitute indices for different gases. See text for the complete pairings. (Adapted from CGA Pamphlet V-1, p 38, Pin-Index Safety System, Compressed Gas Association, Inc., New York.)

Table 8-9. *Pin-Indexed gases*

Gas	*Index hole position*
O_2	2-5
O_2/CO_2 (CO_2 not over 7%)	2-6
He/O_2 (He not over 80%)	2-4
C_2H_4	1-3
N_2O	3-5
$(CH_2)_3$	3-6
He/O_2 (He over 80%)	4-6
O_2/CO_2 (CO_2 over 7%)	1-6
Air	1-5

the total system; but because of overlapping, adjacent holes cannot be used, and there are thus 10 possible combinations, of which nine are now in use. Fig. 8-11 is a composite illustration of the location of all six possible holes and the numbers by which they are indexed. Table 8-9 is based on Compressed Gas Association information and lists the gases now in Pin-Indexed cylinders, with their index positions.

OXYGEN THERAPY

The single most important need of the human organism, as an earth surface dweller, is oxygen; and the therapist, now well versed in the hazards of hypoxia, can understand that the effective administration of oxygen is his most vital function. Indeed, most of the techniques he employs in patient care are designed to facilitate the adequate distribution of oxygen to pulmonary capillary blood. As a technical expert in the clinical use of this essential gas, the therapist should learn as much about it as he can, through independent study; and to give him a start, we will consider some of the basic characteristics of oxygen that specifically relate to its medical use.

In the cosmos as a whole, the three most abundant elements in order are hydrogen, helium, and oxygen; in and about the earth oxygen is the most prevalent and widely distributed. In view of our great dependence upon oxygen, the presence of which we take so for granted, it is interesting to note that countless millions of years ago oxygen was completely missing from the atmosphere of earth. In those first hours of time, earth's atmosphere probably consisted entirely of hydrogen.[171] The evolution of our common air was a complex sequence of physical-chemical reactions spanning eons of time and involving the production and consumption of energy, the magnitude of which defies the imagination. It is theorized that the great energy of the stars was produced by the burning of hydrogen, with its eventual conversion to helium and other elements heavier than itself. Under conditions of extraordinary temperature, helium can transform to carbon and can even react with some of this carbon to produce the element oxygen along with gamma radiation. Such reactions, slowly progressing over millions of years, gradually shifted the composition of the earth's atmosphere, increasing the concentrations of oxygen. Other contributing phenomena included the ultraviolet energy of the sun, which dissociated water into hydrogen and hydroxyl radicals, further breaking the latter into hydrogen and oxygen, and finally, when life on earth was represented by algae in the sea, the significant chemical reactions of photosynthesis. It has been estimated that there was a great increase in the amount of oxygen in the atmosphere about 5.5×10^8 years ago, coincident with a surge in evolution of life forms. As oxygen established itself among the earth's elements, the lighter hydrogen gradually diffused outward into space. Thus, since its origin, earth's atmosphere has been in a process of continuous change; and it is interesting to ask ourselves whether we should consider our present atmosphere any more permanent than the atmosphere of 10 million or 100 million years ago and to speculate that the familiar composition of our air may be but a momentary step in the evolution of nature, gradually to give way to other as yet unguessed at gases. However, faced with survival in a breathing mixture, of which oxygen comprises some 21%, let us examine some of the features of this element and then discuss the therapeutic uses of the "number one medicine."

Characteristics of oxygen

Oxygen is a colorless, transparent, tasteless, and odorless gas occurring in nature as free molecular O_2 and as a component of a host of chemical compounds, both organic and inorganic. It comprises almost 50% of the weight of the earth's crust and occurs in all living matter as water and in combination with elements other than hydrogen. At 0° C and 1 atm pressure, oxygen has a density of 1.429 gm/liter, compared to the density of air, 1.30 gm/liter. It is but slightly soluble in water; at room temperature and 1 atm pressure 3.3 volumes of oxygen dissolve in 100 volumes of water. Nonetheless, this small amount is essential to aquatic life, both plant and animal.

Oxygen does not burn. However, it does support combustion, a matter of considerable importance to its widespread use in hospitals. A minute spark can become a large hot flame in an enriched oxygen environment, or a glowing ember can burst into open flame. The relationship between the burning intensity of a combustible substance and the amount of ambient oxygen is direct but not simple. Burning speed increases with an increase in the partial pressure of oxygen in the environment. Thus, increasing concentrations of oxygen at a fixed total pressure, or an increase in total pressure of a constant gas concentration, both, will augment the kinetics of combustion. However, burning speed will also increase when only oxygen concentrations are raised, and the partial pressure of the various oxygen percentages is kept constant by suitably lowering the total pressure.[172] These data demonstrate that both oxygen concentration and partial pressure influence rate of burning. Another factor to consider in the relation between burning and the amount of oxygen is the self-perpetuating effect of combustion in oxygen. The reaction of oxygen with other elements is markedly enhanced at elevated temperatures, and once combustion starts in a high-oxygen atmosphere, the heat produced potentiates further combustion and is not wasted on the relatively inert nitrogen content of ordinary air.

Although oxygen can be produced by many chemical reactions and the electrolysis of water, as noted in Chapter 1, its main source is compressed air. Under the influence of tremendous pressure followed by the cooling effect of sudden expansion combined with heat exchangers, the components of air are converted to liquid. Through the process of fractional distillation, as the liquefied air is allowed to heat slowly, nitrogen, with its boiling point of −195.8° C (−320.5° F), escapes first; then the trace gases of argon, krypton, and xenon are removed. Standards require that the final remaining oxygen have a purity of at least 99%, a value that is usually exceeded. The liquid oxygen is stored in special containers or converted to gas under high pressure in tanks.

Precautions in the use of oxygen

We have emphasized the importance of oxygen in the treatment of disease and have considered in some detail the seriousness of oxygen deprivation, but it must not be thought to be a completely innocuous agent. The inhalation therapist must familiarize himself with all aspects of the physiologic action of oxygen, the harmful as well as the beneficial. He must be aware of those conditions in which oxygen is not indicated, when it may even be a threat to life, for such caution will make him a safe as well as an effective therapist. Before discussing the equipment and techniques for administering oxygen, we will consider some of the risks of its use and explore a bit its pathologic potential. As a guide, we will take up oxygen-induced hypoventilation, atelectasis, retrolental fibroplasia, and oxygen toxicity, considering these effects only at 1 atm pressure.

Oxygen-induced hypoventilation. This is not a new topic, for in our study of cardiopulmonary physiology we covered it superficially in discussions of ventilatory control, comparing the roles of the cerebral respiratory center and the peripheral chemoreceptors. Here, we will be interested not only in the specific academic relationship between oxygen and the ventilatory control mechanisms but also in the practical clinical use of oxygen in patients suffering from failure of these mechanisms. For example, for the patient who is in ventilatory failure with its accompanying hypercapnia, we may usually assume that oxygen can be safely administered at concentrations slightly above ambient, at 1 atm pressure. Flow rates of 1 to 2 liters per minute carry little risk and can be achieved by techniques to be discussed subsequently. Even so, the arterial carbon dioxide level may rise slightly but, after a period of perhaps 1 hour, will usually plateau at a level still within the bounds of safety. It has often been noted that if the oxygen administration is stopped oxygen tension in arterial blood may fall below pretreatment levels.[173] In such a situation, it is evident that intermittent use of the gas may be dangerous to the patient's respiratory equilibrium and, to assure adequate oxygenation, oxygen should be given constantly with mechanical support of ventilation if necessary. This latter aspect will be dealt with in detail in another chapter.[174] As a guide for the use of oxygen in patients with ventilatory failure, it has been suggested that an arterial oxygen tension of about 50 mm Hg will prevent immediate death from hypoxia while keeping the adverse effects of oxygen to a minimum. This does not imply that such a level is therapeutically desirable as definitive therapy but that this tension will prevent rapid deterioration of the patient's state while other measures are being prepared.[175]

The effect of oxygen administration on ventilation is well documented in a study of several patients with chronic respiratory disease who were tested for their response to concentrations of oxygen in the 90% to 100% range.[176] When a normal subject breathes 100% oxygen, his chemoreceptors remain inactive and, because of the increased oxygen in the blood, there is less reduced hemoglobin available for carbon dioxide transportation and arterial P_{CO_2} tends to rise. To maintain a normal acid-base balance, the increased $P_{a_{CO_2}}$ acting on the cerebral respiratory center, plus the irritating effect of the high concentration of oxygen on the respiratory mucosa, can produce a 5% to 20% increase in ventilation and correct the hypercapnia. In the presence of hypoxia, the arterial unsaturation stimulates the chemoreceptors, and if there is no airway obstruction to carbon dioxide excretion, the augmented ventilation may produce hypocapnia. This reaction is not uncommon in patients at high altitude, with venous-arterial shunts, and with alveolar-capillary block. It would seem that the reactions of the respiratory center to blood carbon dioxide and to the stretch-receptor signals in the diseased lung are still adequate. Of course, this sensitive response implies a normally functioning respiratory center. In contrast, when hypoxia exists with the hypercapnia of ventilatory failure, because the latter denotes an unresponsive respiratory center, oxygen administration suppresses the chemoreceptors and produces a hypoventilation that is not compensated.

It was observed that, on the average, when the arterial carbon dioxide tension was greater than 50 mm Hg the risk of oxygen-induced hypoventilation increased; and this value seemed more significant than the pH level. This substantiates the observation, which the inhalation therapist will have frequent occasion to make, that the obstructed patient with hypoxia presents the greatest hypoventilation risk and that not far behind is the patient whose respiratory center is obtunded by sedation or narcosis.

This hazard of oxygen therapy does not militate against its use when indicated; for the relief of hypoxia is the most critical therapeutic need, and even for the most unresponsive patient, there are methods of giving oxygen. It does mean, however, that the therapist assigned to administer oxygen must never assume such administration to be a "routine" procedure. He should take the time to acquaint himself with the basic disease problem under treatment so that he will be alert to potential danger. This point is important enough that we will return to it again when we specifically discuss the management of ventilatory failure.

Atelectasis. The collapse of alveoli as the result of high concentrations of oxygen in the inhaled air is due to the elimination of nitrogen from the lung and the effect of oxygen on pulmonary surfactant. We will consider the first here, and the second below. Normally, the most prevalent gas in the alveoli is nitrogen, the bulk of which comes from the inspired air, with a much smaller amount coming from the general body metabolism. Breathing pure oxygen depletes the circulating nitrogen within several minutes as each tidal air excursion washes it out of the alveoli, into which the gas has diffused from the blood. The patient who is excessively relaxed and ventilating at a minimal tidal level, especially if he has some degree of airway obstruction as from retained secretions, is liable to suffer ill consequences of 100% oxygen breathing. As the patient breathes the oxygen, should the easy tidal flow be impeded to and from a partially blocked alveolus or one somewhat hampered by a dependent location, the oxygen that gains access to the alveolus may diffuse into the pulmonary circulation faster than it can be replaced by ventilation. This results in a gradual shrinking of the alveolus and, when aided by other factors, may lead to complete collapse. In the alert patient this is not as great a risk, since the natural "sigh" mechanism periodically hyperinflates the lung, ventilating those alveoli that may be considered sluggish in their tidal exchange.

It is of historical interest only that, in the past, the nitrogen-washout effect of 100% oxygen was used to relieve intestinal distension.[177] Nitrogen is one of the major intestinal gases causing distention, especially postoperatively. Because of its diffusibility into the lungs, 100% oxygen was used to remove it from the blood, thereby creating a gradient that allowed the nitrogen to move from the bowel into the circulation, thence to the lung, and out. It was shown that a given amount of nitrogen could be reduced 62% in 24 hours by this method, as against 10% by breathing room air. It is interesting to note that breathing 95% oxygen for no longer than 10 hours was one recommended technique; and we can only wonder how often recovery may have been retarded by pulmonary complications, even though bowel distress may have been relieved.

Retrolental fibroplasia. The term *retrolental* means "behind the lens" and refers to an ocular condition of premature infants associated with oxygen administration. The disease was established as a specific entity in the 1950's, when it was observed that some premature infants given oxygen therapy developed damage to the eyes that was severe enough to produce permanent blindness. The pathology is basically a fibrotic process behind the ocular lenses which impairs light penetration to the retinae. Apparently excessive blood oxygen levels produce retinal vasoconstriction, and if this is severe enough to persist after the cessation of oxygen therapy, permanent damage is likely.[178] This risk poses a serious management problem, for the prema infant is often in great need of supplementary oxygen, and, as in the inf with a lung expansion defect, sometimes large amounts of oxygen are nece sary for survival. Experience has demonstrated that if the concentration c inspired oxygen delivered to the small patient does not exceed 40% the risk of retrolental fibroplasia is significantly reduced. Most incubators, which provide the proper environment for premature infants, have devices that limit the oxygen concentration to 40%. However, more experience will be needed to determine more precisely the critical arterial oxygen tension level that is associated with oxygen damage to the eyes.

Oxygen toxicity. The adverse effects of oxygen described above can be considered local in nature and, although serious, do not cause the widespread destruction that is classified as toxicity. The scope of injury to the organism varies from the mild and transient to the overwhelmingly fatal, and we will describe the more important clinical and pathologic changes characterizing oxygen toxicity. The early signs and symptoms may include substernal distress, paresthesias in the extremities, nausea and vomiting, malaise, and fatigue. It is only under hyperbaric conditions that serious convulsions occur. The onset of discomfort beneath the sternum has been suggested as a significant indication of actual or impending toxicity.[179] The time necessary to produce toxic symptoms in human volunteers breathing 100% oxygen is reported to range from 6 to 30 hours, in one study, with the maximum limit of tolerance at 110 hours.[179] However, the voluntary limit of tolerance to 100% oxygen has been estimated to be between 53 and 75 hours.[180] As a rough guide, it has been suggested in the past that the risk of toxicity was minimized if the partial pressure of the inspired oxygen did not exceed 425 mm Hg, which is the equivalent of an oxygen concentration of 56% at 1 atm pressure. It is now felt that, given enough of a time exposure, toxic symptoms can appear at partial pressures much lower but that, because it is not known at what tension level man has unlimited tolerance, there are no sure rules to follow in the administration of oxygen. These so-called early signs and symptoms may progress to severe structural lung damage and to injury to other systems.

Some idea of the extent of oxygen toxicity in its advanced stages is revealed by the observation that 100% oxygen at atmosphere is able to inhibit the growth of living tissue cultures, apparently by interfering with the synthesis of DNA and RNA. In addition, pure oxygen disturbs many enzyme systems, especially those containing sulfhydril (SH) groups. The exposure of several species of animals to oxygen concentrations above 95% until they succumbed, or to a maximum duration of 240 hours, produced the following pathologic changes: pleural effusions, pulmonary edema, emphysema, dilatation of the tracheobronchial tree, and edema of the walls of airways and large vessels. It was noted that those animals surviving 240 hours of 100% oxygen demonstrated pulmonary edema and other damage to the lung but did not have pleural effusion; no conclusions were drawn from this observation.[181]

In another study, the average survival of a group of dogs exposed to 98% oxygen was 67 hours, and a significant finding was the loss of surface activity of lung extracts, associated with pulmonary damage. This reaction to oxygen became evident after exposure of 54 hours.[182] It has been postulated that high oxygen concentrations inactivate the pulmonary surfactin and do not invariably destroy it; it is felt that perhaps the adverse effect of oxygen is a redistribution of surfactin, removing it from its close contact with alveolar walls. The potential for this phenomenon to produce atelectasis is evident and is probably more important in this regard than the absorption of oxygen from poorly communicating alveoli, although both subject the patient to a double hazard.

We are more interested in the physiologic effect of high concentrations of oxygen in the human than in experimental animals, and several good studies provide the following data on human oxygen toxicity[183-186]: Postmortem examination of lungs of patients who had received intensive oxygen therapy immediately prior to death have revealed some important pathologic changes. The lungs are almost always described as heavy, congested, and "beefy" in appearance on gross examination. Microscopically, there is much capillary congestion, with proliferation (overgrowth) of capillaries. The interalveolar septa are thickened, and there are papillary projections or tufts of proliferated capillaries into the alveolar spaces. Alveolar edema and intra-alveolar hemorrhage are common, in both adults and infants. The interesting observation was made that the damaging effect of oxygen on the lungs tends to be less in patients with well-established lung disease than in those without such intrinsic disease. The implication is that the presence of such pathologic elements as exudate and fibrosis, which might be found in the lungs of patients with chronic bronchopulmonary disease, protects the pulmonary tissue from the assault of oxygen, as opposed to what occurs in the relatively normal lungs of patients receiving oxygen for such nonpulmonary conditions as shock, narcosis, and shunts. Fibrosis was noted to appear after 2 weeks' exposure, but capillary congestion and proliferation in as short a time as 2 days'. It is felt that the capillary "tufts" resolve in patients surviving high-oxygen therapy but, while present, are intra-alveolar space-occupying lesions that have been postulated as a cause of oxygen dependence, which requires "weaning" until they disappear. Infiltration of pulmonary tissue is generally lymphocytic, indicating that the tissue response is not that of an infectious inflammation.

Of great clinical importance is a pathologic phenomenon that deserves individual mention; but to appreciate it clearly, we must digress a bit and describe a pediatric disease relevant to our main topic. Many infants born prematurely suffer from a condition called *hyaline membrane disease,* or respiratory distress syndrome of the newborn (RDS). The major defect in this disease is a severely noncompliant lung, placing a tremendous physical strain on the ventilatory mechanics of the underdeveloped child. Many of these patients succumb in their early postnatal life, and others may survive only after intensive mechanical ventilatory support. The alveoli of the victims are lined with a thin but definite membrane, which because of its clear, transparent homogeneity is referred to as a "hyaline membrane." Such a structure is a normal prenatal component of the lung, but one that disappears prior to birth, and premature birth often does not allow time for its natural disappearance. One of the more serious complications of high concentration–oxygen therapy is the appearance of a hyaline membrane, in adults as well as children. As a demonstration of the ease with which a membrane can be formed 75% of a group of guinea pigs exposed to 98% oxygen at atmosphere from 40 to 100 hours developed such a defect. Interestingly, if a subject survives despite this injury, there is apparently no residual damage. The hyaline membrane produced experimentally with high oxygen concentrations appears to be structurally identical with that which occurs in RDS and seems to be the result of injury to the alveolar duct and terminal bronchiole. If the experimental animal is given high doses of adrenocorticosteroids with the elevated oxygen concentration, it deteriorates rapidly and dies from fulminating pulmonary vascular damage. Human postmortem lung specimens demonstrated reactions similar to the experimental, if the patients had been treated with high oxygen concentrations. The membranes noted consisted of layers of fibrin on the alveolar walls, extending into the alveolar ducts and respiratory bronchioles. Many patients succumbing to oxygen toxicity not only had received oxygen concentrations in the 90% to 100% range but had also had this delivered by mechanical ventilators. However, there is little correlation between the pulmonary pathologic changes and the mechanical ventilation, per se, but there is close correlation with the oxygen therapy. As yet, no dependable safety limits have been determined for oxygen administration, but it is evident that both factors of gas concentration and duration of treatment are critical. There is some evidence that prolonged administration of oxygen concentrations above 70% will increase the risk of membranous toxicity and that levels above 90% are dangerous.

There are important clinical implications in the available data concerning the scope and mechanisms of oxygen toxicity. We frequently encounter patients whose hypoxia demands oxygen therapy, often with mechanically assisted ventilation, but who show a progressive downhill course while increasing concentrations of oxygen are administered in a vain attempt to maintain adequate blood levels. Not only is alveolar-capillary diffusion impaired, but obstruction of small airways and alveoli by edema, hemorrhage, and capillary proliferation produces an increasing venous admixture, demonstrated in the laboratory by a widening alveolar-arterial oxygen tension gradient.[187] We now appreciate that this can be the direct result of the topical action of high-concentration oxygen on the pulmonary tissue, with the creation of a chaotic disturbance of physiology as the lung is beset, simultaneously, with shunting and atelectasis. Because the relation between pure oxygen breathing and absorption atelectasis was recognized before the more deep-seated oxygen damage to the lung was known, it was frequently assumed that the morbidity and mortality of oxygen breathing was associated with atelectasis. On this basis, it has been suggested that prevention of lung injury might be accomplished by alternating periods of oxygen breathing with the breathing of air, permitting expansion of alveoli by the nitrogen content of the latter. Studies of this maneuver, however, have failed to substantiate its predicted virtue.[188] We can summarize the topic of the dangers of oxygen by emphasizing again, strongly, that when oxygen is needed it must be given, even though we recognize the potential risk of toxicity. After all, the patient might not suffer toxic reactions, since these are not predictable with any precision, but failure to supply oxygen may well cause irreversible tissue damage. Nevertheless, oxygen, like any potent medicine, should be used with reason and according to indications. If high concentrations of oxygen are necessary, the duration of administration should be kept to a minimum and reduced as soon as possible. The objective in oxygen therapy is to maintain the arterial oxygen tension between 90 and 100 mm Hg, not 150 or 200 mm Hg. Frequent arterial blood monitoring is a mandatory safety measure when concentrations above 50% are used. Also, the exact concentration of inspired oxygen should be measured, especially when the gas is used in mechanical ventilators; and if air-diluting mechanisms cannot be depended upon to deliver desired concentrations, then premixed gases should be used. The safe and effective administration of oxygen to suit any individual need is one of the most important services that a knowledgeable and skilled inhalation therapist can offer, a service matched by few other technical members of the hospital health team.

Oxygen equipment and techniques

Masks. Oxygen masks are of many different types, varying in style of construction, materials, and specific purpose. Not too long ago most masks were of rubber, but now many are made of plastic and can be discarded after use, minimizing the risk of cross contamination, work of sterilizing, and storage space. Although we will discuss some critical differences among them, oxygen masks have some important common characteristics. The therapist will note variation in the use of masks, as with other pieces of equipment, among the hospitals with which he may have contact; but in general we can say that the oxygen mask is used where oxygen is needed quickly and for relatively short periods of time. It is the emergency equipment of choice, and some type of a mask should be available wherever patients are being treated. A mask may be used for up to several hours, but other techniques are more appropriate for prolonged constant therapy. Masks can be uncomfortable as a result of the frequent need for a tight seal between the unit and the patient's face, and the head strap or harness necessary to hold it in place adds to the discomfort. They are often quite hot, as they confine heat radiating from the face about the nose and mouth. The therapist must ever be aware of the risk of producing pressure necrosis of the skin when he attempts a tight fit of the mask to the face. Constant pressure of the edge of the mask over areas where little subcutaneous tissue separates skin from underlying bone, such as the bridge of the nose and the malar eminences of the cheeks, can readily interrupt cutaneous blood flow. Within a short time the skin may become devitalized, with the risk of permanent scarring. A snugly fitted mask should be removed frequently and dried, and the face should be dried and gently massaged over the pressure areas to stimulate circulation, then powdered to minimize the accumulation of moisture, which tends to soften the skin and to augment danger of pressure damage. An oxygen mask can be hazardous on a patient who is prone to vomit for it can block the flow of vomitus and subject the patient to dangerous aspiration. Because of this risk of aspiration, and the possibility of airway obstruction by a flaccid tongue, a mask should never be strapped onto an unconscious patient. If mask therapy is indicated in such a patient, an oral airway should be inserted to prevent the tongue from retracting into the pharynx, and the oxygen mask should either be held in place by an attendant or loosely set on the face. Finally, the therapist must recognize that by the nature of their construction face masks add dead space to the patient's airway, which may be considerable with some appliances. The space under the mask, about the nose and mouth, is functionally an extension of anatomic dead space and, depending upon the location of the exhalation ports, may cause a significant accumulation of carbon dioxide. Assuming a normally responsive respiratory center, the dead space of many masks produces a hyperventilation that may add to the patient's work of breathing, and in the patient with an obtunded center and hypercapnia, such dead space can be an added hazard. Despite these shortcomings, however, oxygen masks have a wide use in therapy and are often lifesaving. We will describe some of the characteristics of the following five general types of masks: simple, rebreathing, partial rebreathing, nonrebreathing, and venturi.

SIMPLE MASK. The usual simple mask, shown in Fig. 8-12, is a disposable plastic unit with neither valves nor reservoir bag, exhaled air being vented through holes in its body. Generally, it is relatively loosely fitted without the capability of close molding to facial contours possible with more elaborate types. In the event of an interrupted oxygen supply, air is drawn in through the exhalation ports as well as around the edge of the mask. The mask dead space and its "reservoir effect" influence the relationship between oxygen flow rate and the resulting alveolar oxygen concentration.[189] A minimal flow is necessary to flush the dead space for removal of carbon dioxide, but beyond a given flow rate, since the oxygen supply is continuous throughout the ventilatory cycle, the reservoir or dead space is filled with oxygen at the end of exhalation. The oxygen enrichment of inhaled air is dependent upon the balance between the patient's ventilatory need and the oxygen supply during inhalation. The deeper the tidal volume or the greater the inspiratory flow rate of the patient, the more will the oxygen be diluted by supplementary air drawn in through the ports or around the mask, since at any given instant the inspiratory flow rate may exceed many times the delivered oxygen flow rate.

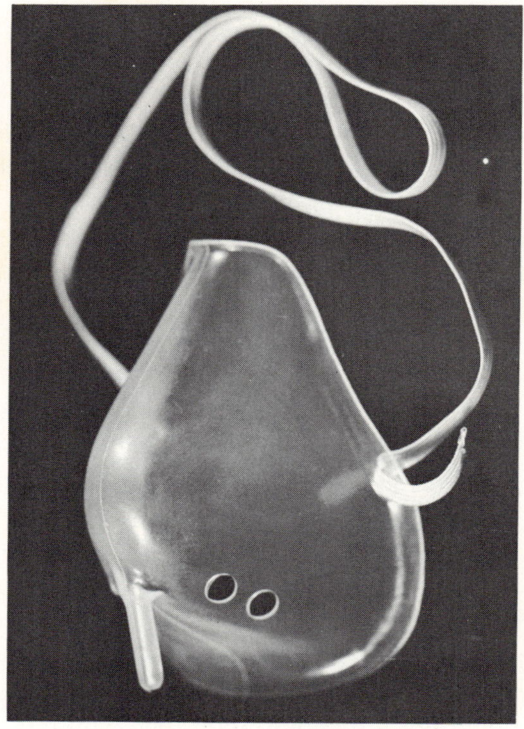

Fig. 8-12. Simple plastic mask with an oxygen inlet and exhalation holes.

The more oxygen supplied during inhlation, the greater will be its alveolar concentration.

Because of its convenience and relative comfort, the simple mask is widely used whenever moderate oxygen concentrations are desired for short periods of time. This includes the postoperative recovery state, temporary therapy while awaiting definitive plans, and interim therapy while weaning a patient from continuous oxygen administration. The crudeness of a simple mask makes it impossible to predict exact amounts of oxygen going to the patient, but in general the delivered concentrations vary from 35% to 55% at gas flow rates of 6 to 10 liters per minute.[190] It must be kept in mind that such values give no indication of the alveolar or arterial oxygen levels.

A special problem is presented by the very small infant, for whom the standard masks are often ineffective. There is available a custom-made and fitted mask that is molded from a very malleable plastic compound inside a shell, contoured like an infant's nose.[191] when partially set, the mask is molded about the patient's nose for a perfect fit, allowed to harden, and then cemented to the face. The dead space of such an appliance ranges from 0.3 to 0.5 ml, as compared to the tidal volume of newborns, which measures from 7 to 15 ml. This mask can withstand delivered gas pressures over 40 cm of water and can

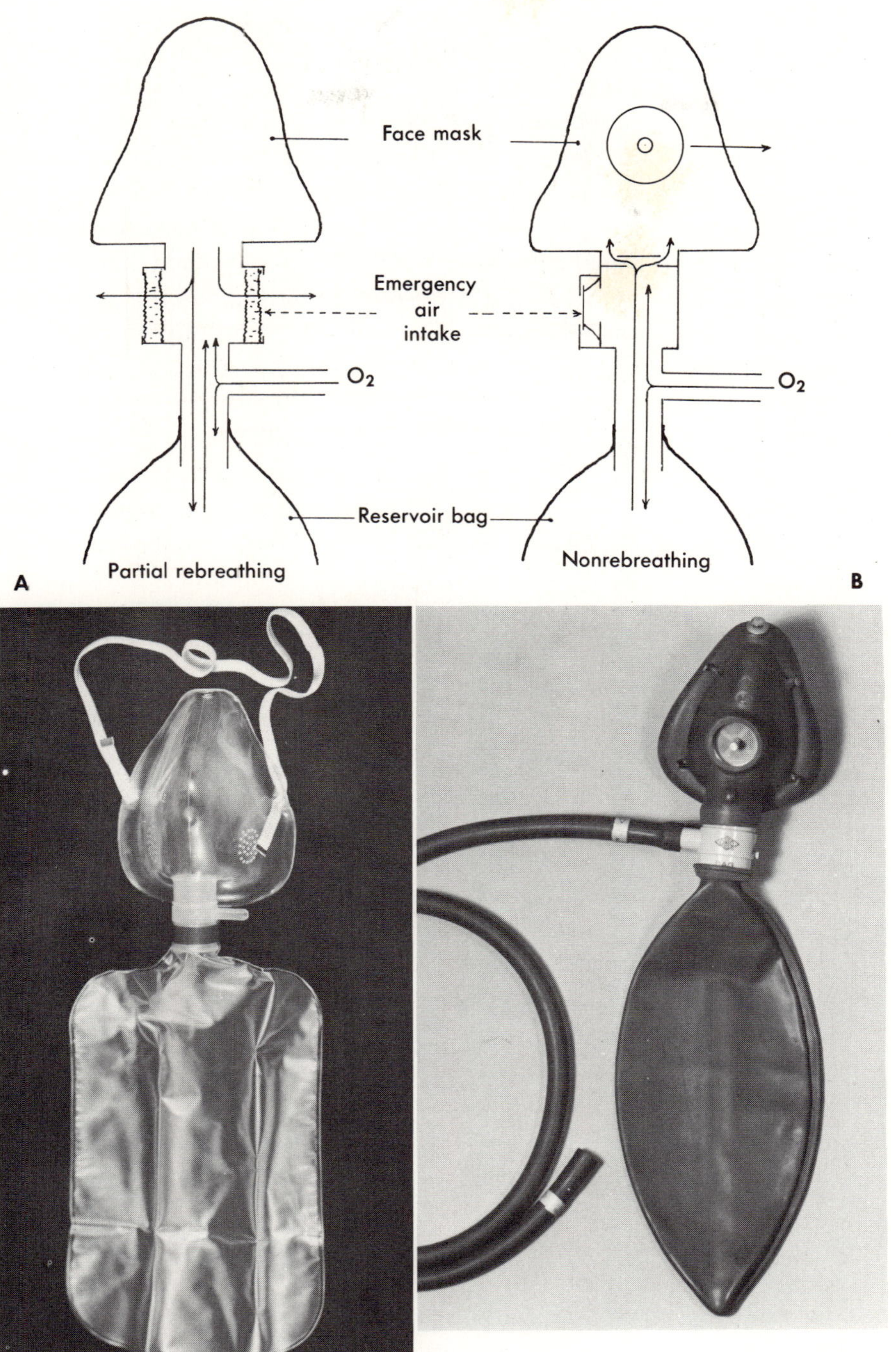

Fig. 8-13. Diagrammatic illustrations of the difference between, **A**, partial rebreathing oxygen mask and, **B**, nonrebreathing mask. In both, oxygen flows directly into the mask during inspiration and into the reservoir bag during exhalation. However, the early portion of exhaled air in **A** returns to the bag to be rebreathed with incoming oxygen in the next breath. Terminal air escapes through exhalation ports. In **B**, all exhaled air is vented through a port in the mask, and a one-way valve between the bag and mask prevents rebreathing.

be used with mechanical ventilators. The infant's skin is reported to be undamaged after the continuous use of the mask for as long as 4 days.

REBREATHING MASK. This unit is not used for clinical inhalation therapy and will be but briefly described. It consists of a mask tightly covering the mouth and nose, with an attached reservoir bag into which the breathing mixture flows and from which the patient inhales. The bag and mask are used in a closed system whereby the exhaled gas is circulated through a carbon dioxide absorber and additional breathing gas is added to replace that metabolized by the patient. The chief use for a rebreathing circuit is the administration of anesthesia, for it prevents waste of anesthetic agents and permits the addition of desired amounts of oxygen to the breathing mixture.

PARTIAL REBREATHING MASK. Like the rebreathing mask, this device is a combined face mask and reservoir bag; but unlike the rebreathing mask, it is an open circuit without a carbon dioxide absorber. The purpose of the partial rebreathing mask is to conserve oxygen by a technique that, as the name implies, permits the patient to rebreath some of his exhaled air. Fig. 8-13, *A*, schematically illustrates the basic parts and function of such an appliance. Source oxygen flows into the neck of the mask and during the inhalation phase passes directly into the mask proper, but during exhalation enters the reservoir bag. As the patient exhales, approximately the first third of his exhaled air is returned to the reservoir bag to mix with source oxygen. This fraction of the exhaled volume essentially represents the pulmonary dead space, which contains mostly oxygen and it is flushed into the bag to be reinhaled. As the bag distends with both source oxygen and exhaled air, pressure in the system then directs the terminal two thirds of exhaled air, with its carbon dioxide load, out the exhalation ports. If the oxygen inflow is adjusted so that the bag does not collapse during inhalation and the rate is over 4 liters per minute, the amount of carbon dioxide contaminating the reservoir is negligible.[192] Some older-style masks employed sponge discs in the exhalation ports, and these readily became waterlogged from respiratory gas moisture, rendering them less permeable to exhaled air and allowing an excess of carbon dioxide to accumulate in the bag. The exhalation ports of many masks are only vents in the face piece, and they also serve as emergency inlets for room air in the event of a failure of source oxygen. With a well-fitted partial rebreathing mask, adjusted so that the patient's inhalation does not deflate the bag, inspired oxygen concentrations of from 35% to 60% can usually be achieved at delivered flow rates between 6 and 10 liters per minute.[193]

NONREBREATHING MASK. Also a mask and reservoir bag device, the name of the nonrebreathing mask indicates that there is no exhaled gas rebreathing. Fig. 8-13, *B*, depicts the essential differences between the partial and nonrebreathing masks. The one major characteristic of the nonrebreathing mask is a one-way valve placed between the bag and the mask. As in the partial rebreather, source oxygen flows either into the bag only (during exhalation) or into the mask and bag (during inhalation). However, the valve between bag and mask prevents exhaled air from returning to the bag and diverts it into the atmosphere through a flap valve in the face piece. Somewhere, either in the neck as illustrated or in the mask itself, flap- or spring-loaded valves permit the intake of room air should source oxygen fail or the patient's needs suddenly exceed the available oxygen flow.

Because the patient inhales only the gas present in the bag, the nonrebreathing technique is the most precise method of administering a specific gas concentration, but to be effective there must be no significant leakage about the face or elsewhere in the system. This is the type of apparatus used to deliver 100% oxygen, or tanked gases of precise composition such as oxygen-nitrogen, helium-oxygen, and carbon dioxide–oxygen mixtures. The nonrebreathing mask is often used with an oxygen diluter ("meter mask") to allow a variety of oxygen concentrations to be administered, illustrated in Fig. 8-14. The diluter is based on the venturi principle and is provided with a sequence of different-sized holes through which volumes of room air can be entrained to dilute the source oxygen. The unit is calibrated to deliver specified concentrations of oxygen at given flow rates, depending upon which apertures are used, and will supply 100% gas when closed. The concentrations

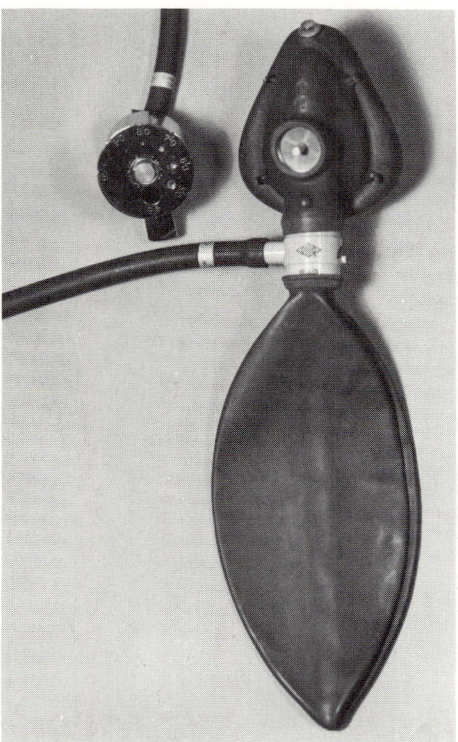

Fig. 8-14. Nonrebreathing mask with an oxygen diluter for varying the concentrations of inhaled oxygen.

are only approximate but are generally adequate for general clinical use. Care must be taken to provide suitable humidification whether the mask is used with or without a diluter, and some reservoir bags have drain plugs for removal of accumulated moisture. By and large, the nonrebreathing mask and bag is one of the most useful and practical tools for short-term precision administration of respiratory gases.

VENTURI MASK. This mask is designed to deliver a relatively low but predictable oxygen concentration, especially indicated in patients suffering from ventilatory failure. The principle behind this therapy is called *high airflow with oxygen enrichment* (HAFOE) and employs the venturi effect of air entrainment.[194,195] In addition to a presumed constant concentration of in-

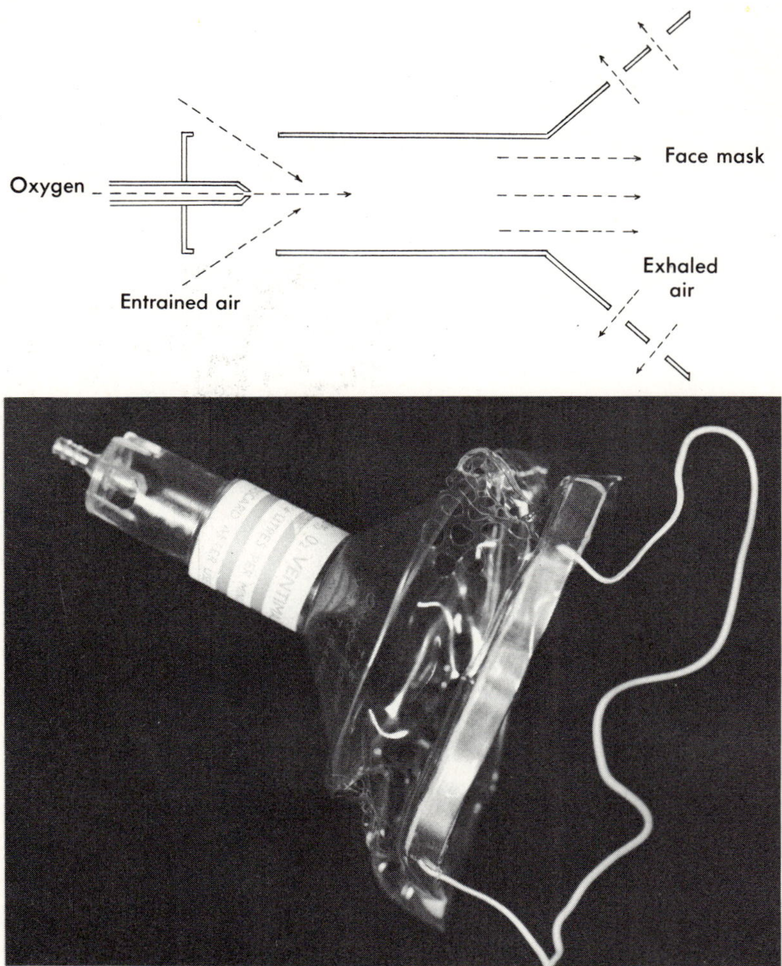

Fig. 8-15. Entrained air mixes with oxygen, which is supplied through the jet of a venturi mask. Construction design maintains a constant air/oxygen ratio, ensuring a fixed concentration of inhaled oxygen over a wide range of oxygen flow rates.

spired oxygen, the venturi provides a high total gas flow that is intended to flush the dead space about the face mask and to prevent the accumulation of carbon dioxide for rebreathing. Construction of the venturi mask is simple, as shown in the photograph and diagram of Fig. 8-15. Oxygen passes through a jet orifice and pulls in room air through the ports in the surrounding cylinder. The total volume of the breathing mixture is far in excess of the patient's ventilatory needs, and the excess, along with exhaled air, is vented out the holes in the flexible plastic face piece.

Table 8-10. *Flow characteristics of venturi masks*[197]

Delivered FO_2	*Air/O_2 ratio*	*Received oxygen flow rate (lpm)*	*Total gas flow (lpm)*
24	20:1	2-4	42-84
28	10:1	4-6	44-66
35	5:1	4-8	24-48

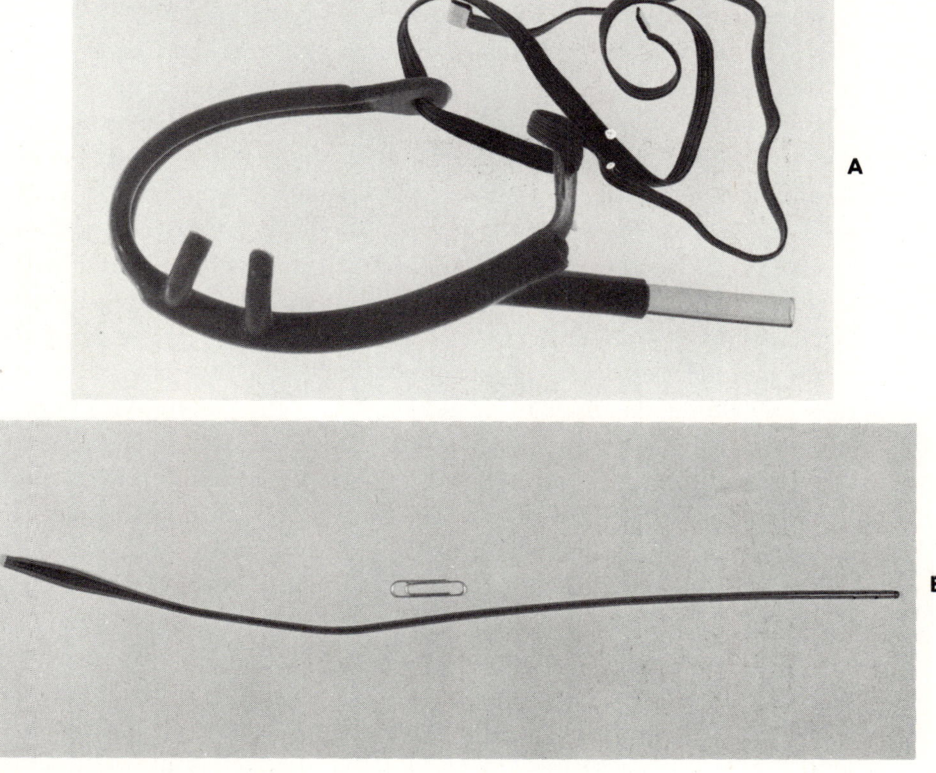

Fig. 8-16. A, Nasal oxygen cannula. **B,** Oropharyngeal catheter.

There are available three disposable commercial venturi masks, which deliver oxygen concentrations of 24%, 28%, and 35% each one designed so that there is a constant ratio of entrained air to source oxygen, even over a wide range of oxygen flow rates.[196] Table 8-10 outlines the flow and concentration data for each capacity mask.

Cannulas and catheters. We will discuss these two similar items together, for their general principles of function are the same. Their proper designations are *nasal cannula* and *oropharyngeal catheter.*

The *nasal cannula* (Fig. 8-16, *A*) is a plastic appliance (formerly made of metal) consisting of two tips about 0.5 inch long arising from an oxygen supply tube and inserting into the nostrils. It can be held in place by head straps or by bows that hook over the ears like eyeglasses. The cannula has the advantages of ease of application, lightness of weight, economy, and disposability. It has the disadvantage of instability, being easily dislodged from a restless or unobservant patient. It is a common experience, while making medical rounds, to note open oxygen flowmeters but cannulas so twisted out of place that the patients could not possibly get any significant therapy. It is also necessary to pay attention to the patient's comfort when instituting treatment, for excessive flow rates (variable among patients) can produce considerable pain in the frontal sinuses. Finally, such nasal pathology as a deviated septum, mucosal edema, mucus drainage, and polyps may interfere with adequate oxygen intake.

The *oropharyngeal catheter* (most commonly called "nasal catheter")is so named because it is placed with its tip in the oropharynx (Fig. 8-16, *B*). Made of soft flexible rubber or plastic, the catheter has several holes in its terminal 1 inch. Success in catheter therapy depends upon its proper insertion and maintenance, techniques with which every inhalation therapist should be familiar. Prior to introduction, the distal third to half of the catheter is lubricated with either a water-soluble lubricant or a thin layer of petrolatum. The latter is a better and longer-lasting lubricant and, if used sparingly, poses little risk of oil aspiration. A low flow of oxygen is started to ensure patency of the tube and its apertures and continued during the insertion. The catheter is gently slid along the floor of either nare into the oropharynx until, in the cooperative patient, direct viewing into the mouth while the tongue is depressed shows the tip of the catheter just below the uvula. It is then retracted out of sight and fastened to the bridge of the nose with adhesive tape. If direct vision is not possible, there are two "blind" procedures that can be used. The catheter can be placed on the side of the patient's face and the distance from the nose to the ear measured off; this length of the catheter is then inserted through the nose into the pharynx. Alternatively, with a moderate oxygen flow, the catheter can be introduced into the pharynx until the patient starts to gulp air, and can then be retracted approximately 1 inch and fastened. Under no circumstances must force be used to advance the catheter through the nose, and if significant resistance is encountered, the opposite nare should be used. Nasal disorders as enumerated above may block passage of the tube, and attempts to ram it through will only produce mucosal edema and worsen the condition. There are patients in whom this therapy cannot be used. Catheters should be removed and fresh ones inserted in the opposite nostril at least every 8 hours since, because they are foreign bodies in the nose, nasal secretions will cause them to adhere to the nasal mucosa if they are not changed periodically and their removal is a painful event. Generally, a well-placed catheter is not uncomfortable and allows at least a bit of bed mobility for the patient. This therapy should be used with some caution in a deeply comatose patient with completely obtunded reflexes and in one who is elderly and debilitated, such as in a post-stroke state. With ineffective epiglottal reflexes or epiglottal paralysis, the administered oxygen stream may be directed down the esophagus and seriously distend the stomach. The risk of gastric rupture is real, and distention will further handicap ventilation that is already impaired. After inserting a catheter in such a patient, the therapist should observe and palpate the epigastrium for several minutes to see whether distention develops and, if present, he should remove the catheter and employ some other technique. Finally, because oxygen is delivered as a blast in the pharynx, its desiccating effect on the respiratory tract must be prevented by adequate humidification. For this, a good humidifier is safe and effective because it provides good water vaporization with a minimal amount of particulate water to deposit in and obstruct the oxygen tubing.

There has been considerable controversy over the relative merits and efficiency of the nasal cannula versus the oropharyngeal catheter. The issue has been clouded by failure of partisan advocates to apply uniform criteria in evaluating these appliances. Some have studied their performance in healthy subjects, others in patients; some have used the delivered oxygen concentration as a gauge, others have used arterial oxygen tension. Nevertheless, there seems to be enough available data to make at least some valid generalizations. With oxygen flow rates up to 6 lpm, concentrations of 40% can probably be achieved with a well-placed nasal cannula; and with flows to 8 lmp, concentrations up to 50% can be delivered by an oropharyngeal catheter. It has been suggested that for the mouth-breathing patient a catheter is preferable to a cannula on the grounds that mouth breathing would dilute the nasal flow of oxygen below a therapeutic level. Studies have shown, however, that the eventual delivery of oxygen to the blood is not significantly different when either a cannula or catheter is used and whether the mouth is open or closed.[193,198] We may conclude, therefore, that the choice between a cannula and a catheter will rest more on convenience than on significant differences in performance. Both techniques are very useful in those instances when low oxygen concentrations are desirable and are thus interchangeable with the venturi mask described above. There is little doubt that the cannula is more comfortable or less of a nuisance than the catheter, but patient acceptance as

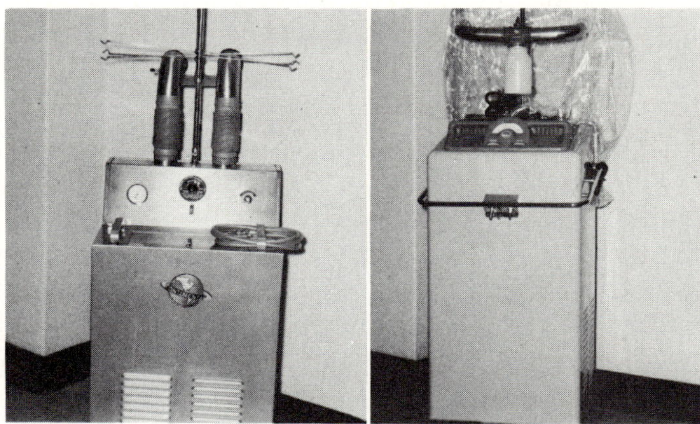

Fig. 8-17. Two typical oxygen tents.

a determinant must be weighed against the reliability of each technique. It might be practical to suggest that a cannula be considered for the cooperative and alert patient who can be depended upon to keep the appliance in its proper position, and the catheter for the restless or less dependable patient.

Tents. Oxygen tents have been used for many years, but technical refinements in modern design have given them capabilities unknown in the original models. There are many styles of tents commercially available, of which two are shown in Fig. 8-17, but we will describe what might be termed a typical unit and emphasize some of the features with which both physicians and therapists should be familiar. The term *oxygen tent* implies an electrically operated, recirculating, canopied appliance designed to provide a patient with an oxygen-enriched, temperature-controlled, humid environment. The mechanism and controls are housed in a console placed by the bedside, attached to which is a plastic canopy enclosing the upper half of the patient's body. A well-maintained and well-operated unit may be expected to provide a canopy atmosphere of no more than 50% oxygen; and, because there are far more economical ways of supplying oxygen, the tent is usually employed where oxygen and humidity, or humidity alone, are the therapeutic needs at a comfortable and constant temperature.

With these general indications for tent therapy as a start and before we consider the more technical aspects of treatment, three precautions should be emphasized. First, along with mechanical efficiency of the tent, success of treatment depends upon the proper application of the tent to the patient. The key is a tightly fitted canopy. The therapist will learn by experience the best methods of attaching a canopy to the patient's bed so that leaks are kept to a minimum. Unless a maximum seal can be attained between canopy and bed, leaks will negate any therapeutic effect. Maintaining a canopy in its proper operational state can be a problem with a restless or uncooperative patient. Second, and related to the first, is the need to leave the patient and his tent as undisturbed as possible. Every time the canopy is opened for any reason, the enclosed atmosphere is disrupted. An informal rule of thumb guide is to reserve the use of a canopy tent for those patients who can be left alone for periods of 3 to 4 hours at a time. If a patient is so ill that medical and nursing attention must be given every 10 or 15 minutes, he will not enjoy the benefits of the tent and will do much better with some other technique of oxygen or humidity administration. Third, if it is ever necessary to operate a canopy tent from cylinder oxygen, the therapist must be sure to have at least two cylinders in manifold and to replace tanks as soon as they are emptied. Should the oxygen supply be depleted, the patient may suffocate in his plastic enclosure.

The canopy atmosphere is recirculated through the console, where excess moisture is removed, and heat exchange keeps it at the desired, thermostatically controlled temperature. The cooling unit is often of the compressor-Freon-12 type, which allows circulation of the canopy air about cooling coils or which itself cools water to circulate through coils in the tent. Removal of carbon dioxide is no problem as long as there is an adequate inflow of oxygen into the tent, for carbon dioxide readily diffuses through the plastic canopy into the atmosphere. All therapists should read the excellent description of gas exchange in oxygen tents by R. E. Jahn.[199] Despite the airtightness of a well-placed canopy, there is a tremendous escape of gas from the tent. This explains why high liter flows are required to maintain a steady concentration although no patient ever consumes more than half a liter of oxygen per minute. Tent oxygen is lost by displacement of incoming gas at junction of canopy and bed and around the console and by diffusion of gas molecules through minute leaks. Formulas are available to allow calculation of oxygen flow into canopies of various sizes that will provide specific oxygen concentrations and prevent the accumulation of carbon dioxide above specific limits. For practical purposes this is not necessary, and with the popular size tents, liter flows of source oxygen of 12 to 15 lpm will keep oxygen concentration to a maximum and carbon dioxide to a minimum. The initial filling of a canopy requires flushing for several minutes with very high flow rates until the desired concentration is reached. For safe operation, the atmosphere of all tents should be measured with an oximeter every 4 hours. This not only monitors the oxygen concentration but also allows the therapist to check the level in the water overflow pan, to look for signs of mechanical overheating, and in general to assure himself of the operating efficiency.

As noted above, an oxygen tent may often be used primarily for the administration of high humidity, and most units have very effective aerosol generators for this purpose. If oxygen is used to power the aerosol generator, the therapist must remember that back pressure of the nebulizer jet may reduce the liter flow into the tent below the safe value to wash out carbon dioxide. A second oxygen line must be attached to the gas inlet to provide the necessary ventilation. If oxygen therapy is not indicated and the tent's aerosol generator is powered by a compressor, canopy ventilation will also be

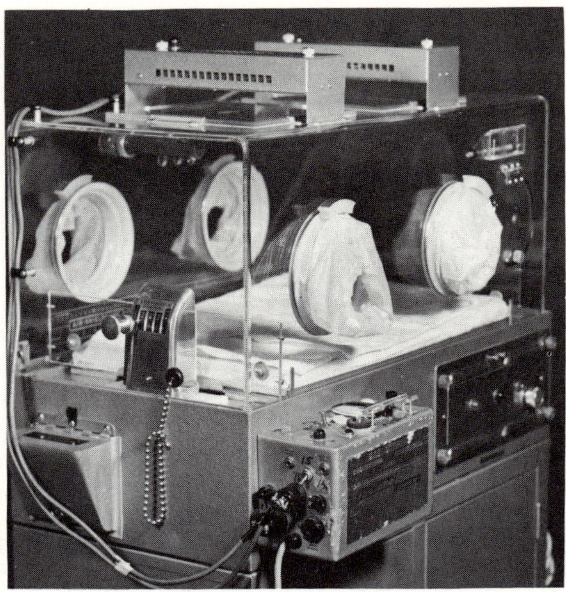

Fig. 8-18. Incubator to provide the premature or newborn infant an environment of controlled oxygen concentration, temperature, and humidity.

inadequate unless the compressor is able to deliver 15 lpm from the nebulizer. With the usual available equipment this will probably not be possible, and another source of ventilation must be provided. Many tents have an air intake venturi as part of the aerosol generator, and with this open, entrained room air will make up the needed liter flow.

There are many variations of the canopy tent designed for pediatric use. The incubator (Fig. 8-18) is a controlled-environment unit with special provisions for steady elevated temperature and humidity. A special feature of the incubator is an oxygen-limiter, which, unless specifically adjusted otherwise, limits the concentration of the oxygen in the unit to a maximum of 40%, as a precaution against the dangers of elevated oxygen in the newborn or premature. Accessories are available to monitor the infant's skin temperature and regulate the incubator accordingly. For the older child, the "croup tent" is frequently used (Fig. 8-19). Designed to be used in a crib or small bed, it provides high humidity through a nebulizer powered either by oxygen or by a compressor. Cooling of the unit is by ice, which lowers the temperature not more than 8° below ambient. A venturi in the aerosol generator circulates the canopy atmosphere through the ice and mixes it with freshly generated aerosol.

Reference was made above to the necessity of frequent measurement of the oxygen concentration of all tents, and it should be obvious that the need is even greater with incubators. The therapist can acquaint himself with the details of testing equipment through information supplied by manufacturers,

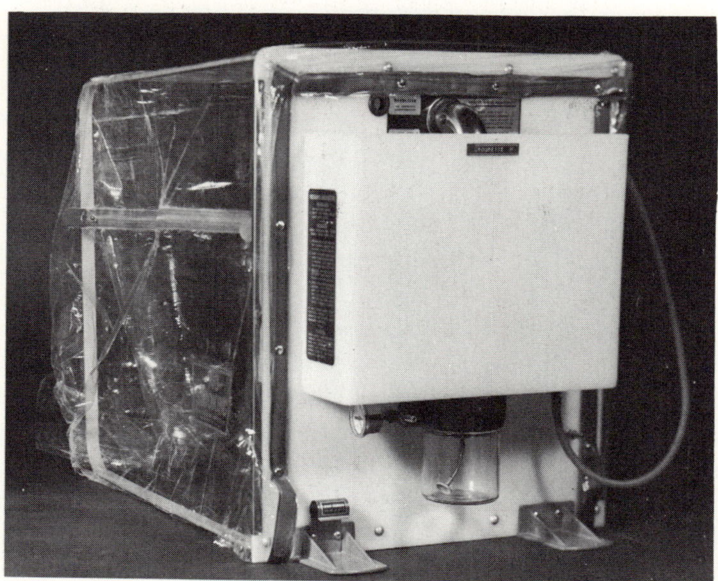

Fig. 8-19. Croup tent, an ice-cooled unit that provides high humidity and aerosolized water, powered either by compressed air or oxygen.

but a brief résumé of the principles upon which the two most commonly used types depend will be noted at this time. The older chemical analyzers have given way to those that operate on either "thermal conductivity" (commonly called electric analyzers) or "paramagnetic susceptibility" (also called physical analyzers).

The *electric analyzer* consists of a battery-powered Wheatstone bridge of platinum wires, two arms of which are subjected to the test gas, the other two exposed to air, functioning as references. The instrument is designed only to measure differences in concentrations in a mixture of oxygen and nitrogen and is *not* to be used with any other gas or gas mixture. A physical property of oxygen is its ability to remove heat from a warmed object faster than can nitrogen, so the higher the concentration of oxygen, the cooler will be the object (the platinum wires in this instance). Since the electrical resistance of a wire varies directly with the temperature, the resistance will reflect the oxygen concentration. The instrument is calibrated before use by the drawing of room air into it and balancing the Wheatstone bridge by adjusting the scale to read 21%. The test gas is then entered, and variations in oxygen concentration will upset the balance of the Wheatstone bridge through the effect on electrical conductivity, an event noted by an ammeter whose indicating needle reads out on a scale calibrated in oxygen percent.

The *physical analyzer* also uses batteries but only to establish an electromagnetic field in which a small glass dumbbell is suspended on a taut quartz fiber. In the absence of oxygen, the forces of the torque of the quartz fiber and the magnetic field are equal and in balance. If oxygen is introduced into the system, because of its unique capability, among all the gases, of being magnetized, it is drawn into and augments the electromagnetic field. This upsets the balance, as the torque of the quartz fiber is overcome, and the glass dumbbell rotates in response to the new magnetic force. A small mirror attached to the fiber reflects a beam of light onto a translucent scale calibrated to translate motion of the fiber into oxygen percent. A major advantage of this oximeter is its ability to detect and measure concentrations of oxygen in any mixture of gases, and the instrument can safely be used with flammable and explosive gases.

A few comments must be made concerning the fire hazard of oxygen tents, a question that the therapist may expect to encounter occasionally. A frequent source of worry is the presence of static electrical sparks often generated by the friction of movements of the patient in bed or by uniforms of personnel rubbing against bed clothing. This subject has been studied in some detail, and the inhalation therapist should be aware of the following data. To start any fire, three conditions must be met: flammable material must be present; oxygen must be present; the flammable material must be heated above its flash or igniting temperature and kept there by some external heat or the heat of its own combustion. Thus, for any spark to ignite flammable material, the spark must be able to generate enough heat energy to start the process. In relation to the patient in bed, it was determined that the maximum energy capacity was to be found in the ungrounded bed itself (estimated to be less than 100 micromicrofarads); and it was further estimated that the electrical potential of a hospital bed is about 20,000 volts. Theoretically, such a combination could produce a spark some 0.7 inch long with a maximum energy of 0.02 joule. The likelihood of a casual, random static spark of this magnitude was felt to be very remote. Under conditions of oxygen concentrations varying from 21% to 100%, sparks exceeding this potential were applied to such fabrics as vinyl plastic canopy material, tissue paper, nylon, wool, cotton, muslin, and dacron-cotton. With a barrage of sparks at a frequency of 60 per minute ignition was achieved with elevated oxygen concentrations, but under no circumstance was a single spark able to produce fire.[200] Further experiments were conducted with fabrics impregnated with petroleum jelly or lanolin, simulating conditions that might be expected in the presence of surgical dressings. Again, even with high oxygen concentrations and frequent sparking, few ignitions occurred. The conservative conclusions were drawn that the overall hazard from static sparks with the fabrics in common use, even in high oxygen concentrations, is very low but not nonexistent.[201] The static sparks just do not have sufficient heat energy to raise the material to their flash points. The minimal risk that may be present can be further reduced by maintaining a relative humidity in the tent of 60% or greater.

It should be strongly emphasized that the above refers only to static sparking, *not* sparks from electrical equipment such as meters or exposed switches, which are very dangerous. All appliances that transmit house current should be kept out of oxygen tents. The energy of battery-operated current, such as might be found in the many appliances being developed for cardiac support, probably is of too small a magnitude to constitute a risk, especially if well grounded; but the specifications of these appliances should include this information. Recording equipment, such as cardiac monitors, are not hazards since they pick up only minute physiologic currents and amplify them for inspection outside the high-oxygen environment. It is expected that the therapist is fully aware of the precautions to take against the presence of open flames about a tent and the prohibition of smoking in the room with an operating tent. One last note of caution should be made, more for completeness than for anything else. With an attached oxygen appliance, an oxygen cylinder should be opened slowly to avoid a rush of gas downstream into the appliance. The heat of compression of rapidly flowing oxygen carries the potential risk of elevating to their ignition points such materials as valve seat packing and contaminants in the system. Gradual dissipation of this heat by slow opening of the valve will avoid this hazard.[202]

Miscellaneous oxygen equipment. Although most therapeutic oxygen is administered by the mask, cannula, catheter, and tent techniques described above, there are a few others that deserve mention. The *face tent* is a popular item for short-term use because it is economical and easy to apply. A plastic enclosure open at the top, the face tent is held by head straps in such a manner that it encompasses a space about the chin, mouth, and nose. By means of a simple attachment at the bottom, oxygen flows into the enclosure supplying a reservoir from which the patient can inhale. Exhalation simply diffuses out the open top. At oxygen flows of 6 to 10 lpm, delivered concentrations up to 45% may be realized. The chief disadvantages of the face tent are, first, the nuisance of the appliance attached to the face and, second, the heat retained about the face by the plastic. The *head tent* is no longer frequently used because of its inherent clumsiness. It consists of a transparent, hard, plastic box without a bottom and with a cutout in one end to fit over the neck. With the patient supine, the appliance covers the entire head. An adjustable vent in the top allows the escape of exhaled air, and an inner receptacle is provided for ice. A modification of this principle is in use, utilizing a container completely open at the top for the removal of both carbon dioxide and heat, with provisions for adequate continual flushing of the unit by oxygen. Finally, oxygen is frequently given by intermittent positive-pressure devices, but these will be dealt with later.

SUMMARY

Because of the wide variety of techniques of administering oxygen, it is obvious that there is no one best method, and although the decision to give oxygen to a patient is a medical one, determined by the physician, it is not always easy for him to know which procedure will be the most effective in a given instance. Clinical observation of the patient, coupled with experience, will often suffice for the physician to initiate treatment, and in the not too distant past these were his only guides. More recently, however, improved technology in both instrumentation and diagnosis have made the therapeutic use of oxygen much more rational and precise.

In our discussion of oxygen equipment, it will be noted that values of oxygen concentration were suggested for each type. Such data certainly have merit, but only in a very general way, for the delivered concentration of gas from any appliance is subjected to many modifying influences such as condition of the equipment, technique of application, cooperation of the patient, and the ventilatory pattern of the patient. It is probably necessary to know only, for example, that the delivery of high oxygen concentrations can best be accomplished by a nonrebreathing mask; intermediate concentrations by a simple mask, tent, or high flows with a cannula or catheter; and low concentrations with cannula, catheter, and venturi mask. It is much more important to recognize that complete relief of hypoxia may be easily achieved by low-flow cannula oxygen in one patient and be impossible by mask therapy in another. Indeed, there may be instances in which, at least for a period of time, full correction of hypoxia may not even be desirable. The point to be grasped here is that the pathology of the disease under treatment is the major determinant of the effectiveness of oxygen administration. Except for short-term therapy, such as prophylaxis, or for conditions felt to be very transient, safe and rational treatment must depend upon the actual measurement of blood oxygenation. At the present time, in view of current techniques, this means the determination of oxygen tension of arterial blood. We have considered the major pathologic and physiologic changes that disease can effect in ventilatory and gas exchange functions of the lung, and it is easy to visualize that there may be little correlation between the fractional concentration of inhaled oxygen and the realization of a normal arterial oxygen content. Unless the initial degree of hypoxia is quantitated by direct measurement and such measurements continued through therapy until stability is reached, treatment can be based on little more than guesswork.

The correction of hypoxia as part of the management of patients with acute or chronic ventilatory failure requires special care because of the disturbance in the acid-base balance. Due to the risk of untoward reactions to oxygen in acute failure, many techniques of oxygen administration have been suggested that are based on the use of low concentrations of oxygen or oxygen with supporting mechanical ventilation. Although the latter is usually required in severe circumstances and will be discussed in detail later, oxygen alone may be indicated. We know the great hazard of hypercapnia if therapeutic oxygen obliterates the hypoxic drive mechanism, and to minimize this risk, the use of cannulas or the venturi mask on continuous or intermittent schedules has had various advocates.[194,197,204,205] Similarly, continuous low-flow oxygen in the treatment of chronic hypoxia has received much attention. However, the criteria for the choice of patients for such therapy, as well as an evaluation of its success, are always dependent upon the effective arterial oxygen tensions achieved and the response of the acid-base balance. Thus, after the degree of hypoxia has been determined, the choice of technique may require some trials and errors, guided by blood oxygen levels, with thought given to patient comfort as well as the avoidance of over-oxygenation.

HELIUM THERAPY

In an earlier chapter, reference was made to the use of helium in the treatment of obstructive disease, and we will now discuss this technique in more detail. Helium is second only to the highly inflammable hydrogen as the lightest of all gases, with an atomic weight of 4.003 and a density of only 0.1785 gm per liter. Limited in supply, the source of most commercial helium is deep mines in the Southwest, produced under control of the Federal Government. Chemically, it is an inert element, and thus physiologically it neither participates in nor interferes with any biochemical process in the body. It is odorless, tasteless, noncombustable, nonexplosive, poorly soluble, and a good conductor of heat, sound, and electricity.

It is the low-density property of helium that makes the gas a valuable therapeutic tool, and its only medical indication is the management of airway obstruction. We know, from previous discussions, that turbulence characterizes the gas flow pattern through an obstruction and that in such a circumstance the most influential property of a moving gas is its density. With no technical background, we should be able to perceive that the less dense a gas is the easier it can negotiate an obstruction; but for clarity let us look at the process from two slightly different viewpoints. First, it should be noted that as a flow of gas passes from a relatively wide passage into one that is relatively narrow, if the driving force is constant, the gas velocity must increase to maintain the same volume leaving as entering the restriction. As Bernoulli's principle demonstrates a decrease in pressure with an increase in gas velocity, there is thus a pressure drop across an obstruction. However, since less driving pressure is required to move a light (low-density) gas than a heavy one, at the same velocity there would be less of a pressure drop. In ventilation this would mean greater efficiency and less work expended in breathing. Second, the movement of a gas through the narrow aperture of an obstruction subjects it to some of the principles of diffusion, or the passage of a gas across an obstruction in response to a pressure gradient. In Chapter 4 we learned that the rate of diffusion of a gas follows Graham's law and is inversely proportional to the square root of the density of the gas. Obviously, the speed (or ease) of such movement is greater for low-density gases than for high.

Currently, helium is the only low-density gas acceptable for medical use, and since it is inert and unable to support life, it cannot be used alone but is always mixed with oxygen. The therapist should keep in mind that helium has no curative properties of its own, in a pharmacologic sense, and that its sole purpose to to lower the total density of any mixture of which it is a part, so that such a mixture can ventilate the lungs with minimal effort. All helium-oxygen mixtures must have at least 20% oxygen to supply basic metabolic needs, and a popular combination is the so-called 80-20 mixture, with 80% helium and 20% oxygen. For practical purposes, such a mixture is comparable to air, with helium substituted for nitrogen. A patient breathing 80-20 helium is not being provided with any more oxygen than would be provided by air, but because of the low density of the helium mixture, he is effectively getting more; the helium more readily reaches the alveoli through obstructed passages and thus more oxygen actually is available for diffusion into the blood. For a more specific comparison, it should be noted that the density of air is 1.293 gm/liter whereas that of 80-20 helium is 0.429 gm/liter. It may be said that with the same effort three times as much of the helium mixture as of air will ventilate the lungs or that the same volume of helium-oxygen ventilation as of air can be moved with one third the effort. In either case, the tremendous advantage of a helium mixture is evident to a patient struggling, often to the point of physical exhaustion, to breathe against severely obstructed airways. It should be noted that the viscosities of oxygen and helium are almost identical, although both are slightly greater than that of air. The mixing of the two gases, therefore, does not alter the laminar flow patterns of pure oxygen breathing, and only insignificantly those of air-oxygen mixtures. Table 8-11 lists the densities and relative diffusibilities of air, helium, oxygen, and certain combinations of these and nitrogen, frequently used in therapy.

Table 8-11. *Densities and relative diffusion rates of selected gases (rate of diffusion varies inversely with square root of density)*[206]

Gas	*Percentage*	*Density*	*$\sqrt{Density}$*	*Relative diffusibility*
Helium	100	0.179	0.423	
Air	100	1.293	1.135	
Oxygen	100	1.429	1.182	
Oxygen-nitrogen	40/60	1.321	1.105	
Helium-oxygen	80/20	0.429	0.655	
Helium-oxygen	70/30	0.554	0.745	
Oxygen / Air	100 / 100		1.135 / 1.182	0.960
Oxygen-nitrogen / Air	40-60 / 100		1.135 / 1.105	1.027
Helium-oxygen / Air	80-20 / 100		1.135 / 0.655	1.743
Helium-oxygen / Oxygen	80-20 / 100		1.182 / 0.655	1.805
Helium-oxygen / Oxygen	70-30 / 100		1.182 / 0.745	1.586

It is possible to mix pure helium and oxygen at the bedside, but the hazards of error and mechanical failure are so great that it is much safer, as well as more convenient, to use commercially prepared cylinders of premixed gases. In addition to the 80-20 combination discussed above, another commonly used mixture is a 70-30. This gives an additional quantity of oxygen, often helpful in correcting severe hypoxia associated with obstruction, and although it does so at a slight cost of low density, as noted in Table 8-11, it is probably the most generally useful mixture.

Completely safe to use, helium-oxygen is one of the most valuable therapeutic tools in the treatment of respiratory disorders and should be available in all hospitals caring for pulmonary patients, even though it may be put to only occasional use. Helium-oxygen is specifically indicated for the patient with diffuse airway obstruction, especially when due to bronchospasm, as in status asthmaticus, or following instrumentation or other traumatic bronchial irritation. It is also useful in obstruction from extensive secretions, although in this case the major effort should be directed toward airway cleansing. More ordinary therapy is usually employed first, to achieve bronchial patency, and then oxygen administration by conventional techniques next, to combat hypoxia. However, if the obstructive process is unresponsive or the patient is in risk of weakening from fatigue, helium-oxygen should be promptly started before the patient deteriorates to a critical state. There are four points of practical importance to consider in giving helium-oxygen:

1. Helium mixtures must always be given in a tightly closed system, because their high diffusibilities will allow them to escape from even small leaks. Tents, catheters, and cannulas are not satisfactory, and the gases should be given by a tightly fitted nonrebreathing mask and bag or through cuffed endotracheal or tracheostomy tubes. They are frequently administered to great advantage by intermittent positive-pressure ventilators.
2. The average hospital gas flowmeter is calibrated for oxygen, and since it depends on the kinetic support of a float by the metered gas, gauge readings will not be accurate for the lighter helium-oxygen mixtures. Special meters, calibrated for the helium mixtures, can be used, but they are not necessary because correction can be made for the scales of the oxygen meters. Table 8-11 shows that an 80-20 helium-oxygen mixture is 1.8 times as diffusible as 100% oxygen and a 70-30 mixture 1.6 times. This means that for every 10 lmp gas flow recorded on the meter, 18 lmp and 16 lmp, respectively, of the above helium gases would flow. To deliver a desired flow rate, the flowmeter is adjusted to a reading equal to the desired rate divided by either 1.8 or 1.6, depending upon the gas mixture being used. Factors for any other combination can be calculated if needed.
3. The low density of the helium mixtures makes them poor vehicles for the transport of pharmacologically active aerosols. Humidifiers, of

course, must be used as with any administered gas, but high therapeutic concentrations of water particles cannot be expected.

4. The only side effect directly attributable to helium is a benign one, but one that should be kept in mind. In the low-density gas the spoken word is badly distorted at a pitch so high as to make it almost unintelligible. This is of importance only to the conscious, nonintubated patient, who should be warned of the phenomenon and reassured that it will disappear within a few seconds of discontinuance of therapy.

CARBON DIOXIDE THERAPY

Paradoxical though it may seem, a gas whose removal from the body occupies much of the attention and efforts of the inhalation therapist is sometimes used therapeutically. The inhalational application of carbon dioxide is not extensive, but the therapist will be called upon to administer the gas frequently enough to necessitate his becoming very familiar with its characteristics.

At normal atmospheric temperature and pressure, carbon dioxide is a gas, colorless, orderless, and about 1.5 times as heavy as air, that will not support combustion or maintain life. Unrefined gas for the commercial production of carbon dioxide may be obtained from the following: combustion of coal, coke, natural gas, oil, and other carbonaceous fuels; by-product gases of ammonia plants, lime kilns, carbide furnaces; fermentation processes; and gases from certain natural springs and wells. From these sources, carbon dioxide is refined to a purity of no less than 99.9%.

For safe administration of carbon dioxide, the therapist should know its physiologic actions:

Respiratory response. Carbon dioxide is basically a respiratory center stimulant, but maximal stimulation is probably attained with the inhalation of a 10% concentration. Higher concentrations depress the respiratory center after initial stimulation.

Circulatory response. Two major effects are recognized.

DIRECT STIMULATION OF THE CARDIOVASCULAR BRAIN CENTERS. This leads to an elevation of the systolic and diastolic blood pressures (up to an increase of 40 mm Hg systolic); an increase in the heart rate of up to 20 beats per minute; an increase in the force of myocardial contraction; contraction of vascular beds supplied by the sympathetic nervous system, thereby diverting blood flow from general body areas to the brain, whose vessels are not sympathetic-responsive; and increasing the cerebral circulation (conversely, hypocapnia leads to cerebral constriction and a reduced flow).

LOCAL VASODILATATION. Increased carbon dioxide at the tissue level dilates the vascular bed, as is found in exercising muscle, producing a more active flow for metabolic needs.

Central nervous system response. Generally, high carbon dioxide concentrations produce CNS stimulation to the point of convulsions, and low concentrations cause depression. It is vital for the therapist to remember, however, that the administration of 5% carbon dioxide may produce severe mental depression, if given for no longer than 1 hour, and 10% may lead to loss of consciousness within as short a time as 10 minutes.

The clinical indications for carbon dioxide therapy antedate the current techniques of inhalation therapy and in general have been replaced by the latter. Nevertheless, because it is being used, we will briefly describe its therapeutic effects. Under *no* circumstance must carbon dioxide be given to a patient unless he is definitely known to have a responsive respiratory center. Failure to be assured of this may produce a fatal hypercapnia and respiratory acidosis.

IMPROVE CEREBRAL BLOOD FLOW. This depends upon the physiologic effect described above and has had long use in attempting to overcome cerebral vascular spasm and to evoke compensatory increased flow following stroke. In general, results have not been spectacular, perhaps largely because many of the patients so treated had associated hardening, or sclerosis, of their vessels, making them impervious to the effect of carbon dioxide. Ophthalmologists sometimes use the gas to dilate vessels in the retina of the eye, when thromboses have impaired the circulation.

OVERCOME HYPOVENTILATION. Especially in the aged, or those physically weakened by serious disease, debility results in a low tidal volume air exchange. Carbon dioxide has been used often to stimulate such patients to deep breathing, effecting a better distribution of inhaled gas. Caution must be employed in such instances to be sure that there is no underlying respiratory dysfunction; for unless the patient is able to respond to treatment by hyperventilation, not only is the therapy of no value but hypercapnia is a certainty. Modern inhalation therapy equipment and techniques can usually perform this function better and safer than can carbon dioxide.

PREVENT POSTOPERATIVE ATELECTASIS. This indication parallels that just described and was often used to stimulate deep breathing in the immediate postoperative state to prevent atelectasis from retained secretions, and to overcome the usual postoperative hypoxia following inhalational anesthesia. As above, better techniques are now generally used.

ASSIST COUGH. Oftentimes effective, although tiring, the hyperventilation of carbon dioxide inhalation can aid in the tussive removal of secretions. Again, the available aerosols and other equipment are more effective and safer than carbon dioxide.

SINGULATION (HICCUP, HICCOUGH). Although there are other methods of treating this very annoying and sometimes serious condition, singulation is one of the most specific indications for carbon dioxide therapy. The hiccup is an abnormal spasmodic contraction of the diaphragm against a closed glottis, under the stimulation of an irritated phrenic nerve. Such irritation can come from a host of conditions, including gastric distention or irritation, toxins, and metabolic upsets, and often it plagues patients who are immediately postoperative as well as those who suffer from debilitating diseases.[207] Prolonged hiccupping can produce severe physical fatigue, interfere with eating, and cause emotional distress. We all know some of the traditional maneuvers for stopping hiccups, such as forced inspiratory breath holding, taking long drinks of water, and breathing into a paper bag. The reason these acts have met with variable success is their one common factor: they all withhold carbon dioxide and produce some degree of hypercapnia. This is what stops the hiccups. Subjecting the respiratory center to excessive stimulation of hypercapnia supposedly initiates a rhythmic discharge of impulses to the diaphragm so strong that they override the interposed spasmodic contractions and restore a normal cycle. The administration of low concentrations of carbon dioxide usually accomplishes this more quickly and smoothly and in most instances is effective in stopping the hiccups. Sometimes simple mechanical stimulation of the pharynx, with a catheter, will stop the attack through a reflex mediated by way of the vagus nerve. This technique has been used with success by anesthesiologists on patients suffering from postanesthesia hiccups. For some patients combined therapy, including tranquilization, is necessary to bring relief.

Because carbon dioxide, like helium, does not support life, it must be used in combination with oxygen. In addition to its action as an asphyxiant, carbon dioxide produces toxic effects in excess dosage, and it *must be given with great care.* During its administration the therapist must remain in constant attendance and watch the patient closely, because there is variation among individuals in their responses to the gas. It is suggested that each department of inhalation therapy establish its own rules governing the use of carbon dioxide and that these include such items as the following: (1) unless otherwise specified, all treatments will use a mixture no stronger than 5% carbon dioxide and 95% oxygen; (2) no treatment will exceed a period of 10 minutes in duration; (3) if higher concentrations or longer periods of treatment are ordered, a physician must be present. The carbon dioxide mixture should be given with a well-fitted nonrebreathing mask and bag, and the mask should be held to the patient's face by an attendant rather than strapped on so that it can be removed in an instant if necessary.

The potential side effects are many and include headache, dizziness shortly after start of treatment as diastolic blood pressure makes an initial drop, dyspnea, nasal irritation, palpitation, dimming of vision, muscle tremors, paresthesias, sensation of cold, and mental depression. The toxic symptoms indicate serious physiologic injury and should be watched for because they can appear any time after 15 minutes of treatment. Toxicity is manifested by severe dyspnea, nausea and vomiting, disorientation, and a dangerous elevation of blood pressure. When the pressure reaches 200 mm Hg, systolic, convulsions and cardiac collapse are apt to occur. It is recommended that carbon dioxide be contraindicated in patients with significant airway obstruction for two reasons. First, it is this type of patient who is most likely to have less than normally responsive respiratory center and run the risk of hypercapnia. Second, with an active respiratory center, the increased work of breathing under carbon dioxide stimulation against obstruction may more than negate any positive value of therapy.

Chapter 9

Mechanical ventilation

It should be emphasized at the start that this chapter is not a technical manual of ventilators nor is it intended to supplement commercial material supplied by manufacturers of equipment. There is an unquestioned need for a well-composed, comprehensive technical textbook, describing structural and operational details of all commonly used ventilators, with emphasis on preventative maintenance and repair. Our objective is to discuss the basic principles of mechanical ventilation, relating them to patient care; and we will note the characteristics of specific instruments, as needed, to illustrate topics under discussion.

To understand the design and function of mechanical ventilators, we must first understand the condition for which they are used—failure of the normal physiologic mechanism to provide adequate respiratory gas exchange. It makes little difference whether we refer to ventilatory or respiratory failure or insufficiency, but for the sake of consistency we will use the term *ventilatory failure.* While recognizing that subtleties and shades of meaning exist in many definitions, to reduce our subject to its most important characteristics, we will define ventilatory failure as that state of impaired breathing accompanied by retention of blood carbon dioxide. The student should recognize that this definition excludes those patients who suffer from breathlessness but who are able to maintain at least near normal blood gas values, often by virtue of heroic efforts; nor does it include those with hypoxic disease whose ventilatory efforts, though inadequate for normal oxygenation, are able to excrete carbon dioxide. The severe physical exertion of breathing experienced by such patients constitutes disability that may be total, but because they are able to keep their blood carbon dioxide at a normal level, they do not fall into our category of ventilatory failure. From our earlier study of pulmonary physiology, it is evident that *alveolar hypoventilation* is the fundamental defect in ventilatory failure, since ineffective tidal rinsing of the alveoli is the only barrier to adequate removal of carbon dioxide from venous blood. In summary, we can consider ventilatory failure as the sequel to alveolar hypoventilation of any cause (reduced total ventilation or increased pulmonary dead space), manifested by hypercapnia and its subsequent physiologic and biochemical effects and usually accompanied by variable degrees of hypoxia while breathing air at atmosphere. It is reasonable to expect that air exchange which is inadequate to remove normal amounts of the readily diffusible carbon dioxide will not satisfy oxygen demands.

Because it is an end result, ventilatory failure is found with a variety of diseases, which can be grossly but practically grouped as follows[208]: (1) *alveolar hypoventilation associated with normal lungs*—respiratory centers damaged by disease, trauma, drugs; paralysis of ventilatory muscles from neurologic diseases; thoracic skeletal deformities such as from kyphoscoliosis, trauma, and mutilating surgery; (2) *diffuse fibrosis or pulmonary granulomatosis*—"stiff lungs" of asbestosis, scleroderma, beryllosis, sarcoidosis, recurrent or chronic infections, and healed destructive tuberculosis; and (3) *chronic bronchitis-emphysema*—combinations of distention, destruction, obstruction, and fibrosis. In the daily experience of general hospital inhalation therapy, probably most of the patients in ventilatory failure will fall in the third group. The severity of failure runs the gamut from questionable to rapidly fatal, and the decision to designate a condition as significant failure is a responsibility of the attending physician, a task that is not always easy. With the contemporary techniques now available to treat this condition, the diagnosis of acute ventilatory failure implies a course of therapy that may be drastic as well as intensive; and yet it is a state that cannot long go unattended without subjecting the patient to increasing risk. Although, as in most aspects of medicine, there are no hard and fast criteria for judging a patient to be in or approaching a critical level of ventilatory failure, there are guidelines available to the physician, with some of which the inhalation therapist treating this type of patient should be familiar. The fundamental evaluation of the patient is a clinical one, involving the physician's knowledge of the patient's past history, physical findings, and careful observation of the disease progress for signs of a compromised ventilatory system. It is important that the physician determine whether his patient's condition can be reasonably explained on a purely respiratory basis or whether it is also influenced by some metabolic disorder. With this background, the physiologic measurements of arterial blood pH and carbon dioxide and oxygen tensions will be meaningful and in most instances decisive in the evaluation. However, even though these laboratory data are objective and accurate in themselves, each physician must interpret them according to his own standards; and although there will be little disagreement with values that are grossly abnormal, those that vary but slightly from normal are often difficult to judge. It has been suggested that acute ventilatory failure is present, and deserving of intensive therapy, if there is clinical evidence for it supported by findings of an *arterial blood pH less than 7.25, arterial blood carbon dioxide tension greater than 55 mm Hg, and arterial blood oxygen tension of less than 60 mm Hg.*[209] Such data are more significant if they represent acute changes, and there could be no criticism of using less severe values than these. This matter is being emphasized to underscore the importance of employing both clinical and physiologic evaluation, for treatment, after all, is directed toward a patient and not a laboratory report.

Objectives of the inhalation therapy of ventilatory failure are thus twofold: first, the improvement of alveolar ventilation, with the return of a normal carbon dioxide blood level and stabilization of acid-base balance, and, second, correction of associated hypoxia. We have discussed the latter in the last chapter and will refer again to oxygen therapy in relation to its role in management of the patient in failure, but our prime attention now will be directed to the correction or compensation of alveolar hypoventilation, using mechanical devices to accomplish that which the patient is unable to do for himself. Mechanical support of ventilation ranges from the relatively simple use of a breathing gas driven by positive pressure, on an intermittent basis, to the full maintenance of a helpless apneic patient; and such support is divided into the two descriptive categories of *assisted* and *controlled* ventilation. For our purposes we will define "assisted" ventilation as mechanically generated airflow that augments the patient's spontaneous, but inadequate, breathing and that is initiated by his own inspiratory effort. "Controlled" ventilation is mechanically generated airflow delivered according to a predetermined cycling pattern, completely without patient influence. It must be used to support an apneic patient; but the choice of either mode is available to the patient with spontaneous breathing, according to clinical need and circumstance. Assisted ventilation may be administered on a continuous or intermittent basis, but controlled ventilation is usually continuous. Therapeutic details will be discussed below, but it should take little imagination for the therapist to appreciate that controlled ventilation imposes an awesome responsibility upon all members of the managing medical team. Whenever he is given such an assignment, the therapist must always be aware that the patient is completely dependent upon the skill and integrity of the medical attendants and the effective function of the equipment used. It is the responsibility of the patient's physician to judge the clinical status and prescribe therapy, but it is the inhalation therapist's responsibility to see that the therapy is properly and safely instituted, maintained, and monitored. Only those therapists with a sound physiologic background and mature dedicated interest are qualified to participate in this dramatic and rewarding aspect of medical care. Finally, it should be recognized by all members of the medical team that *the performance of a ventilator is no better than the skill of its operator.* The simplest apparatus is safer and more effective in the hands of an expert therapist than the most sophisticated in the hands of an amateur.

VENTILATORS: CLASSIFICATION AND PRINCIPLES

Classification of ventilators

There are many available references describing the origin and development of mechanical ventilators, classifying them according to different criteria, structural and functional.[210-212] Such classifications tend to be based on technical characteristics that are not necessarily clinically oriented, and the continued development of ventilators of increasing complexity, with overlapping principles and features, makes classification difficult. Actually, a rigid classification of equipment is not essential, but some type of grouping according to similar characteristics allows an orderly approach to the study of ventilators and helps to keep in mind the physical features by which they function. We will classify ventilators according to characteristics that are easy to differentiate and that lend themselves to description and illustration, using the outline below. Fig. 9-1 shows pictures of several commonly used instruments.

Classification of mechanical ventilators

I. *Negative-pressure ventilators—time-cycled*
  1. Controller
    a. Body tank (iron lung) (Drinker[213])
    b. Cuirass (Monaghan[214])
  2. Assistor-controller: cuirass, modified (Emerson[215])

II. *Positive-pressure ventilators*
  A. Time-cycled—assistor-controller: blower-bellows, double-circuit (Air-Shields[216])
  B. Volume-cycled (pressure-limited)
    1. Controller
      a. Piston, rotary drive, single-circuit (Emerson[217])
      b. Piston, rotary drive, double-circuit (Engström[218])
    2. Assistor-controller
      a. Piston, linear drive, single-circuit (Bourns[219])
      b. Compressor-bellows, double-circuit (Bennett[220])
  C. Pressure-cycled—assistor-controller, pneumatic (IPPV)
    a. Flow-adjustable (Bird[221])
    b. Flow-sensitive, time-cycled control (Bennett[222])

First, it should be noted that some of the ventilators are designated as controllers and others as assistor-controllers. The former are limited only to complete control of the patient's ventilation; if spontaneous respiration is present, it must adjust to the operation of the machine, the machine must be adjusted to it, or the machine may override the patient's voluntary efforts. Assistor-controllers can either assist spontaneous ventilation or control breathing completely, depending upon how they are operated. There are appliances that can be classified as only assistors, but in a practical clinical sense they are not considered as true mechanical ventilators, since they are not suited for maintaining the patient in severe failure; and reference will be made to them later in a discussion of intermittent positive-pressure breathing treatments. Second, the student should note that the ventilators are divided into two major groups—those classified as negative-pressure ventilators and those as positive-pressure ventilators. Fig. 9-2 schematically illustrates the basic difference in function of these two types of machines during the inspiratory phase of airflow. The negative-pressure ventilator generates a negative pressure (more precisely, a subatmospheric or gauge-negative pressure), or suction, on the external surface of the thorax, as shown by the arrows in sketch A. This negative pressure is transmitted to the interior of the thorax, creating a pressure gradient with the atmosphere, and air flows into the lung.

In contrast, the positive-pressure ventilator, using a power source, forces air into the lungs, developing an intrathoracic positive pressure that expands lungs and chest, as depicted in sketch *B*. Perhaps the student will observe that the negative-pressure ventilator is more physiologic in its function than is the positive-pressure since normal ventilation is the product of negative pressure generated in the thorax by the action of the ventilatory muscles. Reference

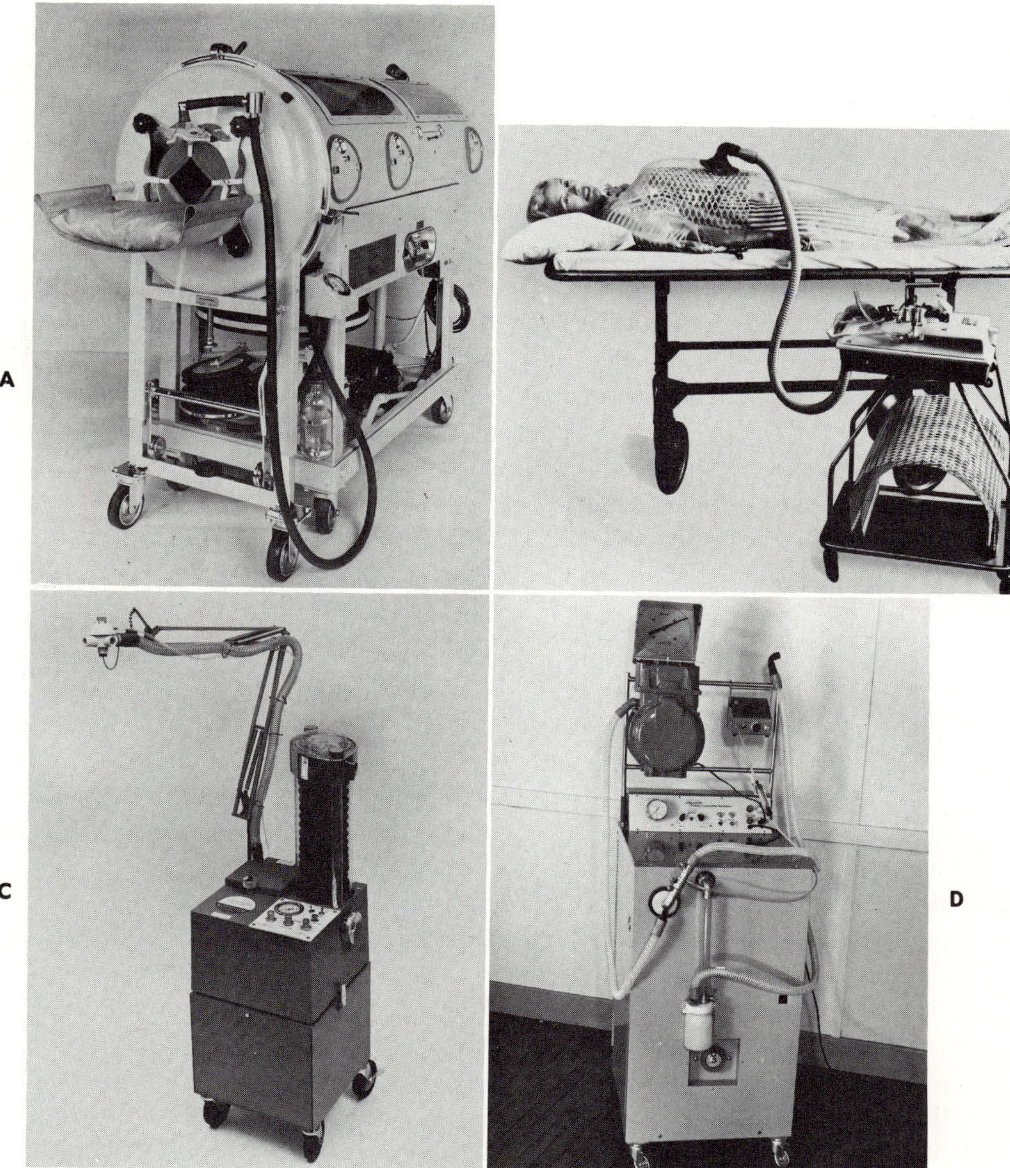

Fig. 9-1. Several mechanical ventilators representing a variety of operating and functional principles, details of which will be discussed in the text. **A,** Drinker. **B,** Emerson cuirass. **C,** Air-Shields. **D,** Emerson Post-Operative. **E,** Engström. **F,** Bourns. **G,** Bird. **H,** Bennett.

will be made to this important point later. Third, attention of the student should be drawn to the three different control modes of ventilators—time cycling, volume cycling, and pressure cycling. It might occur to him that volume cycling, whereby the functioning of an instrument depends upon the delivery of a volume of air to the patient, is the most reasonable since, after all, the act of breathing is designed to bring into the lungs a volume of air

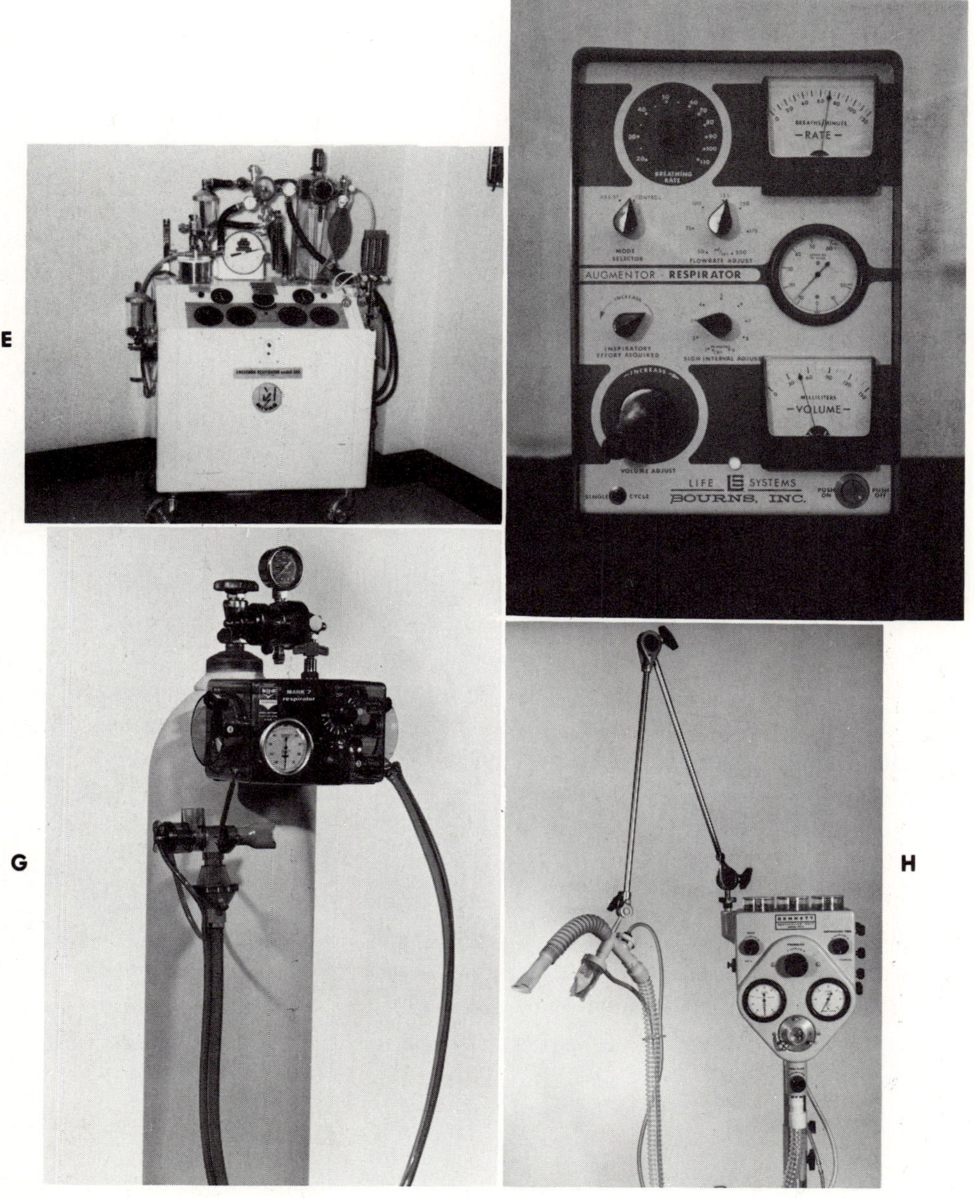

Fig. 9-1, cont'd. For legend see opposite page.

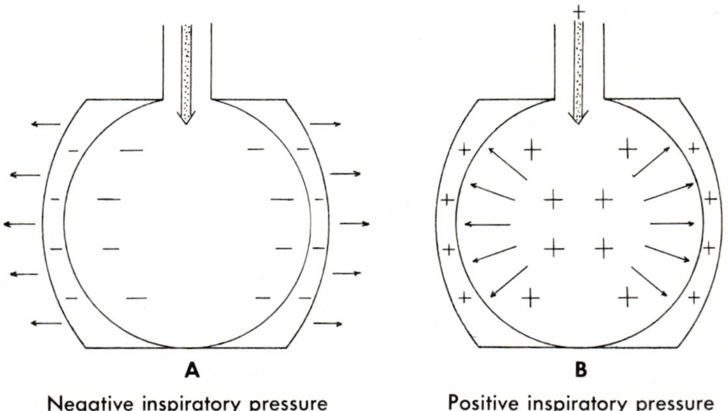

Fig. 9-2. Diagrammatic illustration of the difference between inspiratory forces of, **A**, negative-pressure and, **B**, positive-pressure ventilators.

adequate to satisfy physiologic needs. In other words, we breathe a volume of air rather than a pressure or time. Perhaps the student can see, however, that whether we talk about pressure, volume, flow rate (volume per time), or time we are talking about the same thing. It is somewhat like using any one of several doors to enter a house. Spontaneous ventilation is a summation of the effect of muscular activity (pressure), delivering air at a rapid enough rate, to bring into the lungs the correct volume of air within the time limit set by metabolic demand. A healthy, normally controlled respiratory system is able to integrate all these factors on an instant-to-instant basis to achieve effortless resting gas exchange and to expand this function to accommodate the needs of severe exertion. An appliance that attempts to substitute for the damaged normal mechanism, on the other hand, is limited in its ability to coordinate as efficiently and must confine its operation to one major function. The more sophisticated the apparatus, the better able it is to influence the remaining elements of ventilation. The plain fact of the matter is that there is no "best" mechanical ventilator or else there would not be the large variety now available on the market. Each type or style of machine is an attempt to exploit some facet of physiology that seems to lend itself well to manipulation by a mechanical principle or, conversely, to exploit some mechanical principle that holds promise of better regulating ventilatory physiology. None of them are particularly good, in the sense that they can safely and predictably replace normal breathing; but to the patient in ventilatory failure for whom death is soon inevitable without assistance, they are infinitely better than nothing.

Let us now consider some of the structural and functional features of representative ventilators listed in the table. It is strongly emphasized that the choice of instruments used as a basis for our discussion in no way implies a rejection of competitive models by omission. Those chosen are believed to be such familiar examples of their respective classes that they lend themselves well to description.

Negative-pressure, time-cycled ventilator. The exponent of this type of ventilator is the time-honored body tank respirator, known for so long as the "iron lung." First described in 1929, the tank respirator saw widespread, lifesaving use through many poliomyelitis epidemics.[223] The body respirator is an airtight cylinder that accommodates the patient up to his neck, leaving his head exposed to atmosphere. At the opposite end, or underneath the tank, is a large bellows powered by an electric motor, with a handle for manual operation in the event of electrical failure. Expansion of the bellows creates an intracylinder negative pressure, the magnitude of which is indicated by a pressure gauge calibrated in centimeters of water. Under the influence of the pressure gradient between the interior of the respirator and the atmosphere, air flows into the patient's lungs, and subatmospheric pressures of up to 15 cm H_2O are frequently employed.

This respirator has the advantages of ruggedness and durability and relative ease of operation. However, it has many disadvantages and in most institutions has been replaced by equipment of more recent design. The unit is large and cumbersome, requiring considerable space to compensate not only for its physical size but also for its operational noise. From both nursing and medical viewpoints, it makes patient care difficult and awkward. A patient ill enough to require respirator care generally needs much personal attention, and yet he is isolated from his surroundings, accessible only through arm ports in the wall of the tank or by being removed from the machine for hurried care. Monitoring of physiologic functions and the administration of intravenous infusions are done under handicaps. Even more important than these inconveniences is the inflexibility of the tank respirator's function. It is a controller with an adjustable negative pressure that moves the thorax at set, predetermined intervals, with no provisions for the patient to use whatever spontaneous ventilation he may possess. There is no way of controlling or regulating flow rates—a feature that is less important in ventilating patients with normal lungs, such as those with poliomyelitis (with whom the tank had its initial experience), than it is in ventilating the larger number of patients who are disabled with obstructive pulmonary disease. In the latter, flow rate control may be critical to successful ventilation. A generalization may be inserted at this point by stating that a patient in ventilatory failure, but with normal airways and lungs (neuromuscular or central nervous system disease), can usually be ventilated adequately with any of the standard ventilators now available. It is the patient with obstructive or restrictive pulmonary disease who presents the greatest maintenance problems. Finally, the negative pressure by which the tank respirator functions can, itself, be a hazard to the patient. The negative pressure is applied not only to the semirigid thorax but also to the much more pliant abdomen and is, accordingly, transmitted to the abdominal cavity. Here, it tends to cause the venous blood on its return to the right atrium to pool in the large vascular abdominal reservoirs, with a resulting decrease in venous return and cardiac output. The so-called "tank shock" was not an uncommon complication, as peripheral vascular collapse followed the interference with cardiovascular dynamics. This effect will be dealt with in a little more detail, later in this section, in relation to the physiology of positive-pressure breathing.

In an attempt to retain the benefits of negative-pressure ventilation while minimizing the disadvantages of the large tank respirator, the *cuirass,* a shield-like appliance, was developed.[214] Basically, this consists of a rigid shell (available in a number of sizes) with its edges designed to conform to the lateral surfaces of the thorax, base of the neck, and hip-pubic area. From the top of the shell a flexible hose leads to an electric pump. In operation, the cuirass functions as does the full body respirator, but the negative pressure is confined only to the thorax, avoiding the undesirable effect upon the abdomen, as described above. At the same time, however, it is less efficient than the tank; and with its own inherent deficiencies, it cannot be relied upon to give the support to an apneic patient that is possible with the larger unit. It is frequently difficult to effect the necessary close fit of the shell to the great variety of body contours, and unless it is applied properly, it is undependable. A loose contact between patient and shell not only reduces the available ventilating pressure but can also produce serious chafing of the skin. Like the tank respirator, the cuirass is a controller, and it can "assist" only if its cycling pattern can be adjusted exactly to the patient's spontaneous breathing, although this is not true assisted ventilation by our definition. The main use of the chest respirator, as it is commonly called, is to wean a patient from the body tank. This was especially helpful in the treatment of poliomyelitis, since it allowed access to the patient's extremities for the much needed physical therapy of that disease. Many patients with residual, permanent, partial paralysis of the respiratory muscles who could function adequately during their waking hours have used the chest respirator regularly upon retiring to prevent the occurrence of hypoventilation during sleep.

Although use of the cuirass, along with that of the body respirator, has declined in recent years, an improvement in design has made available a chest respirator that is an assistor as well as a controller.[215] Instead of the heavy and rigid chest piece of the original style, the new model uses a lightweight fenestrated plastic shell that sits loosely over the patient's trunk, with no close skin contact. An airtight seal is achieved by a plastic wrapping that encloses the shell and the patient's back and is snugly applied around the legs. A vacuum cleaner–type power unit supplies the negative pressure and can be adjusted for various settings of the control mode. The major feature, however, is a triggering device that permits the patient to initiate the powered inspiratory phase of ventilation at his own rate and to support his own voluntary breathing. An electronic sensor, attached in front of the patient's nostril, responds with high sensitivity to the slight airflow of the start of his spontaneous inspiration and activates the respirator to assist the rest of inspiration.

We can summarize the status of the negative-pressure ventilators by making a few final comments about the group as a whole. Shortly, we will discuss details of the use of *intubation* of the airway in mechanical ventilation, which entails passing a tube through the mouth and larynx into the trachea or through a surgical opening beneath the larynx directly into the trachea. This is a procedure usually necessary for the application of positive-pressure ventilators but is not ordinarily required for negative-pressure ventilators. The ability to ventilate a patient without the need for intubation is certainly an advantage in favor of the negative-pressure machines, but it is an advantage that must be viewed with some reservation. First, patients with chronic bronchopulmonary disease in ventilatory failure need frequent aspiration of secretions, done most effectively through an airway. Second, many patients in failure without pulmonary disease, in whom pathologic secretions are not a problem, may have paralyzed or obtunded epiglottal reflexes, and normal oral secretions may pool in the mouth or hypopharynx. In such instances, the strong inspiratory suction of a negative-pressure ventilator may draw these fluids into the bronchial tree, with resulting atelectasis or pulmonary infection. Intubation is usually necessary to prevent such complications.

In addition to the problems of size and patient isolation posed by the negative-pressure machines, the much greater versatility of the positive-pressure generators, which have developed in recent years, has placed these machines in the foreground of the therapy of ventilatory failure. The original indication for the big tanks was the large number of patients with bulbar, or respiratory paralytic, poliomyelitis; but effective prophylactic medicine has reduced the incidence of this disease to a negligible quantity. At the same time, there has been a steady increase in the number of patients with failure due to airway obstructive disease, and in this group the negative-pressure ventilators are generally less effective than the positive. Nonetheless, because there are some patients who can benefit from the use of negative-pressure support of their ventilation, and especially if the avoidance of intubation is felt to be advisable for some valid reason, ventilators of this group should be available in hospitals with a heavy load of respiratory care patients.

Positive-pressure, time-cycled ventilator. In contrast to the class just discussed, there are many types of positive-pressure generators, employing drastically different principles to achieve the same results. Regardless of the method used, these ventilators deliver a breathing mixture under pressure to inflate the lungs and expand the chest. A descriptive example of the time-cycled positive-pressure ventilator is the electrically operated blower-bellows, double-circuit assistor-controller by Air-Shields.[216] The power unit is a motor-driven blower that is able to deliver up to 148 liters of airflow per minute into a bellows and to generate pressures up to 55 cm of water. It is referred to as a double-circuit apparatus because the airflow furnishing the power of the

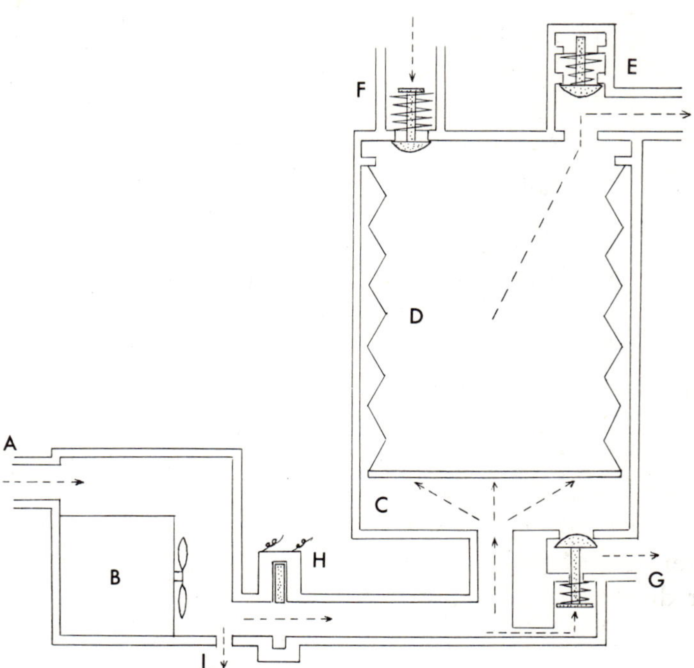

Fig. 9-3. Positive-pressure, time-cycled ventilator. See text for description.

instrument is separated from the ventilating airflow that reaches the patient. Fig. 9-3 schematically illustrates the relationships between the blower and bellows, and the power and patient circuits, during the inspiratory phase. Air is drawn into the power circuit at A and is driven by the motor-blower (B) at various adjustable velocities into a sealed cylinder (C). Here, the forced air acts upon a bellows (D), which with its outflow tract comprises the patient circuit; and the ventilatory gas in the collapsing bellows goes to the patient through the valved outlet (E). During inspiration the patient-gas intake port (F) is closed; and the power-gas pressure closes the cylinder dump port (G). Not illustrated is an inlet provided for the addition of oxygen to the bellows breathing mixture.

At the end of inspiration, the ventilator's electric cycling mechanism closes a solenoid valve (H), which blocks further airflow in the power circuit to the bellows; and the air blown by the continuously operating motor-blower is vented through an escape port (I). Pressure in the circuit is quickly dropped through a bleed-off (not shown) in the solenoid valve, allowing the cylinder dump port to open for rapid emptying of the cylinder. The weighted bellows then falls, opening the patient air intake to fill the bellows, while the outflow valve closes and the machine is ready for another cycle.

The cycling pattern is determined by electrically timing the duration of inspiration, the duration of expiration (total time between the end of one inspiration and the beginning of another), and varying the flow rate of the power circuit. Controls allow considerable variation in both inspiration and expiration so that the best time ratio between the two phases for maximum ventilation can be set for each patient. The volume of air delivered to the patient is determined by the combination of flow rate and time, and a rough measure of its magnitude is indicated on a scale marked on the pressure cylinder, against which the upward excursion of the bellows is read. The volume measurement of tidal air is only approximate because of gas compression, common to all gas-conducting systems subjected to pressure. The volume gauge actually measures the amount of air drawn into the bellows during the patient's exhalation phase, and as such it is accurate. However, because the bellows empties under the pressure of the power circuit airflow and this pressure is in continuity with the patient's respiratory tract, the tidal volume on the bellows is compressed to a smaller volume in its delivery. Volumetrically, therefore, the patient receives less than the bellows gauge indicates. A close estimate of the actual tidal volume can be calculated by using the "compression factor," which is the number of milliliters of gas lost by compression per centimeter of water pressure and must be measured for each gas system. In the ventilator under discussion, the compression factor for the adult bellows is 5 ml/cm water pressure and, for the smaller pediatric bellows, is 2.25 ml/cm water. The product of the factor times the reading of the machine's pressure gauge is subtracted from the volume indicated by the bellows, and the difference is the approximate delivered tidal volume.

In the control mode, then, both inspiratory and expiratory time controls are manipulated to achieve the desired total number of breaths per minute and the phase ratio, whereas the appropriate flow rate is adjusted to deliver the tidal volume prescribed by the attending physician in the time allotted to inspiration. It can be seen that pressure plays no direct role in determining the pattern but is the result of the variables of time and flow. To prevent the development of dangerous pressures, a relief valve will be activated in the neighborhood of 55 to 60 cm of water.

As an assistor, the time-cycled ventilator can be set for triggering by the patient, with an inspiratory effort of as little as 0.5 cm water negative pressure. Once initiated, inspiration continues according to the time duration and flow rate previously established. The expiratory time can be set at a long enough interval not to interfere with the patient's own frequency but at a short enough interval that it will automatically activate inspiration before serious hypoxia develops, should the patient's breathing fail.

This type of ventilator is compact, relatively easy to maintain, and can be provided with a special bellows for pediatric use. Like the body tank, it is especially effective for the patient with relatively clear airways, and its advantages over the tank include, in addition to size, its ability to assist as well as control and the adjustability of ventilatory cycle phasing. Unlike the tank, it does have a wide range of available flow rates to accommodate changes in airway resistance, a point that will be discussed in more detail when we consider the clinical application of ventilators. Like all positive-pressure ventilators, intubation is required for prolonged, effective use; and one of the major weaknesses of this time-cycled unit is its precision solenoid valving system, upon which the unit's function depends.

Positive-pressure, volume-cycled, controller ventilator. The ventilators in this class are electrically operated and depend upon a motor-driven piston to deliver a predetermined volume of air from a cylinder. Volume, rather than time, is the cycling monitor, with pressure, as in the time-cycled machines, exerting a limiting effect beyond an established safety level. Adjustable gearing allows changing the travel distance of the piston to vary the volume of air displaced from the cylinder, and this constitutes the tidal volume delivered to the patient.

This type of ventilator is powered by a wheel-and-piston mechanism that might be called a rotary drive. The electric motor turns a wheel to which is attached a connecting rod, which in turn is attached to the shaft of the piston. Such an arrangement produces forward movement of the piston that can be plotted graphically as a so-called *sine curve*. The student, in his reading of the literature and advertising media, will frequently encounter reference to a

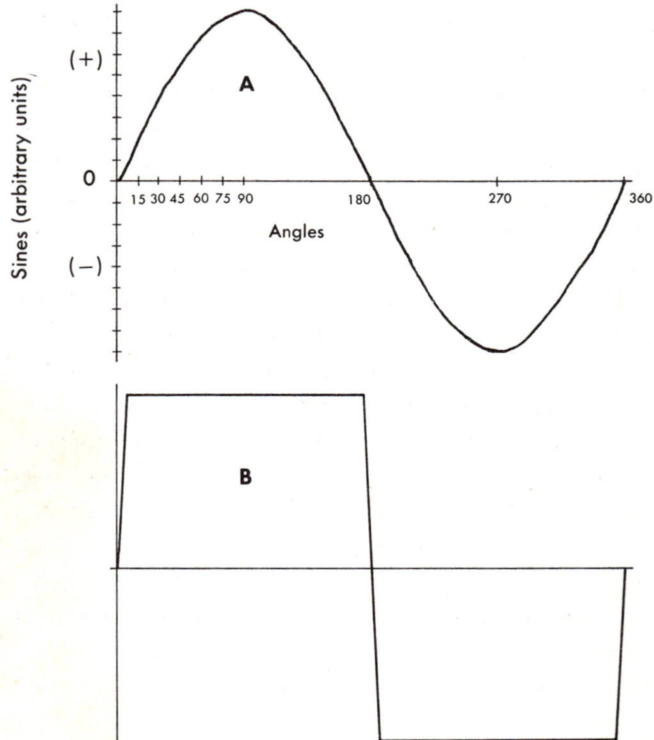

Fig. 9-4. Sketch **A** is a *sine wave*, a plot of a series of angles against their sine values. Note that for angles greater than 180 and less than 360 degrees the curve is negative. Sketch **B** contrasts a "square wave" with the sine. See text for significance of these graphs.

sine curve pattern and certain benefits attributed to it. Although the importance of this phenomenon in the daily practical application of mechanical ventilation is probably overemphasized, the sine curve pattern is at least of academic interest as a characteristic of one type of ventilator; and the student should understand its meaning and the influence it may have in therapy. Without straying too far afield, we can describe a sine curve, which is a trigonometric term, as a graph obtained when one plots the sine values of a series of angles against the angles. A complete sine curve results from recording the values of a full circle of angles, and it has the configuration shown in Fig. 9-4, *A*, an undulating, reciprocal curve with equal positive and negative components above and below a base line. The sine curve is a natural function in that it occurs in many natural phenomena, where it is given the name of periodic or harmonic motion; and it is characteristic of the behavior of alternating electrical current, the vibration of a stretched string, and the movements of electrons within atoms.

The relevance of the sine wave to ventilation may come into focus if we recognize that, as a given point travels around a circle, at any instant its position represents an angle to the center of the circle, for which there is a corresponding sine value. Thus, its circular route can be plotted as the sine wave of an infinite number of angles. Let us now consider the sketch of Fig. 9-7, which schematically represents a wheel driving a piston (not shown), ignoring the legend, which pertains to a later topic. Half the circumference of the wheel is marked off in 18 equal arbitrary units of time (t_0, t_1, t_2, etc.), indicating uniform velocity of the wheel; and the time markers are projected by dashed lines onto the horizontal diameter of the wheel. A connecting rod, from wheel to piston shaft, is attached to the wheel at point A, which corresponds to a time marker; and the diameter of the wheel is divided into 10 equal arbitrary units of horizontal travel of point A, also the travel of the piston. With the wheel turning at a fixed rate, the forward velocity (distance per time) of point A, and the piston, gradually increases from its starting position at distance 0, and time point t_0, to a maximum at distance 5, and time t_9, one quarter of a turn, or 90 degrees of travel. Beyond this, the velocities of point A and the piston decrease to zero again at distance 10. This increase and decrease of velocity is shown by the relative numbers of distance intervals per time markers on the horizontal scale. At both ends there is but a fraction of a distance unit per time, whereas in the center there is almost a one-to-one ratio. In the piston ventilator, the forward motion, delivering a tidal volume, represents the inspiratory phase. Obviously, the distance-time relationships will be the same during the exhalation phase return of the piston to its starting point, but since this half of the cycle does not involve airflow to the patient, we need not consider it at this time.

It is evident that the forward travel of the piston, represented in the sketch by point A, conforms to the first or upright half of the full sine curve shown in Fig. 9-4, A. This is what is meant by the sine wave characteristic of this type of volume-cycled piston ventilator. The significance of the sine wave is related to its effects upon the kinetics of inspiratory airflow. Because the piston gradually picks up speed in its forward motion during the first half of inspiration (90 degrees of travel) then progressively slows down, the gas it delivers into the patient's airways must follow the same pattern. Therefore, from a point of no airflow prior to inhalation, the velocity of the breathing gas increases to midinspiration, then decreases to zero at end-inspiration. The slowly increasing airflow, with its minimal turbulent effect, theoretically is better able to overcome the initial inertia of the lung-thorax system and the resistance of decompressed bronchi than if the flow were of sudden high velocity, following a pattern like that of Fig. 9-4, *B*. The sine wave pattern facilitates maximum flow rate at midinspiration, when the bronchial tree is best able to accommodate it; and finally, toward the end of inspiration, the slowing flow rate supposedly enchances an even distribution of gas among the alveoli.

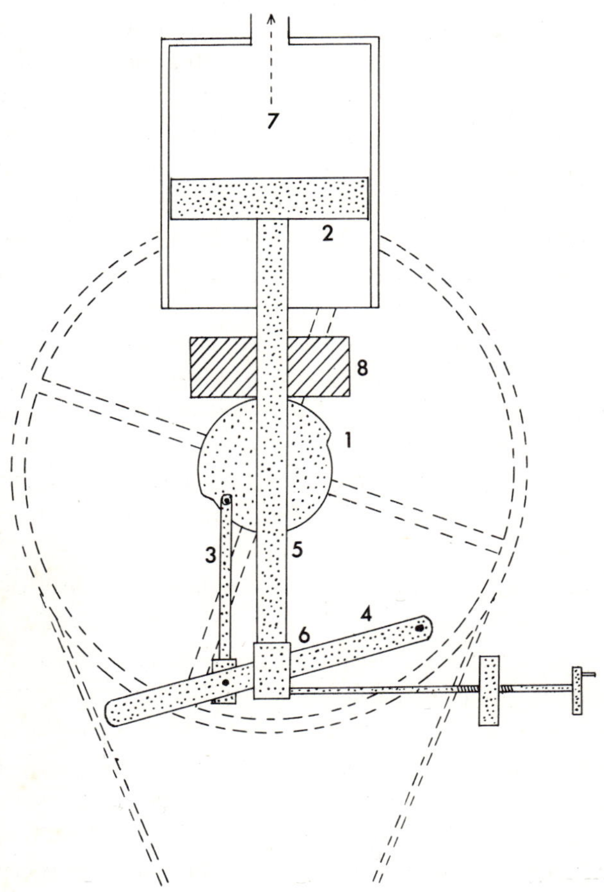

Fig. 9-5. Positive-pressure, volume-cycled, single-circuit, rotary-drive ventilator. See text for description.

Two ventilators of this category will be described—one employing a single gas circuit and the other a double circuit.

SINGLE-CIRCUIT (Emerson[217]). This ventilator is relatively simple in its construction, durable, and easy to use. The essentials of its circuitry are diagrammatically illustrated in Fig. 9-5. The electric motor acts through a belt to turn a large wheel, shown as dashed lines, but the basic parts directly concerned with air delivery are solidly sketched. The piston drive wheel (1) is eccentrically contoured and attached to the hub of the large wheel. It moves the piston (2) through the action of a connecting rod (3) that is fixed to a pivoting arm (4). The piston rod (5) attaches to the pivoting arm by a screw-adjusted slide block (6). It can be seen that the position of the slide block in relation to the pivot point of the arm will determine the extent of the vertical travel of the piston and, thus, the amount of air delivered from the cylinder (7) per stroke. Air intake into the cylinder is not shown, but because the power of the machine is exerted directly on the breathing gas going to the patient, this apparatus is designated as a single-circuit unit.

Phasing of the ventilatory cycle is possible through independent controls of inspiratory and expiratory times, activated by a special switching mechanism (8) and the eccentric drive wheel. Through a mechanical sensor, the wide arc of the wheel triggers the inspiratory cycle, and the narrow arc the expiratory cycle, the timing of both of which can be adjusted by the operator. Humidification, automatic deep sighing, excessive pressure release, and the addition of oxygen are all provided for. Although the screw mechanism that sets the piston to deliver a desired tidal volume has a calibrated scale, the volume must be measured by one of several meters available for this purpose. The measurement of exhaled air is usually accurate enough for clinical purposes and eliminates the need to account for the effect of gas compression in the system. As the student considers the function of this ventilator, he may begin to understand why it is difficult to formulate a hard-and-fast classification of ventilators. Although it is designated as a volume-cycled machine, timing, through phasing control, certainly plays a role in its function. There is no question about its being a controller, for there are no provisions for patient participation.

DOUBLE-CIRCUIT (Engström[218]). Much more complex than the Emerson ventilator just described, the double-circuit time-cycled piston machine embodies the same principles but utilizes them in a more elaborate manner. By its designation, the Engström has separate pneumatic circuits for power and ventilation, somewhat similar to those described in the time-cycled, blower-bellows Air-Shields. A motor-driven piston moves back and forth in a cylinder, alternately creating positive and negative pressure. The cylinder is connected to a large transparent pressure chamber in which is suspended a breathing bag. When negative pressure is generated in the power cylinder, it is transmitted to the chamber and air flows into the suspended bag, which is valved to the atmosphere; during the positive-pressure cycle, pressure transmitted to

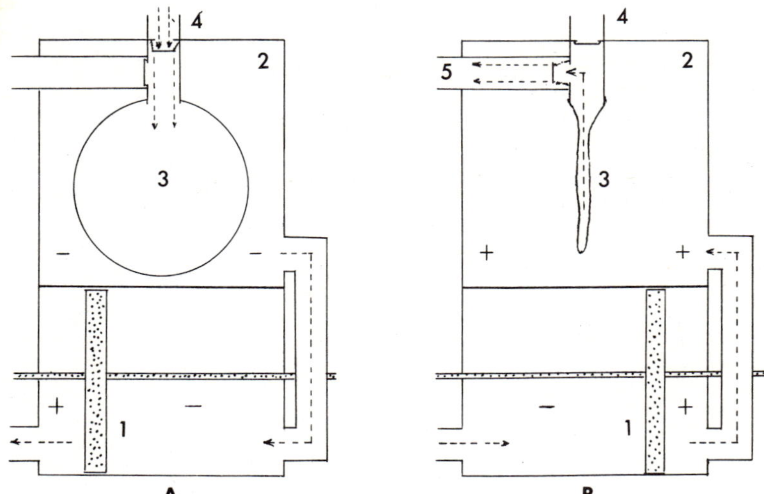

Fig. 9-6. Positive-pressure, volume-cycled, double-circuit, rotary-drive ventilator. During expiration, **A,** travel of the piston, *1,* to the left creates subatmospheric pressure in the chamber, *2,* filling the breathing bag, *3,* with air through the intake valve, *4,* in preparation for the next inhalation. During inspiration, **B,** travel of the piston to the right pressurizes the chamber, driving air from the breathing bag into the patient circuit, *5.*

the chamber empties the breathing bag into the patient circuit. Fig. 9-6 illustrates the general relationships and function of the two circuits and needs little further explanation. Not indicated in the sketch is the safety water lock and the rest of the valve control system, including the manner in which oxygen or anesthetic gases can be added to the breathing mixture. A feature of this instrument not found in its single-circuit counterpart is a mechanism for creating a negative pressure in the patient's airways if desired, the physiologic and clinical indications for which will be discussed in detail later. Suffice to point out here that the intake-output port of the power cylinder can be used to activate a venturi in the patient's exhalation line and drop the pressure in the respiratory tract to subatmospheric.

One of the major characteristics of the Engström ventilator is the pattern by which its flow is delivered to the patient, and to describe it, we will refer to Fig. 9-7. The ventilator has a fixed inspiratory/expiratory ratio of 1:2, which means that one third the total ventilatory cycle is used for inspiration and two thirds for exhalation, regardless of the minute breathing rate. A range of frequencies is available from 10 to 30 per minute, and once a given rate is chosen, the predetermined tidal volume is delivered according to the machine's specifications. To maintain its I/E ratio of 1:2, the ventilator must complete its inspiratory function by the time point A reaches time marker t_{12}, for this represents one third the full cycle. Inspiration is thus completed by the time the piston has reached three fourths its forward stroke distance, for time t_{12} corresponds to 7.5 distance units of a total of 10. Under conditions of normal lung-thorax compliance and minimal airway resistance, the tidal

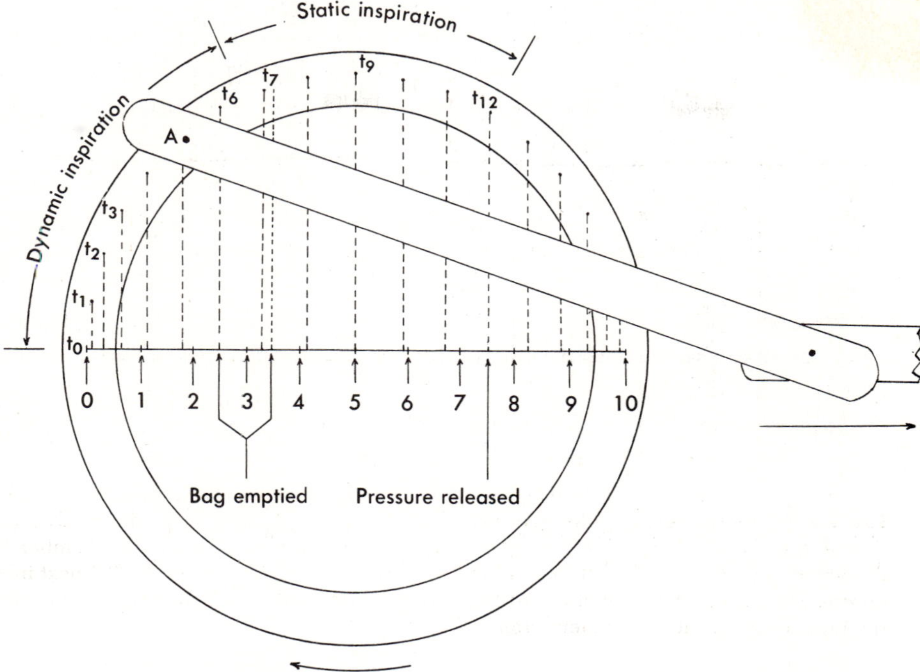

Fig. 9-7. Some inspiratory mechanics of the Engström ventilator are shown in this wheel and piston–drive shaft sketch. Half the circumference of the wheel is marked off in equal *time units,* and the diameter of the wheel is divided into 10 *distance units* of forward travel of point *A.* With a fixed I/E ratio of 1:2, inspiration must be complete when point *A* reaches time marker t_{12}. See text for detailed description.

volume in the breathing bag will empty into the patient circuit while pressure is still developing in the pressure chamber, somewhere between 0.5 and 0.6 of the allotted inspiratory time, or between time markers t_6 and $t_{7.2}$. At the three-quarter point in the piston stroke, a valve in the piston opens to release cylinder pressure and prevent further generation of pressure; and the piston completes its forward travel. Two interesting features should be noted. First, the tidal volume (*patient* inspiration) has been delivered to the patient before *machine* inspiration is finished and while the power unit is still exerting pressure in the chamber containing the breathing bag. Second, expiration begins while the piston is still in forward motion. Obviously, the remainder of exhalation occurs during the return of the piston to its starting position.

There is an advantage to the Engström's pressure-airflow relationship, and it revolves about the slight time lag between the emptying of the breathing bag into the patient's airway and the termination of mechanical inspiration. In the normal respiratory tract, the continued pressure in the breathing bag chamber helps effect the maximum distribution of the inspired gas among the alveoli. In a sense the tidal volume is rapidly delivered to the airways by the pressure of early inspiration and then evenly dispersed throughout the lung by the steady pressure of the few moments until the piston releases its force.

In the event of a drop in compliance of the lung or an increase in resistance, this same time interval is a reserve period during which the continued generated pressure can ensure maximum delivery of the tidal volume. The manufacturer of this ventilator refers to the initial part of inspiration as the *dynamic inspiratory period,* and the last part as the *static pressure period.*

As soon as the power cylinder pressure drops, at one third the cycle, exhalation begins even though the piston is still completing its stroke. This interval comprises what is called *passive exhalation,* and the time of reverse travel of the piston the *negative phase.* During the former, pressures in the circuits are falling toward atmospheric, and no extraordinary influences act upon exhalation; but while the piston is reversing its position, the negative pressure is available.

Like the Emerson ventilator, the Engström is a controller only. At certain times in the cycle the patient may be able to take a spontaneous breath from the reservoir bag, but this does not constitute any sustained effort toward independent breathing. Pressures are adjustable up to 70 cm H_2O, and there are nomograms available to assist in selecting the proper air volumes for both adults and children; and the gas compression effect is taken into consideration in such calculations.

Positive-pressure, volume-cycled, assistor-controller ventilator. There are two commercially available instruments that fit this category, but they differ so in their construction, operation, and indications that little can be said for their common features except that they are volume ventilators and are able to assist as well as control ventilation. It is this latter function that differentiates them from the two described above.

PISTON, LINEAR-DRIVE, SINGLE-CIRCUIT (Bourns[219]). This ventilator is designed only for the premature or term infant and has a maximum stroke tidal volume of 150 ml. A single-circuit device, the instrument is powered by an electrically operated piston-cylinder unit, utilizing a mechanism very different from that of the other piston machines. The Bourns ventilator has a

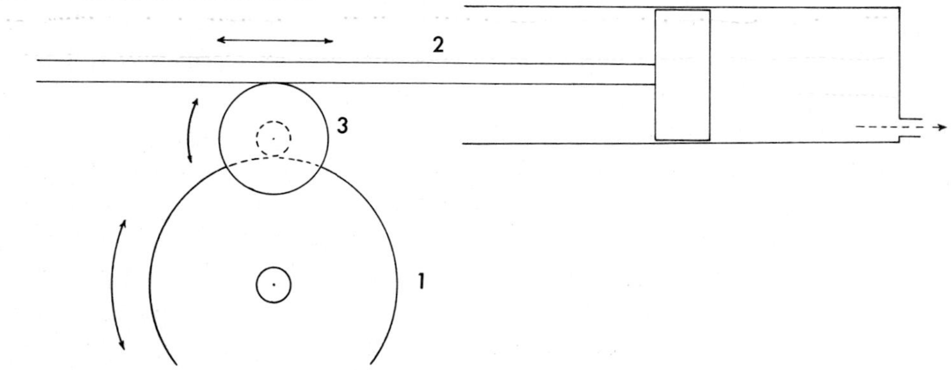

Fig. 9-8. Simplified sketch of the drive mechanism of the Bourns respirator, showing the linear travel of the piston. See text for details.

linear rather than a rotary drive, schematically illustrated in Fig. 9-8. The drive wheel (1) oscillates back and forth and moves the piston drive shaft (2) in a similar fashion through a transmission gear (3). The travel of the drive wheel thus determines the delivered tidal volume. The actual operation of the mechanism is governed by elaborate electronic circuitry through an electromagnetic clutch that has almost instantaneous response. Supplied with the ventilator is a specially designed criblike holder to confine the infant and yet leave him accessible to general care and even permit him to be maintained in an incubator. The patient is most easily connected to the breathing tubes by means of a custom-molded nasal mask[191] or through nasotracheal intubation.

For controlled ventilation, the respirator has adjustments for rate, flow rate per stroke (in milliliters per second), periodic sighing, and stroke volume. The inspiratory/expiratory ratio can be varied and is set by means of selection of the proper flow rate. The principle involves, first, determination of the tidal volume and minute breathing frequency desired, then, adjustment of the milliliter per second flow rate that will deliver the tidal volume in that fraction of the ventilatory cycle allotted to inspiration. The machine, in delivering the calculated flow rate, automatically conforms to the predetermined inspiratory time. For example, if it is desired to deliver a tidal volume of 25 ml at a frequency of 50 per minute and to limit inspiration to 30% of the ventilatory cycle, then a flow rate of approximately 69 ml per second is the only rate that can satisfy these conditions. To avoid the necessity of making this calculation every time the instrument is set up, the manufacturer provides a nomogram to give the required information quickly and accurately. At the same time, compensation must be made for the gas compression effect, for this is a critical value in the small tidal volumes used in infant ventilation.

For use as an assistor, the Bourns respirator has a variable resistance to activation of the machine. For the very weak patient, only a small negative pressure at the start of inspiration will trigger the ventilator, and this can be increased whenever desired to aid the patient in his development of strong inspiratory effort in preparation for termination of assistance. The instrument will automatically take over ventilation if the rate falls below 60% of the established rate, for a period of 12 seconds; and an alarm will indicate this change in pattern.

COMPRESSOR-BELLOWS, DOUBLE-CIRCUIT (Bennett[220]). One of the most comprehensive of ventilators, this unit delivers a determined volume with pressure variable, but with pressure limits available as safety and warning devices. The instrument is compact with a large number of control dials, switches, and signals conveniently mounted on a panel. It is supplied with an adjustable heated humidifier, a monitoring spirometer, and an optional negative-pressure venturi. In addition to the usual controls governing tidal volume and minute breathing frequency, the MA-1 has adjustable maximal pressure limits up to 60 cm H_2O, maximum flow rates from 10 to 100 lpm, oxygen concentrations of five levels from 21% to 100%, artificial sigh with rate, pressure limit, and volume control, and expiratory resistance. The ventilator is powered by the action of a compressor on a bellows, creating a double circuit vaguely similar to that found in the Air-Shields model but more complex in its structure and interacting controls.

When the MA-1 is used as a controller, inspiration is initiated by a timer and is volume limited at end-inspiration unless a preset pressure limit is reached first. Two techniques are available in the adjustment of pressure limits. In the first method, once the observed pressure in the system has been noted, the pressure limit may be set just above this value so that changes in the patient's respiratory system that might produce an increase in pressure will limit the delivered volume and indicate the change by activating a pressure limit signal. This is an effective means of monitoring ventilation. The second method involves setting the pressure limit to the highest range felt to be safe and then letting the ventilator deliver its volume unrestricted, according to changes in patient compliance and resistance. In a manner somewhat similar to the Bourns respirator, the flow rate of the MA-1 governs the inspiratory/expiratory ratio. With a predetermined volume to be delivered under conditions of a fixed frequency, the machine needs enough flow to accomplish its purpose. Guides are available from the manufacturer to initiate ventilation, but adjustments may be necessary as conditions change in the airways. Under any circumstance, should the time of inspiration exceed one half a controlled cycle, a warning light comes on and indicates the need to increase flow rate. This assures that an I/E ratio will never be greater than 1.0. By adjusting the flow rate and carefully timing the ventilatory cycle, the operator can obtain a wide variety of ratios. In addition to negative pressure during exhalation, positive pressure is also available. Other ventilators often use a cap over the exhalation port, but the MA-1 introduces expiratory resistance by an adjustable control dial. The clinical use of the seeming paradox of resistance to exhalation will be detailed later.

This ventilator is easily used as an assistor. A patient-sensitivity control permits a wide range of inspiratory effort to initiate inspiration, but care must be taken to ensure an adequate flow rate for the needs of spontaneous breathing. For the patient with uncertain breathing patterns or who may be subject to fatigue and hypoventilation, the rate control of the instrument may be set to a limit lower than his own, and in the event of failure of spontaneous effort, the ventilator will support him.

Positive-pressure, pressure-cycled assistor-controller (pneumatic) ventilator. Ventilators in this classification, by virtue of their great versatility and wide usefulness, have become some of the most important instruments of the inhalation therapist. We will discuss suitable representatives of this group in greater detail than we have devoted to other types, not only because of their clinical importance but also because they so readily permit a review of certain critical ventilatory relationships and principles. This does not mean that they are the best ventilators for all patients; but they do have the most widespread applicability of all ventilating instruments in the general care of respiratory diseases. They are associated with a general form of therapy popularly called *intermittent positive-pressure breathing* (IPPB), but we are going to discuss them under two headings in an attempt to avoid a confusion of terms. For our purposes in this section, we are interested in the use of these machines as true ventilators and will refer to them as *intermittent positive-pressure ventilators* (IPPV); a little later we will cover other uses of these same units under the title of IPPB. With this specification, we will limit our discussion to only two ventilators as examples of the group, for not only do they have significant differences in their functions, but, for all practical purposes, they are the two most widely accepted total ventilators as well.

There is no need to recapitulate the development of positive-pressure breathing, for there are some excellent reviews in the literature with extensive bibliographies; and the student is encouraged to study the background of this form of therapy in which he is expected to be an expert.[224] We have already described several ventilators, classified as positive pressure in nature; but, as with many expressions in common use, the term *intermittent positive pressure* connotes a certain type of mechanism. The IPPV and IPPB units are pneumatically powered, completely independent of any electrical current, and have a minimum of moving parts, most of which are valves. They are driven by gas pressure of 50 psig, the source of which can be a cylinder, central supply, or a compressor. In addition to a certain safety factor, the lack of need for electrical power affords considerable mobility; and the simpler mechanical structure facilitates maintenance and repair. Finally, the pneumatic positive-pressure ventilators are conveniently smaller and more compact than the electrically operated machines. These features are not necessarily determinants in themselves for the choice of a ventilator or for the evaluation of the performance of any one of them, but they are practical considerations in the management and operation of a busy inhalation therapy department, especially when it is noted that the pneumatic machines are less costly than the other types.

The IPPV reduces the source pressure to a selected predetermined level, on the average somewhere between 10 and 30 cm H_2O, and delivers the breathing gas until equilibrium is established between the patient's lungs and the ventilator. End-inspiration and thus cycling of this ventilator are primarily dependent upon a pressure buildup in the lung rather than upon time or volume, although both time and volume exert influence under certain circumstances. The valving mechanism shuts off the gas flow when pressure balance is reached, and passive exhalation ensues. Whereas the volume-cycled machines deliver a volume at whatever pressure is needed to move it, the pressure-cycled instruments deliver a pressure that will produce a desired volume change. To express this in a somewhat oversimplified manner, we might say that, since every respiratory tract has characteristics that require a certain relationship between volume and pressure (compliance) to move air, theoretically it makes no difference which of the two factors determines end-inspiration; the other will follow accordingly. Based on this premise, the original pressure-cycled instruments were very simple, and pressure generation was directly dependent upon the flow rate of gas introduced into the apparatus from the source pressure. With his background in the physics of airflow, the student should now realize that such a direct relationship between flow rate and pressure cannot be satisfactory because of the pressure effect of increasing flow through a tubular conducting system, an effect that becomes increasingly important and influential in the presence of obstruction. Therefore, the theoretical consideration mentioned above is not valid for real situations, and unrestrained flow rate–generated pressures cannot be depended upon to give us the resulting volume changes we wish. It is obvious that the factor of flow rate is an important one in the effective use of pressure-cycled ventilators; and in order to relate pressure and volume for the purpose of safe ventilation, flow rate control is a necessity. The IPPV units now suited for ventilation provide for this important factor but differ in the principle employed, a subject we will cover in our description of the two major machines.

Before pursuing the technical details further, we should make a point of practical importance. It is the nature of people to be impressed with size and apparent complexity of machinery and instruments, a characteristic that poses a frequent problem with the use of the IPPV. These units are relatively small, make very little noise in operation, and to the uninitiated eye give the appearance of simplicity. As a result, many members of the hospital staff feel themselves qualified to operate the ventilators, with no more preparation than a brief orientation demonstration, perhaps supplemented by a review of the instrument's instructional brochure. Ignorance of the principles and mechanics of the IPPV has given many a distorted or downright erroneous impression of both its capabilities and its limitations, and in some hospitals such equipment is not used properly or for the correct indications, to the detriment of patient care. Far from being simple, except in physical design, the IPPV is a precision instrument based upon some complex fluid-engineering principles; and the realization of its full clinical potential demands more operational skill and knowledge of physics and physiology than do most of the more impressive electrical machines. It is safe to say that, after a didactic introduction to IPPV, a full-time student therapist requires several months to develop the skill and confidence to use it safely and effectively, a fact that is not readily appreciated by many.

The IPPV is an assistor and a controller. To assist ventilation, it is supplied with a demand valve that responds to very slight patient inspiratory effort to activate gas flow. Demand valves differ in structure, but their general functions are the same. Both sides of the valve are at atmospheric pressure just before inspiration, but when the patient makes a small effort to inspire, creating as little as 0.5 cm of water or less subatmospheric pressure, the valve opens to allow the flow of respiratory gas. Inspiration then continues until the preset pressure develops in the respiratory tract, and the absence of a pressure differential across the valve causes it to close. The amount of patient effort needed to start inspiratory flow is variable through a sensitivity control that makes it possible to assist the very weak effort or stimulate independent breathing by imposing a suitable work load on the patient. As a controller, the IPPV is able to cycle according to a rate determined by the operator, initiating inspiration through pneumatic timing devices. Expiration is triggered by pressure, but its length is subject to operator control. The patient control and automatic control abilities of the IPPV can be combined to give a backup assist to a patient with spontaneous but uncertain breathing. The apparatus is adjusted for controlled ventilation at a rate less than the patient's own, and should he become apneic or his rate fall off, the ventilator will take over. Negative pressure during exhalation is available to aid controlled ventilation if desired, activated by a simple venturi that uses source gas to introduce subatmospheric pressure in the patient line.

Although there is much good instructional material available from manufacturers describing and illustrating technical and operational aspects of their products, in conformance with our policy stated at the beginning of this chapter, we will consider some of the features of the two commonly used IPPV's. It is hoped that this will help the inhalation therapist to understand better those mechanisms of the ventilators that are critical to their safe and effective function.

FLOW-ADJUSTABLE (Bird[221]). We will use the Mark 8 model as an example because it embodies the major characteristics in which we are interested. Working off a source gas pressure of no less than 50 psig, the Bird ventilator is a relatively small, two-chambered instrument whose basic operation is illustrated in the greatly simplified sketches of Fig. 9-9. Source gas (A) enters the partition between the chambers, called the *centerbody,* where its flow rate is controlled by an adjustable valve (B), permitting rates from zero to approximately 80 lpm. Calibrations on the external valve knob are for reference only and do not indicate delivered flow. The chamber on the left is called the *ambient chamber* because it is in constant equilibrium with the atmosphere through a filter-equipped aperture (C). Its counterpart is a *pressure chamber,* for this is where therapeutic pressure is developed; it is in direct communication with the patient's respiratory tract through tubing attached to the outflow port (D).

Cycling mechanism. The heart of the cycling mechanism is a sliding valve located in a channel in the centerbody (E). Basically, this consists of a *ceramic cylinder* ground to close tolerance, with a vent through it (indicated by the dashed lines), and at each end of the cylinder an attached metal *clutch plate* (F) and (G). The two illustrations show that the cylinder duct can align with the source gas inflow to allow its passage or can misalign to shut off the flow

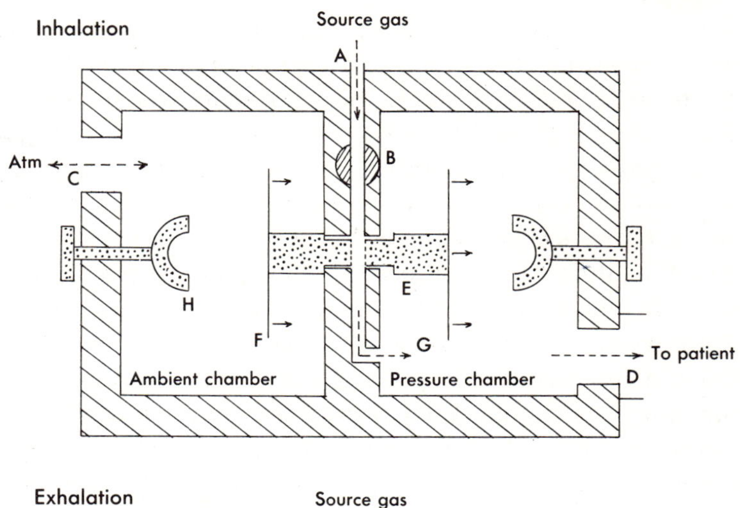

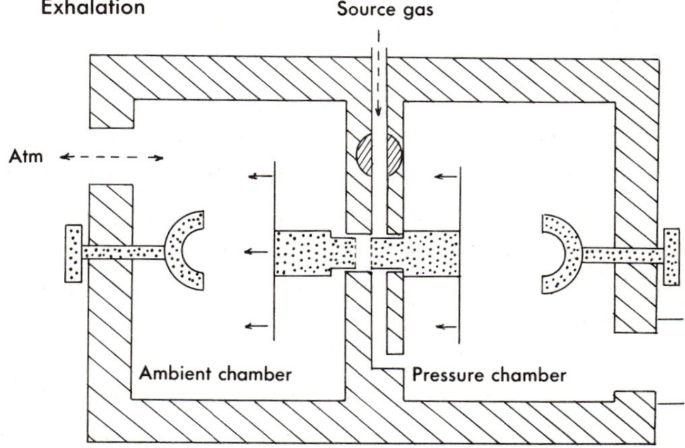

Fig. 9-9. Schematic illustrations of the inspiratory and expiratory mechanics of the Bird respirator. See text for details.

of gas; and it should be noted that inspiratory gas enters the pressure chamber only. Each chamber has a permanent magnet (H) and (I), whose positions in the chamber can be adjusted by an outside threaded control.

A magnet (H), in the ambient chamber, constitutes the *sensitivity control,* so important to the function of the ventilator in the control mode because it determines the inspiratory effort required of the patient to trigger the start of inspiration. The patient is connected by airtight tubing to the pressure chamber, and if he creates a negative intrathoracic pressure through contraction of his inspiratory muscles, this negative pressure will be transmitted back to the pressure chamber of the ventilator. If such pressure is of sufficient force, the pressure gradient between the two chambers will move the ceramic valve toward the pressure chamber, opening up the source gas channel and initiating inspiration. The amount of inspiratory effort needed to open the valve depends upon the proximity of magnet H to metal clutch plate F. Obviously, the closer together the magnet and the plate, the greater will be the negative pressure in the pressure chamber required to move the valve, and the greater will be the patient inspiratory effort. Conversely, if the magnet is withdrawn farther from the plate, its weaker hold on the plate is more easily overcome, and less work by the patient will start gas flow. This control is so sensitive that it can be adjusted to respond to but a fraction of a centimeter of water negative pressure to begin the respiratory cycle.

Once the sliding valve opens, gas flows into the pressure chamber until a preset pressure is reached in the chamber and the communicating respiratory tract; this constitutes the pressure-cycling characteristic of the ventilator. The amount of pressure required to stop inhalation is determined by the *pressure-control magnet* (I), and again, operation depends upon the relationship between magnet I and clutch plate G. The closer the magnet and plate, the greater will be the pressure needed to separate them as the rising pressure in the chamber acts upon the sliding valve. As the adjustable magnet is advanced, higher pressures will build up in the chamber and in the patient's lungs; as it is withdrawn, lower pressures will activate the valve. On the outside of the instrument there is an aneroid manometer that records the pressure in the chamber, and this is referred to as the *system pressure,* the pressure delivered by the machine. It must be clearly understood that this pressure is not the *intrapulmonary pressure,* although the two are obviously related. Because of the nature of the bronchopulmonary tree, there is a pressure drop from ventilator to alveoli; and whereas the pressure in the instrument can be easily measured, that in the alveoli cannot, except indirectly. We can assume that as system pressure is increased pulmonary pressure will follow accordingly; but from our earlier consideration of factors influencing gas flow, we know that increments of increasing pulmonary pressure may get progressively smaller as delivery pressure rises. It is possible to generate pressures up to about 60 cm of water, although such a level is used only in extraordinary circumstances. Calibrations on the pressure-control mechanism are helpful in setting a desired pressure, but final adjustment is made by observing the actual pressure recorded on the manometer. In Fig. 9-9 the exhalation sketch depicts the movement of the ceramic valve toward the ambient chamber, with interruption of gas flow; exhalation then proceeds passively, as air escapes from the patient through a special valve located at his end of the gas tubing in the breathing head assembly.

Exhalation valve. The breathing head assembly, at the patient end of the gas delivery tubing, consists of several components. Here, the *mouthpiece,* or an adapter to fit an intratracheal tube, delivers the breathing gas to the patient. In the unit also are the *exhalation valve,* a *nebulizer,* and the *negative-pressure venturi,* when used. Source gas is tapped from the main channel, below the cycling valve and carried by small-bore tubing to both the exhalation valve and the nebulizer. As shown in Fig. 9-10, the exhalation port is fitted with a spring-loaded plunger that acts against a caplike "gate," supplied

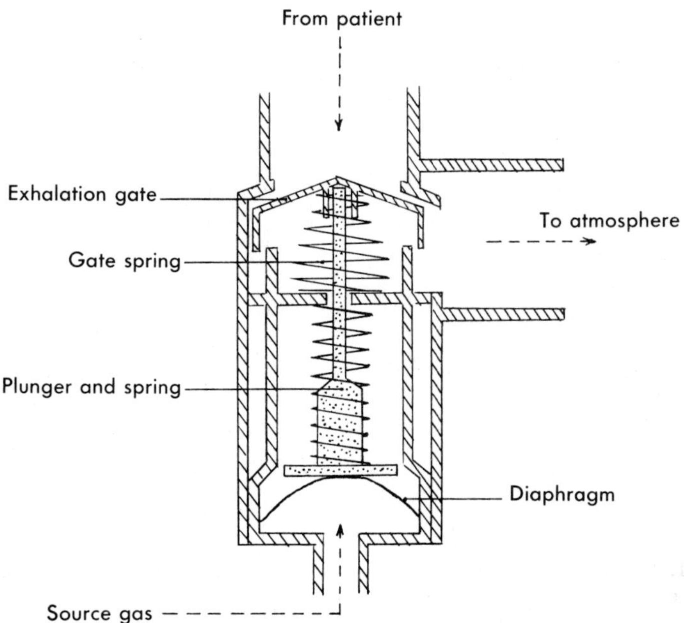

Fig. 9-10. Exhalation valve of the Bird respirator, diagrammatically simplified. See text for description of parts.

with its own fine, weak spring. During inspiration the source gas pressure against the plunger forces the gate into the valve seat and closes the port. As soon as end-inspiration is reached and source gas flow ceases, the plunger retracts by its spring tension, allowing the port to open for instant exhalation. The gate spring, through its gentle action, offers very slight resistance to the outflow of gas, permitting the gate to open smoothly in response to the expiratory flow rate and pressure. It should be pointed out here that one of the most common causes of air trapping, especially in patients on controlled ventilation, is a failure of the gate spring. After considerable use, with frequent disassembling and handling for cleaning purposes, this fine spring often becomes stretched. Its tension and resistance to exhalation increase, impeding the passage of the terminal portion of exhaled air and retaining it in the airways. This event will be manifest by failure of the pressure manometer needle to return to atmospheric zero, leaving it "hung up" in the pressure zone of the gauge. Although there are other causes for this phenomenon, as soon as the therapist notes it, he should check the exhalation valve by inserting a pencil tip into the outflow port to see whether the trapped pressure can be released by freeing the gate. Should this be the problem, the gate must be replaced at once by one equipped with a good spring.

Nebulizer. The same source pressure supplying the exhalation valve is used to power the medication nebulizer, another component of the breathing head assembly. Either sidearm or mainstream nebulization can be used, and because the power gas flows only during inspiration, there is no nebulization

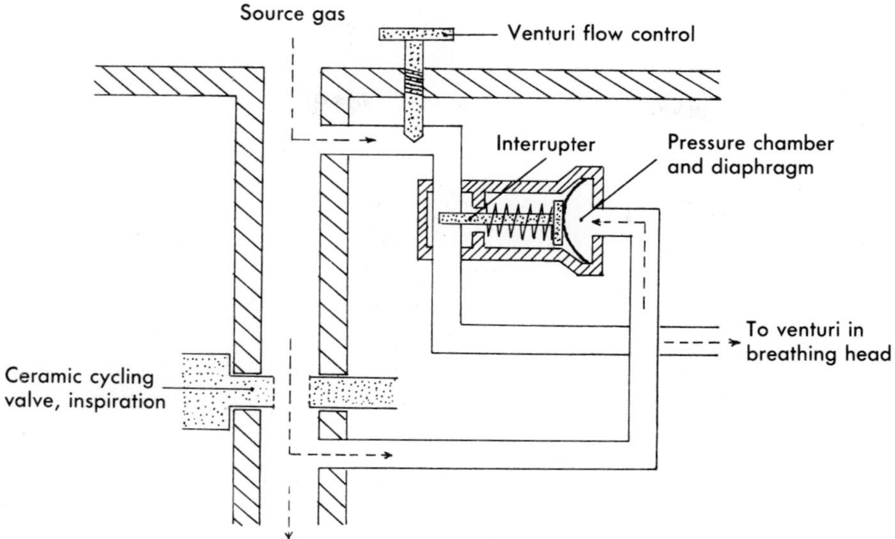

Fig. 9-11. Diagram of the control mechanism for the negative-pressure venturi of the Bird respirator. Details are described in the text.

during exhalation. In addition to supplying medication, the nebulizer plays an important role in determining the composition of inhaled gas and will be considered further a bit later.

Negative pressure. If negative pressure during exhalation is desired, an adapter allows a venturi to be added to the breathing head assembly directly opposite the gate of the exhalation valve, in the passage designated "From patient" in Fig. 9-10. The power for the venturi is derived from a tap line of the source gas above the cycling valve, diagrammed in Fig. 9-11, the flow through which is controlled by a needle valve, adjustable from the outside of the instrument. The force of negative pressure generated by the venturi is dependent upon the flow permitted by this control valve. Inside the ventilator there is a pressure cartridge with a spring-loaded *interrupter valve* in the venturi tap line, distal to the needle control valve. The small pressure chamber of the cartridge, however, is powered by a tap from the source gas after the cycling valve. During inspiration, as gas flows through the ceramic valve, it exerts pressure in the cartridge, forcing the spring-loaded interrupter to block the passage of gas from the needle valve to the venturi; but as soon as exhalation begins, the cessation of gas flow to the cartridge releases the pressure on the interrupter and the latter springs back, allowing source gas to activate the venturi. Employing the usual principle of air entrainment, the fast flow of power gas through the venturi jet pulls into its stream air from the respiratory tract, creating an intrapulmonary subatmospheric pressure of −1 to −5 cm of water. The mixed gas escapes through the exhalation port with a distinctive sound.

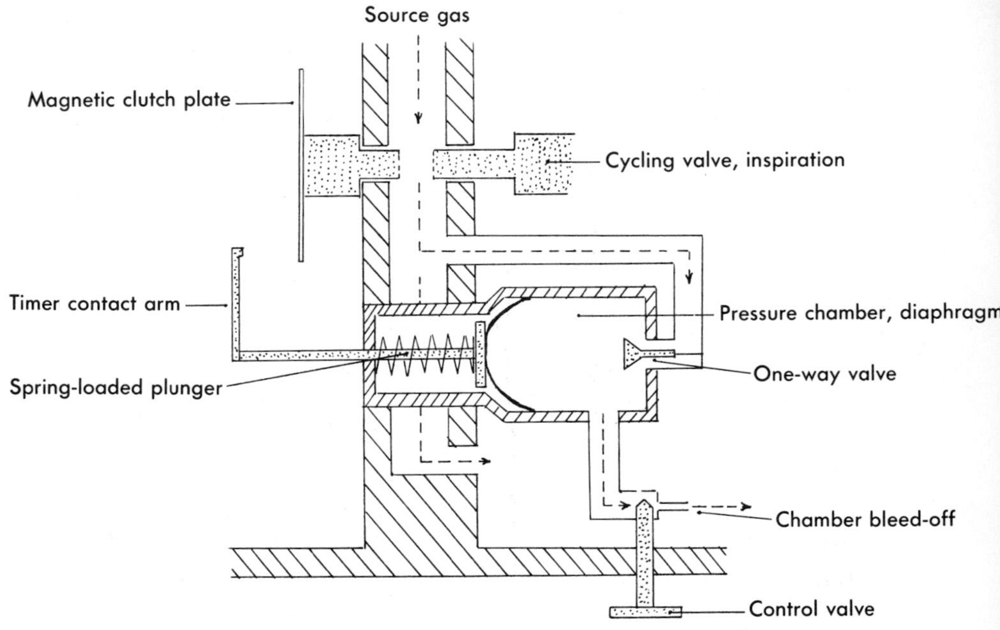

Fig. 9-12. Diagram of the expiratory timer of the Bird respirator. See text for details.

Expiratory timer. When the Bird respirator is used as a controller, the length of exhalation can be varied within a wide range through the action of an *expiratory timer,* housed in a cartridge in the instrument. Like the exhalation and interrupter valves just described, the expiratory timer employs a pressure chamber to activate a spring-loaded plunger. Fig. 9-12 diagrams the parts of the expiratory timer and shows their interrelated functions. For the sake of simplicity, the events of the inspiratory phase are illustrated, despite the fact that the unit influences exhalation; but it is easier to depict the mechanics of preparation graphically and describe the final action. The pressure chamber, separated from the spring-loaded plunger by a diaphragm, is supplied by a tap line of the source gas below the ceramic cycling valve so that flow to the timer is limited to the inspiratory phase. During inspiration, then, the diaphragm compresses the plunger spring, extending the plunger into the ambient chamber of the ventilator. The pressure chamber has an outlet, the flow through which is controlled by a needle valve adjusted from the outside of the instrument and which terminates in a restricted ostium functioning as a bleed-off. If the timer control valve is closed, the unit is nonoperational; and the pressure chamber is, in a sense, a dead-end street. For the expiratory timer to be activated, the control valve must be opened to allow gas to escape from the bleed-off; and the degree to which the valve is opened will determine the speed with which pressure is released from the chamber. When expiratory time control is started by opening the control valve, gas escapes from the bleed-off continuously, even while the pressure chamber is filling during inhalation; but its loss is small in comparison to the higher flow filling the chamber and does not interfere with diaphragmatic activation of the plunger. At end-inspiration, source gas is abruptly shut off to the pressure capsule, and a one-way valve in the capsule closes to prevent a retrograde loss of pressure through the source gas tap lines that supply the nebulizer and the air-mix venturi (to be described below). The bleed-off reduces chamber pressure at a rate determined by the control valve and allows a gradual return of the plunger. The distal end of the plunger is supplied with a right-angle extension, and as the plunger returns to its starting position, the extension contacts the magnetic clutch plate in the ambient chamber, pulls it away from its magnet, and initiates the next inspiratory cycle. Thus, in summary, the duration of exhalation depends upon the speed with which the control valve allows retraction of the spring-loaded plunger and its contact arm, tripping the cycling valve to start the next inhalation. Because the mechanism in no way interferes with the operation of the cycling valve, a patient may spontaneously initiate inhalation with his own effort; and Fig. 9-12 makes it clear how readily the ventilator will adjust to the new cycle.

Air-mix venturi. The last of the major mechanical features of the Bird respirator to be discussed is the *air-mix* and the *main venturi* of the instrument, and anyone operating the ventilator must understand the workings of this system. In the preceding paragraphs we have referred frequently to the source gas of the ventilator without further specification as to its composition. As long as there is an adequate pressure available, any gas can be used to power the machine; but the ready accessibility of oxygen makes this the most commonly used of gases; and in everyday hospital practice, it is usual to connect the ventilator to the nearest oxygen outlet. We have already been exposed to the risks of prolonged use of pure oxygen, so it is reasonable that provisions be made for reducing the concentration of source gas oxygen to safe levels for final delivery to the patient. This is the function of the air-mix control and the main venturi, and it is with this function that we will now concern ourselves.

In principle, the operation of the air-mix is very simple, as inflowing source oxygen is directed through a venturi, where it entrains air from the ambient chamber of the ventilator. The resulting mixture of less than 100% oxygen passes into the pressure chamber and on to the patient. Before considering the actual operation of the air-mix and the concentrations of oxygen it produces, let us look at the mechanism involved. Fig. 9-13 schematically shows the relationships between the components, sketch *A*, with the air-mix control in the "in" position, and *B*, with the control in the "out" position. The source gas is channeled into a narrow chamber with two outlets misaligned with one another, and in the chamber is the plunger of the air-mix control. We can see that, depending upon the position of the plunger, its two baffles will direct the flow of source gas to one or the other outlet. With the plunger pushed in, source gas escapes undiluted into the pressure chamber of the

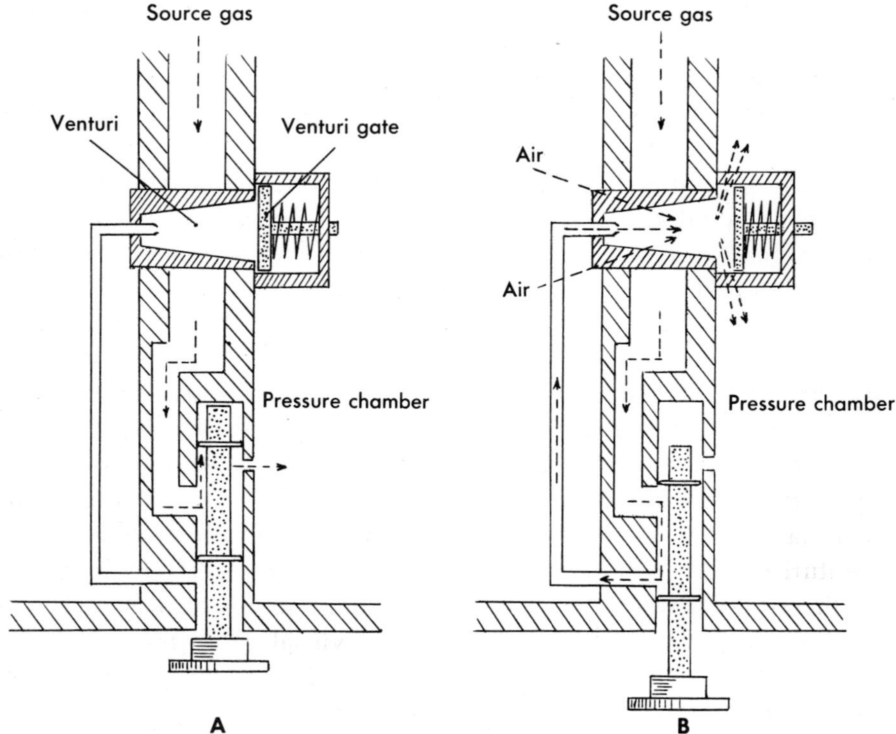

Fig. 9-13. Diagram of the air-mix venturi complex of the Bird respirator. In **A,** the air-mix is in the "in" position, delivering pure source gas to the pressure chamber, bypassing the venturi. In **B,** the air-mix is in the "out" position, diverting source gas through the venturi, where it is diluted with entrained air. A further description of this mechanism, along with the important pneumatic clutch action of the venturi, is found in the text.

ventilator for direct administration to the patient. Obviously, with oxygen as the power gas, the patient will receive 100% oxygen with the control in this position. When pulled out, the air-mix control shunts the source gas to the lower tap line, where it passes through a jet orifice in the venturi. Here, as shown in sketch *B*, air from the ambient chamber of the ventilator is entrained by the source gas jet stream and enters the pressure chamber subject to the influence of the spring-loaded venturi gate. As a result of this action, the breathing gas is a mixture of the source gas and room air. To avoid cluttering the illustrations, we have omitted two items from the air-mix control. One is a small metal flap over the source gas ostium to the pressure chamber, which acts as a one-way valve to prevent backflow of gas or loss of pressure through the tap lines, as described for the expiratory timer above. The second is a small opening from the distal end of the plunger chamber into the pressure side of the ventilator. This acts as a pressure equalizer to prevent a cushion of gas from being trapped in the blind end of the plunger chamber to interfere with advancing the plunger and to prevent a vacuum in the same area from hindering withdrawal of the piston to the "out" position.

The function of the air-mix venturi mechanism is a dual one, for not only does it influence the oxygen concentration of the breathing gas, but, equally as important, it also determines the characteristics of the ventilator's airflow pattern. The two roles are interrelated and together constitute one of the main mechanical features of this ventilator. We will consider this aspect in detail because of its great importance. The structure of the venturi comprises what is termed a *pneumatic clutch,* and according to the manufacturer, it permits the volume of gas going to the lung, and its flow rate, to vary independently throughout the inspiratory cycle, mimicking the accelerations and decelerations of gas flow characteristic of normal spontaneous breathing.[225] In essence, the clutch action is designed to modify the flow characteristics of inhaled gas according to the resistance and compliance status of the respiratory tract. The actual clutch action is the result of the combined operation of the venturi and its gate. As pulmonary resistance and compliance change in the expanding lung, these changes are reflected backward into the pressure chamber of the ventilator. Here, they act upon the venturi gate held in the outflow of the venturi by a sensitive spring, and the gate responds to increasing resistance in the ventilator's outflow tract by reducing the venturi output. By referring to the illustrations in Fig. 9-13, one can visualize pressure in the pressure chamber gradually building up during the inspiratory phase, this pressure slowly closing the gate to retard the flow rate of gas entering the chamber and, consequently, the flow of gas ventilating the lung. Thus, as inspiration proceeds and the resistance of end-inspiration increases, the impedance to airflow produces a back pressure that closes the venturi gate slowly and facilitates the maximum terminal flow of gas to the lung. The student may recognize that the principle of the pneumatic clutch in this version of the pressure-cycled ventilator is designed to achieve the same objective as the sine curve we discussed in relation to the wheel and piston volume-cycled ventilator. We pointed out there that some importance was attached to a slow initial, as well as terminal, flow rate, best afforded by the rotary drive mechanism. The pressure-cycled ventilator starts inhalation with a substantial flow rate but slows down the flow as distal pressure develops. Some degree of the effectiveness of the pneumatic clutch may be demonstrated by comparing the relationships between gas flow rate and distal pressure of the Bird ventilator operating off 100% oxygen as source gas, both without and with the air-mix in use.

To understand better the difference between these two conditions, the student should be aware of an entirely different classification of ventilators, based upon flow and pressure qualities.[211] Two basic types of ventilators are recognized—*flow generators* and *pressure generators,* differentiated as follows: Since the purpose of a mechanical ventilator is to inflate a flexible lung through a fairly rigid conducting system of constantly changing proportions, the ventilator must force air under pressure against the back pressure of airway and elastic resistance. The two factors involved that are determined by the ventilator are the flow rate and the delivery pressure (pressure at the mouth as opposed to alveolar pressure), and any given machine controls but one of these. In the presence of such changing lung characteristics as increased resistance and decreased compliance, if a ventilator at a given pressure maintains a constant flow rate of delivered gas, not influenced by the status of the lung and not hampered by increasing back pressure, the instrument is called a *flow generator.* On the other hand, if the machine holds the delivery pressure at the mouth constant while the flow rate responds to the lung characteristics by gradually diminishing in the face of back pressure, the ventilator is called a *pressure generator.* Knowing the relationship between flow rate and obstruction to gas flow, we know that to reach anything close to a pressure equilibrium on both sides of an obstruction (or, back pressure, generally), we must have a reduction in flow rate. We can visualize a flow of gas building up a pressure proximal to an obstruction in an airway much faster than in the airway distal to the obstruction; such a condition can cause a pressure-cycled ventilator to terminate inspiration before enough gas has reached the partially blocked alveoli to satisfy respiratory needs. The advantage of a pressure generator over a flow generator in ventilating a diseased respiratory tract is evident.

The basic original IPPB instrument was a flow generator with the delivered flow rate dependent upon the source pressure applied; but as its use increased and its greater potential was recognized, as noted earlier in this section, the need for flow rate control became clear. The introduction of a manually variable flow rate adjustment, as in the Bird ventilator under discussion, represented a significant development in IPPV and materially increased both its effectiveness and its safety. Although it remained fundamentally a flow generator, because flow was still constant at any given combination of pressure and flow rate, the ventilator could be manually set, by trial and error and clinical observation, to accommodate a much wider variety of bronchopulmonary abnormalities. A further refinement of the pressure-cycled ventilator was the addition of the venturi apparatus, and we shall see shortly that this feature imparts to the instrument some of the characteristics of a pressure generator.

Let us first consider the operation of the Bird respirator with its air-mix control "in," eliminating the venturi. Now the instrument functions as an adjustable flow generator with independent pressure and flow settings. Source gas passes unmodified through the instrument inflow tract into the pressure chamber, where it develops the preset delivery pressure regardless of either static or changing conditions in the respiratory system that it is ventilating. Not only is the ventilator unable to vary its flow in response to developing impediments, such as accumulations of bronchial secretions, but also its flow rate remains linear and unchanged in the face of the normal resistances characteristic of the inspiratory phase. In other words, when once set for a given pressure-flow pattern, the instrument is inflexible in its opera-

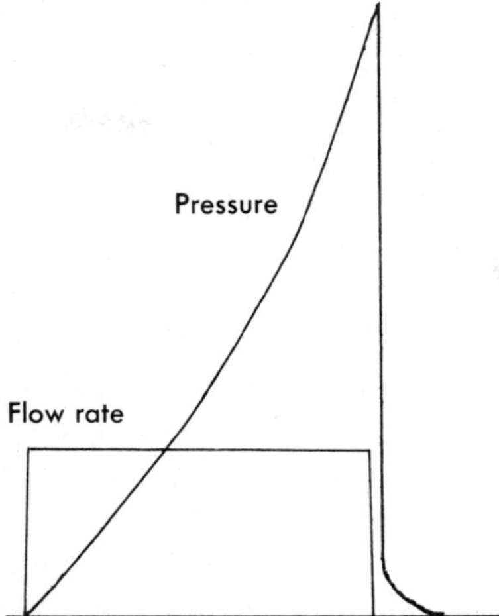

Fig. 9-14. Relationship between ventilator flow rate and pressure when these two factors are independently adjusted. At any given setting the flow remains constant even though resistance increases. (Adapted from Edwards, W. L., and Sappenfield, R. S.: Pressure-cycled ventilators and flow-rate control, Anesth Analg **47**:77, 1968.)

tion. An excellent mechanical study of the performance of this ventilator emphasizes this facet of its performance, and Fig. 9-14 is diagrammatically adapted from one of the recorded pressure-flow relationships of that study.[226] At the outset of inhalation, gas flow rapidly reaches its maximum (as opposed to a sine curve flow) and maintains an unwavering rate throughout inhalation, despite the steadily rising pressure. It must be borne in mind that the amount of pressure recorded reflects airway back pressure against which the machine is working and yet the flow of gas makes no adjustment to this resistance. It can well be imagined that with such a constant gas flow rate, the pressure drop along airways may so increase that alveolar ventilation, dependent upon pressure delivered to the alveoli, may be quite inadequate. Certainly, skillful operation of such a ventilator depends upon the ability to drop the constant flow to a level that will make possible the maximum alveolar ventilation consistent with the estimated resistance or compliance, but every such change must be manual and in response to airway conditions gross enough to be observed.

Activation of the venturi gives to the ventilator considerable versatility in coping with the characteristics of the airways. Source gas no longer enters the pressure chamber directly but is first used to power the venturi where it pulls in and mixes with air from the ambient chamber as described and illustrated in Fig. 9-13. Let us understand that the venturi does not make of the ventilator something it is not for it is still basically a flow generator with the need to employ adjustable flow rate control; but the additional service of the venturi enhances the performance of the machine and supplements the action of the flow control. We have just seen that without the use of the air-mix, the instrument is an adjustable flow generator with a rigid flow rate whereas the function of the venturi modifies it to what might be termed an adjustable flow generator with a flexible flow rate; and for a given manual pressure-flow setting, the ventilator behaves somewhat like a pressure generator. The key to the successful function of the venturi lies in the performance of its gate, separating the mixed gases from the pressure chamber. The spring-loaded gate, acted upon by the outflowing gas on one side and the developing pressure of the pressure chamber on the other, adjusts the venturi outlet to permit that flow of gases which will best compensate for the growing pressure. The sensitivity of the gate's responsiveness can be clearly seen if the outlet of the breathing head is alternately blocked and unblocked by the hand during gas flow. The gate is seen to open and shut in proportion to the applied obstruction and can be made to oscillate back and forth with rapid pressure changes. When the ventilator is cycling, the venturi gate can be seen to open abruptly with the start of inhalation, then gradually close as the cycle progresses. Fig. 9-15 is another adaptation from the same study of ventilators referred to above and shows the effect of the pneumatic clutch on airflow. Graphically evident is the immediate drop in flow rate accompanying the rise in pressure for the first half of inspiration, after which the flow levels off until cycling pressure is reached. This response by flow rate to mounting pressure is called *flow sensitivity* and is the primary characteristic of a pressure generator. Because the Bird respirator is not a pressure generator, the flow sensitivity is not complete and it does not continue to the termination of flow, but for each manually set combination of pressure and flow rate, there

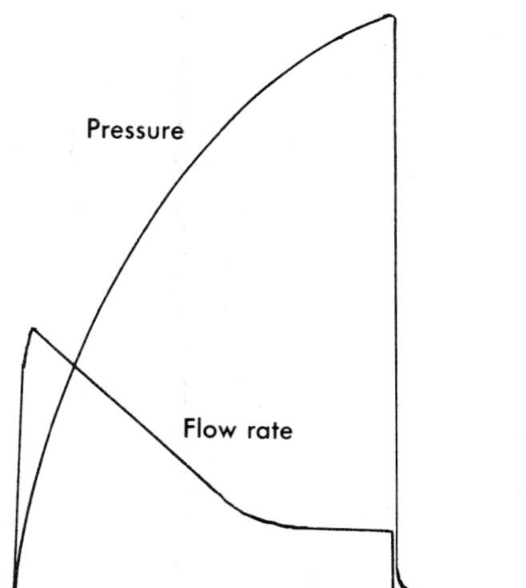

Fig. 9-15. Relationship between ventilator flow rate and pressure when pneumatic clutching is active. With rising pressure, flow initially decreases, then levels as cycling pressure is reached. (Adapted from Edwards, W. L., and Sappenfield, R. S.: Pressure-cycled ventilators and flow-rate control, Anesth Analg **47**:77, 1968.)

is a significant degree of such sensitivity. We will describe more effective flow sensitivity when we discuss the next ventilator.

We cannot separate the pneumatic clutching action of the venturi from its oxygen-diluting function, for the two are interdependent. With the air-mix "in," the breathing gas is 100% oxygen, if that is the source gas; and with the control retracted, the concentration is something less than 100%; but the question is how much less. When the venturi principle came into popular use, there was an unfortunate lack of clear understanding of its operation, and assumptions about its diluting action were accepted that have since been proved false. Although corrective action has been taken, manufacturer's specifications originally gave the impression, still persistent in some minds, that the air-mix venturi automatically produced a breathing gas with an oxygen concentration of 40%. Analyses of delivered gas, on the contrary, have frequently demonstrated oxygen concentrations over 90%; and in clinical use one rarely if at all finds the concentration less than 50%. Thus, although the venturi may be designed to produce a 40% air-oxygen mixture during unrestricted flow, when it functions against a resistance, its performance is completely changed. The major influence on the venturi is the factor of pressure, mediated through the venturi gate, and itself subject to the influence of flow rate. With the venturi output dependent upon so many variables, which themselves are interrelated, it is no wonder that we encounter a bizarre fluctuation of delivered oxygen concentrations that seem to have no rhyme or reason. However, we can get a clue to the relationships of these influences if we conduct the simple experiment of measuring the delivered oxygen concentration of a base line pressure–flow rate setting and then determine the concentration as pressure and flow rate are each individually increased and decreased. This will show us that if the original pressure–flow rate setting is changed so that pressure increases relative to flow rate the resulting F_{O_2} will rise. This change in the ratio may be either an actual increase in pressure or a decrease in flow rate. Obviously, a converse effect on the ratio will decrease the subsequent F_{O_2}; but the clinical situations to which we will be most frequently exposed usually involve pressure increases, so we will use this orientation for our discussion. Finally, a proportionate increase or decrease in pressure and flow will not significantly alter the oxygen concentration, since no ratio change will result.

Let us see how pressure can be so influential in determining the delivered oxygen content and how it uses the venturi gate. In our earlier description of the gate, we were concerned only with the general manner in which it acted as a clutch to compromise gas flow with opposing pressure and did not intimate that it might not be active throughout the entire inspiratory phase. Actually, the gate does not necessarily remain open until end-inspiration and indeed can do so only under a given circumstance. Regardless of the time interval of inspiration, the venturi gate closes when the system pressure reaches somewhere between 10 and 15 cm of water pressure. This is felt to be a reasonably accurate range because the actual closing pressure of a given gate depends upon its physical state. Should it be worn or contaminated with foreign matter of adhesive nature, its closing point can be altered. Especially important in this regard is the condition of the gate spring, normally under a tension of 2 cm of water but which may be weakened by use or handling during maintenance or may be under increased tension after replacement. As we have done frequently throughout these pages, we will make a recommendation to the alert inhalation therapist and urge him to check the function of this important part, if through no other way than observing the gross action of the gate to see whether it is responsive or sluggish or, indeed, whether it is functioning at all and to take corrective action. This limitation on the activity of the gate was designed to permit it to exert its most effective clutching function when confronted with the usual flows and pressures encountered in clinical medicine. Now that we have established that increasing the ventilator pressure in relation to its flow rate will elevate the delivered oxygen concentration and have described the pressure point at which the venturi gate will close, let us see how these two mechanisms cooperate to influence the percentage of oxygen. There are two reasons why oxygen concentrations are unstable.

First, after the venturi gate closes, the *only* gas flow to the patient to complete his ventilation is *pure oxygen* through the medication nebulizer by way of the nebulizer tap line from the ventilator oxygen inflow tract. This gas, which has been activating the nebulizer since the beginning of inspiration, continues to flow into the patient until the preset system pressure is reached in the patient's airways, equilibrating with the ventilator to terminate inspiration by the cycling mechanism described earlier. Thus, the longer inhalation lasts after closure of the venturi gate, the more oxygen will flow undiluted through the nebulizer line and the higher will be the concentration of oxygen in the inspired mixture. This is why any change in the pressure-flow relationship that favors pressure, as noted above, will increase F_{O_2}. If pressure is increased while flow rate is kept constant, longer time will be required to reach the preset pressure, the postclosure time of the venturi gate will be lengthened, and nebulizer oxygen will raise the inspired oxygen concentration. If flow rate is reduced while pressure remains constant, the same circumstances will prevail and the actual flow time of nebulizer oxygen will be lengthened. If the cycling pressure set for the ventilator is less than the gate closure pressure, the gate will remain open throughout inspiration; and not only will the oxygen concentration be at its lowest, but variations in the pressure/flow rate ratio (below the closure point) will effect little significant change in concentration.

Second, in addition to the nebulizer flow, another source of oxygen has been found that significantly increases its concentration in the inspired gas.[227] After the venturi gate closes, oxygen still flows into the venturi through its jet and, denied egress through the gate, backflows from the venturi into the ambient chamber of the ventilator. Here, the oxygen concentration may rise as high as 60%, and during inspiration the oxygen flow to the venturi is diluted, not with supposed atmospheric air but with air already highly enriched with oxygen. We can summarize the action of the air-mix and the venturi in controlling delivered oxygen by comparing the sources of gas available during the initial and terminal portions of inhalation, with 100% oxygen as the source gas. With no dilution (air-mix control closed), both early inspiration and late inspiration are supplied by source oxygen and nebulizer oxygen; with dilution (air-mix control open), early inspiration is supplied by source oxygen, ambient chamber gas, and nebulizer oxygen; and late inspiration by nebulizer oxygen only.

There are many modifications of the flow-adjustable, positive-pressure pneumatic ventilator embodied in various accessories and models of the basic instrument, designed for such special purposes as minimizing dead space, adding a supplementary source of oxygen, correlating machine cycling with chest expansion, and accommodating the needs of the infant. Since it is not the purpose of this text to serve as a technical manual, we have limited our discussion to the fundamental principles that will be found in all variations of the ventilator; and it is felt that the student, through his clinical experience and personal investigation of equipment, should be able to apply his understanding of these principles to any specific instance.

FLOW-SENSITIVE (Bennett[222]). We will describe the PR-2 respiration unit, for it is the most sophisticated and complex, not only of all the Bennett models but of all pneumatic positive-pressure ventilators; and if the therapist understands its functions, he will have little difficulty with the others. Like the Bird respirator, the PR-2 operates from a gas source pressure of 50 psig and exerts a pressure to inflate the lungs, but here the similarity ends. The physical design and the principles upon which the Bennett works are radically different from those of the Bird, and for this reason we will not follow the same descriptive format of the past few pages since it will not be possible to compare the two instruments item for item. Although we have included the PR-2 in the class of pressure-cycled assistor-controllers, we will have to expand this a bit to accommodate all its functions. To be all-inclusive, we should describe the machine as a positive pressure-cycled, time-cycled, flow-sensitive, assistor-controller, a cumbersome designation but accurate. When used as an assistor, the PR-2 is pressure cycled, and patient triggered by subatmospheric pressure. When it is used as a controller, end-inspiration is cycled either by preset pressure or by time, depending upon which factor is activated first. Because the manufacturer has made available an adequate operating manual and some excellent teaching aids, we will not go into a minute description of the ventilator, but we will discuss some of the details that are unique to its function and with which all operators should be familiar.

General features. Unlike the Bird respirator, the PR-2 is not a chambered instrument but basically consists of a system of very complex pneumatic circuitry that intermittently feeds the breathing mixture to the patient under rigid control. Gas flow is regulated by one central valve, aided by several other automatic and manually operated controls, and three ingenious cylindrical pneumatic timing devices that integrate the functions of the components into the total output of the instrument. As source gas enters the machine, that which is to ventilate the patient passes directly to a unit which may be called a regulator-diluter. Here, the gas is reduced from its source pressure to the working range of 0 to 45 cm of water by the adjustable manual pressure control, the exact level being determined by the ventilatory needs of the patient. This mechanism, unlike that in the Bird, which uses a movable magnet, is very similar in its action to the adjustable cylinder gas–reducing valve described in an earlier chapter, in that it employs a control attached to a spring-loaded diaphragm to oppose the incoming gas and limit its pressure. The regulator also contains a balloon that, when inflated, shuts off the outflow of gas from the regulator; and we shall see later that this works in conjunction with the timing mechanism to help establish ventilatory patterns. Pure source gas may be delivered to the patient, or a manually operated venturi may be activated to dilute the gas with atmospheric air. This venturi functions only as a diluter and plays no part in modifying the airflow pattern. As in the Bird respirator, the Bennett venturi is designed to dilute source oxygen to a 40% concentration when operating with an unrestricted flow. However, during inspiration as obstruction to flow is encountered, the efficiency of the venturi decreases and the concentration of oxygen in the delivered gas increases above 40%. Additional oxygen mixes with the breathing gas through the nebulizer, described below. The instrument also contains another pressure regulator, called the unit regulator, that reduces source pressure to about 60 cm of water. Its function is to distribute gas to power several of the automatic components and has no direct communication with the patient. Still other components work directly off source pressure without reduction. The adjustable pressure delivered by the patient regulator (regulator-diluter) is recorded on the face of the ventilator by a gauge calibrated in centimeters of water and labeled "control pressure." Adjacent to this is another similar gauge designated "system pressure," and the two must be differentiated. The control pressure is the pressure delivered by the patient regulator to the flow-control valve and is the pressure that will be reached in the outflow tubing and that will terminate inspiration if the ventilator is pressure cycled. The system pressure (often called mask pressure) records the actual pressure reached distal to the flow-control valve, or at the patient's mouth. For reasons we already know, it does not indicate patient alveolar pressure. Under most circumstances, the two gauges will record the same peak, but perhaps the student can already see that in the control mode in the face of significant airway resistance, because of the optional time-cycling capability of the PR-2, inspiration may end before the mask pressure has had time to reach the set control-pressure value. The careful observation of these two gauges is an important function of the inhalation therapist in the management of his patient.

Before describing the interesting details of the flow-control and cycling mechanisms, we shall enumerate the additional manual controls available on the PR-2 so that we will be familiar with them when we refer to them later in the discussion. Nebulization can be individually adjusted for either inspiration or expiration, or it can be activated continuously. Nebulization during exhalation enables the maximal amount of medication to be delivered to the patient since aerosol fills the breathing tubes during this phase and is immediately available in quantity as soon as inspiration starts. The nebulization unit is powered by direct source gas pressure, but its phasing with respiration is dependent upon an inflatable valve activated by gas at control pressure, tapped after the cycling mechanism. Respiratory rate can be adjusted from 1 to 45 breaths per minute, obviously only applicable when the machine is functioning as a controller. The regulating mechanism assures that expiration will never be less than 1.5 times the duration of inspiration, the physiologic reason for which we will learn later in this chapter, although circumstances may reduce the 1:1.5 ratio. Expiratory time can be prolonged, changing the I/E ratio, always favoring a lowered ratio such as 1:2, 1:3, etc. As with all patient-activated assistors, the sensitivity of the start of inhalation is adjustable over a wide range. Negative pressure during exhalation can be applied to the patient's airways by opening a venturi that works through the nebulizer control unit directly from source pressure. Peak and terminal flows are adjustable, and their functions will be discussed below. The student should note that we have not mentioned a manually operated flow rate control, which was so important in the Bird respirator. One of the major features of the PR-2 is the automatic regulation of flow, at any control-pressure setting; and we will now describe the mechanism responsible for this quality of flow sensitivity.

FLOW-SENSITIVE VALVE. Described by the manufacturer as the "valve that breathes with the patient," the Bennett valve is further affirmed to open with slight inspiratory pressure to permit a flow of gas that varies according to the balance between the delivered control pressure and the total resistance of the patient airways, and to close automatically when the flow of gas through the valve reaches a low terminal point.[228] The Bennett valve is housed in the respirator in a horizontal position, front to rear, and is pictured in Fig. 9-16. It is a metal cylindrical drum, approximately 36 mm long by 26 mm in diameter, penetrated by two large and one small apertures, called windows. Eccentrically placed near the cylinder's wall, a rod runs lengthwise of the drum to function, as we will see, as a counterbalance. Projecting from the front end of the valve is a small lever that allows manual operation from outside the housing. Finally, attached to the outer surface of the valve are two rectangular vanes. The valve and its housing are precision made, and the cylinder is suspended with very close tolerance by jeweled bearings, front and rear.

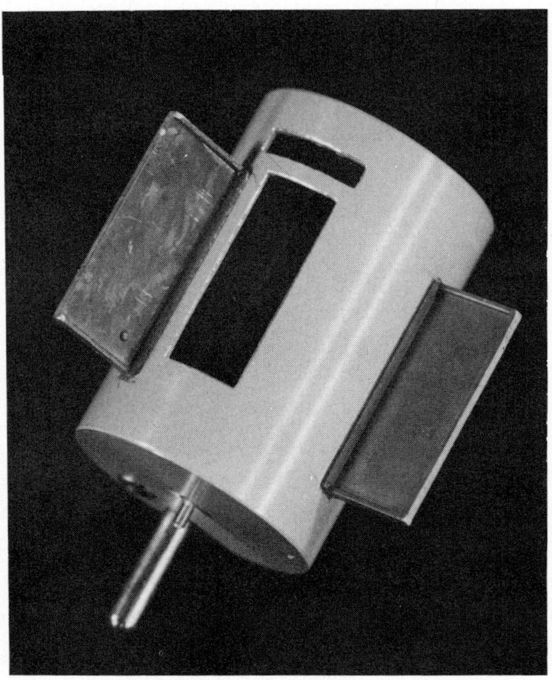

Fig. 9-16. Bennett valve drum, showing two of its windows, the vanes, and the projecting lever for manual operation.

We shall use four illustrations to show the basic function of the valve, of necessity simplifying both graphic and verbal descriptions. The sketches show a longitudinal section through the drum and its housing, exposing the major gas channels and showing the relative positions of the vanes, windows, and the counterbalance rod. In Fig. 9-17 the valve is in the resting state, as during the exhalation phase. Attention is drawn to the configuration of the drum housing with its three ports, 1, 2, and 3. Port 1 is the entry for the main gas flow, which may be either pure source gas or an air mixture, coming directly from the regulator-diluter through the main inflow tract (4). Port 2 is a vestibule leading into the outflow tract (5), to which is connected the patient tubing, and port 3 is the site of action of the inspiratory sensitivity control. The drum housing, more detailed than indicated in the illustration, is provided with many small-caliber channels that receive gas from the various controls noted above or allow the escape of gas to them, all as part of the functioning of this critical center of providing just the correct character of flow, breath by breath. This view of the drum shows a cross section of the counterbalance rod and the position of the two large windows and the vanes in the resting state. Neither window approximates a major gas channel, and vane 2 (in port 2) is against the upper wall of its port, as is vane 3. At this moment, no gas is moving in the valve mechanism. The outflow tract (5) is provided with an adjustable restriction (6), called the peak flow control, that obstructs

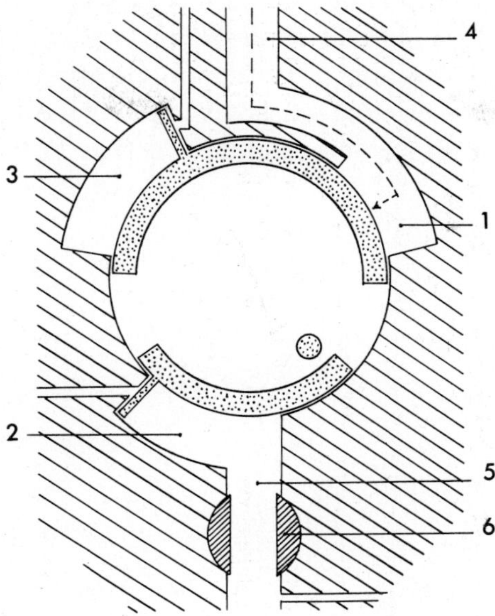

Fig. 9-17. Bennett valve in resting position. See text.

the gas flow to the tubing. Its operation will be described with a subsequent illustration, as will the purposes of the three small channels connected to ports 2 and 3 and the outflow tract.

Fig. 9-18 depicts the events of immediate pre-inspiration, just before inspiratory gas starts to flow in assisted ventilation. The negative sign in port 2, with the airflow arrow directed toward the tubing, represents the negative inspiratory pressure exerted by the patient in an effort to trigger the cycle. This negative pressure draws down vane 2, giving the drum a counterclockwise rotation. We know that the instrument has a sensitivity control to aid the patient in this effort, and its action is evident in port 3, where a flow of gas is seen moving down channel 7 into the port. Such a flow exerts a positive pressure on the upper side of vane 3, forcing it downward, again urging the drum in counterclockwise motion. The dual action of the negative and positive pressures on the two vanes rotates the drum with a minimum of work on its jeweled bearings, and by varying the gas flow to the upper vane, the cylinder can be rendered responsive to the weakest inspiratory effort. During controlled ventilation, without spontaneous patient effort, gas is supplied to vane 3 by the rate-control mechanism through the pneumatic timers mentioned above but yet to be described. Thus, whether assisted or controlled, inspiration is initiated, either in part or in total, by nudging the upper vane with a flow of gas to set the drum in motion. Care must be taken in assisting ventilation not to set the sensitivity flow too high or cycling may be initiated without the patient's help and disturb the breathing pattern.

As the drum continues to rotate to allow inspiratory gas flow, we can illustrate an imaginary moment in midinspiration with Fig. 9-19. Movement of the cylinder has brought one window opposite port 1 and the other opposite port 2, effectively opening direct communication between the main inflow and outflow channels so that gas flows to the patient. It is at this time that the flow sensitivity of the valve is manifested. The exact position of the valve is

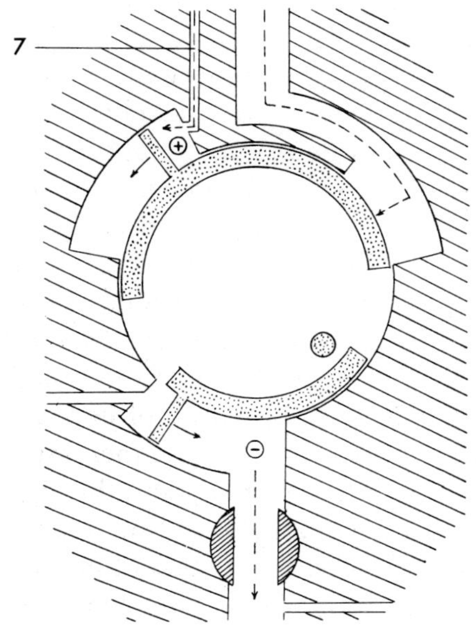

Fig. 9-18. Bennett valve just before inspiratory gas flow. See text.

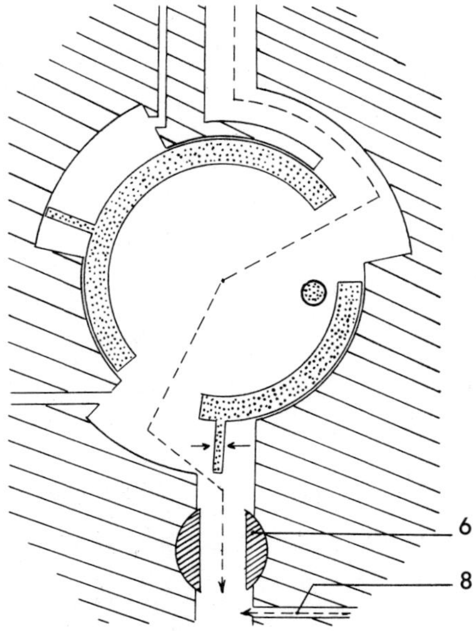

Fig. 9-19. Bennett valve in midinspiration. See text.

determined by the resistance-compliance characteristics of the airways and lungs downstream, and in our illustration ports 1 and 2 are not fully opened. The two small arrows on each side of vane 2 indicate opposing forces responsible for the delicate balance of the drum. The arrow on the right represents the back pressure of downstream resistance whereas that on the left reflects the force of the flowing gas. As resistance to flow develops, back pressure on the vane rotates the drum, reducing the flow rate through the valve to a level that still permits a flow adequate to ventilate alveoli. This mechanism prevents a rapid buildup of pressure that could otherwise cycle the ventilator into exhalation before sufficient volume reached the lung and, by slowing the flow rate, allows the maximum volume of gas to navigate restricted airways. Such a flow-sensitive response achieves automatically that which requires manual operation on flow rate–controlled ventilators. In order to compare the flow sensitivity of the PR-2 with the Mark 8, Fig. 9-20 is adapted from the same source as Figs. 9-14 and 9-15.[226] Sketch *A* shows the very clear response of flow rate to steadily rising pressure, continuously to the end of inspiration, and demonstrates the gradual closure of the vaned drum as airway resistance increases. In sketch *B*, the real virtue of flow sensitivity is evident as flow through an obstructed passage meets an increase in resistance, with an ensuing sudden rise in pressure. At this point, the Bennett valve abruptly retards flow rate to allow gas to ventilate the distal passage.

Terminal flow. Earlier we stated that in the assist mode end-inspiration is cycled by pressure; although this assertion is essentially true, it must be slightly modified. The instrument is basically a pressure-cycled machine, but the actual closure of the valve is dependent upon a *terminal flow point* of

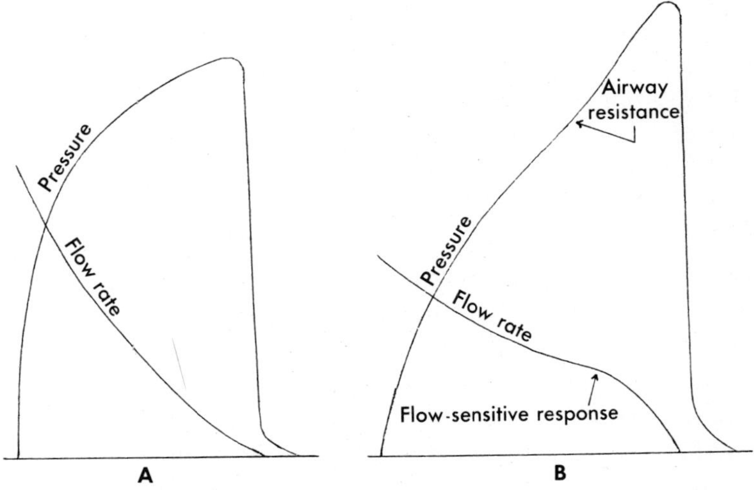

Fig. 9-20. Relationship between ventilatory flow rate and pressure in response to automatic flow-sensitivity control. See text. (Adapted from Edwards, W. L., and Sappenfield, R. S.: Pressure-cycled ventilators and flow-rate control, Anesth Analg **47**:77, 1968.)

1 liter per minute, which means that the valve will not close until the flow through it drops to 1 lpm, when with the aid of the weight of the counter-balance rod, the drum rotates fully clockwise and all flow stops. The terminal flow characteristic of the valve does not mean that it is not pressure cycled, because terminal flow, control pressure, and resistance are all related; but it does mean that the valve is so constructed and mounted that the driving pressure of gas will keep flow active until the developing back pressure has retarded the flow to 1 lpm. To put it another way, as long as gas flow is in excess of 1 lpm, inspiration will not cycle off. It is apparent that when the machine is pressure cycling the presence of a leak in the delivery system will let gas flow continuously without subsiding to the terminal flow point and inspiratory flow will not stop. Under certain circumstances, leaks are difficult to avoid, especially if the respirator is used with a face mask or an intratracheal tube; but the instrument provides a means to compensate for such a loss of gas. The terminal flow control is a manually operated adjustment that introduces a flow of source gas at source pressure into the outflow tube below the peak flow control (8), as shown in Fig. 9-19. When the control is activated, gas is introduced through the same mechanism that regulates the inspiratory nebulizer, so it flows only during inspiration. The gas added to the Bennett valve's output by the terminal flow control in a sense "feeds" the system leak and allows the flow through the valve to drop to the terminal shutoff level of 1 lpm, even though the total output of the ventilator is greater than this. The same procedure for managing a leak can also be used during controlled ventilation, although in this situation compensation for gas loss can be achieved by varying the rate to give a longer time for lung inflation; often the latter is used as a backup for the terminal control technique, as a safety measure.

Peak flow. The peak flow control (6, in Fig. 9-19) is a manually adjustable variable restriction in the gas outflow passage that merely reduces the diameter of the lumen. Its name derives from its ability to regulate the maximum flow rate that is available to the patient, reducing it from a high of 80 lpm when fully opened to approximately 10 lpm when completely turned. The restriction, when activated, creates a back pressure on the Bennett valve, preventing the drum from opening widely. It serves two purposes. First, it reduces the initial blast of air striking the patient's airways as inspiration starts, sometimes a matter of discomfort about which the therapist should always inquire of the conscious patient. Second, if there is significant downstream obstruction, it prevents the development of sudden back pressure, which will result from the force of high-velocity gas. Thus, the more restriction applied to the gas flow, the more gradual will be the rise to the peak of the control pressure. To a considerable degree, the Bennett peak flow control resembles, in its end result, the manual flow control of the Bird ventilator; but it is applied after the cycling mechanism instead of before and functions cooperatively with the flow-sensitive valve.

Negative pressure. The final sketch of the Bennett valve (Fig. 9-21) shows

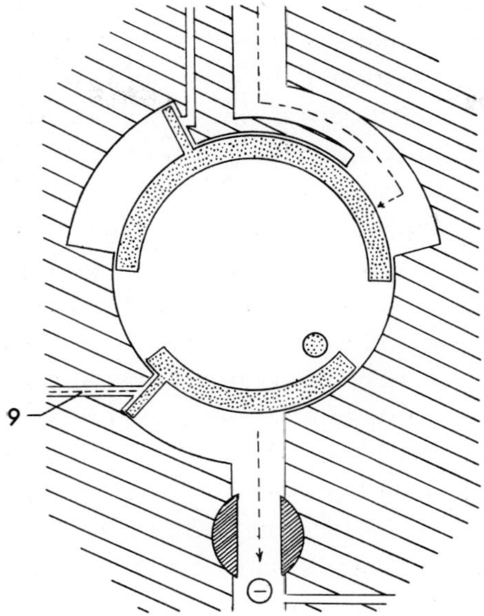

Fig. 9-21. Bennett valve during expiratory negative pressure. See text.

the valve closed during exhalation, for it has rotated back to its starting position. However, instead of this exhalation phase's being passive, it is subjected to a negative pressure for the therapeutic effects of that pressure, a function we have noted in connection with other ventilators previously. A control knob on the instrument regulates a flow of source gas at source pressure from the expiratory nebulization mechanism to a venturi located beneath the body of the machine. From the venturi two lines extend to the circuitry. One goes to a special exhalation valve manifold at the patient end of the gas flow tubing. The Bennett exhalation valve consists of a small balloon that inflates by gas flow from the cycling valve during inspiration to close an aperture to the atmosphere and collapses during exhalation to allow the escape of exhaled air. The negative-pressure venturi line enters the manifold between the balloon and the patient, and when the venturi is activated, negative pressure is generated in the entire conducting system, from the cycling valve to the patient's alveoli. Subatmospheric pressures down to -6 cm of water are available, depending upon the extent to which the control is opened; and the negative force ceases as soon as inspiration begins. In the illustration the system negative pressure is indicated by the negative sign in the outflow tract at the tip of the dashed arrow. The second line (9) from the negative-pressure venturi is connected to the blind end of port 2 (Fig. 9-21). We know that patient cycling of inhalation is achieved by creating a small negative pressure in port 2, so we can understand that an uncontrolled negative pressure of the degree generated by the venturi would rotate the drum wide open as soon as end-inspiration had been reached and the venturi set into action. To prevent this serious interference with cycling, the same amount of negative pressure applied to the exhalation manifold is applied to the upper surface of the vane in port 2. This perfect balance of forces across the vane keeps the drum closed during the negative-pressure phase, and because of this balance, the same small inspiratory negative-pressure effort will trigger inhalation and shut off the venturi.

Timing accumulators. The timing mechanism of the PR-2 is composed of three interconnected and interrelated piston-in-cylinder devices known as *timing accumulators,* plainly visible protruding from the top of the instrument, one or all three of which are in motion whenever the ventilator is operating. It would be unnecessarily time consuming and needless to diagram in its entirety the circuitry joining these units with one another and with other components of the machine. Such information is available through instructional material; yet we should not pass over these interesting and vital mechanisms without at least describing their general structure and functions.[229] The three timing accumulators are identical in design and consist of spring-loaded grooved pistons, topped by inflatable balloons, and they ride in vertical cylinders supplied with a number of gas inlets and outlets. Fig. 9-22 is a schematic representation of one of the units, not to scale and not showing the exact relative positions of the gas connections since it is a two-dimensional projection of a three-dimensional object with radially placed outlets; but it does show the functioning parts that are responsible for the smooth operation of the respirator. The upper, visible portion of the cylinder (1) is transparent, and through its wall can be seen the upper end of the piston (2) with its recoil spring (3), surmounted by a collapsed balloon that is supported by a metal disc (4). The lower part of the cylinder is narrow, pierced by six pairs of small

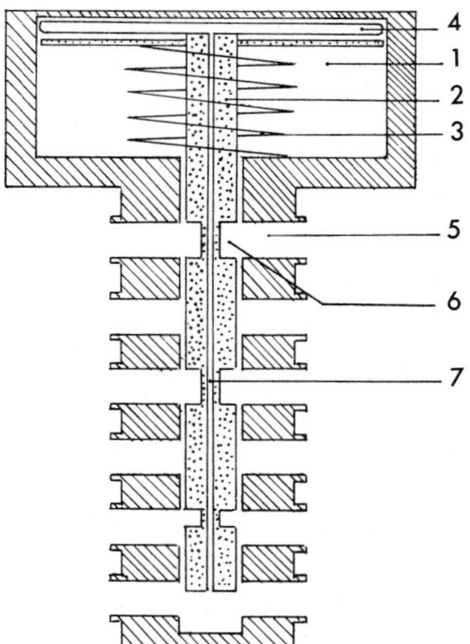

Fig. 9-22. Diagrammatic sketch of a Bennett timing accumulator. See text.

gas conduits (5), and that part of the piston in the narrowed cylinder has three circular grooves cut into it (6). Finally, a narrow channel runs the length of the piston, open at its lower end and communicating with the balloon at its upper (7). The paired openings in the cylinder are connected in an intricate fashion among the three accumulators—the sensitivity, rate, and expiratory time controls; the Bennett valve; and the gas outflow tract.

Each accumulator functions as a multiple-action valve, dispatching gas flow according to the position of its piston. When the piston grooves are aligned with gas channels in the cylinder, gas flows across the unit; and when they are misaligned, flow is blocked. The changing patterns of valvular action result from gas moving up the narrow channel at the core of the piston, inflating the balloon. As the balloon swells, the piston is forced downward, changing the lineup between its grooves and the gas passages; and it is returned to its resting position by the action of its spring when freed of the driving gas pressure.

If we orient the three accumulators from a front view of the respirator and designate them as left, middle, and right, we can briefly describe the principle role played by each. During ventilatory assistance, only the *middle timing accumulator* is operating, and it functions in this circumstance as a regulator of the inspiratory sensitivity mechanism. Opening the sensitivity control allows gas to pass from the unit regulator through an open channel across the cylinder of the middle timer to port 3 of the Bennett valve housing via gas line 7 (Fig. 9-18). Here, it helps the patient initiate inspiration, but once flow starts, a gas line from the outflow tract back to the bottom of the middle accumulator inflates the middle accumulator's balloon, depressing the piston and terminating flow to the Bennett valve. During exhalation, the accumulator's balloon deflates and the groove realignment readies flow to the drum vane for the next cycle. When the instrument is used for respiratory control, all three timing accumulators function; and although to the casual observer their action may appear to be random in nature, they are actually performing with split-second precision. The *middle timer* now acts to coordinate the action of the other two by blocking and releasing gas flow to their balloons in the proper timing sequence, correlating this with the flow rate leaving the vaned drum through its communication with the outflow tract. Thus, it senses the start and stop of airflow and prepares the circuitry of the other accumulators for suitable response. The *left timing accumulator* is activated by the rate control and starts inspiration by sending gas to the same vane on the Bennett valve as does the sensitivity control. The breathing rate is determined by the length of time devoted to exhalation, and the more gas sent to the left accumulator balloon by the rate control, the shorter will be exhalation and the faster this timer will open gas flow to the vaned drum from the unit regulator. The left accumulator acts in concert with the right timer to maintain and I/E ratio of 1:1.5 at any rate by taking proportionately more time to line up its channels than does the right. In addition, gas to the left accumulator balloon from the rate control can be retarded by the expiratory time control, prolonging the time it takes to align its flow passage and, thus, extending the expiratory time. When this occurs, the I/E ratio is reduced to 1:2, 1:3, etc. The *right accumulator* starts exhalation by terminating inhalation. During inhalation, the middle timer directs gas to the balloon of the right timer, and this opens a circuit through the right timer from the unit regulator to the balloon in the patient regulator, which inflates and shuts off inspiratory flow. The hazard of describing individually several concomitant functions is to give a picture of intermittent action. In reality, all the interrelated movements of the timing accumulators noted above are smoothly integrated into a continuously repetitive cycle but one that can be modified at will by the trained operator and that will also respond to spontaneous patient effort.

In summary, the Bennett PR-2 is a versatile instrument that can deliver either assisted or controlled mechanical ventilation, or a combination of both, to allow the patient spontaneous assisted breathing with backup control in the event of recurrent failure. It is a pressure generator since it delivers gas at a preset pressure, and its flow rate varies according to resistance in distal airways through the operation of an automatic flow-sensitive outflow valve. Because of this mechanism, manual adjustment of gas flow into the ventilator is not necessary for most circumstances; but to overcome severe obstruction, the gas leaving the valve for the outflow tract can be retarded so as to delay the point of time in inspiration that peak gas flow will be reached. In the assist mode the instrument is pressure cycled, but inspiration will not terminate until the flow rate through the valve drops below 1 lpm. When used as a controller, the PR-2 is time cycled through the action of the timing accumulators, which allows the determination of total ventilatory rate and the I/E ratio, not to exceed 1:1.5. However, should conditions permit the buildup of control pressure in the airways before the end of the preset inspiratory time interval, the machine will pressure cycle. Because of the ease with which the drum valve operates, a controlled patient can take a spontaneous breath at any time; and the accumulators immediately rephase themselves to continue control as soon as spontaneous effort ceases.

PHYSIOLOGIC EFFECT OF MECHANICAL VENTILATION

Mechanical ventilation cannot be used either safely or effectively until those responsible for it are knowledgeable in its effect upon the physiology as well as proficient in its mechanics. When artifically ventilating a patient, we deliberately attempt to change a physiologic condition, hopefully from a poor to an improved status; but we are nonetheless interfering with a level of function, even if that function is pathologic. It is vital that we know what effect our therapy is likely to have on the patient, not only in terms of the objectives we are trying to achieve but also, equally as important, in terms of the effect upon organs or systems not directly related to the primary disease and in terms of unwanted adverse sequelae. It is a safe generalization to state that a form of treatment potent enough to alter or correct the progress of a disease is most apt to have some accompanying side effects that may be undesirable. We have already noted with emphasis the caution needed in the administration of oxygen and will now consider the physiologic responses, good and bad, to mechanical ventilation. The comments that follow will apply primarily to positive-pressure breathing, except where otherwise noted, and especially, although not exclusively, to the pneumatic, pressure-cycled type. For convenience, we will discuss separately the effects on *ventilation, circulation,* and *metabolism.*

Effect on ventilation

With assisted mechanical ventilation we can generally expect an improvement in total ventilation manifested by an increased minute breathing volume, improved alveolar ventilation, a better distribution of inspired gas, a normalization of blood gases, and a reduction in the patient's work of breathing. It should be apparent to the student that these responses are interrelated and dependent upon one another but that the degree to which any given one is favorably effected will be determined by the underlying disease and the effectiveness of the ventilator. It is most usual to expect an increase in minute volume and tidal volume, which are dynamic compartments of the total lung volumes, whereas changes in static volumes, the functional residual capacity and the residual volume, are more variable, depending upon the bronchopulmonary condition.[230] Theoretically, all five of the functions noted above should be improved or stimulated by mechanical assistance; and if they are not, the cause will be one of the following: (1) The respiratory tract may present a severity of obstruction or a reduction in compliance beyond the ability of the ventilator to surmount. We have described enough of the principles and characteristics of ventilators for the student to accept the fact that such instruments are too severely limited in both scope and flexibility to compensate for all types of failure. (2) Most instances of inadequate mechanical ventilation in daily hospital practice are the result of the wrong choice of instrument for a given circumstance or improper technique in its administration. Both of these responsibilities require in-depth experience in assisted ventilation but are critical to successful therapy. It can be assumed as obvious now that the beneficial effects of mechanical ventilation can be realized only when consideration is given to the establishment of breathing rates and the use of flow rates consistent with the conducting potential of the airways, coordinated with just the proper delivery pressure. If the student looks into the growth history of positive-pressure breathing, he will encounter strong opposing views of its efficacy and safety, especially reported during its early years of use. There is little doubt, in retrospect, that many of the unfavorable opinions originated from failure to achieve satisfactory ventilation because the disease was untreatable with available equipment, the equipment was ill chosen, or especially because the equipment was not effectively used.

The relationship between the distribution of inspired gas in the lung, alveolar ventilation, and the correction of abnormal blood gases and pH is apparent; and in these areas positive-pressure breathing performs some of its most important functions. For the overall stabilization of ventilation, it is not enough merely to increase the gas flow to alveoli already ventilated if there are alveoli persistently nonventilated. A major contribution of PPB is its ability to effect a more normal and uniform distribution of inspired gas to all lung areas by opening up to gas exchange lobules and other pulmonary units that have been nonparticipating. This claim for PPB is made notwithstanding some opinions to the contrary. A study was made of voluntary hyperventilation and IPPB in normal subjects and patients with emphysema.[230] In the normals, essentially equal increases in tidal volume were recorded during both hyperventilation and PPB assist, but in the patient group the increase in tidal volume was significantly greater with mechanical aid. In all subjects experiencing an increase in tidal volume, alveolar distribution of air was improved by the nitrogen-washout test; and it is interesting to note that this distribution was improved in patients who could not hyperventilate spontaneously but needed the PPB assistance. In more precise physiologic terms, there was an implied improvement in the ventilation/perfusion ratio. On the other hand, another group of patients was reported to show increases in alveolar-arterial oxygen tension differences during positive-pressure breathing.[231] This suggested that the inspired air was not normally distributed among the alveoli in relation to the alveolar perfusion; and it was concluded that, since emphysema is characterized by an abnormal $\dot{V}/\dot{Q}$, PPB might not be expected to improve this relationship in lungs so diseased. However, in comparing divergent results, it is often difficult, if not impossible, to determine how uniform were the techniques employed; and unless comparable equipment is used and close attention given to rates, flows, and pressures, comparison is on shaky ground. Many years of clinical observation substantiate the view that an improved $\dot{V}/\dot{Q}$ ratio incident to better alveolar distribution of inspired gas is a significant result of properly applied PPB.

Thus, improvement in alveolar ventilation, the major objective of the therapy of respiratory failure, coincides with bettering the $\dot{V}/\dot{Q}$ ratio. More effective alveolar ventilation is evidenced by a decrease in arterial blood carbon dioxide tension and an elevation of arterial blood pH. It must be noted that the effect of PPB on carbon dioxide and pH, well documented and universally accepted, does not necessarily depend upon its ability to expand the general distribution of inspired gas, discussed above. Such changes may be accomplished by the hyperventilation of existing functioning alveoli, taking advantage of the easy diffusibility of carbon dioxide. However, it has been aptly demonstrated that not only does PPB decrease the carbon dioxide but it also elevates the arterial blood oxygen tension of hypoxia, even when ambient air is the source gas without added oxygen.[232,233] This was taken as evidence of an increased uniformity of alveolar ventilation and an improved $\dot{V}/\dot{Q}$ ratio.

Last, but by no means least, an important physiologic service of positive-pressure breathing is a significant reduction in the work energy expended by the patient in labored breathing. The inhalation therapist will have frequent occasion to see the gratifying physical relaxation enjoyed by a patient as a mechanical ventilator assumes a major portion of his work. This response to assisted ventilation not rarely is sought to prevent a patient, still compensating, from slipping into failure from the cumulative effect of respiratory fatigue. Again, it must be strongly emphasized that merely subjecting a patient to mechanical ventilation does not assure him relief from his struggle to breathe; for unless properly administered, ventilatory "assistance" may seriously handicap him further. Obviously, to aid the patient and lessen his work, ventilation must be adequate for his needs. Although this may appear to be so basic as to be redundant, it is an aspect that must be carefully considered to prevent the spontaneously breathing patient from "fighting" the machine. Unless the ventilator can deliver inspired air rapidly enough, the patient will work harder to augment the gas from the instrument; and if flows are too rapid or forceful, the patient may oppose the gas with expiratory efforts. It has been noted that with pressures in excess of 25 cm of water, and with unadjusted flow rates, alveolar hypoventilation may persist; and the resulting struggle of the patient to get air can increase the work of breathing 250% without benefit.[224] An excellent investigation into the work of breathing explains how effective ventilation helps the patient.[231] We will recall that carbon dioxide is metabolically produced by contraction of muscles, including the muscles of ventilation. Indeed, in severe respiratory disability the energy of all the muscles brought into use to move tidal air may account for a major portion of the carbon dioxide production as well as the oxygen utilization. In short, most of the patient's work may go into driving the machinery that supplies the body's energy fuel, leaving little for other activities. Also relevant to the discussion is the note that the more efficient is a muscle the less carbon dioxide it produces per unit of work performed as compared to a less efficient muscle.

The level of arterial carbon dioxide tension is dependent upon both the production of carbon dioxide by the body and the effectiveness of alveolar ventilation and can be expressed in the following proportionality:

$$P_{a_{CO_2}} \cong \frac{\dot{V}_{CO_2}}{\dot{V}_A}$$

Reduction in the carbon dioxide tension is thus the result of increasing the alveolar ventilation or limiting the CO_2 production. In severe airway obstructive disease voluntary hyperventilation is not apt to decrease the arterial CO_2 tension significantly because the uneven alveolar ventilation accompanying obstruction prevents the deep breathing from improving the alveolar ventilation. If, by a strenuous effort, the patient is able to effect a better alveolar ventilation, the work involved will increase the CO_2 production simultaneously to maintain the same general proportion in the above equation. It has been determined that the muscles of respiration use one third less oxygen when passively moved; and thus, positive-pressure ventilation increases the alveolar gas exhange, with less patient work, and without raising the CO_2 production.

Effect on circulation

With the close functional and anatomic relationship between the respiratory and circulatory systems, it is not surprising that interference with the performance of one of them will affect the other. The great potential hazard of circulatory response to mechanical ventilation makes it mandatory for the therapist to understand fully what does and can happen to cardiovascular function when a patient is artificially ventilated.

In our study of the physiology of ventilation we learned that ventilatory muscle contraction expands the diameters of the thorax, lowering the intrathoracic pressure so that ambient air flows into the lung. The pressure within the thoracic cavity is never above atmospheric with quiet breathing but rather is slightly below even at the resting level, and it exceeds atmospheric only during forced exhalation as the expiratory reserve volume is moved. This is illustrated in the balloon-in-box sketches of Fig. 3-5, which depict the fluctuations of intrathoracic pressure from its average resting value of about −5 cm of water, with ventilatory excursions. The cardiovascular system is designed to function with its central power source, the heart, in a subatmospheric pressure; and, as noted in Chapter 5, the "thoracic pump" is necessary for venous return to the heart and for an adequate cardiac output. Thus, airflow into and out of the lungs and the circulation of blood to and from the heart are both accomplished most efficiently when the ventilatory cycle starts with a subatmospheric pressure that increases in negativity during inhalation and decreases during exhalation but never exceeds atmospheric except under conditions of stress. Obviously, this normal intrathoracic pressure environment is reversed when positive-pressure ventilation is employed, as inspiratory gas under pressure inflates the lung, raising the intrapulmonary pressure, and is then transmitted through the lung into the pleural "space" to elevate the intrathoracic pressure during inhalation. Passive exhalation returns the pressure only to atmospheric so that, in contrast to natural breathing, the pressure in the chest is never subatmospheric. Fig. 9-23 is a schematic example of two tidal volume curves, comparing the pressure relationships between normal spontaneous breathing and pressure ventilation. Here, the resting level of voluntary ventilation is shown as −2 cm of water, and as air enters the lung, the pressure drops to −7 cm of water, a net pressure change of 5 cm of water; but the pressure at all points is below atmospheric. In contrast, the ventilated lung starts its cycle from a resting level of atmospheric pressure because the subject's airways are a closed system with the instrument, and the instrument

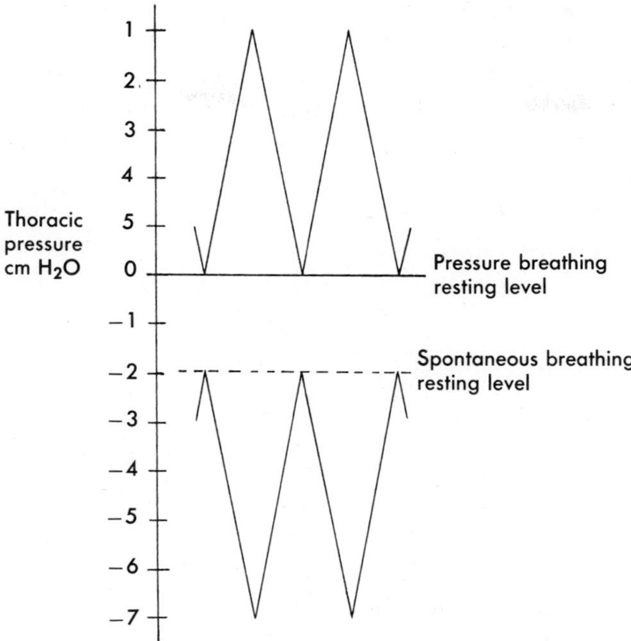

Fig. 9-23. Comparison of the pressure relationships between positive-pressure and spontaneous tidal ventilation.

returns to atmospheric pressure at the end of each cycle. The same driving pressure of 5 cm of water causes the intrathoracic pressure to fluctuate between atmospheric and atmospheric plus 5 cm of water, and at no point is the pressure subatmospheric.

The significance of intrathoracic pressure deviations in their effect on cardiovascular function is one of the most important clinical aspects of mechanical ventilation. During all phases of normal or abnormal pulmonary airflow, those elements of the circulatory system that are located in the thorax, especially the heart and large veins, are subjected to the ambient pressure generated in the thorax; so let us describe details of the circulatory response to both normal and pressure ventilation. The fall in intrathoracic pressure that accompanies a normal spontaneous inspiration enhances the flow of venous blood to the thoracic vessels and hence into the right atrium, increasing the right ventricular output and flow to the lungs. Temporarily, less blood moves from the lungs to the left atrium as the intrathoracic negative pressure fills up the pulmonary vessels, and left ventricular output falls. During passive exhalation, the events are reversed as the increasing (although still subatmospheric) intrathoracic pressure dampens venous return and right atrial filling and output but, at the same time, in a sense, squeezing blood from the pulmonary vessels to increase left atrial filling and left ventricular output. When the lung is ventilated under positive pressure, venous return, right atrial filling, and pulmonary blood flow are impaired; but the pressure squeezing the lung, now during inspiration, increases left heart filling and output. However, this lasts for but a few heart strokes, and if the pressure is continued, flow to and from the left heart falls. Exhalation lets the intrathoracic pressure return to atmospheric, encouraging venous return and an increase in pulmonary flow but retarding left ventricular output. Let us compare these sequences in natural and pressure breathing. During normal spontaneous ventilation, the fluctuations in intrathoracic blood flow are rhythmically synchronized with the breathing pattern, a decrease in one component during inhalation increasing during exhalation, and so on. Thus, whereas venous return accelerates in inhalation and left ventricular output falls, both are reversed in exhalation; and the net result, cycle after cycle, is a smooth-flowing circulation. The same description can be given of pressure breathing, with the time sequences of the kinetics turned about; but the efficiency of the net result is markedly modified by one significant factor—a steady atmospheric or supra-atmospheric pressure. Several excellent studies have clarified the effect of positive pressure on circulation to explain why such pressure interferes with cardiac function, and we will consider the relevant data.[234-239]

It is necessary to understand the concepts of *mean pressure* and the *pressure-time relationship*, for they are the keys to the problem. Fig. 9-24, *A*, is a biphasic sine-like curve, plotting positive and negative pressures against arbitrary units of time, first traveling from its starting point to a peak pressure of 20 and back to zero pressure in 5 time units, then dropping to −20 units of pressure and back in another 5 time units. For the first 5 time units, positive pressure is being exerted; and for the last 5, negative pressure of the same magnitude. As we look at the curve, our common sense tells us that the net or final result of these two opposing pressures will be to negate one another since they will average out to zero. The *mean* pressure of the entire cycle then will be zero, for mean is an arithmetical average. Each half of the curve has its own mean pressure, which is easy to visualize because of the regularity of the curve, but this is not so in curves with changing contours. The mean value of any curve is the average of an infinite number of points along the curve (a, b, c, d, etc., in Fig. 9-24, *A*), and although we cannot measure an infinite number of values, the more that are measured, the more accurate will be the calculation. In practice, the calculation of the mean of an irregular curve is done by methods of mathematical calculus or with accurate and rapid electronic calculators, necessary instruments in the modern laboratory. It is obvious in our illustration that the mean pressure of the terminal half of the curve is the same as that of the first but with the opposite sign. If we refer back to Fig. 9-23, we can see that the mean pressure of the upper, positive ventilatory pattern is 2.5 cm of water whereas that of natural breathing is −4.5 cm of water (the resting level is already at −2 cm H_2O). The *pressure-time relationship* is the length of time that a pressure is active and refers to the duration of a mean pressure. For example, in the first half of Fig. 9-24, *A*, the pressure continuously changes from time 0 to time 5, but its represents a mean

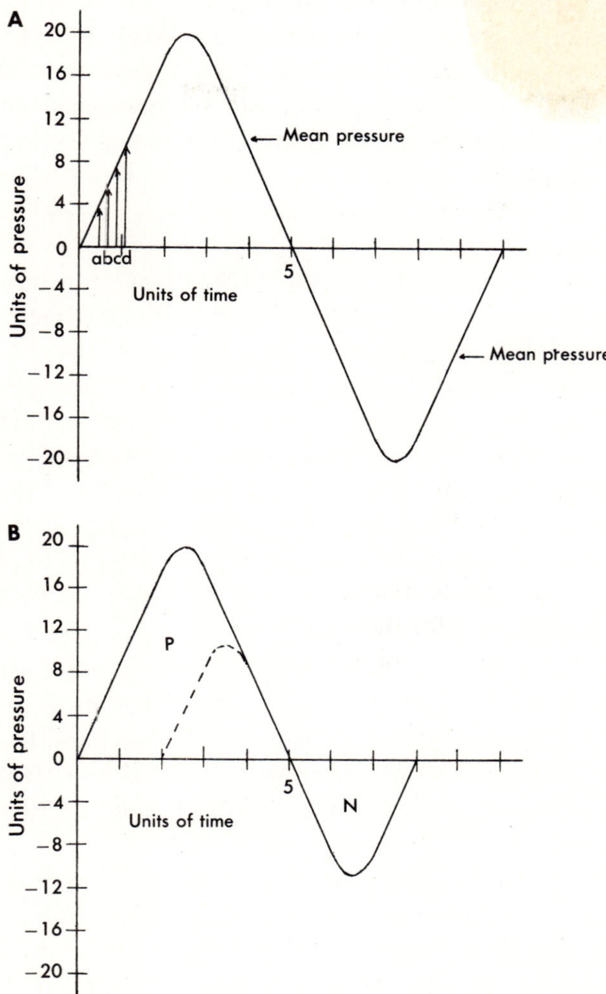

Fig. 9-24. Illustrations of the concept of mean pressure and the relationship between pressure and time. Sketch **A** is a sine curve, and **B** an asymmetrical biphasic curve. See text for detailed description.

pressure of 10, for 5 time units; and the second half of the curve represents a mean of −10 units of pressure for another 5 units of time. The same interpretations can be derived for the tidal excursions of Fig. 9-23.

It may be evident at this stage that whatever effect pressure will have on circulation will be directly related to the mean pressure to which the circulation is exposed and to the time of this exposure, or in other words, the pressure-time effect. In ventilation the time interval is the duration of the respiratory cycle, or its components; and the pressure is the intrathoracic, which, in clinical practice, must be measured indirectly. It was noted in the earlier discussion of the lung-thorax relation and compliance that to avoid the risks of a direct measurement of intrathoracic pressure, esophageal pressure is often used since it reflects changes within the chest; but the student will frequently see reference to *mask pressure* and *mouth pressure* in relation to the kinetics of mechanical ventilation. They refer to the pressure of the ventilating gas as measured at the subject's mouth or administering appliance or the pressure in the trachea of patients who have been intubated. Although the mask pressure is not quantitatively the same as the intrathoracic pressure, the mean values of both are linearly related and thus can be used interchangeably to monitor qualitative changes.

Let us direct our attention to Fig. 9-24, *B*, and consider the positive segment to represent the pressure-time curve of a positive-pressure ventilator generating an arbitrary maximum mask pressure over a 5-unit time period. Regardless of what the mean pressure might be, in a general way the area under the curve (P) can be thought of as proportional to the pressure-time effect of the ventilatory pattern, for it represents the total pressure for the total time. The larger the area under a given pressure curve, the greater potential effect it will have on circulation. Let us now imagine a subatmospheric pressure applied to the subject's airway during exhalation that lowers the mask pressure as indicated by the last part of the curve, enclosing pressure-time area (N). The net circulatory effect of the pressure over the entire cycle will be proportional to the difference between the areas P and N, graphically depicted by superimposing N on P, with the dotted outline. The mean mask pressure for the whole ventilatory cycle has been lowered from that of the inspiratory phase by the addition of terminal negative pressure, proportionately reducing the effect on circulation that would be expected from the original pressure.

At this point we might pause and summarize our information on the circulatory response to positive intrathoracic pressure. We can say that the determining factor is the relation between the height of the mean intrathoracic (or mask) pressure and the duration of pressure; and we know that the total mean cycle pressure can be kept low by the addition of negative mask pressure during exhalation. In our above description of the circulatory sequences through the natural or pressure-generated ventilatory cycle, we noted the different effects on right and left hearts, depending upon the respiratory phase. However, the picture can be simplified and the "meat" of the matter illustrated in its crudest form as shown in Fig. 9-25, where the sketches demonstrate the basic relationship between intrathoracic pressure and the circulation. The thorax is represented by a box with a gas inlet, containing the heart and major vessels. To avoid clutter in the illustration, the lungs are not included although this does not imply that they play no role. It is assumed, however, that whatever pressure is delivered to the lungs is readily and fully transmitted to the thoracic cavity. Both diagrams depict inhalation (A) during natural spontaneous breathing and (B) during positive-pressure ventilation. Despite the circulatory fluctuations during each ventilatory cycle, the mean intrathoracic pressure of natural breathing is subatmospheric; and thus the

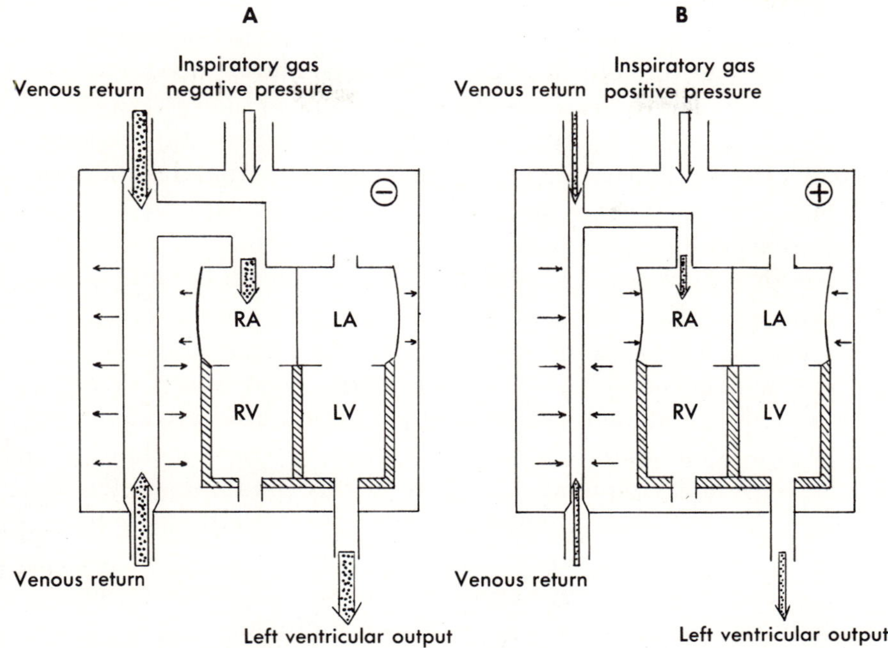

Fig. 9-25. Relationship between intrathoracic pressure and cardiac output in, **A**, negative-pressure and, **B**, positive-pressure breathing. Details are explained in the text.

net pressure effect on blood flow is that of low pressure. This is indicated by the negative sign within the chest cavity and the effect of this *mean negativity* on circulation. Venous return is enhanced, and the negative pressure is shown as dilating the intrathoracic veins and encouraging filling of the atria. In contrast, positive-pressure inhalation produces an overall positive mean intrathoracic pressure, the net circulatory effect of which is just the opposite of natural breathing. The continuous *mean positivity* in the chest depresses venous return by blocking its flow into the thoracic veins. The student is encouraged to consider the conditions demonstrated in sketch *A* as the normal status, the natural environment in which the heart and supporting vessels developed and grew. In this environment the circulatory dynamics of both inspiration and expiration are such that the body's needs are most efficiently met. It is not so much that the mean negative pressure of spontaneous breathing excessively encourages venous return and a subsequent increase above normal of left ventricular output as it is that *deviations* from the normal mean intrathoracic pressure adversely affect the circulatory efficiency. Therefore, in the positive-pressure breathing of sketch *B*, regardless of whether the left heart filling and output may be temporarily increased by the rising pressure in the thorax, the net effect of subjecting the heart and its tributary veins to an abnormally high mean pressure is to impede venous return and to reduce the arterial blood supplied to the systemic circulation.

When venous blood flows toward the heart from the peripheral areas of the body and encounters an abnormally high pressure as it attempts to enter the thoracic vessels, portions of it will pool in vascular reservoirs, mostly in the huge network of veins and capillaries of the abdominal organs.[240] This can effectively remove from circulation a volume of blood large enough to reduce the left ventricular output, as noted above, and constitute a serious potential danger to the hypoxic patient by reducing his cerebral blood flow and further compromising the oxygen supply to his brain. Lesser degrees of the effect of excessively high intrathoracic pressure on cerebral blood flow can be demonstrated in the normal subject by voluntary breath holding at end-inspiration while exerting a strong expiratory effort against the closed glottis. Impaired venous return is manifested by distended neck veins, suffusion of the facial skin, and eventual loss of consciousness or at least faintness. In the mechanically ventilated patient, continued interference with venous return and left ventricular output can lead to a full-blown state of clinical shock, with all the signs and symptoms described for this condition earlier. When precipitated by mechanical ventilation, such vascular collapse is termed *respirator shock.*

So far we have been concerned only with the mechanisms responsible for the physiologic influence of intrathoracic pressure on the circulation, but let us now see how important all of this is in clinical medicine to which the inhalation therapist is exposed. Data from the references cited at the beginning of this discussion, as well as from the observations of those who have managed patients under mechanical ventilation, attest to the reality of this phenomenon. When the mean mask delivery pressure exceeds 7 cm of water, there is a measurable decrease in the left ventricular output, although it need not be clinically evident.[234] In relaxed patients without specific bronchopulmonary disease who were ventilated at a fixed tidal volume and rate, measurement of the mean intrathoracic pressure showed an elevation above normal, ranging from 3.5 to 6 cm of water.[235] The degree to which circulation is impaired and the risk there is in store for the patient are dependent upon three modifying factors in addition to the mere level of pressure.

Cardiac status. The integrity of the heart and circulatory system is an important influence on the effect of an increased intrathoracic pressure. As noted above, even small pressures interfere with cardiac output; and it can be anticipated that anyone subjected to pressure will be so affected. However, the normal healthy heart has a great functional reserve and can tolerate considerable resistance to its action. There is no rule to follow to estimate the risk of circulatory depression from pressure breathing, and the large majority of patients so treated suffer no apparent ill effects. Some have been supported on positive-pressure ventilation for several consecutive weeks without evidence of a compromised circulation. There is no doubt that the patient with overt or potential cardiac disease is a high-risk candidate for trouble. Part of the management of the ventilated patient is a close surveillance of his cardiac condition, with appropriate measures taken to support a failing heart so that the needed ventilation can be carried out. Certainly, a circulatory complication might be considered a more likely possibility in an elderly patient than in a young one or in a patient with long-standing pulmonary disease than in one with a new, acute disease. It is this varying response of each individual and the uncertainty of his reaction to the pressure of mechanical ventilation that make skillful and intelligent management the keys to successful therapy.

Pulmonary status. Positive pressure generated in a ventilator flows into the alveoli and from there is transmitted across alveolar walls to the thoracic cavity. The ease and the degree to which such transpulmonary transmission of pressure occurs are a function of the physical state of the lung. The more compliant the lung, the more readily will intrapulmonary pressure carry into the thorax since the flexible lung easily responds to pressure applied to it. The patient with normal bronchi and lungs who needs mechanical ventilation for nonpulmonary hypoventilation is the most apt to demonstrate circulatory interference, a risk greatly enhanced, of course, by concomitant heart disease. In contrast, the patient whose disease has left his lung relatively stiff, with marked loss of compliance, is least apt to transmit intrapulmonary pressure to the thoracic cavity. His lungs can tolerate high positive pressures and need such force to move an adequate tidal volume of air. On the other hand, should the compliance of the chest wall, rather than the lung, be reduced, there will be a rapid transmission of pressure to the thorax as expansion of the latter is limited. Perhaps the therapist can visualize the difficulty in ventilating a patient with basically normal lungs but whose chest wall is partially immobilized by pain or injury or even extensive postoperative dressings. The compliant lungs and noncompliant rib cage will combine to generate the maximum intrathoracic pressure for any given mask pressure. Finally, allied to the reduced chest wall compliance just described is the resistance to ventilation of the agitated or unrelaxed patient who may have no intrinsic thoracic disability. The patient who "fights" the instrument because poor technique denies him an adequate flow or who is wittingly or otherwise uncooperative will have increased transmission of intrapulmonary pressure. His muscular activity prevents the necessary chest wall (and diaphragmatic) flexibility for compliant submission to a developing intrathoracic pressure.

Ventilatory pattern. The pattern by which positive-pressured air is delivered to a patient incorporates the concept of the pressure-time effect, recently discussed, but applies it to the practical use of mechanical ventilation. Attention was drawn to the importance of pattern when it was observed that a rise in intrathoracic pressure during positive-pressure breathing could be kept minimal if the inspiratory phase was limited to no more than one third the total cycle time. When we now relate pressure and time to the physiologic process of ventilation, the matter is not as simple as our definition and graphic representation of peak and mean pressures, and it becomes evident that an effective ventilatory pressure-time pattern must be more complex than those used in Fig. 9-24.

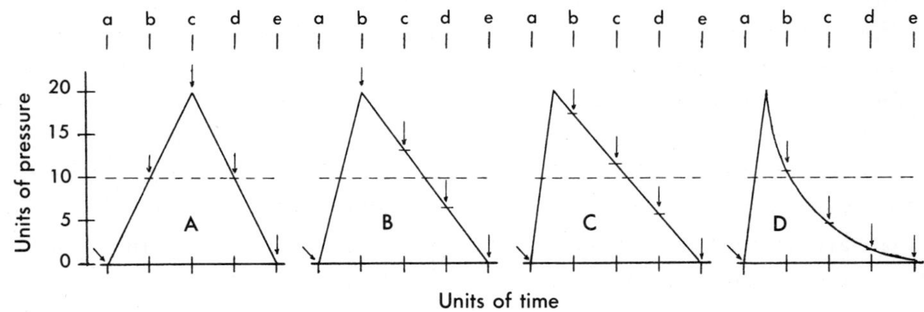

Fig. 9-26. Diagrams illustrating the effect of the relationship between cardiac diastoles and the intrathoracic pressure curve of positive-pressure breathing upon the resulting mean pressures affecting cardiac output. See text for details.

The immediate effect of elevated intrathoracic pressure is to interfere with right atrial filling and subsequently to reduce left ventricular output. Thus, each atrial diastole is a point of time during which pressure may exert its influence on venous return, and we have another important relationship to consider, that between cardiac rate and the pressure-time curve. Fig. 9-26 is designed to demonstrate the potential differences in cardiac response to various combinations of the cardiac rhythm and pressure. The vertical bars at the top of the sketches indicate the times of atrial diastole in a heart with a rate of 60 per minute, the small arrows showing where each atrial diastole falls in the ventilatory cycle. For the sake of comparative uniformity, the oblique first arrow represents the last atrial diastole of the previous ventilatory cycle; thus each cycle is correlated with four diastoles. Generation and degeneration of pressure follow linear paths in the three triangular ventilatory patterns of *A*, *B*, and *C*, and the mean pressure of each is necessarily 10 units, since the range is from 0 to 20 units. In curve *A*, the final mean pressure effecting the four diastoles is the same as that of the total cycle—10 units—and even though inspiratory time is reduced in *B*, the pressure mean of the points of diastole is unchanged. Because of the relationship between the heart rhythm and ventilatory time intervals, the student who remembers his geometry can see that the diastolic pressure means in both these sketches must be identical. A further, sharp reduction in the inspiratory time of *C*, however, changes the diastole-pressure relation; and the mean of the pressures coinciding with the diastoles has here dropped to 8 units. Careful examination of these illustrations should make it apparent that when diastole occurs with the peak pressure the mean will be the same as the mean of the cycle. This clear-cut relationship is easy to see in the examples used, the data for which were chosen for simplicity; but with any combination of cardiac rate and ventilatory cycle, it can be demonstrated that the average of diastole-associated pressures will be lower if a diastole does not coincide with peak pressure and if a maximum number of diastoles fall in low-pressure areas of the cycle. This view of the relation of positive intrathoracic pressure and heart action is more of academic interest than anything else, for it is not practical to attempt to correlate the two clinically; but it does give emphasis to the fact that mechanical ventilation has a significant effect on circulation.

The next step in our discussion is of great clinical importance, however. Fortunately, passive exhalation does not follow the simple linear deceleration of the sketches used so far but has a configuration more like that of Fig. 9-26, *D*, somewhat exaggerated.[18] The curved contour of exhalation makes for an early drop in pressure and a reduction of mean pressure during exhalation. Although the mean *inspiratory* pressure of *D* is 10 units, as in the other patterns, more of the *exhalation* curve lies below the 10 units pressure line, showing that mean exhalation pressure is something less than 10. It is not necessary mathematically to try to calculate the mean of the curved pressure-drop line, as long as the ventilatory and circulatory advantages of this configuration are appreciated by the student. The projections of diastoles c and d fall well below the 10 units pressure level, so that mean intrathoracic pressure effecting atrial diastolic filling is the least in *D* of the four patterns illustrated. The student should note that the time relationships of *C* and *D* are the same and that the projections of the atrial diastoles of *D* onto the lower pressure levels are due entirely to the curved shape of the exhalation line. Apart from changing the diastole-pressure relation, the transformation from a straight to curved exhalation line decreases the important pressure-time relation, since the area under sketch *D* is less than the area of the others; and for all practical purposes, this is the major contribution of such a ventilation pattern. Modern mechanical ventilators allow the operator great flexibility in determining the most advantageous pressure-time curves for each patient's ventilatory and cardiac status, which is a critical consideration in managing the patient in failure. The curves in Fig. 9-27 illustrate three clinical points. The patient ventilated by curve a experiences a rapid buildup in his intrathoracic pressure, which is held as a plateau for a major portion of his cycle before falling precipitously to atmospheric. The area under this curve is extensive, implying the prolonged exposure of the intrathoracic circulatory system to the steady effects of a high mean pressure. Maximum interference with venous return and consequent left ventricular output can be anticipated from such a pattern. Later we will describe a clinical condition for which such a pressure-time curve is highly therapeutic, but for our present purposes we can consider it a serious hazard. Pattern b demonstrates a marked modification of pattern a. The inspiratory time is slightly prolonged but is still less than one third the cycle, and it delays somewhat the initial exposure of the circulation to high pressure. The key difference in these two patterns is the immediate drop in pressure as soon as peak has been reached and the rapid falloff to the end of exhalation. The effect upon the circulation of curve b would be less than that of curve a to the same degree that the area under b is smaller than the area under a.

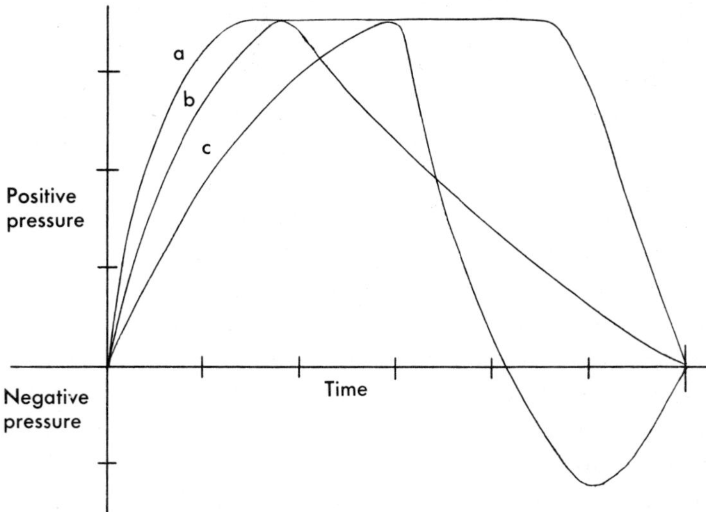

Fig. 9-27. Three pressure-time ventilatory patterns with the same range of positive pressure. Curve *a*, with its sustained peak pressure, has the greatest total pressure effect on circulation. Curve *b* reduces pressure-time by a slower rise and immediate descent. Curve *c* uses terminal negative pressure to offset some of the positive-pressure effect.

There are occasions when inspiratory needs cannot be fulfilled in the early third of the cycle because factors of obstruction and low compliance necessitate longer inflationary periods. If possible, duration of exhalation is increased accordingly to maintain a favorable I/E ratio of 1:1.5 or 1:2 to keep the mean pressure down, but sometimes in assisted ventilation the patient will not tolerate the resulting reduction in ventilatory rate. In such a case, should the prolonged inspiration pose a threat of reduced cardiac output, terminal expiratory negative pressure can be introduced into the system, as in curve c. Such a precaution is also applicable to any situation in which, even with a well-balanced ventilatory ratio, cardiac action is embarrassed from other causes. The rapid drop in pressure to below atmospheric increases the venous return during exhalation to make up for a deficit incurred during inspiration. Employing the concept of net pressure referred to earlier, we see that the final effective mean intrathoracic pressure of this type of curve is proportional to the difference between the areas under the curve, above and below the atmospheric zero line.

Let us summarize the physiologic effect of positive-pressure ventilation on the circulatory system from a clinical viewpoint. Although the primary objective of mechanical ventilation is to ensure an adequate tidal alveolar air exchange, the therapist must always be aware of the side effects of such treatment, especially on cardiac function. When considered over cycle after cycle, the continuous supra-atmospheric pressure generated in the patient's chest retards the return of venous blood to the right atrium. The important consequence of this is a drop in the cardiac output, with eventual reduced circulating systemic flow that may develop into a full-blown circulatory collapse or shock. The normal heart can tolerate the restrictive action of high mean intrathoracic pressure for prolonged periods of time, but a heart actually or potentially weakened from disease or one subjected to excessively high pressure may be seriously affected. The degree to which venous return is impeded is proportional to the height of the mean pressure developed in the thorax and the length of time such pressure continues. This gives rise to the concept of the pressure-time relationship, which, in a given circumstance with available data on instant-to-instant pressure and time, can be graphically expressed as a curve by plotting pressure against ventilatory cycle time.

The inspiratory-to-expiratory time ratio is an important factor in assuring adequate ventilation while minimizing the adverse circulatory effects of positive pressure. In general, if an I/E ratio is established so that expiration is longer than inspiration, the mean intrathoracic pressure will be lowered to a level of relative safety. The setting of an I/E ratio requires skill, understanding, and patience of the operator, for the final ventilatory pattern must be able to satisfy inspiratory needs while keeping inspiratory pressure time to a minimum. In our discussion of ventilators, we described the mechanisms for adjusting inspiratory and expiratory times in some of them and found that others had fixed I/E ratios.

Negative pressure during exhalation is available to produce the maximum reduction of mean intrathoracic pressure. Generated by a venturi, 3 to 5 cm of water subatmospheric pressure applied to the airways, when used with a favorable I/E ratio, can reduce the mean pressure in the chest almost to atmospheric. For reasons to be noted below, negative pressure in exhalation should not be used on a routine basis but reserved for those patients in whom peripheral cardiovascular collapse is an immediate or actual threat. Its use is monitored by close observation of heart rate and blood pressure, and elevation of the first with depression of the second in a patient maintained on positive-pressure ventilation is a most probable indication for instituting negative pressure, regardless of the cause of cardiac dysfunction. Although all other appropriate measures to combat shock are also used, it is not uncommon to observe how easily the stability of the blood pressure can be manipulated by varying the combination of positive and negative pressures.

Artificially induced subatmospheric airway pressure is not without its own inherent hazards, and because it entails a calculated risk its use is restricted to the support of failing circulation only. The two potential dangers of negative expiratory pressure are *air trapping* and *pulmonary edema.* Fig. 6-2 can be used to illustrate the risk of air trapping if we visualize the ventilatory pressures as intralumenal, with positive pressure inflating the alveolus and negative pressure deflating it. The illustrated bronchiolar collapse due to extralumenal positive pressure would then be caused by intralumenal negative pressure. This hazard is especially great in patients with chronic bronchopulmonary disease, in whom diseased airways are a major characteristic and many of the smaller passages lack enough connective tissue support to maintain their integrity in the face of subatmospheric pressure. The therapist can understand the seriousness of further restricting the alveolar gas exchange in a patient already in ventilatory failure by cutting short his exhalation with airway collapse, retaining air in his lungs and significantly elevating his functional residual capacity. This is why it is necessary to reject the temptation to use negative pressure as a means of aspirating secretions or overcoming airway obstruction, for the suction needed to accomplish these objectives is just as apt to have the opposite effect. The risk of air trapping can be minimized by introducing subatmospheric pressure gradually and limiting it to the least that will achieve the desired purpose.

Negative intrapulmonary pressure also subjects the patient to the danger of pulmonary edema. Like the effect of positive pressure on venous return, the probability of circulatory harm from negative pressure is dependent upon the general health and stability of the pulmonary circulation. Venous return is greatly enhanced during the negative-pressure phase of exhalation as the mean intrathoracic pressure precipitously drops and the pulmonary vasculature fills with blood, creating at least a temporary state of pulmonary congestion. Should some defective function of the left heart make it slow to accept the pulmonary venous outflow, pulmonary vascular hydrostatic pressure will rise and the gradient between the high intravascular pressure and the subatmospheric intra-alveolar pressure will force blood water into the alveoli. The same condition can prevail without an undue rise in hydrostatic pressure if there is an abnormal increase in the permeability of the pulmonary capillaries so that the usually well-tolerated capillary to alveolar–pressure gradient is enough to move fluid from circulation to alveoli. The therapist working in a hospital with a busy pulmonary service will occasionally encounter one of the most difficult patients to ventilate because of a serious physiologic paradox. This is the patient with severe obstruction or impaired compliance who needs relatively high pressure for alveolar ventilation but who has concurrent heart disease, often with myocardial damage from an inadequate coronary artery circulation. Because of the unstable cardiovascular system, not only do high ventilatory pressures easily embarass venous return and precipitate respirator shock, but the corrective measure of expiratory negative pressure induces pulmonary edema. In an extreme example of such a patient, the adjustment of the negative pressure within the range of but a few centimeters of water may find a dropping blood pressure and dry lungs replaced by a rising pressure but accompanied by the wet lungs of edema. The careful and delicate titration of positive and negative pressures against alveolar ventilation and circulatory stability requires the ultimate in physiologic understanding and technical proficiency.

Our discussion of the effect of mechanical ventilation on circulation would not be complete unless we commented on this relationship in *negative-pressure* breathing, for comparison. After the above discussion of the action of positive-pressure ventilation, the student may be surprised to be told that the same deleterious effect can be found in the patient treated by a tank respirator. In our description of this instrument, we noted that chest expansion and subsequent pulmonary inflation result from the action of subatmospheric pressure upon the external surface of the thorax; and the comment was made that this principle is more nearly like that of natural breathing than is positive-pressure breathing. This was a valid observation since, with this technique, intrathoracic pressure never exceeds atmospheric; but there is another factor. If we refer to Fig. 3-14, we will see that in the body respirator negative pressure is applied not only to the thorax but to the rest of the body as well, with the exception of the head and neck. However, because of the relative flexibility of the abdomen as compared to the chest, the pressure is readily transmitted into the former; and this is not physiologically similar to natural breathing when inspiration generates positive intra-abdominal pressure. The drop in abdominal pressure destroys the normal gradient from abdomen to thorax that aids the return of venous blood to the heart. In consequence, there is a dilatation of the vast network of abdominal capillaries, as described above in reference to positive-pressure breathing, and pooling of venous blood. Just as with positive-pressure ventilation, the pooled blood is effectively removed from circulation, reducing right atrial filling and ventricular output. Thus, the same hazard of circulatory failure is encountered in both types of ventilation. During the years of the poliomyelitis epidemics, when body respirators were extensively used, the circulatory depression caused by distal venous pooling was called "tank shock." With the large number of patients so treated, this complication would undoubtedly have been more prevalent than it was except that most of the patients were young, with good cardiovascular function. The student can now see an advantage of the chest cuirass other than convenience, for with subatmospheric pressure applied only to the thorax, the circulatory insufficiency produced by both intrapulmonary positive and body surface negative pressures is circumvented.

Effect on metabolism

In this context, *metabolism* is used to include the function of systems other than the cardiorespiratory system and responses of that system other than those included in the above discussion. An acute and progressively deteriorating state similar to the respiratory distress syndrome in infants has been described in some patients supported by continuous positive-pressure ventilation.[241] Affected patients demonstrate severe dyspnea, tachypnea, cyanosis refractory to oxygen administration, a large alveolar-arterial oxygen tension gradient, a loss of pulmonary compliance, and a chest x-ray picture identical to that seen in acute pulmonary edema. We have considered the damage sustained by the lung after exposure to high oxygen tensions, but in the patients under discussion, unusually high concentrations of oxygen were not used and oxygen toxicity was not considered the cause. With a variety of underlying diseases necessitating mechanical ventilation, it was postulated that damage to pulmonary surface-active material might be responsible for the precipitous loss of lung function. A comprehensive study was made of this condition, reviewing the pulmonary and metabolic status of 100 patients undergoing prolonged mechanical ventilation.[242] In addition to the signs and symptoms noted above, 19 of these patients exhibited a significant retention of body water and either a weight gain or failure to lose weight as anticipated. Also, they showed a drop in concentration of serum sodium (hyponatremia) and a reduction in hematocrit, both consistent with an increase in blood volume (hypervolemia) due to retained water (hydremia).

An association between pressure breathing, both positive and negative, and kidney function has long been recognized. A normal subject under continuous positive-pressure breathing may experience a reduction in urinary flow as much as 50%, attributed to a reduced renal blood flow, whereas negative-pressure breathing induces an increase in these functions.[243,244] It was suggested that renal circulation is at least temporarily compromised to compensate for circulatory deficiencies during the stress of positive-pressure ventilation and that one of the mechanisms involved may be an alteration in the so-called *antidiuretic hormone* (ADH). This is a substance secreted by the pituitary gland that is instrumental in regulating body fluid content and concentration by appropriate adjustment of urinary output. By virtue of its name, one can see that the more hormone present the less excretion of urine there will be and the greater retention of water. The relation of the action of ADH to the patient undergoing mechanical ventilation may lie in the experimental observation that vagal reflexes from the cardiac atria seem to influence ADH activity in response to pressure changes in the atria; and we now know that positive-pressure ventilation markedly alters right heart blood flow and pressure.[245]

Thus, as pointed out in the study noted above,[242] a potentially serious physiologic effect of mechanical ventilation may be the disturbance of the usual body fluid–ADH balance and the selective accumulation of abnormal amounts of water in the lungs, since peripheral edema is not noticeable in the absence of frank cardiac failure. The latter cannot always be ruled out, but the degree of pulmonary fluid appears out of proportion to the sparse indications for heart failure. Certainly, the interference with pulmonary function in these patients can reasonably be attributed to pulmonary congestion and edema, an interpretation confirmed by the often rapid and dramatic improvement in the clinical condition and the x-ray picture of the lungs following the administration of a diuretic. It is obvious that management of the ventilated patient must include close attention to maintaining a safe balance between fluid intake and output; for although dehydration must be avoided, so must the risk of overhydration in the event of an increase in ADH activity. The therapist may feel confused by the apparent paradox of positive-pressure breathing acting to limit the blood volume of the lung as described under its circulatory effects and also precipitating pulmonary edema as just noted. In our first consideration of the physiologic action of positive-pressure breathing, we described the usual, or expected, effect of pressure, whereas the hazardous metabolic disturbances accompany long-term ventilation, during which many of the body's reserve functions and compensations become depleted. This underscores the lability of physiologic response, especially under the stress of severe disease, and emphasizes the need for intelligent observation of the patient, with an awareness of the possible complications that may develop.

Chapter 10

Inhalation therapy management of ventilatory failure

Ventilatory failure is a multisystem derangement even though it focuses so dramatically on the function of the lung, and its successful management involves several facets of therapy. In patients with inadequate ventilation, good nursing is a critical factor, nutrition and fluid needs must be met, the control of infection may determine the eventual prognosis, and special care must often be given to cardiac function. Our interest is limited to those aspects of treatment that directly relate to the responsibility of the inhalation therapist. However, he must be aware of and understand the purpose of the efforts and the concern of other medical disciplines involved. Cooperation among members of the medical team is essential, and the rapport among themselves is as important as that between them and the patient. We will discuss such aspects of the management of failure as *airway patency, selection of ventilators, ventilatory patterns, monitoring ventilation,* and *positive-pressure breathing.* Unavoidably, there will be repetition and many references to material previously discussed in other chapters as well as cross-references among the subtopics themselves. However, we will use this to good advantage and summarize and correlate many principles of physiology and therapy and show their practical application to patient care.

IMPORTANCE OF PATENT AIRWAYS

By now we have been well oriented toward the great hazard of airway obstruction and its pathologic origins and can justifiably relate it to the problems of assisting the patient in ventilatory failure by the following dictum: *The effectiveness of mechanical ventilation is directly proportional to the patency of the airways.* The importance of the health of the bronchial tree gives it priority in our discussion. Airway obstruction is a major obstacle to ventilation and an almost constant challenge to the skill of the inhalation therapist—obvious in the patient suffering from chronic bronchopulmonary disease or insidiously developing in a patient otherwise afflicted. Not only is the attempt to administer artificial ventilation against severe obstruction usually futile, but the efforts may be demonstrably harmful. Such an attempt may cause a serious increase in dead space ventilation and reduce effective alveolar tidal exchange, as the mechanically driven air rapidly generates back pressure to shorten inspiratory time. It may also encourage air trapping, with a subsequent increase in functional residual capacity and an elevation in the resting level, further burdening a lung that may already be abnormally distended.

Before instituting ventilation, the therapist should make an estimate of the status of the patient's airways. This in no way conflicts with the role of the attending physician nor does it usurp any of his function, for since the therapist is to carry the burden of supervising therapy, it is both his right and his obligation to acquaint himself with the problem he faces. The therapist should learn something of the patient's background, either from the physician directly or through a study of the clinical chart, to determine whether airway obstruction has been a clinical feature. A significant smoking history may be a valuable warning clue in the patient with no apparent current obstruction; it should caution the therapist to be on the alert for a later complication. At the bedside, the experienced therapist can listen for telltale gross wheezes or rhonchi; and if in doubt, he can use the stethoscope for better evaluation. Once therapy is under way, indications of obstruction should always be sought. Periodic observation of the assisted patient's ventilation is helpful to note whether exhalation is unduly prolonged or effortful, whether the pattern is irregular, or whether the rate significantly increases. In the assisted or controlled patient, obstruction may be evidenced by marked shortening of inspiratory time, noted by listening to the cycling of the machine. Air trapping can often be detected by slowing of a tidal volume–metering device to reach its end-expiratory base line or by an elevation of this base line.

The pharmacologic agents most frequently used in the treatment of airway obstruction were covered in earlier pages, and we will now consider the mechanical techniques available that may be used before the start of ventilation or introduced into the program at any time needed. The three important procedures with which we must be familiar are *bronchoscopy, intubation,* and *tracheobronchial aspiration.* The first two are performed by physicians; the last is an important function of the inhalation therapist.

Bronchoscopy

Bronchoscopy is a procedure that is both therapeutic and diagnostic, requiring the services of a skilled and experienced physician, usually a specialist in the fields of either otorhinolaryngology (diseases of the ear, nose, and throat) or thoracic surgery. It is extensively used for direct visual examination of a suspected lesion in the bronchial tree or of one previously noted by x-ray; and if the lesion is available to the bronchoscopist, he can often remove a small specimen (biopsy) for histologic examination. The procedure is usually performed in a room provided for it, although in extraordinary emergency situations it can be done at the bedside. The pharynx and larynx are locally anesthetized and, with the patient supine and head hyperextended, the operator introduces a long, lighted telescopic tube into the bronchi. Each side is examined in turn, and as the instrument is advanced deep into the main bronchi, the orifices of the branches are visualized. A long metal aspirator is inserted down the tube and secretions are sucked out; often large plugs that may have obstructed large bronchi are removed. The value of bronchoscopy in treating and preventing serious atelectasis is obvious. Because the procedure is carried out under sterile precautions, the secretions obtained can be cultured to determine the extent of any infectious process that may be active. In many patients suffering acute obstruction from secretions, a single drainage by this technique is often adequate; but if the disease is extensive enough to require repeated suctioning, other methods to be described below are preferred. Certainly, bronchoscopy is the most direct approach to the problem of excessive secretions, but it has little if any value in diffuse bronchospastic obstruction. Indeed, the mechanical irritation of the procedure itself may precipitate or worsen bronchial spasm. There are varying degrees of patient discomfort, both during and after the procedure; and many patients complain of soreness of the throat for several hours. The introduction of the instrument into the respiratory tract constitutes an obstruction to breathing, and this can be a serious hazard to the patient already markedly hypoxic. Finally, when rapid relief of acute obstruction is needed, the responsible personnel may not be immediately available for the most opportune use of bronchoscopy, and delay may not be justified. Nevertheless, when used for the proper indications within its limitations, it is an excellent procedure that may not only help correct an existing obstructive problem but may also forestall serious progressive buildup of secretions and prevent atelectasis.

Intubation

We will explore intubation in considerable detail because it is almost a standard procedure in the patient with severe ventilatory failure, and the therapist will work extensively with patients so treated. In contrast to bronchoscopy, which is a short-term technique, intubation is the placing of a rigid or semirigid tube in the respiratory tract and leaving it for varying periods of time, from a few hours to permanently, to assure patency of the upper airway. The following points should be noted about intubation: First, the tube itself is space-occupying in the airway, and its use constitutes somewhat of a compromise in that the tube reduces the caliber of the natural lumen although it ensures that the narrower passage is clear. Second, intubation is indicated for the access it provides to the bronchial tree for the aspiration of secretions (to be described in detail below). Third, it is a means of administering mechanical ventilation. Under certain limited circumstances, pressured air may be given to a patient by means of a face mask; but a moment's reflection will bring to mind several practical inadequacies of such a measure. (1) Because of the great variations in contours of the human face, a secure fit between mask and face is difficult to achieve; and if delivered pressure is to be responsible for ventilation, a leak in the system is hazardous. (2) With the best-designed face mask, considerable pressure must be applied to hold it in place to prevent slippage as well as leaks. The dependability of head straps or a harness is highly questionable, and, with the force required, the risk of pressure necrosis of the skin is very real. The alternative method of the therapist manually holding the mask in place can be effective sometimes for very short periods but is obviously impractical for prolonged supportive therapy. (3) There is a great risk of oropharyngeal obstruction by the lax tongue in the unconscious patient, a complication that is often precipitated by the supine position and the pressure of a mask. In such circumstances, a mouth airway must always be used to hold the tongue out of the way and to provide a good channel for the delivered air. (4) In the presence of significant airway resistance, the flaccid cheeks may absorb enough of the ventilating pressure that pulmonary ventilation is compromised. Thus, except for short-term emergency treatment, the use of face masks is not suitable for positive-pressure ventilation; and a substantial airway must be provided.

For this last indication the tubes are almost always "cuffed." The cuff is a rubber balloonlike item that fits over the lower end of the airway tube and has a narrow rubber tube extending outside the body by which the cuff can be inflated with air. The simple illustration in Fig. 10-1 shows the general relationships of the parts involved. As the cuff distends with air, it seals the airway to prevent the retrograde flow of gas cephalad under pressure. Thus, all gas movement is through the indwelling tube. The outer end of the inflating tube has a small pilot balloon that distends with the cuff and serves as a monitor, for should the cuff develop a leak, the pilot balloon will also deflate. The cuff is usually filled with air by a syringe, and a clamp is placed proximal to the pilot balloon. More details of cuffs and their management will be covered later under the discussion of tracheostomy.

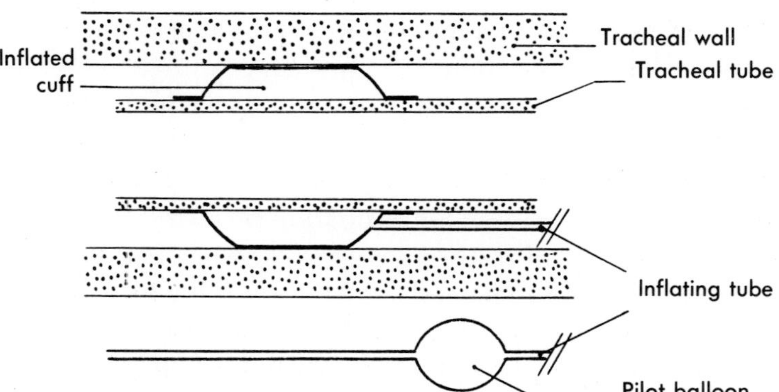

Fig. 10-1. Sketch of intratracheal tube with inflated cuff in place, in longitudinal section of the trachea. Air is introduced into the cuff through an inflating tube, which extends through the surgical incision to the outside. A pilot balloon warns of accidental deflation of the cuff after a clamp is placed distal to it on the inflating tube.

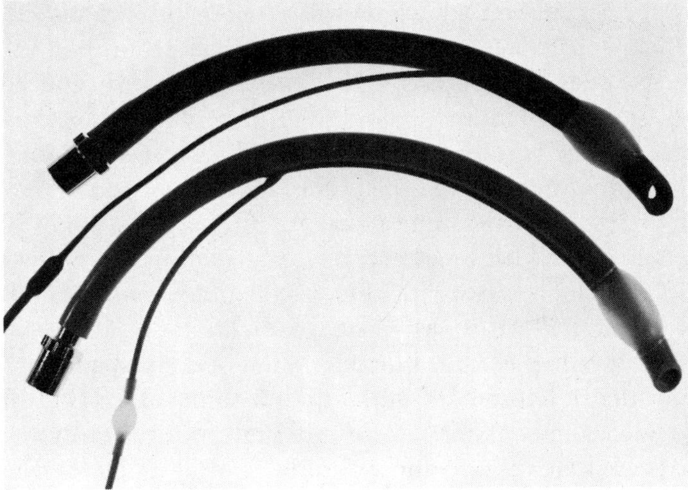

Fig. 10-2. Endotracheal tubes with inflated cuffs and pilot balloons.

There are three types of intubating tubes in general clinical use—the *oral endotracheal tube,* the *nasotracheal tube,* and the *tracheostomy tube.* The individual features of each will be described, but characteristics common to all and the general principles of intubation and patient care will be discussed with the tracheostomy as the model.

Oral endotracheal intubation. Endotracheal tubes are of rubber or plastic and come in a variety of sizes from 12 cm long with an inside diameter of 2.5 mm to about 38 cm long and 11 mm inside diameter. They are curved to facilitate introduction into the respiratory tract and are available with attached cuffs, as shown in Fig. 10-2. Oral endotracheal intubation has long been used to maintain an open airway during surgery, usually instituted after induction of the anesthesia; but with the increasing incidence of pulmonary diseases, it has become an important part of medical management of the conscious or unconscious patient in ventilatory failure.

The base of the tongue, the pharynx, and the larynx are rendered insensitive with local anesthetic nebulized or directly applied to the area and sometimes infiltrated into the larynx by injection. With the patient in the supine position, the way is readied for intubation by introducing a laryngoscope into the pharynx. This is an instrument consisting of a handle containing batteries and small bulb at approximately right angles to which is a blade that may be straight or curved. Thus, under direct lighted vision, the tip of the laryngoscope blade displaces the epiglottis and exposes the larynx. The endotracheal tube can then be inserted between the vocal cords through the larynx into the trachea just far enough that the cuff clears the larynx. A small oral airway or some other effective "bite block" is fastened between the patient's teeth to prevent accidental compression of the tube by closure of the jaws.

The question frequently arises as to whether endotracheal intubation should be part of the responsibilities of the inhalation therapist, and at this particular stage in the evolution of inhalation therapy, the general answer should be a firm no. The procedure, for the most part, is a fairly simple one, but it carries serious potential risks. At the outset, there is the possibility of an adverse reaction to the local anesthetic, a great hazard to any patient but more so in one with defective ventilation. The larynx is a sensitive organ and often responds to irritation or trauma by becoming spastic, completely occluding the airway; and attempts to force the tube may seriously damage the vocal cords. It is important that every effort be made to pass the cords on the first attempt, for repeated probing will stimulate an almost immediate edema of the cords, markedly hampering the procedure and risking the life of the patient. Intubation should be considered a medical procedure, not a technical one; and its responsibilities entail such legal and ethical considerations that its use must be reserved for the professionally trained physician, usually an anesthesiologist. There is no doubt that a good therapist could be trained to perform intubation, but the skill and finesse with which it is done are directly proportional to the frequency of its performance. Even though it is widely used in patients receiving inhalation therapy, the actual number of times per week or per month that the average therapist would have occasion to intubate is negligible when compared to its frequency in the daily work of the anesthesiologist. It is recognized that there may be circumstances in which trained professional personnel are not readily available, and emergency intubation must depend upon the therapist. However, it is most probable that a hospital with an inhalation therapy department potentially able to assume the duties of intubation would have a general work load necessitating an active anesthesiology service. In summary, each hospital must work out its own solution to providing emergency intubation; but, whenever possible, a trained physician, especially an anesthesiologist, should be on first call. It should be remembered that even the most skillful operator is at a serious disadvantage when faced with the task of intubating a larynx already spastic and edematous from a bungled earlier unsuccessful attempt.

The advantages of oral endotracheal intubation are summarized in a study of this technique.[246] As noted above, a good airway can be obtained by an expert operator in a very short time without the risk and inconvenience of a surgical procedure, as is necessary for tracheotomy. There is no tissue destruction or scarring and no anatomic distortion, so that a repeat intubation can be done whenever necessary. Extubation (removal of the tube) time was found to be shorter than with a tracheostomy because there seemed to be less patient and physician dependence upon nonsurgical than on surgical intubation. Of great significance was the observation that the return of an effective cough was almost immediate following extubation whereas there is always some delay after surgical violation of the trachea. Finally, the prior oral intubation of the trachea makes much safer and easier a subsequent tracheotomy, a point that will be emphasized below in the discussion of the latter procedure.

In comparison, the disadvantages of oral intubation are of less significance. The most important is some degree of patient intolerance to the awkwardness and inconvenience of the large tube through the mouth. Frequently, much continuous assurance must be given the patient, supported by sedation to allay his apprehension and reduce discomfort, obviously not a problem in the unconscious or mentally obtunded patient. Occasionally an agitated patient may pull out the tube, but after replacement, proper restraint will prevent recurrence. Laryngeal edema may be troublesome in the post intubation period, but this has not proved to be a serious hazard, and reintubation can always be done if needed. Until fairly recently it was almost a dictum that oral endotracheal intubation be terminated at 48 hours and that if further therapy were necessary tracheotomy be done. With increasing experience in its use, the duration of intubation has been greatly expanded, and in the study referred to above, tubes were left in place for periods ranging from 21 to 171 hours, with no ill effects.

Nasotracheal intubation. The objectives of this technique, as well as the tube employed, are similar to those of oral intubation. In this case, however, the tube is introduced first through the nose rather than the mouth and then into the trachea. Although "blind" passage of the tube through the larynx can be attempted, it is much safer to use the same direct visual approach as with oral intubation once the tube has passed the nasal cavity. Nasotracheal intubation has been most extensively used in children but is now finding increasing favor in treating adults; and a study compares its effectiveness with that of tracheostomy in the latter group.[247] With a variety of underlying conditions necessitating intubation, nasotracheal tubes were used for periods ranging from 12 hours to 14 days. The advantages of this procedure are the same as those described for oral intubation with the additional feature of better patient tolerance and less discomfort since the mouth is free of the large tube. Similarly, the disadvantages are basically those noted above with the possible additional risk of some kinking of the tube as it navigates the tortuous nasal passages.

The opinion is frequently heard that a nasotracheal tube must be smaller than an oral or tracheostomy tube and that resistance to airflow will be accordingly increased. The report cited above disputes this, implying that there need be no difference between the oral and nasal tubes, although it would seem reasonable that unfavorable nasal conditions might limit the size of tube that could be effectively used. It further states that despite its greater length, the nasotracheal tube may be less resistant than a loosely fitted tracheostomy tube. It is interesting to note that the survey of the oral endotracheal technique referred to earlier found the use of nasotracheal tubes in adults much less satisfactory than the use of oral tubes and was accompanied by a sharp difference in patient survival. In all probability, the differences in opinion reflect the results of personal experiences and interest in one technique over the other rather than any significant inherent difference in these two similar procedures. The therapist will perhaps note that just as we were unable to describe one best mechanical ventilator, endowed with all virtues and no vices, so there is no single intubation technique to satisfy all needs.

Tracheostomy intubation. The greatest portion of our discussion on airway patency and intubation will be devoted to the intubation of the tracheotomized airway, for this is the standard against which all other techniques are evaluated. Let us first define two terms widely used, often erroneously interchangeably. *Tracheotomy* is a surgical procedure that produces an opening in the trachea (the suffix *tomy* means "a cutting or incision"), and a *tracheostomy* is the opening so made in the trachea (the suffix *stomy* coming from the Greek *stoma,* "mouth"). A *tracheostomy tube* is therefore a tube designed to be placed in the trachea through a tracheostomy. This technique has been a lifesaving procedure for some three centuries, to and including the present, and is the most precise and definitive way to establish and maintain a free upper airway. Many of the comments to be made will apply to both oral and nasal tracheal intubation as well, and to avoid unnecessary repetition, the reader will be left to relate them in his own mind.

The indications for a tracheostomy can be enumerated as follows: (1) to establish and/or maintain a patent and accessible airway after endotracheal intubation or when the latter is not considered desirable; (2) with a cuffed tube, to prevent aspiration of regurgitated gastric contents or blood from facial or oral trauma, as in a comatose patient or one with obtunded reflexes; (3) to permit the aspiration of bronchopulmonary secretions, a maneuver somewhat easier through a tracheostomy tube than through the longer endotracheal tube; (4) to reduce the anatomic dead space and relieve the work of breathing. By short-circuiting the nasal, oral, and pharyngeal passages, the tracheostomy tube affords the spontaneously breathing patient less distance to move air from atmosphere to alveoli. Reference will be made to this again later, but it should be observed that the cost of reducing the dead space is a reduction in the lumen of the upper airway since the tracheostomy tube itself is an obstruction. It has been shown that resistance to breathing does not drop significantly below normal in the adult patient until the internal diameter of the tube exceeds 9.5 mm, and this is larger than the three most commonly used tubes[248]; (5) with a cuffed tube, to permit long-term positive-pressure mechanical ventilation.

THE TRACHEOTOMY. Tracheotomy itself is not to be taken lightly, for it is a surgical procedure carried out on a patient with a severely compromised major system. Emergency tracheotomies have been performed under a variety of circumstances, and many will be, of necessity, in the future. However, every attempt should be made to see that conditions for it are as ideal as possible, and in the modern hospital the bedside tracheotomy is denounced. Even in the most critical situations, tracheotomy should be an elective procedure, done in the operating room with due regard for preparation and careful technique. With the recognition of airway obstruction severe enough to warrant mechanical interference, the patient should immediately be intubated endotracheally to assure his survival; supportive therapy should be given, and surgery performed, when both the patient's condition and the operating facilities are at their best. The techniques of tracheotomy may vary, but in general the incision into and through the skin and subcutaneous tissue is made high enough that the trachea can be entered at the level of either the second or third cartilage. This site is essential so that the tip of the tube will not impinge on the carina. Selection of a tube of proper size and shape is critically important, for the tube must be neither too tight nor too loose if the complications that will be described later are to be avoided. Once firmly in place, the tracheostomy tube is secured by a fabric tape around the patient's neck. Tracheotomy carries with it definite surgical risks; the mortality directly attributed to the procedure, as opposed to the underlying disease, is estimated at 3% and serious complications at nearly 50% in some series.[247] The three most important immediate surgical complications can be classified as follows.

Bleeding. This is an exceptionally potential hazard, for not only is the involved anatomic area naturally very vascular, but congestion in the vessels is often increased as a result of the hemodynamic changes incident to both pulmonary disease and supportive ventilation. Every bleeding source must be meticulously attended, for these patients can ill afford the stress of excessive blood loss.

Tissue emphysema. The great variety of neck contours seriously challenge the surgeons, and the probing and dissection in some patients hold the risk of invading the apices of the lungs with subsequent pneumothorax. Not rarely, air escapes from the opened trachea and works its way through exposed tissues to accumulate under the skin of the face, neck, and thorax, a condition known as *subcutaneous emphysema.* More serious is the movement of air along the paths of the major airways into the mediastinum, *mediastinal emphysema,* where it builds up in response to the negative pressure of the patient's inspiratory efforts and may embarrass the intrathoracic cardiorespiratory mechanics. Fortunately, most of the time such events are correctable or tolerated by the body, but since they can occur even when tracheotomy is done with operating room care, the therapist can understand the risk of operating in haste.

Cardiovascular collapse. There are two types of adverse cardiovascular reactions to the tracheotomy procedure itself, similar in their end results but differing markedly in their mechanisms. First, one of the immediate hazards is acute cardiac arrest, most often encountered during a hurried tracheotomy but fortunately becoming less frequent with adherence to currently accepted practices. At one time believed to be due to some vagal reflex accompanying the trauma of surgery, arrest is now attributed to a severe and sudden hypoxia superimposed on the hypoxia of the underlying disease, as ventilation is impaired during the manipulations of the procedure. This is the major reason for prior intubation and efforts to improve oxygenation before surgery and for maintaining good mechanical or manual ventilation until the new airway is adequately functioning. Second, cardiovascular, and sometimes respiratory, collapse may be the paradoxical result of rapidly achieving a good airway during tracheotomy.[249] Shortly after the airway is secured and secretions cleaned out, the patient may become acutely hypotensive and pulseless and go into complete apnea. This reaction is believed to be due to the sudden washout of accumulated carbon dioxide from the body as alveolar ventilation is precipitously increased and the respiratory acidosis reversed. Such a rapid swing in acid-base balance is known to produce arrhythmias and hypotension. The accompanying apnea is the sequella of cerebral blood flow reduction from both the circulatory failure and vascular dilatation of sudden hypocapnia. Before, during, and immediately after tracheotomy, the patient's blood pressure should be checked frequently and vasopressors kept close at hand to prevent the shock from becoming irreversible.

It might be of interest to note that a secondary, but definitely helpful, benefit of preoperative intubation is the increased ease of locating, mobilizing, and handling a trachea already identified and supported by an indwelling tube. In summary, we can say that the incidence and seriousness of tracheotomy complications are inversely related to the degree that the procedure is performed under elective, controlled conditions.

TUBES AND CUFFS. There are many types of tracheostomy tubes now available. For many years only silver tubes were used, but disposable plastic has now become a popular material and the general structure of all is similar. The tubes are curved to accommodate the anatomy of the trachea and to facilitate introduction and removal, varying from an outside diameter of 3 mm and a length along the outside of the curve of 1.75 inches to an outside diameter of 14 mm and a length of over 4 inches. Unfortunately, sizing of tubes involves at least two scales and mixes metric with English units of measurement. It is not critical that the inhalation therapist be familiar with the details of such data, for he will have available for his purposes a large enough variety of adapters that he will be able to service any tracheotomized patients under his jurisdiction; but if he is interested, equipment catalogues are available with specifications of the many types. The tracheostomy tube is basically a cannula within a cannula, as shown in Fig. 10-3. The outer cannula maintains the patency of the airway, whereas the inner is removable for cleaning to prevent secretions from obstructing the tip. If there were but a single tube and it became plugged with secretions, it would have to be removed, thereby disrupting the entire surgical area. This is avoided by the removable inner cannula. The stylus-like accessory is called an obturator, and it is used only for the initial introduction of the outer cannula to prevent scraping of the tracheal wall. Once the outer cannula is in place, the obturator is withdrawn and the inner cannula

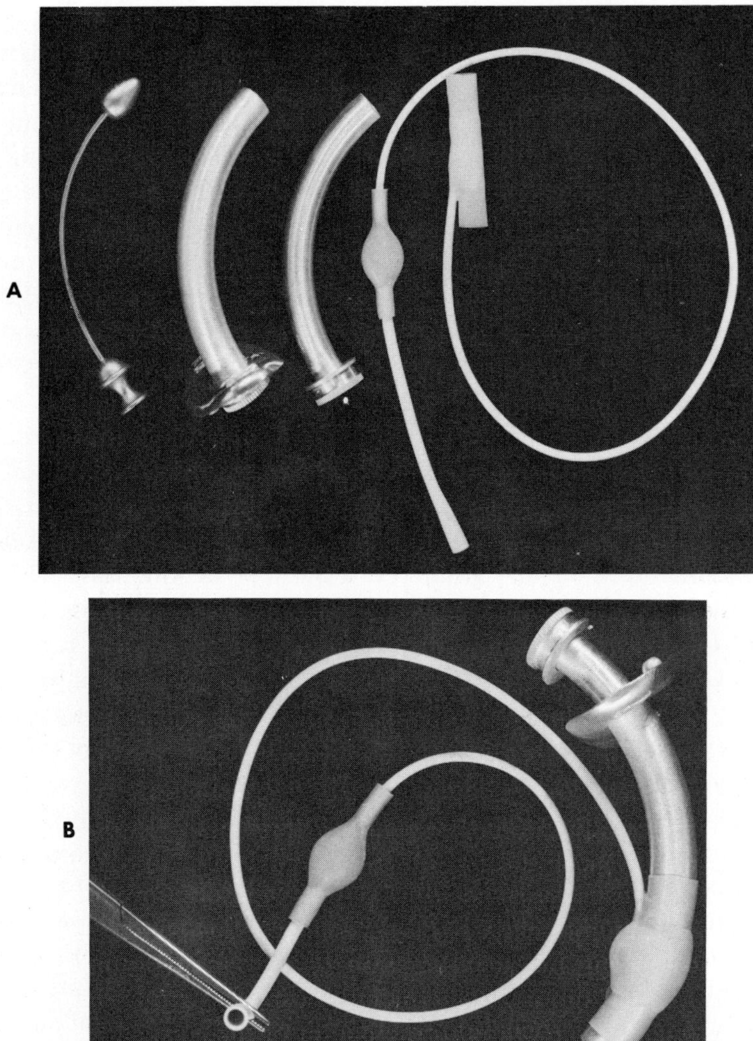

Fig. 10-3. A, Components of a dissembled silver tracheostomy tube. On the left is a stylus, or obturator, used only during insertion of the outer cannula, followed by the outer and inner cannulae, and a cuff. **B,** The cuff is in place and inflated, and the inner cannula is seen protruding slightly from the outer tube.

inserted. The two cannulae are held snugly together by a locking mechanism on the metal units or by friction on the plastic. The head of the inner cannula is designed to accept adapters that permit the attachment of ventilators to the system.

We have made frequent references to the cuffs used on intubation tubes, and because of their importance in making effective ventilation available to patients, we shall describe them in a bit more detail. Some plastic tracheostomy tubes have built-on or bonded cuffs, but with other tubes the cuff must be put on according to the size of the tube. Such separate cuffs vary in size from 4 mm to about 13 mm, and success of subsequent ventilation may depend upon the proper application of the proper size cuff. As shown in Fig. 10-3, the ends of the cuff are narrower and less elastic than the easily distensible midportion. The tight fit of the ends of the cuff holds it in place on the outer cannula of the tube, to prevent both leakage and slippage; and a special cement is often used for additional support. A very informative and practical study of tracheostomy cuffs describes two basic types, the single-lumen and the double-lumen.[250] The single-lumen cuff is a simple tube of thin rubber with snug ends and a distensible body supplied with an inflating tube. It distends evenly in all directions, exerting pressure equally on all mucosal contact points, and it holds the tracheostomy tube in the center of the trachea; but it tends to leak air and to ride up and down on the outer cannula as it is subjected to the motion of the patient and manipulation of attached equipment. The double-lumen cuff is double walled. As it is inflated, the inner wall is compressed against the outer cannula, securely holding the cuff in place while the outer wall distends to occlude the airway between the tube and trachea. A disadvantage of the double-lumen cuff is its tendency to bulge mostly in one direction, opposite the attachment of its inflating tube. Not only does this create unequal pressure on the inner tracheal wall, but it also displaces the cannula from the center of the airway to an eccentric location. In spite of these undesirable characteristics, because of its stability, the double-lumen cuff is probably the more desirable of the two. One popular brand of plastic tube has no inner cannula and is supplied with two attached single-lumen cuffs. The cuffs are inflated alternately to minimize the risk of prolonged pressure against a single segment of the tracheal mucosa, as described below. Inflation of either type of cuff is the same. With the cuffed cannula in place, approximately 5 ml of air are injected into the end of the inflating tube by means of a syringe or a syringe and needle through a plug supplied on the ends of some inflating tubes. The exact amount needed in each instance is determined by listening for leaks. If a ventilator is to be used, the machine is started and the amount of air in the cuff adjusted to make the system airtight. A clamp is then placed on the inflating tube distal to the pilot balloon.

MANAGEMENT OF THE INTUBATED PATIENT. The management of the tracheotomized patient mechanically ventilated through a cuffed tube constitutes one of the inhalation therapist's greatest responsibilities. It can be flatly stated that no member of the hospital team is as qualified or as able as a trained and mature inhalation therapist to supervise the ventilatory care of such a patient. There is as yet not universal agreement on this point, and some conflict is evident between nursing and inhalation therapy services. For the most part, this is understandable, stemming from the facts that inhalation therapy is new, it involves patient care to a degree formerly reserved for nursing, and there is a shortage of therapists to meet hospitals' needs. Because of the intense care required for these patients, there is need for both nursing and inhalation therapy working cooperatively, and in those hospitals where inhalation therapy functions at its highest level, conflicts dissolve as each service concentrates on its contribution to overall care.

There are several factors which the therapist must bear in mind in addition to the attention he directs toward the efficient functioning of his ventilator. He must remember that the patient is entirely dependent upon all medical and nursing attendants and can do little for himself. If the patient is alert, he will initially be apprehensive and may justifiably be greatly frightened. Reassurance by the therapist through word and action is a *critical* part of therapy, for the patient's emotional status may markedly influence his breathing pattern or his acceptance of mechanical ventilation. The therapist must create an atmosphere of calmness and confidence for the patient, aware that the patient watches every move and listens to every word. It must be remembered that the cuffed patient cannot talk because his vocal cords are bypassed by the tracheostomy tube. He can speak only after disconnection from the ventilator, deflation of the cuff, and obstruction of the outer opening of the tube, so that exhaled air can leak around the tube through the larynx. This may be tiring and should be reserved for those instances when the patient desires to communicate or when it is necessary to get information from him essential to therapy.

It was noted above that adapters are used to attach the ventilator to the end of the inner cannula. For the most part, these are plastic and come in sets to accommodate all sizes of tubes. They are generally held into the inner cannula (a further reduction in the caliber of the airway) by friction, connecting the airway to the machine by a flex tube. It is important to adjust this joint in such a manner that there is a minimum of strain on the connector to reduce the risk of accidental dislodgment, which would completely separate the patient from his major, if not only, source of ventilation. There is available a very secure threaded swivel connector that permits patient mobility without loosening.

The inflated cuff is a potential danger to the respiratory tract because of its constant pressure on the tracheal mucosa, which may cause areas of mucosal necrosis. To avoid this possibility the cuff should be deflated for approximately 5 minutes every hour; but if the patient's ventilatory status is so critical that he cannot tolerate this length of time, then deflation should be done more frequently for shorter periods. Whenever the ventilator is not in operation, the cuff should be deflated. Because some cuffs are defective and may break, the therapist must be on the watch for evidence of a leak, the first instance of which may be the failure of end-inspiratory cycling of a pressure-cycled ventilator or the prolongation of inspiration if the leak is relatively small. The ear of an alert and experienced therapist will pick up changes in the cycling patterns of his equipment, but these warnings will be absent in time-cycled ventilators. The pilot balloon is usually a reliable indication of the inflation of the cuff, but on occasion the inflation tube may become pinched at the tracheal stoma so that the pilot balloon remains filled even after collapse of the cuff. In the event that a defective cuff is detected or suspected, the therapist should notify the responsible physician at once.

The constant potential hazard to the intubated patient, as noted frequently, is obstruction, especially from accumulated secretions. One of the safeguards against this is effective aspiration, the technique of which will be described separately below. In addition, the inner cannula should be removed and cleaned every 4 hours, or more frequently if needed; and for long-term care, the entire tube should be removed and changed weekly, even in the absence of malfunction, a responsibility of the physician who did the original surgery.[251] The final protection against secretion buildup is adequate humidification; and we do not exaggerate when we say that not only will intubation fail to achieve its purpose but it may be positively harmful to the patient if humidity is lacking. While the patient's dead space has been reduced by tracheotomy, so has his natural humidification mechanism been bypassed; and little can be more detrimental to this respiratory hygiene than a flow of dry air or gas (even room air) directly into his trachea. While the patient is being ventilated, humidification will be provided by the many effective devices available as attachments; but humidification must not be overlooked when the patient is removed from the machine for significant periods of time. A tracheostomy mask or collar that conveniently fits over the opening of the cannula is satisfactory if it is used with a good humidifier. The ultrasonic humidifier has been found to be effective, although the better jet units are probably adequate. It is felt by many that secretions will not usually be a serious problem if the patient is supplied with adequate vapor and water aerosol for most secretions will be wet enough to be easily aspirated. Water in the inspired gas serves another purpose than maintaining general health of the respiratory tract. No matter how good is the fit of a tracheostomy tube, there is always some motion of it in response to respiration, patient activity, and handling of the attachements; and a bit of excess water in and about the tube acts as a lubricant to minimize its frictional damage to the local mucosa.

Many of the patients who are intubated need supplemental oxygen therapy. Our concern here is not with the indications for or the hazards of oxygen per se, for we have already considered these factors earlier and will discuss them again later on; our concern, rather, is with the method of administration. As in the case of humidity mentioned above, during mechanical ventilation oxygen will be provided as needed through the instrument; but a word is in order concerning its use when the patient is not being ventilated. The safest technique is the use of a tracheostomy mask, which can combine both oxygen and humidification. Unfortunately, there is an old technique still in use that is to be condemned. This is the insertion of an oxygen catheter directly into the tracheostomy tube. Although arterial oxygen levels can be increased, such a procedure offers a significant resistance to exhalation with a potential danger that outweighs any benefit. This subject was studied with convincing results of the ventilatory burden it imposes.[252] We have already indicated that the tube itself increases the airflow resistance in the respiratory tract; and it is reasonable that the introduction of a catheter, no matter how small, will further increase such resistance. When to this is added the resistance of an oxygen flow directly opposing the passive outflow of air, we can only wonder that such a procedure was ever considered safe. The study logically concluded, but with quantitative proof, that peak expiratory resistance increased as the size of the tracheostomy tube decreased, as the size of the oxygen catheter increased, and as the oxygen flow rate increased. Should a therapist encounter this procedure in use or being contemplated, it is hoped that he will use his greatest diplomacy and tact in suggesting an alternate technique.

COMPLICATIONS OF TRACHEOSTOMY. In addition to the hazards of the surgical procedure of tracheotomy and the clinical precautions to be considered in the management of a tracheotomized patient, there are complications that can be attributed to the presence of the tracheostomy tube itself. Although the medical care of such complications is a responsibility of the attending physician, the inhalation therapist should be acquainted with them, for he may be the first to note their onset and so stimulate immediate corrective action. Some latitude may be expected in determining what phenomena constitute complications due to a tracheostomy, but we will include the most important in the following classification.

Obstruction

FROM SECRETIONS. This has already been discussed and is repeated only for emphasis of its importance, but it most certainly is a direct result of the aggravation of preexisting secretions by intubation.

FROM THE CUFF. A loosely fitted single-lumen cuff may partially or completely slip off the end of the cannula, obstructing the airway locally or in either main stem bronchus. This is most apt to occur following rupture of the cuff after it has been in operation, during manipulation of the cannula with the cuff deflated, or during removal of the tube. Clinical and mechanical signs and symptoms of airway obstruction accompanied by inability to inflate the cuff should bring this probability immediately to mind. Because of its better grip on the cannula, a double-lumen cuff is not too apt to become completely dislodged, even when deflated; but it may herniate or hang over the end of the cannula. When it is then inflated, it will occlude both the trachea and the tracheostomy tube as it distends freely across the opening of the cannula. The resulting severe dyspnea in the spontaneously breathing patient will be relieved by deflation of the cuff, and the obstructive response of an attached ventilator will be replaced by evidence of a leak. In such a condition, a probing suction catheter will encounter the obstructing inflated cuff but will pass freely when the cuff is emptied of air.

FROM THE CANNULA. Should the tracheotomy incision be placed too low or too long a tube be installed, the tip of the cannula may impinge on the carina, with resulting severe obstruction. When intubation has been completed and mechanical ventilation started, the attending physician or the responsible therapist should always check to be sure that the cannula is not directed down one or the other main stem bronchi. Should this occur, all the ventilation will go to one lung whereas the other will become severely atelectatic from complete deprivation of its air supply. Suspicion of this complication should be aroused by the inability to achieve satisfactory ventilation with the respirator (due to the reduced volume of but one functioning lung) and is confirmed by the lack of breath sounds in the bypassed lung as the chest is examined by stethoscope. Immediate correction is mandatory, for this is life threatening.

FROM ABRADED MUCOSA. It has been suggested that many of the instances of obstruction following tracheal intubation may be the result of what has been termed the "snowplow effect" of the tracheal cannula.[253] While the rigid tube remains fairly stable, the respiratory tract moves with the breathing cycle, riding upward during exhalation and downward during inhalation. As a result, if the tube is not centered in the airway and its tip is allowed to rest on the inner tracheal wall, the cephalad expiratory movement scrapes the tracheal mucosa against the unyielding edge of the cannular opening. Debrided epithelium, mixed with secretions, has been demonstrated to form a mass of significant size to obstruct a bronchus and require bronchoscopic removal. Selection of tubes of the proper length and, if necessary, supporting them by packing about the tracheotomy opening will minimize this traumatic risk.

Hemorrhage

FROM THE INCISIONAL SITE. Inadequate hemostasis (control of bleeding) during surgery may allow a recurrence of bleeding from the operative site after therapy has been started. The danger of brisk bleeding is obvious; but even a hidden slow oozing of blood is hazardous, for blood may accumulate about the upper part of the cannula in the trachea and be aspirated into the bronchi when the cuff is deflated during routine care.

FROM TRACHEAL TRAUMA. Erosion of the tracheal mucosa as described above with "snowplowing" can produce surface bleeding, with subsequent aspiration. Less common, but far more serious, is a frank perforation of the tracheal wall by the indwelling cannula, with damage to a neighboring artery. This may lead to rapid and fatal exsanguination.

Tracheal pressure necrosis. Briefly alluded to earlier, pressure of a distended cuff on the tracheal mucosa impairs the local epithelial blood supply, which can lead to necrosis (tissue death) and the development of mucosal ulcers. The significance, or even the incidence, of this damage is difficult to evaluate; but based on postmortem examinations, it has been suggested that some degree of necrosis is probably present in all intubated tracheas.[254] Such trauma carries the risk of localized edema, posttracheostomy scarring and stenosis, and providing a port of entry for infection. During the process, the patient may complain of a feeling of tightness in the throat or localized pain. Tissue damage can be kept to a minimum by frequent decompression of the cuff.

Tissue emphysema. The escape of air into body tissues during surgery has already been noted when intrathoracic negative pressure can draw air through the planes of exposed cut tissues, letting it migrate to the mediastinum and subcutaneous areas. During positive-pressure ventilation this is unlikely unless the patient is "fighting" the machine because it is not meeting his needs, in which case his inspiratory efforts may suck air into the tissues around the incision. However, should there be damage to the airway below the level of the tracheal cuff (as from the end of the cannula), positive-pressure ventilation may force air into the tissues, producing extensive subcutaneous emphysema.

Infection. Some feel that infection is the most troublesome, if not the most significant, of tracheostomy complications.[255] It may range from a relatively minor wound sepsis to an overwhelming pneumonia. A frequent major problem is differentiating the infection due to invasion of the respiratory tract through a tracheotomy from that of the underlying pulmonary disease; and at times this is not possible to do with certainty. Many patients have preexisting bronchopulmonary infection at the time of their tracheotomies, and, indeed, such infections may be prominent etiologic factors in the obstructions for which the tracheotomies are performed. There can be little doubt that intubating the trachea increases the possibility of infection, with the deliberate perpetuation of an open wound into the air passages, bypassing the natural filtering mechanism of the upper tract. Handling the cannula, frequent introduction of a catheter into the trachea, attaching ventilators to the tube, and serous seepage about the incision all contribute to the risk of infection. However, even positive bacterial cultures of aspirates or wound discharges are not conclusive evidence of a clinical infection; they may be from local contaminants. For the diagnosis of a significant infection, there must be signs and symptoms other than just bacteriologic. Despite the increased chances for sepsis through a tracheostomy, it is not rare to note rapid clearing of a pulmonary infection following the establishment of good bronchial drainage and the aspiration of obstructing secretions.

Especially troublesome is the bacterium *Pseudomonas aeruginosa,* about which the therapist will hear many references. Its frequent culture from tracheotomized patients and their equipment is a constant cause for concern. Because it thrives in dampness, it is a frequent contaminant of equipment and utensils; but an unusual overgrowth of the organism in a patient weakened by disease can be pathogenic in its own right, a serious hazard to the already handicapped patient. Meticulous care is necessary for the tracheotomized patient, and attention to his wound or his tube should be only under conditions of surgically sterile technique. The incision should be treated as any surgical site, with cleaning and asepsis as indicated; and it should be kept dressed as sterile as is consistent with its use. An awareness of the risk of infection in the patient in ventilatory failure will help all attending personnel to exercise caution and avoid carelessness.

SUMMARY. The importance of tracheostomy therapy justifies a summation of its place in the management of ventilatory failure. If at all avoidable, tracheotomy should never be done as a hurried emergency procedure, for such a circumstance carries with it high mortality and morbidity. Prior intubation should be performed to secure a good airway; for not only does it give technical assistance to the operating surgeon, it also prevents the serious hypoxia that is so apt to damage the patient, even to the point of triggering cardiac arrest. At the same time, overventilation must be avoided or the patient is subjected to the risk of acute alkalosis with cardiovascular collapse and cerebral hypoxia. These two seemingly paradoxical precautions point up the great skill needed to safeguard the patient during the procedure. During follow-up management, medical attendants must watch especially carefully for cuff failure and take all necessary care to prevent tracheal damage. In general, the tracheostomy must be treated like the surgical site it is, to minimize bleeding and infection.

Tracheotomy is surgery performed on a physiologically unstable patient in critical condition, and, in a real sense, it is chosen as the lesser of two evils. The fatality rate among tracheotomized patients has been reported as high as 38% in one group of 300.[256] This is not an indictment against the therapy but rather reflects the gravity of the diseases making it necessary. On the other hand, after a careful review, it was estimated that a similar 38% of over 400 patients survived their illnesses because they did undergo tracheotomy.[255] In addition to the advantages of airway suctioning and the ability to assist ventilation, tracheotomy carries a physiologic benefit of its own, as shown by a study of the character of spontaneous breathing in a group of emphysematous patients.[257] The subjects experienced a reduction in total ventilation, attributed to a reduction in the volume of the dead space, which was more than enough to offset the increased resistance afforded by the tracheostomy tube, as compared to the resistance of mouth breathing. That this was true was indicated in the lowered oxygen consumption, showing a significant reduction in the physical work of breathing. Because less oxygen was needed for ventilatory efforts, arterial oxygen saturation rose, probably aided by a concomitant improvement in the alveolar ventilation-perfusion relationship.

Tracheobronchial aspiration

Aspiration is such an important part of tracheostomy care that it warrants special discussion, for upon its effectiveness may rest the success of the tracheotomy and all other associated therapy. Unfortunately, aspiration, or as it is sometimes called, "bronchial toilet," is a facet of patient care that is frequently done ineffectually and harmfully. Except for other specially trained personnel, such as those employed in intensive-care units, aspiration of the respiratory tract is best done by the experienced inhalation therapist, for he is able to correlate the procedure with the operation of a ventilator or oxygen therapy equipment. Even more significant, his training has impressed upon him the importance of maintaining a free airway, on which the successful performance of his work depends. Aspiration is not satisfactorily left to the general ward nursing staff, who, shorthanded and pressed for time, may delegate it to nonprofessional nursing personnel; and at best, the instruction and experience in bronchial suctioning vary greatly among nursing school curricula. It is not a difficult task, but it does require understanding of its objectives and hazards and great care. We will discuss it in terms of the equipment used, the preparation, and the details of the aspirating technique.

Equipment. A special catheter with a perforated tip through which secretions may be drawn is used to pass into the respiratory tract. It may be of rubber, but many hospitals have found disposable plastic to be more practical and convenient. No matter which type is used, the catheter must be smooth along its length and at its tip; and one that has been cut to leave a rough or sharp distal end should never be used. The catheter must be fully sterilized according to standard procedures, and because the ventilated patient will probably need frequent attention, many should be immediately available. For this reason, the individually packed, sterile, disposable units have become popular. If rubber is preferred, several can be stacked in layers, separated by toweling, and made up in a sterile pack to be left at the bedside where they can be uncovered individually as needed. For each patient, the diameter of the intrabronchial catheter should be no greater than half the diameter of the tracheostomy tube so that aspiration will not generate dangerous intrapulmonary negative pressure.[258] This is especially important to protect the easily compressed airways of children and the diseased bronchioles of emphysematous patients.

As shown in Fig. 10-4, a collecting bottle for the bronchial secretions is attached to the suction source by suitable tubing and the bottle in turn connected to the stem of a glass Y-tube connector. The catheter is attached to one arm of the Y-tube, the other arm left free. After each episode of suctioning the airways, the catheter is discarded, either in the trash if disposable or in a container to be cleaned and sterilized if of rubber. Gone are the days of the single catheter used repeatedly time and again, often left lying on the bedsheet, even dangling to the floor, or futilely immersed in a "germicidal" solution. Examination of such solutions have demonstrated that they very soon become cesspools of bacteria. Once common practice, such mishandling of catheters is inexcusable in the modern hospital.

Preparation. The therapist must carefully open the wrapping of a catheter, making sure he does not touch it with the bare hand, letting it rest on its sterile covering or some other sterile surface. He must then thoroughly wash his hands, preferably scrubbing them with a brush and antiseptic soap,

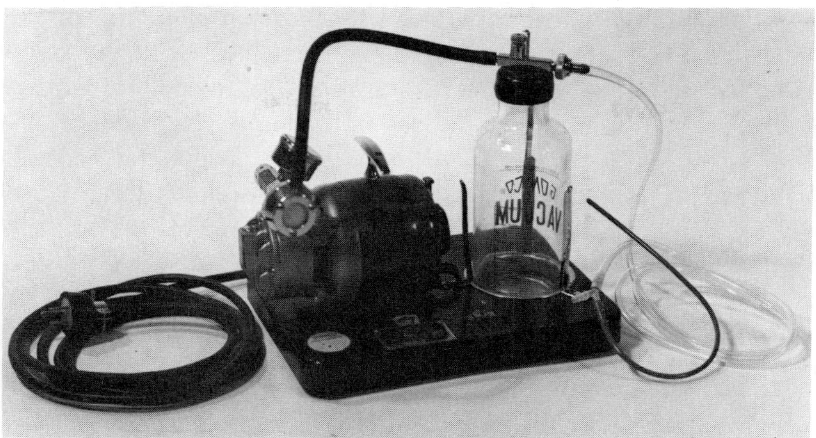

Fig. 10-4. Tracheobronchial aspiration set-up using a suction pump. The aspirating catheter is connected to one arm of a Y-connector, the other arm left free for thumb-controlled suction. Aspirate is collected in a jar located between the Y-connector and the pump.

dry them with a sterile towel, and put a sterile glove on his dominant hand. With the unsterile hand the therapist holds the Y-connector and, with the gloved hand, attaches the catheter to one arm of the Y-tube. The ventilator can be disconnected from the tracheostomy tube by an associate, or if the therapist is alone, he can do it with his uncovered hand. He will take this opportunity to deflate the cuff, both to relieve tracheal pressure and to provide the spontaneously breathing patient some additional airway during the aspiration. If advisable, according to the schedule established for the individual patient, he or his helper can remove the inner cannula for replacement by a fresh sterile one following suctioning. Removal of the ventilator, deflation of the cuff, and removal of the inner cannula can be done by the unaided therapist before scrubbing if the patient is able to tolerate the time off assisted ventilation. Finally, the suction is turned on, and the procedure is ready to begin.

We have described the classical aseptic technique, proper performance of which is universally accepted. However, it is time-consuming and awkward without assistance, and often the clinical situation demands faster, more efficient action. An alternative technique that has proved to be safe and effective omits the hand scrubbing and sterile glove. Instead, the operator manipulates the catheter into and out of the airways with a surgical clamp. When not in use, the clamp is kept in a cylindrical container of an effective chemical sterilizer, and its tip rinsed in sterile water before the catheter is picked up.

Aspiration. No one without a clear understanding of the anatomic structures of the respiratory tract and a responsible appreciation of the vital role played by the bronchial mucosa in protecting the body from infection should be permitted to aspirate the airways. All instrumentation of the tract is traumatic to its delicate lining, and the utmost gentleness is required to keep injury to a minimum. The operator's sterile hand holds the catheter, and the unsterile hand holds the glass Y-tube connector; with the free end of the Y-tube left open so that *no suction* is applied, the operator gently introduces the catheter into the trachea and one of the main stem bronchi as far as it will easily go. Since both lungs will be aspirated, it generally makes no difference which is treated first, but the catheter will readily enter either bronchus if the patient's head is turned to the opposite side. As soon as the catheter's progress has stopped, the therapist occludes the open end of the Y-connector and applies suction for 2 to 3 seconds. Aspiration is stopped by releasing the Y-connector, the catheter is withdrawn a short distance, and aspiration is again activated. This procedure is repeated in two to four steps until the catheter is in the trachea, at which time it is then withdrawn. The following must be remembered: *The catheter is never moved along the axis of the airway while suction is being applied.* While it is stationary and aspirating, the catheter may safely be gently rotated by an easy twirling motion to allow maximum exposure to secretions. It must *not* be plunged up and down in the bronchial tree, for it will then ream the respiratory mucosa and denude the airways of much of the all-important cilia. Following vigorous and injurious ramrodding of the bronchi, histologic examination of sediment from the collecting jar has often revealed large sheets of respiratory epithelium with cilia that have been stripped from and sucked out of the airways. Should additional aspiration be needed, the catheter is reintroduced and the sequence repeated; but once withdrawal has started, it should be completed with intermittent suctioning along the way. The opposite lung is then attended, preferably with a new sterile catheter.

The intervals between aspirating sessions will necessarily vary from patient to patient according to need, but aspiration should be carried out routinely at least every 30 to 60 minutes. The duration of each aspiration will depend upon the patient's tolerance but should not be prolonged beyond 15 seconds even though the patient does not appear adversely affected. Many patients suffer severe apprehension over the procedure, viewing it with great dread and fear; and in some it precipitates distressing coughing and choking. The patient must be closely observed during suctioning because cardiac arrest can occur, especially if the procedure is prolonged. It is felt that arrest is the result of severe hypoxia resulting from the loss of oxygen and lung volume through the catheter.[254] The therapist must remember that he is suctioning not only secretions from the lungs but also lung air, reducing the oxygen available to the patient and shrinking the volume of the lungs.

To make the most of bronchial aspiration, the therapist should mobilize the secretions as much as possible by humidification. We have adequately emphasized the importance of aerosolized moisture in the breathing gas, but if the secretions are still excessively viscid, they may be rendered more fluid by using a steady intratracheal saline drip in the patient not on a ventilator.

When this is not feasible, the instillation of 10 to 15 ml of saline directly into the tracheostomy tube prior to suctioning may increase the aspirate yield. If secretions are predominantly purulent, preaspiration injection into the airways of either *N*-acetylcysteine or pancreatic dornase is a helpful preparation for suctioning.

As noted above, the introduction of an aspirating catheter may reveal an obstruction above the carina. Difficulty in passing the catheter may be the result of its impingement against the tracheal wall, a dislodged or herniated cuff, or dried secretions occluding the distal end of the cannula. If the cuff is at fault, the entire tube must be removed and completely replaced. The therapist should be alert to these possibilities, for he may note their presence during routine aspiration before they have had a deleterious effect on the patient.

Finally, aspiration through an endotracheal or nasotracheal tube follows the same basic principles described for a tracheotomy. The added distance of the indwelling tube through which the catheter must be passed makes the procedure more awkward and probably a bit less effective. Generally, smaller catheters must be used because of the reduced lumen of the tube and the need to avoid serious additional obstruction by the catheter. For the maintenance of clear airways in the intubated patient whose major problem is not obstructive, aspiration through the tube will usually be satisfactory. If secretions are an important pathologic factor and need frequent attention, the patient should be tracheotomized for the assurance of maximum airway clearance.

MANAGEMENT OF THE VENTILATED PATIENT

Because he is among the most critically ill in the hospital, the patient being supported for ventilatory failure ideally should be treated in a specialized area limited to intensive care. The same effort is possible on a general medical division, but the activity attendant upon the patient's care may seriously disrupt the division's routine, to the detriment of other patients. Less than efficient therapy may result from flow of equipment and personnel into and out of a room not designed to accommodate them all, and the additional numbers of therapists and equipment needed to care for scattered patients are uneconomical.

The patient on a mechanical ventilator requires constant close attention and observation by both nurses and inhalation therapists who are knowledgeable in the clinical aspects of inadequate ventilation. As has been pointed out before, the ventilated patient is dependent for every breath on his respirator and the skill of his attendants. The possibility of mechanical failure and the sudden changes that may develop in the patient's physiology make it mandatory that he not be left alone for an instant. It is not enough to have people around; they must be people who know how to respond to the patient's needs and to any emergency that may arise. This obviously leads to the conclusion that the management of the ventilated patient must be delegated only to those with special training in respiratory care at medical, nursing, and technical levels.

The physician ultimately responsible for the therapeutic details must be experienced in clinical chest medicine and versed in basic cardiopulmonary physiology and pulmonary function evaluation. This extent of preparedness often requires the combined efforts of the patient's attending physician and a specialized consultant. An insight of the interacting physiologic and biochemical forces active in respiratory failure comes only with prolonged exposure, and even the most competent general physician usually does not have enough constant experience with this condition to be fully confident in its management, at least during the most acute phases. Certainly, a new house staff should not be given responsibility for the care of respiratory failure without close supervision, for at the present time, undergraduate medical education does not give these people adequate preparation. From a teaching point of view, the consolidation of respiratory patients in a special-care unit provides an unparalleled opportunity to train young physicians in this field and give them the basic knowledge and experience in the minimum time to make them proficient in respiratory care.

General nursing education usually includes pulmonary physiology and respiratory diseases only as segments of overall comprehensive courses, and the nurse who will care for ventilatory failure patients must have additional training. In hospitals with effective inhalation therapy departments, this should be easily accomplished; and it is the responsibility of such departments to make available to all nurses who are interested a course of instruction in the principles and practices of inhalation therapy, with emphasis on acute care.

Let us now consider some of the practical aspects of supporting the patient with a failed ventilatory system.

Choice of a ventilator

General factors in selection. We have established that there is no single best ventilator, that there are several machines which are good, with qualifications, yet each has its champions; and we are accustomed to hearing debates extolling the virtues of one over another. The personal preferences among physicians and therapists alike are based on many factors, among which are experience with one type of ventilator, confidence in one over the others, admiration for a particular mechanical principle, and economy. All of these are important considerations but are dependent more upon whim than upon the specific objectives sought in each individual patient being ventilated. It can be emphasized again that generally the skill and experience of the operating therapist are more important than the specific type of respirator used; but in our discussion of the principles of the various units in common use, we indicated features both favorable and unfavorable. Some of the characteristics that we would like to see in a ventilator would certainly include at least the following: (1) The machine should be able to operate for long periods with a minimum of servicing and maximum freedom from the risk of mechanical breakdown. (2) There should be provisions for operating the instrument on room air, pure oxygen, a variable mixture of both, and any other gas desired. (3) Whether the ventilator is basically pressure cycled or volume cycled, there should be dependable control over, or a safe limit to, the generated pressure. (4) Especially important and strongely emphasized earlier, there should be a variable flow control, either manual or automatic. (5) Desirable, but not always essential, is a combination of both control and assist capabilities or greater versatility in handling the changing patterns of breathing so commonly encountered. (6) Negative pressure during exhalation should be available for the patient undergoing prolonged controlled ventilation. (7) There must be provisions for adequate humidification of inspired gas, a need upon which the patient's survival may depend. (8) For the patient under controlled breathing, there should be means of adjusting the inspiratory-to-expiratory time ratio or at least a provision to assure that inspiration does not exceed expiration. (9) There should be available some means to monitor the delivered tidal volume. This is not an exhaustive list, and the therapist can probably add several more criteria he would like to see met before he would have full confidence in any machine. In summary, we may state that the choice of a ventilator will often depend upon which one of all those available in a given hospital is felt to be the safest and most effective for a given patient with due regard for the number, skill, and experience of the therapists who will be responsible for its operation. This choice will be made from among the groups described in the classification of Chapter 9, negative-pressure versus positive-pressure, assistor versus controller, and electric versus pneumatic.

As a recapitulation of some of the features of the major ventilators, Table

Table 10-1. *Adjustable, variable, and fixed functions of controllers*

Ventilator	*Tidal volume*	*Pressure*	*Flow rate*	*Minute rate*	*I/E*
Tank	V	A (neg)	V	A	V
Chest	V	A (neg)	V	V	A
Air-Shields	V	V	A	V	A
Engström	A	V	V	A	F
Emerson	A	V	V	V	A
Bourns	A	V	A	A	V
Bennett MA-1	A	V	A	A	V
Bird M-7, 8	V	A	A	V	A
Bennett PR-2	V	A	A†	A	F‡

*A = adjustable; V = variable, depending upon A, other variables, and condition of machine-patient circuit; F = fixed by machine.

†Flow rate self-adjusting, with additional modification by rate control.

‡Fixed at a maximum but may be lowered by expiratory timer.

10-1 compares their adjustable, variable, and fixed characteristics while operating as controllers.

Clinical guides to selection. Let us now consider the possible clinical indications that might favor one type of ventilator over another, grouping patients according to normal lungs, restrictive disease, and obstruction, understanding that in actual practice individual circumstances are often complicated by a combination of these factors.

PATIENTS WITH NORMAL LUNGS AND THORAX. This group usually includes those with neurologic or muscular pathology interfering with ventilation. The generalization may be made that a patient in ventilatory failure who has a normal lung-thorax and clear airways can be adequately ventilated with any of the standard respirators, since the only problem is the simple transportation of air into the alveoli against no abnormal barriers. If the removal of bronchial secretions or the risk of aspiration of oral or regurgitated gastric contents is not a clinical consideration, intubation may be avoided and the patient ventilated by the negative-pressure body respirator. The elective use of the tank implies the need for minimal medical and nursing attention and the ability to control rather than assist the patient's breathing. It is in this group of patients, also, that the chest respirator has its greatest application, especially in those being weaned from the large tank or who need support of their own spontaneous breathing, such as during the sleeping hours. The respirator chosen for such patients is, therefore, based on convenience and comfort rather than on the need to combat a physiologic limitation to gas exchange. Although the management of ventilation is fairly easy, it is not without its hazard, for, as will be emphasized below, the risk of serious overventilation is great.

PATIENTS WITH RESTRICTIVE LUNG DISEASE. Restriction that limits ventilation may be due to involvement of the thorax, such as trauma, as well as the pulmonary parenchyma. The primary ventilatory problem in this case is the markedly reduced lung-thorax compliance, which necessitates high driving pressures to deliver adequate tidal and minute volumes. In this circumstance, many physicians and therapists favor the use of a volume positive-pressure ventilator that is able to deliver the necessary tidal volume at whatever pressure is required. The obvious disadvantage of the pressure-cycled respirator is premature end-inspiratory cycling before delivery of the tidal volume if the pressure needs of air delivery exceed the capability of the machine. On the other hand, to expand restricted lungs with a volume ventilator may require setting the pressure-limiting device, or relief valve, to very high levels or the tidal volume still will not be delivered. The factors that will determine whether a volume or pressure ventilator will be necessary are the degree of restriction and the skill of the inhalation therapist. Pressure-cycled ventilators can be successfully used against a considerable loss of compliance and in many patients with chest injury, but success depends upon close attention to the pressure-time relationships of the mechanical adjustments by a patient and experienced therapist. Two observations may help to clarify this problem for the student. First, regardless of the instrument used, the patient with severe restrictive disease is faced with the hazard of the deleterious effects of high intrathoracic pressures that we have already considered in detail; and because of this and progressive loss of compliance, some patients just cannot be sustained with any equipment or techniques now available. In such patients it is more academic than realistic to debate the virtues of delivering air at almost unlimited pressure if the therapy itself puts the patients under increasing risk. Second, in patients with "pure" restriction, the volume-cycled ventilators can support all but those noted above and are probably preferred, especially when there is anything less than ideal technical supervision. However, except in such diseases as the respiratory distress syndrome of the newborn and a few fibrotic or granulomatous conditions of the adult, restriction is frequently associated with obstructive disease, to be described next; and in this case the ventilator preference may be reversed.

PATIENTS WITH OBSTRUCTIVE DISEASE. By and large, most patients in this category present the dual problems of increased airway resistance and reduced compliance and may confront the therapist with his greatest technical challenge. The chief prerequisite of a respirator to manage the obstructed patient is variable flow control, reasons for which have been adequately covered earlier. There is widespread disagreement on the efficacy of pressure versus volume ventilators, but it is futile to engage in debate. With a mechanically dependable instrument that has flow control, the clinical results obtained depend entirely upon the skill and experience of the operator. Theoretically, it makes little difference whether a ventilator is volume cycled or pressure cycled if it possesses flow control, but, practically, this reduces the selection to the IPPV type. It is true that the Engström respirator has a sort of "automatic" flow control, in a sense, active during its so-called "static pressure period" to allow the gas flow to accommodate to resistance. However, at the usual ventilatory rates, this time interval is less than 0.75 second. In contrast, the IPPV's have direct or indirect control over flow rate. Reference to Table 10-1 shows that four respirators have manually adjustable flows, one of which is also self-adjusting, and another modified by manipulation of its I/E ratio. With pressure and flow rate critical factors in the kinetics of ventilating obstructed airways, only two have the distinct advantage of independent control over these two parameters. We should point out here that for the inhalation therapist who understands basic pulmonary physiology and mechanics as well as the detailed functions of his equipment, it makes little difference whether a volume is delivered to a patient at a required pressure or a pressure is delivered to achieve a desired volume, as long as the flow rate of the gas can be adjusted to ensure its delivery. It is the responsibility of the therapist to determine, in his own mind, what variables will respond to changes in adjustable controls for each ventilator he is expected to use. The opinion is expressed here that in the face of the unstable and interacting forces of obstruction and loss of compliance, the patient whose ventilation fails due to chronic obstructive disease can best be managed by a ventilator which gives independent control over pressure, flow rate, and I/E ratio. Both skill and patience are needed, for frequent resetting of controls assures the maintenance of ventilation through the shifting course of the disease; but maximum flexibility is thereby available to the therapist who is able to give tailor-made treatment to his patient.

Summary. To summarize the criteria for respirator selection, we must first observe that opinions today may be outmoded tomorrow as new and improved equipment is made available. The following suggestions are made to guide the therapist until his own thoughts are crystallized by experience: First, in the interest of the many factors noted above, basic reliance should be placed on the flow-adjustable, pressure-cycled ventilator (Bird, Bennett-PR) for all-around use, especially for its efficient, quick adaptation to emergency situations and for its versatility in ventilating serious airway obstruction. Second, for the less urgent patient and when normal or noncompliant lungs are to be ventilated rather than obstructed airways, consideration should be given to the use of positive-pressure, volume-cycled ventilators, although not to the complete exclusion of the IPPV. Third, negative-pressure ventilators should be limited to the relatively uncommon patient described above who is unobstructed and in whom intubation is to be avoided or who needs nocturnal support. Finally, an assistor-controller has the great advantage of facilitating gradual transition from controlled to assisted to independent breathing with a minimum change of equipment.

Instituting and maintaining ventilation

Most of the comments in this section will refer to the patient who is apneic or whose breathing is weak and ineffective and who thus needs complete ventilatory control. It will usually be obvious where they also apply to the assisted patient, but where necessary, this will be stipulated.

Tidal volume and rate. The first problem to be faced by the respiratory-care team is the determination of a suitable tidal volume and rate. For the adult patient with no spontaneous breathing, a rate is generally established somewhere between 15 and 20 breaths per minute, although this decision may have to be modified by tidal volume needs. Because of the great variations in body mass among the many patients being mechanically ventilated, the choice of tidal volume can be a difficult one. Obviously, an attempt is made to establish a pattern of breathing that will give the patient the best alveolar gas exchange, and the *only* way this can be determined is to measure arterial oxygen and carbon dioxide tensions and pH. We will emphasize a little later the necessity of this technique throughout the entire management period, but it should be stressed here that in many instances ventilation cannot be delayed while waiting for laboratory data. Often the initiation of artificial ventilation must rely upon clinical evaluation, and especially upon a background of extensive experience in treating respiratory failure. The highly skilled therapist will base his judgment upon the size of the patient, the depth and ease of chest movements during ventilation, and the many combinations of pressures and volumes that he has had occasion to use in the past. It is quite remarkable how effective this clinical approach can be when later confirmed by blood gas determinations.

The therapist is not without some assistance in setting combined tidal volumes and rates, as there are available nomograms to use as initial guidelines to get ventilation under way. Two such are provided for use with the Engström respirator, one each for children and adults.[259,260] These are complex charts based on a series of mathematical equations that consider such factors as estimated basal alveolar ventilation, body surface area, sex, age, breathing frequency, and tubing size. More applicable for general use is the Radford nomogram, a reproduction of which will be found in Appendix 13.[261] It should be clearly understood that no nomogram or formula for determining tidal or minute volumes is precise. The nomogram is used only to suggest a reasonable starting point with a minimum of delay, with necessary modifications as indicated by clinical observation or physiologic data. However, the Radford nomogram is useful because of the ease and speed with which it can be used, factors of great importance in the often hurried atmosphere of the failing patient. This chart bases its values on the three parameters of weight, respiratory rate, and sex; but it is vitally important to understand that the data refer to *basal* requirements in *healthy* subjects. This means that the chart is composed of information obtained from large numbers of healthy individuals, of a variety of sizes and ages, of both sexes, at complete rest, with all bodily functions at a minimal level of activity. Obviously, then, the direct information provided by the nomogram does not apply to the patient whose physiologic disturbance of his disease may raise his metabolic activity far above the basal level. To compensate for such effects of illness, provisions are made to adjust the nomogram values by specific percentages, according to the clinical situation. The effect of a tracheostomy on ventilatory needs is illustrated in the chart of nomogram corrections, permitting the reduction of basal tidal volume by a significant amount. Also, the adjustment referred to as the dead space of "anesthesia apparatus" reflects the anesthesia orientation of the nomogram but can equally be applied to a ventilator. When the nomogram is used for the apneic patient, respiratory frequency must be established that is consistent with the age as well as the tidal volume. If the patient has spontaneous breathing, the tidal volume actually moved by him is measured and compared with that predicted by the graph to see whether air movement is adequate or intervention is indicated. If the limitations of this nomogram are kept in mind and the therapist has good clinical understanding and judgment, he will find the chart useful. It should not be used by inexperienced personnel as a substitute for a clear understanding of the principles of mechanical ventilation.

Table 10-2. *Estimated basal tidal volume by age, weight, and sex*

Age (yr)	Normal frequency	Average weight (lb)	Tidal volume (ml)	
			Male	Female
Newborn	30-40	8	18- 22	18- 22
1	25-35	22	55- 70	55- 70
2	±28	27	80	80
3	±25	32	100	100
4- 6	20-25	36- 44	125-150	125-145
7- 9	20-25	50- 65	160-180	155-175
10-14	20-25	65-100	200-265	185-245
15-16	16-18	100-115	300-330	280-300
Adult	12-18	120	350	320
		130	370	340
		150	400	360
		175	450	400
		200	500	440
		225	540	460

On the basis of information from many sources as well as personal experience, the average basal tidal volumes by age, weight, and sex, from birth through adulthood are summarized in Table 10-2.[261-267]

It might be added that the tidal volumes of premature infants can be as low as 6 ml, making necessary the use of respirator exhalation heads that have as close to no dead space as possible. There is no value in the student's memorizing the above table, for it is intended only to emphasize the tremendous variation in tidal volumes with which he has to contend; and with continued experience, he will become familiar with a few key values that will enable him to start safe therapy while awaiting more specific guides.

The ventilatory pattern. We will be concerned not with theoretical pressure or flow curves but rather with those factors that contribute to establishing a pattern of breathing most helpful to the patient, emphasizing the clinical problems faced by the therapist.

RELATION OF PRESSURE, FLOW, VOLUME, AND RATIO. Once the desired frequency and tidal volume have been determined, volume-cycled ventilators are preset and activated and the actual delivered volume measured by a suitable meter. Slight adjustments are often necessary since the volume controls are not perfectly precise. If a pressure-cycled ventilator is used, a moderate to low starting pressure is chosen to initiate ventilation and is gradually increased to deliver the desired volume. Whatever instrument is used, an attempt is generally made to keep the pressure below 40 cm of water to minimize interference with the circulation, although this may be difficult in the presence of a significant reduction in compliance. To illustrate this with an oversimplified example, let us assume that we wish to deliver a tidal volume of 400 ml at a frequency of 16 breaths per minute but find that a pressure of 50 cm of water is needed. Because we know from our earlier studies of physiology that compliance tends to vary inversely with respiratory frequency, we will slow down the controlled rate and see whether ventilation can be accomplished with less force. Perhaps we will find that at a rate of 12 per minute the ventilator can deliver 533 ml of air at a pressure of but 40 cm of water, in which case we will provide the same total minute ventilation. Whether this increase in tidal volume is to the patient's advantage will be a matter of medical judgment to determine, but this fictitious example is presented to demonstrate the need for versatility by both therapist and ventilator in accommodating the requirements of respiratory failure.

Frequently patients will have spontaneous breathing but of a character too weak, rapid, or irregular to effect adequate alveolar gas exchange. In a clinical and physiologic sense, such patients are in failure as defined earlier, and it is often possible to "override" such spontaneous breathing with a volume ventilator. If complete control cannot be achieved at once over a rapid rate, the volume ventilator is adjusted to the patient's frequency and then attempts are made to reduce the rate of the instrument gradually, allowing the patient to accommodate to the slowing pace, which relieves him of much of the effort of breathing. The power of the volume-cycled respirators tends to discourage patient competition unless the spontaneous drive is strong, and in such instances safe ventilation may not be possible without modifying the patient's pattern, to be described below, or switching to a different type of ventilator. Semicontrolled ventilation may be achieved with a pressure-cycled machine in a patient with rapid but weak spontaneous breathing. This technique assists the patient's breathing rather than taking complete control over it but at the same time modifies its pattern. The instrument is adjusted for automatic controlled breathing at a rate less than the patient's own, and he is allowed to override the ventilator. If the patient is rationally responsive as he benefits from the assist to his breathing, he can sometimes be encouraged to relax his efforts and give in to the control of the respirator, letting his rate subside to a more efficient level. Even when the patient cannot be brought under full control, continued reassuring support by the therapist will often help the rapid breather to slow his efforts so that satisfactory, restful, assisted ventilation will assure good tidal air exchange. No matter what the technique, the object is to relieve the patient of excessive work, to reduce frequency to the normal range for his age and size, and to deliver to him an adequate tidal and minute volume.

There are no shortcuts to setting up a safe and effective respirator. Although the pressure-cycled machines are the most versatile and sensitive with the potential for fine control if properly used, they require the most skill and experience. It must be repeated here for emphasis that in the hands of the untrained such ventilators may constitute in themselves a serious hazard to the welfare of the patient. During fully controlled ventilation, attention must be given to the inspiratory-to-expiratory time ratio, the rationale for which has been sufficiently covered in previous discussions. Inspiratory time must never exceed expiratory, and in most instances a ratio of 1:1.5 or 1:2 will be safe. The surest way to establish the ratio is to use a stopwatch, but many experienced therapists have so trained their ears that they are remarkably accurate in balancing the respiratory phases merely by listening as they adjust the controls. This important step is not always easily or quickly accomplished, and the manner in which it is done depends upon the instrument used. With some, the matter is simply the adjustment of control switches (Air-Shields, Emerson); with others, it is dependent upon regulating the flow rate control (Bourns, Bennett MA-1); and with yet others, the ratio is machine fixed (Engström, Bennett PR-2). However, we know that even with the PR-2 the ratio can be modified, so that it is not entirely nonadjustable. On the other hand, the Bird respirator, because it is so amenable to custom setting, offers a good example to use for reviewing the intricacies of the I/E ratio. Fundamentally, controlled inspiratory time depends upon the flow rate at a given pressure setting, whereas expiration is regulated by its own mechanism; and the student must remember the interrelationships between flow, pressure, time, and frequency. For convenience, these are summarized in Table 10-3, which does nothing more than compact in columns what we have already described in some detail. The table compares the effects of various combinations of pressure and flow rate on inspiratory time and frequency. Horizontal arrows mean no change; double arrows imply a greater response than a single. For example, increasing the pressure while decreasing flow rate increases (prolongs) inspiratory time more than if flow were kept stable.

Once the desired combination of mask pressure and tidal volume has been established, the I/E ratio is adjusted by individually timing inspiration and expiration, while still maintaining a constant frequency. Let us suppose that we have set a Bird-type ventilator so that a delivery pressure of 30 cm of water provides the tidal volume we feel the patient needs and we wish the breathing pattern to be one of 20 breaths per minute with an I/E ratio of 1:2. This means that each breath will be of 3 seconds' duration, of which inspiration

Table 10-3. *Relationship between P, V, inspiratory time, and frequency*

	P↑			P↓			V̇↑			V̇↓		
P							→	↓	↑	→	↓	↑
V̇	→	↓	↑	→	↓	↑						
Inspiratory time	↑	↑↑	→	↓	→	↓↓	↓	↓↓	→	↑	→	↑↑
Frequency	↓	↓↓	→	↑	→	↑↑	↑	↑↑	→	↓	→	↓↓

will comprise 1 second and exhalation 2 seconds. We will first adjust the control that regulates the time interval between inspirations to get our expiratory time. This will remain independent of other controls since it is activated by end-inspiration, and its duration is determined by the speed of its bleed-off. The 1-second inspiratory phase will be set by appropriately changing the flow rate, increasing it to reduce inspiration and decreasing to prolong it. In the absence of any variable factors that might change the dynamics of ventilation, we should now have set the respirator to deliver our predetermined tidal volume at a safe pressure, at a frequency consistent with the size and age of the patient, and with a phase ratio that we feel will protect the patient from harmful pressure effects.

However, if our patient has chronic bronchopulmonary obstructive disease, we must be prepared to make frequent readjustments because the compliance-obstruction status of his airways changes frequently. In addition to bronchospasm, which may well be present, the shifting of secretions in the respiratory tract and their periodic removal by therapeutic aspiration will keep the status of the airways in a state of continual flux. This is why the obstructed patient in failure must be kept under constant observation and the controls of his respirator frequently changed to maintain as constant ventilation as possible in the face of an unstable tract. Such a patient may put the inhalation therapist's skill to a severe test and often requires his full-time services. Let us now imagine that the compliance drops in the patient we attended in the preceding paragraph. We will find that our machine can no longer deliver the required tidal volume at the initial pressure of 30 cm of water; to restore this volume, we must increase the system pressure. As soon as we do this, we note that the inspiratory time increases since more time is required to transmit the higher pressure to the patient's lungs at the original flow rate. With a prolongation of inspiration, not only is the I/E ratio disturbed, but the total frequency drops because the expiratory time is unaffected and remains unchanged. Obviously, to restore the initial ventilatory pattern, we will have to increase the flow rate accordingly and bring the inspiratory time back to its original value. If our patient's problem is primarily one of loss of compliance, we can continue to increase both pressure and flow rate to deliver a constant tidal volume, up to the limits of the ventilator or to the limit of physiologic safety for the patient. On the other hand, if varying degrees of airway obstruction complicate the condition, our task will be much more difficult.

We are well aware of the problems of ventilating an obstructed passage with pressure-driven air and the great need to be able to vary the flow rate to compensate for such obstruction. If our patient suddenly reduces the effective caliber of his bronchi by spasm or an outpouring of secretions, the back pressure so generated will match the system pressure and cycle end-inspiration before delivery of the full tidal volume and, in this instance, inspiratory time will be markedly shortened. We have a choice of two maneuvers to try to restore tidal ventilation. First, we can increase the system pressure as we did with the compliance defect above, which will prolong the inspiratory time; but our knowledge of gas kinetics tells us that to overcome the pressure drop due to obstruction by this method will probably elevate the intrathoracic pressure to dangerously high levels. Second, we can make use of the variable flow control of our ventilator and drop the flow rate, which will significantly reduce the pressure gradient across the obstruction and deliver a larger pressure (and gas volume) distally with a minimum system pressure and prolong inspiratory time. The response of inspiratory time to both these combinations of pressure and flow are indicated in Table 10-3. However, merely slowing the delivered flow will not necessarily be satisfactory, for overcoming the obstruction may require an inspiratory time so long that the reduced minute rate will prevent an adequate minute alveolar ventilation despite the desired pressure and tidal volume. Also, if the inspiratory time is too prolonged, it can seriously upset the optimum I/E ratio. When faced with this problem, the therapist must be prepared to spend a considerable period of time trying to achieve a compromise balance between the many factors involved because there is no standard procedural guide to follow. He will probably find that a combination of lowering the flow rate and elevating the pressure in gradual steps will give him the best control over the ventilation. In addition, he may find that he will have to settle for a reduced frequency to accommodate a necessarily prolonged inspiratory time and then will try to increase the tidal volume enough to assure a safe minute volume. At any rate, he will be aware that a change in either pressure or flow rate will change the entire balance between pressure, flow, inspiratory time, and frequency; and he will soon develop the patience required to reset controls as he finds it necessary to keep up with ventilation needs. His goal will be the lowest system pressure at the lowest flow rate that will deliver the desired tidal volume at a normal frequency and with a safe I/E ratio.

Reference should be made here to the automatic flow adjustability of the Bennett PR respirator. The sensitivity of the main valve slows down gas flow in the presence of distal obstruction but allows flow to continue to the patient as long as it is in excess of 1 liter per minute. The pneumatic timers prevent the I/E ratio from exceeding 1:1.5. In this instrument some manual influence over flow can be achieved by reducing machine output through use of the peak flow control, and, of course, the delivered pressure can also be adjusted. The automatic responsiveness of the Bennett does not mean that it is a simple instrument to operate, for its safe and effective use requires a full understanding of the mechanical relationships of its parts. It is again emphasized that the choice between these two major positive-pressure ventilators is a matter of the operator's preference for either partial automatic function or freer control over each variable setting.

PERIODIC HYPERVENTILATION. If the student will observe his own quiet breathing during a prolonged period of bodily relaxation, as during a reading session, he will note a phenomenon so natural that he is usually unaware of it. Every now and then he will unconsciously sigh, often rather deeply. The significance of this act and its importance to mechanical ventilation became clear with the rapid increase in use of ventilators. During periods of physical inaction, as metabolic needs approach basal levels, depth of ventilation decreases and the distribution of intrapulmonary inspired air becomes irregular. Some pulmonary units are poorly expanded by the low level of ventilation and get less than adequate air exchange. This sets up localized areas of decreased ventilation-perfusion ratios, which actually constitute small physiologic shunts. In the normal subject, with active respiratory control mechanisms, this presents no hazard because the natural periodic sigh hyperinflates the lung, expanding and aerating all segments. It had been frequently noted, however, that patients maintained on supposedly adequate mechanically ventilated patterns often suffered deterioration of their pulmonary status and became progressively more difficult to ventilate. A detailed study on anesthetized patients demonstrated the cause for this unfavorable response.[268] Ventilatory and physiologic studies showed that prolonged artificial ventilation at an unvarying tidal volume level leads to a gradual and progressive atelectasis. As increasing respiratory units become airless, significant arterial-venous shunting, or venous admixture, develops; and the pulmonary compliance steadily drops. Further, it was found that this phenomenon could be both prevented and corrected by periodic hyperinflation of the lungs, the introduction into the breathing pattern of an artificial sigh.

Part of the management of the ventilated patient on complete control is the use of the periodic sigh, and some respirators have a mechanism to accomplish this automatically—notably the Emerson volume ventilator and the Bennett MA-1. Controls allow one or two deep breaths to be delivered at preset intervals. With other instruments it is advisable to hyperinflate the lungs with two deep breaths at least every half hour. Manual sighing can be done with the Bird respirator by holding open the cycling valve, for which purpose a rod is provided that extends to the outside of the instrument from the ambient end of the valve. The Bennett PR ventilators can be used to sigh the patient by holding open the rotating valve with a finger on its small projecting rod and increasing the terminal flow. Clinical judgment dictates the hyperinflating volume to be so used, but the short duration of the maneuver holds little risk for the patient.

SUSTAINED HYPERVENTILATION. The student and the practicing therapist may sometimes find in the medical literature opinions and recommendations advising that hyperventilation of the apneic or hypoventilating patient is advisable to avoid the ill effects of hypoventilation. This principle employs a philosophy of overcompensation, holding that excessive treatment is safer than undertreatment; but it is a belief that is completely unacceptable to the modern, rational treatment of respiratory failure. In earlier chapters we discussed the response of the acid-base balance of the body to ventilation and the hazards of respiratory alkalosis accompanying hyperventilation. It should be readily appreciated that the patient in respiratory failure is already severely ill and that there is no justification for subjecting him to additional physiologic trauma; for the consequences of ventilator-induced alkalosis are potentially grave. The patient may suffer tetany, convulsive spasms due to marked increased reactivity of muscles. A warning of this impending condition may be jumpiness of the patient in response to ordinary stimuli or may be elicited by tapping the patient's cheek and noting a spasmodic contraction of the facial muscles of the tested side. Especially hazardous is an interference with cerebral blood flow, about which more will be said in detail below. A fall in the concentration of serum potassium has been frequently noted in respiratory alkalosis, believed to be due to movement of potassium ions from the serum into the cells to replace hydrogen ions that are depleted because of the alkalosis. The hypokalemia (low serum potassium concentration) renders the myocardium susceptible to arrhythmias, especially if the heart is already hypoxic or if it is under digitalis treatment. In the latter instance, digitalis toxicity may be precipitated. Finally, alkalosis produces an unfavorable shift in the oxygen dissociation curve, impairing the cellular uptake of oxygen.

The greatest caution must be exercised in ventilating the patient with normal lungs, for he is the easiest to ventilate. It was noted above that in the absence of obstruction or loss of compliance, almost any standard respirator can be used effectively. With such a patient, however, there is the ever-present risk of overzealous therapy, especially true if the therapist is simultaneously supervising the management of a patient who is hard to ventilate.

Let us consider the patient with chronic bronchopulmonary disease who is in respiratory acidosis with characteristically elevated arterial carbon dioxide tension and low pH. It is natural that all members of the medical team are anxious to restore the blood values to normal as soon as possible, for this gives reassurance of effective treatment and subsiding danger; but it is not necessary to bring down the carbon dioxide level precipitously. This is especially true if the hypercapnia is of significant duration and less important if it is acutely elevated. Thus, if the hypercapnia has suddenly risen, it can be more safely corrected rapidly than if it gradually rose over a long time. There are two physiologic reasons for this differentiation—one somewhat speculative, the other positive. First, with vascular dilatation of the cerebral circulation as a major response to high levels of carbon dioxide, any increase in cerebral blood flow due to sudden hypercapnia in all probability is somewhat "extra," being superimposed on whatever has been the usual perfusion of the brain in the given subject, and the removal of this additional flow by rapid excretion of carbon dioxide returns the cerebral blood flow to its own normal. In contrast, prolonged hypercapnia may condition the cerebral circulation to an increased level of perfusion and when suddenly reduced will produce an ischemia of the brain by deprivation of its usual blood supply. This reaction may manifest itself as a period of mental sluggishness or confusion or may produce the signs and symptoms of an acute stroke, with characteristic speech difficulties or muscular weakness, depending upon the location of the brain area affected and the severity of the condition. By and large, chronic hypercapnia is more apt to be found in advanced-age patients since respiratory failure may develop only after many years, whereas sudden, acute uncompensated hypercapnia is more prevalent in the younger patients subject to chest and head trauma, narcosis and anesthesia, and central nervous system infectious diseases. Thus, the patient with acute failure superimposed on chronic hypercapnia often has a preexisting compromised cerebral circulation due to degenerative vascular disease, and his brain is more sensitive to alterations in its circulation than is the one with normal circulation.

We are most commonly concerned with the second reason, which is related to the acid-base status of the body. The more acute the hypercapnia, the more uncompensated is the acidosis, simply because there has not been time for the body to meet the challenge by increasing its available supply of buffering bicarbonate. Basically, the problem in this instance is one of a suddenly high carbon dioxide tension and low pH, and if the excess carbon dioxide can be excreted by the ventilatory route, the acid-base balance will readily return to normal. Much more treacherous to manage is the patient with a chronic but low-grade hypercapnia due to long-standing disease in whom a respiratory infection, for example, has acutely depressed ventilation, pushing him into overt failure. This patient may have as high a carbon dioxide tension in his blood as the one cited above, but his pH will not be as low because he already has an increased bicarbonate accompanying his chronic hypercapnia and is thereby in partial compensated respiratory acidosis. If the excess carbon dioxide should be rapidly depleted, and it need not even reach a normal level, large quantities of extra bicarbonate will be left circulating and the pH can easily jump from a severe acidosis to an iatrogenic alkalosis of serious proportions. As an example of the tremendous acid-base swing that can result from overly aggressive treatment, there is the recorded instance of an arterial pH that leaped from 7.10 to 7.80 in 10 minutes.[269] One can only speculate what effect this must have had on the cerebral circulation and the conductivity of the myocardium. The therapist must keep in mind that in many, if not most, patients, intensive therapy can lower the carbon dioxide tension fairly readily; but accumulated bicarbonate can be removed only by renal excretion, and it may take a normally functioning kidney 2 to 3 days to rid the body of an excess load of the antacid. Since many patients in respiratory failure have imperfect renal function, the result of either hypoxia or other accompanying disease, it is easy to see how they may be driven from the frying pan into the fire in terms of their acid-base balance if they are not treated prudently.

The use of buffers poses another ventilation problem with which the therapist should be familiar because it may compound the effect of the elevated bicarbonate of metabolic compensation in respiratory acidosis. There has been a great deal of disagreement over the use of buffers in respiratory acidosis, stemming mostly from a failure to appreciate the physiologic differences between respiratory and metabolic acidosis. For years, part of the standard treatment of metabolic acidosis has been the intravenous administration of sodium bicarbonate (or sodium lactate, which is metabolized in the body to produce bicarbonate) to neutralize excess acid according to the following nonspecific reaction:

$$NaHCO_3 + HA \rightleftharpoons NaA + H_2CO_3$$
$$H_2CO_3 \rightleftharpoons H_2O + CO_2\uparrow$$

Success of this reaction depends upon the ability of the body to remove, by blowing off through the lungs, the carbon dioxide formed. The patient with metabolic acidosis, as from the accumulation of organic acids accompanying diabetes or renal failure, can readily remove large volumes of carbon dioxide if he has no associated pulmonary disease. Indeed, one of the clinical characteristics of such a patient is severe hyperventilation. However, the student will recall that metabolic acidosis disturbs the Henderson-Hassalbalch equation by decreasing the numerator as the normal body bicarbonate is depleted by the abnormal circulating acids. In such a circumstance, it is logical to replace bicarbonate therapeutically and so restore normal balance. The biochemical situation is different in respiratory acidosis, especially if it is chronic. In the first place, if we substitute for acid *HA* in the above reaction the characteristic acid of respiratory failure, H_2CO_3, the added $NaHCO_3$ merely builds up to high levels because the inherent disability of respiratory acidosis is the inability of the body to blow off even normal amounts of carbon dioxide. Second, when we view respiratory acidosis in terms of acid-base balance, we find it is the result of an increase in the denominator of the H-H equation, not fundamentally a deficiency in bicarbonate. In short, we come back to the basic principle of therapy of respiratory acidosis—acid-base balance can be restored only by actively ridding the body of excess carbon dioxide, not by adding increasing amounts of bicarbonate. Suppose a patient has the extreme physiologic values we used earlier in Table 4-6 to illustrate acid-base balance, with a bicarbonate–to–carbon dioxide ratio of 24/2.4 mM/liter and a pH of 7.10. Even if we add enough bicarbonate to the patient's blood to raise its level to 48 mM/liter, restore a 20/1 ratio, and bring the pH up to 7.40, we still will not correct his basic defect. As long as his CO_2 remains elevated, he will be in severe failure although temporarily compensated.

Since it is established that mechanically ventilating the patient in respiratory failure is the fundamental treatment, let us return to our subject of hyperventilation and see just what are its risks. We will use as examples two fictitious treatment situations as shown in Fig. 10-5, making certain assumptions for the sake of clarity. Let us imagine a patient before respiratory failure with the blood findings of box A, the acid-base ratio expressed in millimoles per liter with the equivalent carbon dioxide tension, and the pH consistent with the ratio. Let us now assume our patient develops respiratory failure

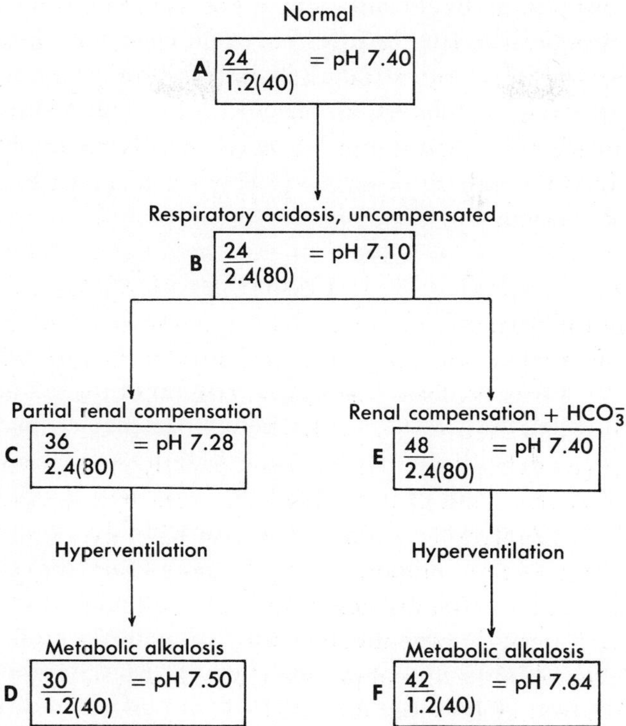

Fig. 10-5. Schematic outline of the hazard of deliberate hyperventilation in the treatment of respiratory acidosis. The mechanisms by which metabolic alkalosis can be induced are described in detail in the text.

(box *B*) with no evident compensation at this stage and a subsequent marked drop in his pH. At this point we can permit normal renal compensation to do what it can to minimize the acidosis (box *C*), or we can actively assist this function with the parenteral administration of bicarbonate (box *E*). If we follow the first course, we may find that the physiologic conservation of bicarbonate will elevate the numerator of the H-H equation, let us say for example, to 36 mM per liter and partially relieve the acidosis by raising the pH to 7.28. Because the carbon dioxide tension is still high and, thus, the underlying hypoventilation uncorrected, we place the patient on a mechanical ventilator and, in our enthusiasm to restore his carbon dioxide to normal, overventilate him. After a few hours of therapy we may find that we have completely corrected his hypercapnia but, because renal bicarbonate excretion lags behind carbon dioxide removal, perhaps the patient's bicarbonate has dropped only to 30 mM per liter and we have now pushed the patient from a severe respiratory acidosis to a moderate metabolic alkalosis. Although a metabolic swing of this magnitude may not be of any great significance in most patients, it may be in some; and it indicates the ease with which therapy can overcompensate. Let us now consider the possibilities if we follow the second course and give the patient bicarbonate because it seems reasonable to treat acidity with an antacid. The combination of renal compensation plus administered bicarbonate (box *E*) may effect rapid and complete ratio balance and quickly restore the pH to normal. Assisted ventilation will still be necessary, of course, and the student should realize that starting with a higher bicarbonate level in this instance, with effective ventilation, will make it difficult, if not impossible, to avoid leaving the patient with a significant bicarbonate excess. Box *F* assumes a response similar to that described in the first course, namely a rapid removal of carbon dioxide but with a concomitant reduction in bicarbonate of only 6 mM per liter, giving the patient a severe metabolic alkalosis.

With the above discussion as a background to impress upon the student the need for caution in establishing the depth of mechanical ventilation, let us now consider what role, if any, buffers can play in managing respiratory failure. To begin with, the student may wonder why there should be a controversy over a procedure that apparently holds so much risk. Until the tremendous development of interest over the past two decades, in pulmonary diseases and their physiologic effects, the training of most physicians oriented their views of acid-base disturbances as being metabolically generated. The physician was well versed in recognizing acidosis and alkalosis resulting from metabolic, gastrointestinal, and renal diseases and the surgical and postoperative states, to mention a few of the common conditions. He was thus used to treating acidosis, generally, with bicarbonate replacement; and it has been difficult for him to accept the concept of "acidosis" where this was not an immediate need. Naturally, as chest medicine has become an increasingly important specialty, there has been a growing understanding of the influence of pulmonary physiology on the acid-base status; and successive groups of young physicians are becoming more skilled in respiratory management. Perhaps the student can see for himself where the judicious use of bicarbonate may contribute to the overall treatment of respiratory failure. It is indicated in those patients who have severe acidosis, with a reduction in pH to levels that are a hazard to cellular survival, in whom there has been a negligible metabolic compensatory response. This is exemplified by the patient who does not have chronic hypercapnia due to long-standing bronchopulmonary disease and in whom there is no chronically elevated bicarbonate but who, for one reason or other, develops sudden carbon dioxide retention. To avoid the damage to this patient's enzyme systems and other cellular functions by subjecting them to a severely acidotic environment, *partial* neutralization of the patient's acidosis by increasing his store of bicarbonate is justifiable. Partial neutralization is further indicated in patients with a combination of metabolic and respiratory acidosis, for in them the ventilator therapy will not correct the underlying metabolic disorder; and the careful use of both modalities will maintain the smoothest acid-base balance. However, such therapy is acceptable only if the physician recognizes it as a stopgap measure to be employed until results can be obtained from definitive assisted ventilation and if he is fully aware of the potential risk of overcompensation. In contrast, the use of supplemental bicarbonate in the patient with an already elevated bicarbonate from renal compensation is extremely hazardous, and the development of a metabolic alkalosis is almost inevitable. It is a wise precaution for the therapist asked to set up mechanical ventilation to inquire of the medical attendant whether the patient has been given bicarbonate.

As a point of interest to the therapist, although not as relevant to his function as is bicarbonate, is the occasional use of a buffer known as tris-buffer, or THAM. Not a true buffer in the sense that a buffer is a substance which, when added to a solution, resists changes in hydrogen ion concentration with the further addition of acid or alkali, THAM is a hydrogen ion acceptor. Chemically known as tris(hydroxymethyl)aminomethane, in the presence of an acid THAM will form a salt. Given by infusion, it has the advantages over bicarbonate of not producing carbon dioxide that must be exhaled, of containing no sodium, which is undesirable in the presence of edema, and of having diuretic properties. On the other hand, it is slow acting, produces a drop in blood sugar, causes a loss of potassium, can be excreted only by the kidney, and, most importantly, causes hypoventilation. Its acceptance in respiratory care has not been wide, although it has been more extensively used in metabolic disorders; and the feeling seems to be that, since the patient must be ventilated to counteract its hypoventilating effect, THAM probably has little to offer except to elevate a severely depressed pH during acute failure, as noted above for bicarbonate.

We can summarize our comments on the risks of hyperventilation by stating that although the primary need of the patient in respiratory failure is a mechanically increased alveolar ventilation, such ventilation must be done cautiously and carefully. Especially must judgment be used in treating the patient with chronic hypercapnia and superimposed acute failure, for too great enthusiasm can easily precipitate a potentially harmful metabolic alkalosis to replace his acidosis. Supplemental systemic buffers must be used with great reservation, if at all, and every member of the therapeutic team must be aware of the risk involved. The final objective of mechanical ventilation is to return carbon dioxide tension and pH to as close to normal as possible, not to overcompensate. There are times when the so-called normals for a given patient may not be identical with the normals associated with a healthy subject. In some patients with chronic hypercapnia and with adequate compensation prior to acute failure, it may be satisfactory to return carbon dioxide levels to those with which they have become adjusted. The therapist can be assured that his treatment is safe and effective if he first stops the rise in carbon dioxide tension and drop in pH and then notes that both are beginning to return to normal. From then on, as long as the progress is steady, it makes little difference how long the treatment takes; and it is safer to bring down a very high carbon dioxide over a period of 2 to 3 days than in a matter of hours.

Suppression of ventilation. It may be impossible to ventilate adequately a patient with strong spontaneous breathing no matter what instrument is used. Although machine override is often possible, a pattern of breathing that is rapid and shallow or grossly irregular may be forceful enough not to submit to the drive of a preset ventilator. In addition, the patient may "fight the machine," consciously or otherwise, because he is severely hypoxic, is fearful or apprehensive, or is mentally unable to cooperate. In such a patient, to continue to assist him is only to perpetuate his pattern, leading to a steady deterioration of his respiratory status. Most often the patient will be breathing very rapidly with shallow tidal volumes and is subjected to the following two hazards: First, the tremendous amount of physical work expended in rapid breathing will gradually deplete his energy. Second, rapid shallow breathing is essentially dead space breathing, and although at great energy cost the patient may move large minute air volumes, all that he accomplishes is ventilation of his dead space, leaving his alveoli relatively unventilated. If he is responsive to metabolic oxygen needs, the resulting hypoxia will continue the ineffective, tiring respiratory pattern. As a general rule, this risk is not great in adults until the frequency exceeds 25, and then, depending upon the conductance (opposite of resistance) and compliance of the lung-thorax, rate increases are apt to be accompanied by reduced tidal volumes.

The condition of the patient with strong, ineffective spontaneous respirations who cannot be brought under at least partial control is a grave one, and his very survival may depend upon the ability of the medical team to correct the deficiency. As soon as it becomes evident that effective assistance or conformance to control is not possible, there is nothing to gain and much to lose by further delay. The decision must be made to abolish the patient's own breathing and place him under complete ventilator control. This is a responsibility of the patient's attending physician, although the technical management will fall upon the assigned therapist. The responsibility that this technique entails cannot be emphasized too strongly, for when we decide to interfere with natural processes as vital as breathing, thus asserting that we can do better for the patient than he can do himself, we are assuming a great burden. The therapist should appreciate that this is not exactly the same as attempting to restore to a patient a function that he has lost completely through injury or disease. Instead, it is the use of our judgment as to the quality and performance of the patient's ability to provide his basic physiologic need, deciding that he is inadequate in this function, destroying it, and supplanting it with an artificial substitute of our choosing. This statement is not intended to overdramatize a procedure for which there is no alternative if the patient is to survive, but it is important that the therapist realize the full depth of his commitment to the patient who is completely helpless and totally dependent upon his medical attendants. Respiratory suppression should be undertaken only where facilities are adequate for complete care and in the physical presence of a responsible physician and inhalation therapist. We will describe the three common techniques currently used—suppression by oxygen, by morphine, and by neuromuscular blocking agents.

OXYGEN SUPPRESSION OF BREATHING. This procedure is especially effective for the patient with long-standing chronic hypercapnia, whose ventilation has been dependent to a considerable degree upon the hypoxic drive that has replaced the damaged function of his respiratory center. It is of interest that in this instance we employ, as therapy, a technique we strongly condemn otherwise. Earlier we discussed in detail the role played by chemoreceptors in the event of respiratory center failure accompanying progressive and chronic pulmonary disease. We stressed the great hazard in administering oxygen promiscuously to such a patient for fear of satisfying hypoxia, thus inactivating the hypoxic chemoreceptor drive and rendering the patient apneic. Now we do exactly that—inactivate the hypoxic chemoreceptor drive—so that we can eliminate the patient's own breathing and ventilate him artificially. The patient is given 100% oxygen through the assisting ventilator or by means of a tracheotomy mask, if he is so intubated, for a period not to exceed 10 minutes; results should be realized in that length of time if at all. As he becomes hypopneic and his respiratory energy decreases, he is put on ventilator control and the oxygen concentration is reduced to a safe level. Close observation must be maintained to ensure that the patient remains under adequate control and does not return to his previous pattern. If this procedure is not successful, then one of the following must be employed.

MORPHINE SUPPRESSION OF BREATHING. Morphine sulfate is a potent addicting narcotic with the ability to relieve pain, produce lethargy, and induce a deep to stuporous sleep. One of its most specific activities, however, is its depression of respiration by directly suppressing the activity of the medullary respiratory center. Like high concentrations of oxygen, morphine is contraindicated in general medical use in any patient with compromised breathing; and many deaths have been attributed to it in patients with asthma, chronic bronchopulmonary disease, and cerebral injury. The respiratory depressant effect of morphine is directly related to dose and is evident to slight degrees even with small doses given—for example, for pain relief. The respiratory response is a decrease in both frequency and tidal volume.

When used to stop spontaneous breathing, morphine can be best controlled if given by intravenous injection. By this route, maximum respiratory depression for a given dose occurs within 10 minutes, as compared to 1 hour or more if given intramuscularly. There are no hard-and-fast rules for its administration, but a good basic program is 5 mg intravenously, repeated every 10 minutes until the desired effect is realized, to a maximum of 20 mg for the series. In most patients, if morphine is to be effective, it will be before this amount of the drug has been used. For maintenance, 2 to 3 mg can be given as needed to keep the patient well relaxed. The duration of morphine therapy is usually too short to warrant concern over addiction, but there are occasional side effects that can prove troublesome. Among the most common are nausea and vomiting, which sometimes preclude further use of the drug. Occasionally morphine causes hypotension and must be used very cautiously, if at all, in the patient in insipient or overt shock. The automatic movements of the intestine, or peristalsis, are retarded or stopped by morphine; and this can lead to gaseous distention of the bowel severe enough to impair diaphragmatic motion and interfere with ventilation. The patient's face and neck may appear flushed, and he may complain of itching of the skin or nose as the effects of the drug subside. Generally speaking, the intravenous administration of morphine is a safe and effective method of suppressing unwanted spontaneous ventilation and relaxing the patient so that he may be ventilated effectively. It has often been lifesaving.

NEUROMUSCULAR BLOCKING AGENTS TO SUPPRESS BREATHING. A neuromuscular blocking agent is a drug that blocks the transmission of motor nerve impulses to skeletal muscles, effectively paralyzing those muscles. They are widely used in surgery to gain maximum muscular relaxation along with anesthesia, making manipulation of muscular tissues much easier by eliminating their normal tonal contraction. For suppression of respiration, total body paralysis is not usually necessary, only enough relaxation to allow overriding of spontaneous ventilation. With minimal side effects, they are rapid in action and effective but must be used only under the closest supervision. There are two preparations in common use—*d*-tubocurarine and succinylcholine.

d-Tubocurarine. This is a plant alkaloid whose paralyzing action has been known for centuries and which has been widely used in anesthesiology for many years. Although large doses may precipitate hypotension, the major hazard of *d*-tubocurarine is respiratory paralysis, the object of our interest in it. When given intravenously, the route of choice, its action is evident in 3 to 5 minutes, lasting about 40 minutes; and doses of 15 mg may be used almost as needed until the desired effect is reached. In case of a mishap or overdosage, neostigmine methylsulfate should be available as an antidote.

Succinylcholine (Anectine). Although a neuromuscular blocking agent like *d*-tubocurarine, succinylcholine differs chemically and in its mode of action. Also given intravenously, it starts acting in less than 1 minute, reaches its maximum in 2 minutes, and disappears within 5 minutes. It has been used in general surgery to provide rapid relaxation for short procedures such as instrumentation. For respiratory suppression, a single dose of 20 mg may be given to test the patient's response or to initiate ventilation and may be repeated as needed until a good ventilatory pattern is established. A smoother response will accompany its prolonged administration in an intravenous infusion, as a 0.1% solution, run at a rate of 2 to 3 mg per minute. By this method, because the action is so short, very close control over the depth of paralysis can be maintained merely by adjusting the infusion flow rate.

Correcting hypoxia. The general subject of oxygen therapy was covered in Chapter 8, and we will only attempt to correlate certain aspects of it with mechanical ventilation and some specific needs of respiratory failure. Most of the emphasis in our discussion of ventilators centered about the importance of alveolar ventilation and the removal of carbon dioxide, but we must not forget that the most pressing need of the patient in failure is the correction of hypoxia. Unless our ventilation can assure him a viable level of arterial oxygen, our efforts will be of no avail. In most instances of significant respiratory failure, we will have hypoxia and hypercapnia as simultaneous problems with which to contend; and our thinking must encompass both when planning management.

We have been almost dogmatic in our insistence that oxygen administration in ventilatory failure be accompanied by assisted ventilation to avoid the potential hazard of worsening the patient's ventilatory drive, but now that the fundamental precautions of such therapy are well understood, let us examine the state of failure to see whether any modifications are justified. Obviously, we are not concerned with the risk of apnea in all hypoxic patients, and if we feel that a given patient has an adequate alveolar ventilation, we do not hesitate to give him oxygen as needed. Perhaps there are patients with some degree of hypoventilation who also can be treated with oxygen unsupported by mechanical ventilation. There are many who feel that a trial of oxygen therapy may safely be given when hypercapnia and acidosis appear to be less a risk to the patient than his hypoxia, thereby hopefully avoiding the need for unnecessary intubation and the additional risks inherent in artificial ventilation. This has been studied by many authors, and the following program is suggested as one way to institute therapy[205]: Arterial blood gas values are obtained as soon as possible while the patient is breathing room air. If the oxygen tension is less than 60 mm Hg (some use 50 mm Hg as the limit) and the pH is above 7.30, the patient is started on a very low oxygen flow, usually by catheter. Since the method employs trial and error, follow-up blood studies are essential; and if a given level of oxygen flow maintains the blood values within the limits specified above, it is continued. If hypoxia is still not corrected, the oxygen flow is increased by very small increments until an arterial oxygen tension of at least 60 mm Hg is reached, provided the pH does not fall at the same time. Should it not be possible to oxygenate the patient without the development of progressive acidosis, then the patient is intubated and given supported mechanical ventilation. This is a conservative approach and, if followed under careful observation, may be expected to be successful in many patients whose ventilatory defects are due to readily reversible conditions. If oxygen is given by oropharyngeal catheter, 2 to 3 liters per minute often suffice for moderate hypoxia and are not apt to cause alarming elevations in arterial carbon dioxide tension unless the ventilation-perfusion balance is seriously disturbed.[270] Unfortunately, many patients with ventilatory failure due to chronic bronchopulmonary disease have such a ventilation-perfusion imbalance as a major contributor to their disability. The venturi mask lends itself well to this type of therapy, for it will deliver a prefixed and relatively stable oxygen concentration at high enough flows to satisfy almost any ventilatory demand; but, of course, it does not guarantee any specific blood oxygen level.[194, 195, 203]

If mechanical ventilation is necessary to prevent progressive hypercapnia and respiratory acidosis, the therapist will have to use the ventilator as a medium to supply oxygen. In Chapter 9 he learned how unreliable is the oxygen diluter on the pressure-cycled machine, and yet he is aware of the need to avoid the delivery of high oxygen concentrations because of the risk of fatal lung damage with prolonged administration. He also has learned that the ventilatory problem he is trying to solve may make it difficult to avoid high inspired oxygen concentrations if he is using a pressure-cycled ventilator in the face of reduced pulmonary compliance. The relationship between the prolonged inspiration often necessary to ventilate stiff lungs and the subsequent rise in oxygen in the inspired air makes it difficult to control the oxygen delivered to such a patient. In the absence of significant loss of compliance, it is somewhat reassuring to note that the short inspiratory phase best suited to circulatory stability also helps to maintain minimal oxygen concentrations with an open air-mix in an IPPV.

There are steps to take to control the delivered oxygen concentration, depending upon the type of ventilator used. It is fairly simple in the volume ventilator by adding oxygen to the air that is the basic gas used by the machine. The structure of the volume machine makes available a chamber in which the gases can readily be mixed, and for each instrument there is provided by the manufacturer either a guide table or a mechanical control by which to adjust the oxygen flow rate to obtain a given concentration under specific operating conditions. It is still necessary to analyze samples of delivered gas to determine the exact concentrations in case of malfunction or maladjustment of the diluting mechanism. The problem is a bit more complicated in the pressure-cycled ventilator, and there are three general ways it can be met. First, it is often satisfactory to operate the ventilator off a source of compressed air, a compressor, central supply, or a cylinder and to add oxygen to the patient-supply circuit. A large humidifier is a good place to accomplish this. Such a method is strictly trial and error, and the mixed gas must be measured for its oxygen content. Changes in the breathing pattern, especially in the assist mode, can change the balance between source and added gases, necessitating frequent examination of the delivered gas in order to maintain any stability in oxygen delivery. Second, a tank of a prepared known concentration of oxygen can be used as the power source gas, a popular mixture being 40% oxygen in 60% nitrogen since this concentration of oxygen is generally safe and effective. There are some practical disadvantages to this technique, however. Prepared cylinder gases are expensive, and they are cumbersome to move and store in the patient's room, especially where the inhalation therapy service is adjusted to a central oxygen supply. More important is the need to operate the respirator on the so-called

"100% oxygen setting," since dilution of the source cylinder gas by entrained room air will defeat the purpose of its use. For the Bird respirator, this means the loss of one of its most valuable characteristics, pneumatic clutching, which depends upon activation of the venturi by an open air-mix control, as explained in Chapter 9. Third, dependable mixing valves are available that can mix source oxygen with air to deliver predetermined oxygen concentrations.[271] They are designed to maintain constant concentrations at all available flow rates, as long as the mixed gases have similar densities, as do oxygen and air. These appliances are useful for volume ventilators as well as for the therapeutic administration of unassisted oxygen but present the same difficulty for the Bird respirator as does the cylinder gas.

The use of helium-oxygen mixtures will be noted only in passing because of its detailed coverage in Chapter 8. Helium-oxygen should always be considered when oxygenation of a mechanically ventilated patient is unsuccessful because of severe diffuse bronchial obstruction. A pressure-cycled ventilator is a good vehicle for the administration of the mixture if the patient has a well-cuffed airway tube, but it must be operated with its air-mix closed.

Monitoring mechanical ventilation. The need for close observation of the mechanically ventilated patient has been amply emphasized, as has the value of a respiratory care unit for this purpose. No matter the physical circumstances under which treatment is being given, there are certain things for which the therapist looks and which he checks and procedures which he follows that experience has shown to be necessary for the patient's safety. We will describe three types of monitoring—clinical, physiologic, and mechanical—although there are overlapping areas among them.

CLINICAL MONITORING. This involves observing the patient and evaluating his condition and the effectiveness of his ventilation based on signs and symptoms and the therapist's critical knowledge of the physiology of the disease and the expectations of therapy. No sophisticated diagnostic equipment is used. The therapist is interested in the physical and mental comfort of the patient, for the patient's attitude is vital to his recovery. Since the intubated patient cannot speak, the therapist must be on the watch for signs of pain, restlessness, and apprehension. Often communication can be established through the use of pencil and paper, and although too frequent annoying questions are to be avoided, the therapist should inquire periodically of the feelings of the patient. The alert and observant therapist soon learns the characteristics of his patient and how best to manage him. The patient's color should be watched and both cyanosis and pallor noted. We know that cyanosis is but a crude quantitative gauge of hypoxia, but it is a good determinant of changes in oxygenation. Excessive pallor, especially if accompanied by cold moist skin, may indicate developing cardiovascular collapse.

Much valuable information concerning the work of breathing and the effectiveness of therapy can be obtained by noting the muscular components of ventilation. This is especially true before the start of treatment in the patient being assisted in his breathing rather than controlled and during breaks in controlled ventilation, as when the patient is being aspirated or equipment is being serviced. Increasing or decreasing use of the accessory ventilatory muscles is noted and is an excellent indication of the energy used by the patient. The therapist should frequently observe the mobility of the upper abdomen, or epigastrium, both when the patient is on and when he is off the ventilator. To do this properly, he should expose the upper half of the patient's abdomen and kneel by the side of the bed so that he can sight across the patient at the abdominal level. Retraction of the epigastrium during the inspiratory phase and protrusion during exhalation constitute paradoxical breathing, described in Chapter 6, and indicate a severe disturbance in the efficiency of ventilation. If present while the patient is being mechanically assisted, they mean that he is completely uncoordinated with the instrument, is working against it, and that therapy is worsening rather than helping him. The degree to which the epigastrium rises during inhalation is a function of the descent of the diaphragm and a rough indication of the tidal volume. Like the evaluation of cyanosis, the volumetric implication of epigastric movement is valuable as a monitor of changes rather than a quantitative measurement. To appreciate the abdominal motion, the therapist should lay his hand gently on the patient, between the xiphoid cartilage and the umbilicus, and observe as well as feel the movement of his hand. In the obstructed patient with spontaneous breathing, assisted or unassisted, the therapist may be able to feel the expiratory contraction of the abdominal wall as the patient works to express air against heavy resistance. Finally, in addition to judging the muscular aspect of ventilation, the therapist will be able to ascertain by inspection and palpation of the abdomen whether there is abdominal distention. The accumulation of intestinal gas postoperatively and the swallowing of air by a dyspneic patient given short-term ventilatory assistance through a face mask or mouthpiece can produce serious distention of the abdomen. Not infrequently distention builds up an intra-abdominal pressure so great that it seriously interferes with the inspirational descent of the diaphragm. In such an instance the therapist will observe the abdomen to be rounded, its skin stretched smooth, and the wall tense to the touch. A gentle but sharp slap will elicit a tympanic, or drumlike, response. If the therapist notes such distention, he should bring it to the attention of the attending physician or nurse, for unless it can be relieved, it may make effective ventilation impossible.

Auscultation of the chest is an examination of the breath sounds through a stethoscope and is a technique with which the therapist should become familiar. It should be clear to him that his use of a stethoscope is limited, for diagnostic auscultation is a fine art employed by a physician and takes many years to develop to a point of proficiency. However, the use of a stethoscope will enable the therapist to evaluate the distribution of air in the patient's chest and to evaluate the degree of obstruction. When the venti-

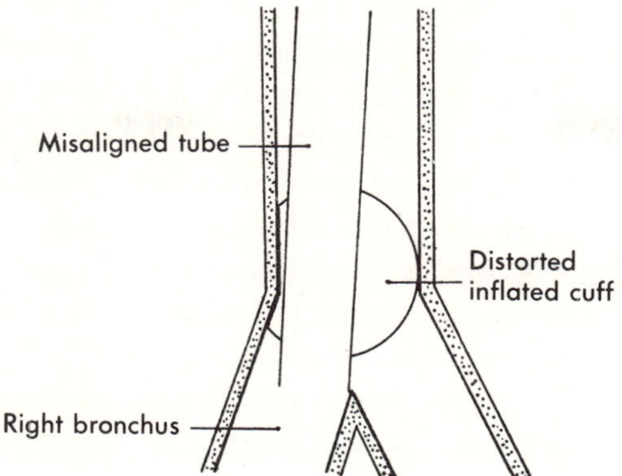

Fig. 10-6. Low position of tracheal tube so that its tip enters one main bronchus. The inflated cuff effectively occludes the other air passage, limiting ventilation to but one lung.

lator has been set up to the therapist's satisfaction, he should listen to the chest with the scope—anteriorly, posteriorly, and in the axillae—comparing the sounds in related areas of both lungs from the apices to the bases. Closing his eyes for maximum concentration, he listens for the intensity of airflow to determine whether there are areas that are not being adequately ventilated. Since many of his patients suffer severe obstruction and have mobile secretions, it is not uncommon to find areas of lung poorly aerated and patterns of air distribution that change from hour to hour. In this regard, special mention should be made of a hazard of intubation referred to earlier in this chapter and illustrated in Fig. 10-6. This is the placement of a tracheal tube too low so that its tip passes the carina into one or the other main bronchi. This is usually the result of a hasty insertion of an endotracheal or nasotracheal tube, intubation by unskilled personnel, or the use of too long a tracheostomy tube. With most if not all the delivered gas directed into but one lung, the serious disturbance to the ventilation-perfusion balance is obvious. Severe physiologic shunting can increase the venous admixture to the point that hypoxia may be fatal, and in the obstructed patient the resistance to the total airflow's diversion to one lung will prevent compensation for the hypoventilation of the blocked lung, and hypercapnia is probable. Usually the clinical appearance of the patient will warn of this complication, but if the occlusion is not complete, the ineffective ventilation may be attributed to underlying disease and correction attempted by such irrelevant measures as increasing airflow, the use of bronchodilators, etc. Thus, in an intubated patient, signs of sudden disruption of ventilatory pattern, accompanied by auscultatory signs of refuced airflow to one lung, should raise the immediate suspicion of a misplaced or slipped tube or a displaced cuff and the responsible physician alerted at once. Last, with experience, the therapist will be able to differentiate the breath sounds encountered in obstructive disease and described in Chapter 6. This will help him in evaluating the status of the airways by recognizing obstruction as primarily due to bronchospasm rather than to secretions; and the better his understanding of the patient, the better will be his services.

With his knowledge of the effect of mechanical ventilation on circulation, the therapist will want to keep himself informed on his patient's cardiovascular status by frequent checking of heart rate and blood pressure. Although these parameters are traditionally the responsibility of the nursing service, there need be no conflict. Indeed, this is a function whereby cooperation between the nurse and the therapist will be to the advantage of the patient. In a special-care unit, rates and pressures are recorded frequently; and the therapist may not need to do the measurements routinely. However, the therapist is aware of the speed with which the ventilated patient's condition may change, and he should monitor these values as often as he feels necessary, and especially if he finds it necessary to increase inspiratory pressure to a high level in an unstable patient or one receiving prolonged therapy. There is no rule to follow, but in the patient whose cardiac condition is in doubt or who has known cardiac weakness, heart rate and pressure may have to be recorded as often as every 15 minutes until stability is assured and then at least hourly thereafter. At any time the therapist feels there is a progressive or significant rise in heart rate or a drop in pressure, the attending nurse or physician or the medical director of the inhalation therapy department should be immediatly notified. If the responsible physician decides that cardiac output is falling and shock developing, he will start corrective measures; and although the therapist knows the role played by expiratory negative pressure in this situation, the physician is the one to order it. However, the tactful therapist may offer his services to adjust the ventilator for negative pressure, thus reminding the physician of the availability of this effective measure. If the physician gives approval, it is then the responsibility of the therapist to reevaluate the ventilatory pattern in terms of the I/E ratio and extend the expiratory time as long as is possible, while reducing inspiratory pressure as much as is consistent with ventilatory needs. If cardiac rate, dropping blood pressure, and other signs of shock, as described in Chapter 5, are unrelieved, negative pressure during exhalation should be introduced. The physiologic rationale for this maneuver as well as its own risks were detailed in Chapter 9. Let us only repeat here that negative expiratory pressure should never be used indiscriminately and only for correction of reduced cardiac output resulting from positive-pressure ventilation. The hazards of air trapping and pulmonary edema must be watched for closely. Negative pressure should be started very gradually, balancing its effect against the blood pressure, and usually 3 to 5 cm of water are adequate. To maintain the same alveolar ventilation as before the introduction of subatmospheric pressure, the therapist may have to increase the tidal volume to make up for additional air removed by expiratory suction at the expense of the functional residual capacity,[272] since in a sense this amounts to increasing the physiologic dead space. Skill is needed to use expiratory pressure safely and effectively, for the procedure entails balancing the negative pressure necessary to protect the cardiac output against a possible increase in positive pressure (if a pressure-cycled machine is being used), to maintain ventilation in the face of the negative-pressure effect on lung volume, and still realize a net drop in intrathoracic pressure.

PHYSIOLOGIC MONITORING. In contrast to clinical observation, physiologic monitoring refers to the laboratory measurements of the physiologic responses to disease and treatment. One does not supplant the other, for laboratory findings are of but limited value unless interpreted in the light of what is actually happening to the patient as a whole; but at the same time clinical examinations cannot give us the precise information we need of what is happening inside the patient. The current therapy of ventilatory failure is predicated on the availability of facilities to give us this physiologic insight, and the use of modern respirators in controlled treatment is dangerous guesswork without such information. Thus, the hospital that is to treat failure must have not only good inhalation therapists but also a pulmonary function laboratory. The organization of such a facility and its relationship to the inhalation therapy service will be noted in the final chapter, but let us say here that, whatever the structure needed to meet the needs of an individual hospital, the pulmonary function laboratory must work closely with inhalation therapy and its findings made readily available to the therapists. Although the services of such a laboratory may be diverse, in our concern with management of ventilatory failure, physiologic monitoring, for the most part, means measurement of arterial oxygen and carbon dioxide tensions and pH; and by this time the therapist's orientation to his work should be firmly fixed on the importance of these values.

In all probability, before the therapist is called to attend a patient, the diagnostic workup will have included blood gas studies on the basis of which, with clinical findings, the decision to institute therapy was made. Frequently the therapist will see a patient admitted as an emergency, obviously in need of ventilatory assistance; and we commented earlier in this chapter on the therapeutic approach while awaiting physiologic data. Whatever the situation, arterial gas values constitute the basis for definitive therapy and should be obtained as soon as possible. The question is frequently raised concerning the frequency of blood gas examinations during therapy, and for this there can be only one answer—as often as is necessary to assure the most effective and safest ventilation. Not rarely is it needed every 15 minutes until the medical team feels confident that its management is proper. When the response to therapy is satisfactory, clinical and physiologic signs of stability become evident; and the frequency of blood gas determinations can be gradually reduced. For the sake of safety, once the acute phase has passed and the patient can be considered at a maintenance plateau, or recovering, gas tensions and pH determinations should be done at least twice daily. Often this can be modified, however, if hypoxia is felt to be permanently corrected and monitoring is reduced to carbon dioxide tension and pH measurements. The therapist must keep in mind that, no matter his skill or the sophisitication of his equipment, the adequacy of his patient's alveolar ventilation can be ascertained only by these last two values.

The therapist might wonder why venous blood cannot be used for monitoring since it is considered more readily attainable. The basic objection to venous blood is that, because it is usually drawn from an extremity, it reflects the local metabolic activity of the area drained by the vein chosen and in a sense tells us what is left over after perfusion of local tissues. Arterial blood, on the other hand, shows us directly the ability of the lungs to effect gas exchange before any extraction of oxygen or addition of carbon dioxide by the tissues. If venous blood is withdrawn after a needle has been left in the vein without a tourniquet about the extremity for 1 minute, there will be some correlation between venous and arterial carbon dioxide tension and pH but none for oxygen tension. Further, there is another technique that makes dependence upon questionable venous blood unnecessary and that is of great value to the management of prolonged ventilation from two viewpoints. First, in most hospitals at the present time, both arterial and venous punctures must be done by physicians or specially trained nurses; and although there is no reason other than legal liability why trained technicians could not be given this task, until such restrictions are lifted in the future, it is prohibited. Second, repeated arterial punctures carry a potential risk of damage to the vessel, although this is extremely rare; but at the very least it is a parenteral procedure and an inconvenience. To obviate these two drawbacks, a technique utilizing "arterialized" capillary blood has become popular and practical. Commonly known as a "finger stick," this procedure consists of puncturing the end of the finger (or toe or heel of an infant) with a sharp blade to obtain a free flow of capillary blood. Prior to puncture, the hand is immersed in hot water for 10 minutes, a technique that has been demonstrated to render blood in the capillaries similar in its characteristics to arterial blood. The blood is collected in a glass capillary or a properly prepared small syringe and analyzed in the same manner as arterial blood. For some time this technique has been considered satisfactory for carbon dioxide tension and pH, but many questioned its reliability for oxygen tension. More comparative experience with it, however, has indicated that all three capillary parameters correlate well enough with arterial blood to be clinically accurate.[273] Acceptance of this technique has made physiologic data readily available, for this is a procedure that can be done by the laboratory technician or inhalation therapist as often as necessary to monitor mechanical ventilation while at the same time sparing the patient repeated arterial punctures. The reliable inhalation therapist may be given freedom to obtain and examine arterialized capillary blood according to his own judgment to fulfill his responsibility for maintaining ventilation. He is thus aware of the condition and needs of his patient at all times.

In an attempt further to simplify the physiologic monitoring of the ventilated patient as well as evaluate the efficiency of ventilation, in general, a technique has been developed that estimates only the arterial carbon dioxide tension.[274] In the normal lung, with an even intrapulmonary distribution of inspired air and a normal ventilation-perfusion ratio, measurement of the carbon dioxide tension in the very last portion of exhaled air, the so-called end-tidal sample, would very accurately reflect the gas tension in arterial blood after alveolar equilibration. This simple procedure is of no value in the patient with abnormal lungs and abnormal V/P ratios. The technique advocated recognizes the unreliability of end-tidal sampling but still uses the principle of the equilibration of carbon dioxide between alveoli and blood. The patient is given an 8% mixture of carbon dioxide in oxygen to rebreathe for 1 minute from a reservoir bag, during which time carbon dioxide is either added to the bag or taken from it by the patient, depending upon the level of the arterial gas tension at the start of the test. A special chemical carbon dioxide analyzer is used to measure the amount of gas in the bag sample after 1 minute and convert it into the tension. When compared to simultaneous arterial blood analyses, the rebreathing method was reported to have a standard error of 4.6 mm Hg. There are two primary advantages of this procedure. First, it avoids needle punctures and is relatively free of discomfort. Second, it uses equipment that is infinitely less costly than that required for blood studies. At the same time, it has two disadvantages. First, although the standard error is less than 5 mm Hg, some would not accept this as insignificant; and because it is a standard error, for a given test in a given subject, the actual error may be much greater. This means that over a long period of time the difference between the test and actual gas tensions may average out to less than 5 mm Hg but at any point in patient management one could not be certain that the error was not in excess of this. Second, management of ventilation should not be done without simultaneous carbon dioxide and pH measurements because of the possible combination of acid-base balance disturbances, with which the therapist is already acquainted. This bloodless test may have value during postventilation recovery to assure the stability of ventilation.

Although the attending physician will often use additional laboratory data to evaluate his patient, the blood gases are the only ones of major concern to the therapist. The physician may want to know the electrolyte status, especially the levels of sodium and chloride and potassium. The relation of these to respiration was touched upon in Chapter 4 and may be of enough interest to the therapist to stimulate him to pursue their study on his own.

MECHANICAL MONITORING. Somewhat limited in scope at the present, *mechanical monitoring* refers to the use of devices to measure the various parameters of ventilation. For the most part, this resolves into the use of spirometers to measure tidal and minute volumes. Some ventilators are equipped with such meters, but they often give only an approximation of the amount of air delivered. Very useful is a portable meter, the Wright respirometer.[275] With a face the size of a small clock, the instrument is a flowmeter constructed as a small air turbine with one dial calibrated in liters up to 100 liters and a second dial calibrated in 10 ml increments up to 1 liter. Its minimum flow response is less than 2 lpm, but it should not be subjected to flows exceeding 300 lpm. It is easily adapted to the exhalation port of any ventilator to measure the exhaled air as a gauge of tidal volume, a practical but not always accurate assumption. Obviously, it cannot be so used with expiratory negative pressure. The meter can give rough but usable information about three characteristics of ventilation. First, severe airway obstruction will cause the small needle to "hang up" in response to interference with exhaled flow rate. Second, in controlled ventilation, if the needle finishes its rotation before the next inspiration begins, it indicates terminal air trapping. Third, if the ventilator pressure and metered tidal volume are noted simultaneously, a working compliance can be calculated; and although not of diagnostic accuracy, this compliance is of importance in monitoring changes in the lung during prolonged ventilation.

Electric monitors are available that will emit visible and audible signals if preset ranges of rate or phase are not met or are exceeded and if the ventilator fails or disconnects from the patient.[276,277] Such instruments have a definite but limited value, and with the current interest in instrumentation in so many fields of medicine, there will doubtless be other developments in monitoring respiratory function as there have been for cardiac function. Any assistance that gives support to the patient is desirable, but mechanical or electronic monitors must not be relied upon as a substitute for the personal attention of a skilled therapist. A monitor will not correct a deficiency, and its value depends entirely upon the capability of the personnel responding to its call.

Weaning from the ventilator

As with all the other aspects of ventilator care, the process of weaning, or gradual removal of the patient from his respirator, must be tailored to the needs of each patient; and only general suggestions can be offered. The therapist must accept the fact that supported ventilation, and especially controlled ventilation, is a harrowing and frightening experience for anyone, accompanied by much psychic trauma. During the course of therapy, the patient develops an understandable dependence upon the machine that was responsible for his survival. No sooner has the successfully treated patient survived the terror of breathlessness, able to relax with the support of his ventilator, than he hears his medical team discussing the possibility of taking it away from him. The thought may panic him, for he is far from sure that, since he needed mechanical help so recently, he is able to do without it now. Two dicta of weaning may be stated together. Remove the patient from his ventilator as soon as possible, but prepare him for it carefully.

In general, the longer a patient is ventilated, the more difficult and the longer is the weaning period. In addition, the state of intubation with power-induced ventilation is both unnatural and unphysiologic and carries the risk of secondary infection and injury to the lung the longer it persists. The objective of mechanical ventilation, therefore, is to support the patient through acute respiratory failure, control or improve the etiology of the failure, and restore the patient to spontaneous unassisted breathing as soon as possible. Conditioning of the patient for this move should start well in advance, not by telling him that he will be taken off the ventilator on a given day so that he will anticipate it fearfully, but by giving him encouraging reports of his progress while he is still supported. From the earliest moment in therapy he should be told repeatedly that mechanical ventilation is a temporary measure, designed to give him rest from the stress of breathing until he is better. Many factors will determine the decision to wean. Obviously, the blood gases and pH should be in normal, or preventilator, ranges. Infection should be controlled and the patient's mental attitude one of cooperation. It is very helpful to watch carefully the patient's behavior when he is removed from the ventilator for the short periods required for aspiration or servicing his tracheostomy tube or ventilator, and if spontaneous breathing is evident at these times, some estimate of its adequacy can be noted. Certainly, such spontaneous breathing must return before weaning can even be considered, and it is often helpful to ask the patient to take an occasional breath while still on control to see whether he can override the machine. He may have to be urged to this effort, for it is so easy for him to conform to the ventilator that he may not exert himself to see whether he can breathe unless encouraged to do so. For short periods of time the patient can be put on assisted ventilation, with take-over control at a lower rate, and the explanation can be given that he must exercise his ventilatory muscles, which have become weak from disuse. Most patients accept as reasonable this need to try breathing on their own, and such periods can be extended to as long as is acceptable to them. The therapist should keep reassuring the patient that, should he tire or even fall asleep, the ventilator will automatically start to function.

Once a patient's spontaneous breathing has been demonstrated to him, he is ready for the next step. While disconnected from the ventilator for tracheostomy care, the patient can be asked whether he would like to breathe on his own for a few minutes with the therapist in attendance, and he should be provided with a tracheostomy mask for the delivery of humidified oxygen or air. Supported ventilation should be resumed before the patient tires, but these intervals of spontaneous breathing are gradually increased until he is breathing on his own most of the time, with occasional periods of restful support. It may be necessary to provide assisted ventilation during the sleeping hours for a little longer. Before removing the tracheostomy tube, the therapist may find it helpful to obstruct the tube with a cap provided for this purpose, always deflating the cuff first. Some difficulty in breathing may be anticipated, at least initially, for the tube constitutes a considerable airway obstruction itself. It is also wise to ambulate the patient, before extubation, to evaluate his walking tolerance. Except for such periods of exercise, humidification must be provided to the tracheostomy at all times. If the weaning schedule has been gradual, the eventual removal of the tracheostomy tube will present little difficulty, and the wound will heal in a few days.

The process of weaning just described is oriented to the patient with a tracheostomy tube, for most patients undergoing long-term ventilation for whom weaning is an important event are so intubated. The removal of an endotracheal or nasotracheal tube that has been in use for a few days presents less of a problem and can usually be removed with little if any preparation. The risk of premature removal of these tubes is less than in the case of a tracheostomy tube, for an endotracheal tube can readily be replaced if necessary with a minimum of trauma.

INTERMITTENT POSITIVE-PRESSURE BREATHING

Until now, we have discussed the use of intermittent positive pressure in the delivery of assisted or controlled ventilation for the patient with inadequate breathing, and we will now consider IPPB as a treatment entity for less acute conditions. IPPB has come rapidly onto the medical scene, enjoying both widespread use and acclamation and considerable condemnation. As with many innovations, pressure breathing suffered from initial overuse without due regard for proper indications or technique, and when expectations that were never claimed for it did not materialize, many users became disenchanted with it. Much, if not all, of the controversy over the value or harm of IPPB was the result of lack of clear understanding of its capabilities and what can be expected of it. In addition, the advent of IPPB preceded the development of inhalation therapy as a skilled technical specialty, and pressure breathing was used by many people with little concept of its objectives or knowledge of the mechanics of the instruments or their physiologic effects. It is little wonder that results were less than spectacular and the treatment blamed rather than those treating. Now, through the rational use of IPPB by knowledgeable physicians and its administration by competent therapists, it has earned an established place in the overall therapy of chest diseases.

Equipment

Most IPPB instruments function according to the principles described for IPPV's, and although the ventilators themselves can be used for intermittent therapy, there are units much simpler in structure designed just for this purpose. Without the need for the many critical controls of ventilators, treatment instruments are generally smaller in size, and many are portable, independent of gas cylinders or centrally supplied air with their own built-in compressors. One of the most recent innovations in IPPB instrument design deserves special mention because of the unique principle that sets it apart from the others. Typical of several units now available is the RETIC automatic respirator, which makes use of the Coanda effect, fluid control principle.[278-280] Almost

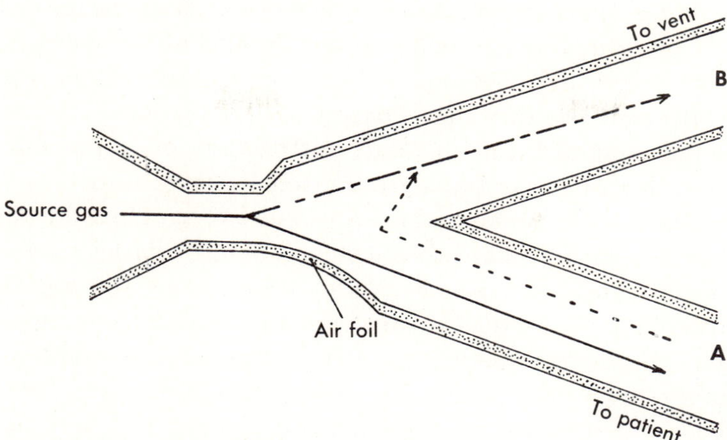

Fig. 10-7. Simplified illustration of the operating principle of a fluid-control system respirator. Source gas enters a divided passage and, because of the air-foil contour of one wall, is pulled into channel *A*. End-inspiratory back pressure breaks the air-foil lock on the gas stream, shifting it and exhaled air to channel *B*, where it is vented to the atmosphere. Ventilatory cycling is thus achieved without moving valves.

uncanny in its operation, it has no moving parts, yet without a cycling valve it is able to initiate and terminate ventilatory phases with flow-sensitive characteristics, powered by an electric gear-type blower. Although it is precision designed for sensitive operation, its basic principle is crudely illustrated in Fig. 10-7. A jet of air upon entering a divided channel will preferentially enter one or the other branches, depending upon certain physical features, one of which is operating in the illustration. The contour of the wall leading to channel A pulls the airstream in that direction and "locks" it against the wall of the channel (solid arrow). This is the Coanda phenomenon, and the stream will stay in this pattern until some force changes it. If channel A represents the flow to the patient, at end-inspiration back pressure of exhaled air (dotted arrow) changes the dynamics of the system by blocking channel A, diverting the entire flow, input and exhaled air (broken arrow), to an atmospheric vent through channel B. At end-expiration, the flow automatically reverts to its original pattern for the next respiratory cycle. Experience will determine the long-range practicability of this type of pressure unit, but its freedom from maintenance problems and the use of fluid control systems in other engineering fields give it promise.

Indications for IPPB

Pressure breathing is generally used for its following physiologic effects: (1) to increase alveolar and total ventilation, (2) to elevate arterial oxygen saturation, (3) to reduce arterial carbon dioxide tension, and (4) to reduce cardiac output. The special use of the last effect will be discussed separately below. Its indications include many clinical entities, such as bronchial asthma, acute and chronic bronchitis, pulmonary emphysema, bronchiectasis lung abscess, postpneumonia, and pre- and postoperative states, to list the most common.

IPPB is indicated for two broad clinical objectives. First, it is used to improve the general intrapulmonary distribution of inspired air, thereby restoring a disturbed ventilation-perfusion balance to as near normal as possible, eliminating venous admixture and lowering carbon dioxide tension. Pressure breathing is especially valuable in preventing postoperative atelectasis by assuring adequate lung expansion during the recovery period. Its judicious and energetic use may prevent potential hypercapnia and subsequent respiratory failure in a susceptible patient, such as one with emphysema who is the victim of trauma or a respiratory infection. Second, IPPB is widely used as a vehicle for deep pulmonary aerosol therapy, because it will effect maximum aerosol distribution. It is valuable in the treatment of bronchospasm and as an aid to the removal of secretions, and it can be used to deliver any of the aerosols discussed in an earlier chapter. In this regard, surgeons have found it valuable preoperatively, to assure maximum airway clearance for the prevention of postsurgical atelectasis and infection, especially in those with known bronchial disease or who are heavy cigarette smokers.

Technique of IPPB administration

IPPB is useless, or even harmful, if not done correctly. The experienced inhalation therapist may feel that simple pressure breathing treatments are pretty routine, lacking the glamour of managing controlled ventilation; but this is only because of his familiarity with it. It still remains one of his most valuable contributions to medicine and deserving of his skill and attention as any other procedure. He must remember that, routine though it may be to him, it is far from routine for every patient subjected to it for the first time. Before initiating therapy on a new patient, if meaningful communication is possible, the therapist must be absolutely certain that he explains to the patient what is going to be done. Without delivering an academic lecture, he should tell the patient the nature of the treatment and in a general way what is expected of it. Resistance or hostility of a patient toward therapy is usually due to one or more of the following: (1) he is irrational from illness or age; (2) he is expressing fright through hostility; (3) he does not understand what is expected of him. A few moments of reassuring explanation will make the treatment helpful for the patient and easy on the therapist.

For best results, the patient should be seated upright in a relatively straight chair, although we realize that this is not always possible for the hospitalized patient. Nevertheless, every effort should be made to avoid a slouched position, which will hamper diaphragmatic mobility. A mouthpiece is preferred to a mask, and at first a noseclip is best, although this can often be omitted shortly. The edentulous patient presents a problem in achieving necessary airtightness, but a trial of several mouthpieces of different shapes, especially with flanges, will generally locate one that is satisfactory. These appliances should be fitted so that the patient can get acclimated to them before the start of treatment. All initial control settings will be tentative, but sensitivity should be relatively free and pressure started somewhere between 10 and 15 cm of water. The control of flow-adjustable instruments can be set somewhere in the middle of the available range.

As treatment is begun, the patient is instructed to breathe slowly and easily and encouraged to allow the machine to do the work. There is a tendency for respiratory frequency to increase, and the patient often appears to be chased by the respirator so that the therapist may have to urge the patient to maintain a normal rate. Especially is the anxious patient or the patient trying hard to please apt to overbreathe, and this must be prevented because it is easy for him to become alkalotic. Pressure and flow rate may have to be adjusted often during an initial treatment until the patient's pattern stabilizes, but most patients do well quickly, reassured by the therapist's relaxed and confident manner. It is prudent to inquire after the patient's feelings to determine whether he is experiencing dizziness or getting tired. Water, or medication to be aerosolized, must be in the nebulizer at all times, and the treatment never given dry; and if medication is used, the patient should be instructed to hold his breath momentarily at end-inspiration to permit maximum particle distribution.

Once the patient appears at ease with the procedure, if he is obstructed, he should be encouraged to prolong his exhalation within the limits of comfort. If he has difficulty doing this himself, the therapist can put a *retard cap* over the exhalation port of the instrument. This is a cap that has a number of holes of different diameters to provide varying degrees of back pressure for slowing down and prolonging exhalation. It is especially useful when air trapping due to bronchiolar collapse is a problem, for the back pressure developed at the port will help to maintain airway patency to end-expiration. The therapist should also teach him to aid exhalation by abdominal contraction. This is often difficult for the patient to grasp, but it will be easier for him if the therapist will demonstrate on himself in front of the patient. Then, with his hand on the patient's epigastrium, the therapist can exert gentle but firm pressure during the terminal third of exhalation, pointing out to the patient how this increases the removal of air. Finally, the patient is allowed to try epigastric retraction himself, but he will need close supervision and must not be allowed to tire himself with this maneuver. For the patient with a severe obstructive problem, there is available an inflatable swath-like belt that can be fitted about his middle and upper abdomen. Coordinated with the ventilator, the belt inflates during exhalation, exerting a forceful squeeze on the abdomen. It does not take the place of active exercise of the abdominal muscles, but it is helpful in instructing the patient in the purpose of forced terminal expiration and demonstrating to him what can be accomplished.

Generally, an IPPB treatment of 20 to 30 minutes is sufficient at a frequency of three to four times daily, although it is obvious that the schedule must be fitted to each patient's needs. However, the indications for treatment are usually such that an intensity of this degree is necessary, at least at first. Care must be taken not to let IPPB become so routine that all patients are treated alike. On the other hand, both the patient's attending physician and the inhalation therapist need some sort of a working standard procedure to present to a patient for whom therapy is proposed. To answer a patient who inquires how long he will need treatments, it is probably safe to tell him that he will need them every day while in the hospital and as an outpatient for up to 2 weeks, at which time his condition will be reviewed. Thus, outpatient services must be available, and in many hospitals they may carry the burden of IPPB therapy. An obvious problem arises in this case, for it is rarely possible for a patient to return to the outpatient service three to four times daily unless there are provisions for all-day care at the hospital. The desirable will have to be compromised for the feasible, and if only one treatment can be given, it is definitely better than none. For the patient previously treated more intensively as an inpatient, once a day is probably satisfactory; and for the outpatient starting therapy, it may be the only arrangement possible. Careful evaluation by both physician and therapist is needed to determine when therapy should be stopped, and to follow a tapering schedule is often better than to stop abruptly.

An increasingly popular solution to the outpatient problem is self-administered home therapy, with the patient borrowing, renting, or purchasing his own IPPB unit; and many instruments are manufactured just for this purpose. Home therapy can be satisfactory if it is subject to certain conditions. First, a series of treatments should be given by a trained therapist in either the inpatient or outpatient service until such time as the therapist is confident that the patient knows the procedure well. There are some patients who never can treat themselves safely or satisfactorily, and the therapist should frankly make this known to the responsible physician. Second, before the hospitalized patient takes his instrument home, the therapist should go over it carefully with him, reviewing the technique of its use, showing him how the components operate, and instructing him in its care and cleaning. The outpatient should bring his machine to the ambulatory service for the same purposes, and often arrangements can be made to have the patient's unit delivered to the hospital so that he can be instructed when he picks it up. It is a responsibility of the patient's physician to follow the progress of home care and, if necessary, to send the patient back to the therapist for an occasional checkup on technique. Experience has shown that many patients on home-care programs are forgotten and tend to become negligent in their treatment.

Treatment of acute pulmonary edema

The student is advised to review the causes and clinical picture of pulmonary edema as discussed in Chapter 5. Its treatment is included here because of the importance of IPPB, although the overall management will be described briefly to familiarize the therapist with this condition which he will be called upon so frequently to treat. The following is modified from a previously published discussion of pulmonary edema.[40] In the management of full-blown acute edema, speed is essential; and treatment can be considered in four categories: (1) physical and mental relaxation, (2) improvement of cardiovascular function, (3) relief of hypoxia, and (4) retardation of venous return.

Physical and mental relaxation. This is a responsibility of the attending physician rather than the inhalation therapist. The patient is allowed to assume a position of comfort, which is usually sitting because of his severe dyspnea. Many patients are extremely apprehensive, and morphine sulfate is the drug of choice to relieve anxiety and promote muscular relaxation. Not only is the patient's mental state improved, but morphine reduces peripheral vascular tone through suppression of vasomotor centers and thus directly affects an underlying mechanism responsible for the edema. If circulation is adequate to ensure absorption, the narcotic can be given subcutaneously in doses of 10 to 15 mg at 30-minute intervals to a total of four doses if necessary. Should shock be present, reducing tissue perfusion, intravenous administration will be necessary, if the drug is given at all. Ventilation must be observed closely, for a respiratory center already depressed by the hypoxia accompanying acute edema will be seriously aggravated by morphine. Also, since wheezes may be present in both acute pulmonary edema and such obstructive bronchial diseases as asthma and bronchitis, it is important that the latter diagnoses be excluded, for the use of morphine could be catastrophic. Should serious hypoventilation or apnea follow the drug, such morphine antagonists as levallorphan tartrate (Lorfan) or nalorphine (Nalline) and respiratory stimulants such as ethamivan (Emivan) or nikethamide (Coramine) may be necessary, in addition to artificial ventilation.

Improvement of cardiovascular function. A critical part of the physician's evaluation of pulmonary edema is his determination of whether the condition is due to cardiac failure, for if it is, successful therapy will depend upon restoring compensation. Digitalis, or one of its analogues, is specifically indicated for cardiac failure, either causing or complicating pulmonary edema; but it has no value in the absence of such failure. The physiologic effects of digitalis, even when given intravenously, are not evident for at least 15 minutes; and thus it does not rank in priority over the use of morphine for the treatment of hypoxia. It should also be remembered that the initial response of digitalis may be an aggravation of symptoms as a result of the marked increase in pulmonary vascular pressure due to digitalis action. It is often better to withhold use of digitalis until the acute emergency has passed or is well under control. Aminophylline is useful in relieving the bronchospasm that is often present and in lessening pulmonary-capillary transudate. For prompt effect it is given intravenously in doses of 500 to 700 mg at a rate not to exceed 20 mg per minute. Intravenous mercurial diuretics are of value only when congestive heart failure is present and have little effect on pulmonary edema per se.

Relief of hypoxia and retardation of venous return. These two objectives will be discussed together, for they are managed simultaneously. The treatment of hypoxia is of the highest priority, and a significant increase in alveolar oxygen tension is necessary to increase diffusion across the fluid barrier of edema. The very first move is to give the patient 100% oxygen while readying other measures, preferably by means of a nonrebreathing mask; and oxygen therapy will be continued during the next step of retarding venous return. For many years the reduction of pulmonary blood volume has been recognized as a prime objective in the relief of the acute phase of pulmonary edema, and there are three techniques that will reduce the volume of blood returning to the right atrium.

PHLEBOTOMY. The physical removal of blood from circulation will certainly reduce the pulmonary blood volume, and it was customary in the past to withdraw up to 500 ml rapidly. This can be hazardous, however, for if acute edema has already precipitated circulatory collapse, blood loss will further aggravate shock. This technique has largely been abandoned.

TOURNIQUETS. Applied to the extremities, tourniquets will effectively reduce venous return and are much safer than phlebotomy. Rubber straps or blood-pressure cuffs may be used and are applied with a force greater than that of the estimated venous pressure but less than the arterial diastolic pressure. Peripheral pulses must be palpable at all times to avoid the risk of ischemic necrosis. Only three extremities are occluded at a time, and the tourniquets are rotated so that each extremity is free, in sequence, for 20 minutes. When the acute phase is over, the restrictions are released, one at a time at 20-minute intervals, to avoid flooding the pulmonary circulation with a sudden return of flow. This technique is safe and effective and should be used while waiting for and during the next maneuver.

INTRAPULMONARY PRESSURE. Pressure-controlled inflation of the lungs is more rapid and effective than either phlebotomy or tourniquets, and its administration by IPPB is an important function of the inhalation therapist. As noted earlier, this is an instance in which the usually undesirable generation of high intrathoracic pressures may be lifesaving rather than a hazard. Instead of regulating his ventilator to minimize its circulatory effect, the therapist does just the opposite. He uses pressures up to 40 cm of water or higher and flow rates high enough to reach peak pressure in the shortest possible time. This allows the maintenance of a plateau of high pressure at end-inspiration and blocks the return of venous blood into thoracic vessels. To a considerable degree, the volume of blood so retarded can be regulated and controlled in a manner not possible with phlebotomy or tourniquets. In the acutely ill patient, almost a breath-by-breath adjustment of the IPPB unit will be required because of the rapid and difficult breathing; but the great assistance the patient receives from the ventilator gradually eases his work of breathing, reducing frequency and increasing tidal volume. Oxygen is now given through the ventilator, so that hypoxia, pulmonary edema, and congestion are effectively treated together. It is common practice to nebulize 20% to 50% ethyl alcohol during treatment, taking advantage of its antifoaming properties to mobilize the edema froth as well as to benefit from the systemic effects after absorption into the circulation. The patient with combined shock and edema is a difficult one to treat, for positive pressure is a hazard to one, and negative pressure a hazard to the other. Still, by progressing cautiously, the therapist can provide relief of hypoxia from oxygen administered by gentle pressure breathing and may reverse circulatory collapse and reduce edema. The combined judgment and talents of physician and therapist may determine the outcome. In summary, it can be stated that acute pulmonary edema is one of the specific indications for IPPB and IPPB has become an accepted part of its treatment.

Chapter 11

Chronic care and rehabilitation of respiratory failure

The steadily improving care of patients with acute ventilatory failure is presenting its own problem. As more survive the acute phases of respiratory disease, there is an increasing population of people with chronic pulmonary insufficiency, displaying a wide spectrum of disability. It makes little difference whether they were originally diagnosed as pulmonary emphysema, fibrotic tuberculosis, chronic asthma, or any of several other conditions, for in their chronic state they have one thing in common—the inability to move to and from their lungs sufficient air for physiologic needs, without being distressingly conscious of the physical effort required. The high incidence of repeated hospitalizations and the progressive disability of these patients make necessary all-out efforts to set up purposeful and supervised chronic-care programs for them, to include not only supportive measures but also vigorous efforts to rehabilitate those with significant cardiopulmonary reserve. This is long-term therapy, for which both trained personnel and physical facilities are in short demand. Many chronically handicapped patients require daily care, some of which can be provided in ambulatory centers; but desperately needed for pulmonary rehabilitation are hospitals primarily intended for the chronic respiratory patient. Only the barest beginning of chronic care can be given in the average general hospital, both the philosophy and cost of which prohibit significant follow-up.

The overall objectives of pulmonary rehabilitation are not different from those of other disabling diseases—to increase the patient's physical comfort and performance and help him maintain or regain economic productivity or improved self-care. There is not yet a solidly based therapeutic pattern for such goals, but the following outline gives the needs that should be considered and provided for rehabilitation.

Rehabilitation of chronic bronchopulmonary disease

A. *Medical therapy*
   1. Control of respiratory infection
   2. Maintenance of clear airways
      a. Aerosol therapy
      b. Assisted ventilation
      c. Postural drainage exercises

3. Correction of inefficient ventilation—ventilatory exercises
4. Improvement in ambulation
   a. Graded walking exercises (with or without oxygen)
   b. Physical conditioning exercises
5. Psychosomatic support
   a. Group therapy
   b. Individual therapy as indicated
6. Evaluation of cardiopulmonary function

B. *Economic and social adjustment*
1. Occupational retraining and placement
   a. Work classification
   b. Employer support
2. Family counseling
   a. Education
   b. Home planning

We will not consider in detail all the items listed, for some are self-evident and others have already been adequately covered. There is no need, for example, to comment further on the control of infection other than to say that its importance is reflected in the position it occupies in the total program and to emphasize that unless it can be achieved none of the other measures will be of much avail. Aerosol therapy and assisted ventilation (IPPB) have been considered in depth relative to their uses in acute medicine, but they are just as important in chronic care, employing the same techniques already described. General physical conditioning is still mostly the responsibility of the physiotherapist, even though, as we shall soon see, other physical techniques are very much a part of the inhalation therapist's services. Comments will be made later on some of the other aspects of rehabilitation, but we will first discuss inhalation therapy procedures that are usually employed in the postacute state, for either immediate recuperation or for prolonged care.

Although the role of the inhalation therapist may seem more dramatic in the care of the patient in acute respiratory failure, it is no less valuable after passage of the crisis. Many of the same therapeutic and diagnostic techniques will apply then as before, but there are some reserved mostly for the convalescent period. We tend to sigh with relief when respiratory compensation is restored to a patient in failure and perhaps congratulate ourselves for normal blood gas values. However, as far as the patient is concerned, this may mark only the start of a long period of disability, threatened with unpredictable relapses and characterized by frustrating physical disability. We are still responsible for the patient, but our aims are somewhat different now, and from here on we will try to accomplish two things simultaneously. First, we will attempt to restore as much function as possible to his ventilatory mechanism; and, second, we will try to keep him out of further episodes of failure. Both are large tasks.

To begin our discussion, let us define the inhalation therapy of chronic respiratory care as those measures intended to improve respiratory performance rather than to save an acutely threatened life. The chronic state can develop gradually according to its own progression, or it may follow an acute illness; but the management will generally be the same. Chronic care may be started in the hospital as an outgrowth of acute care, or it may be initiated in the ambulatory patient who has never been hospitalized. We will discuss techniques that theoretically and traditionally belong to physiotherapy but that have become not only useful adjuncts to inhalation therapy, but an integral part of it. These techniques apply specifically to the treatment of diseases of the chest and, in the United States at least, have been less emphasized by physiotherapists than have other aspects of their field. However, the emerging inhalation therapist found these physically oriented procedures of great interest and use to him, and in the natural evolution of inhalation therapy, they have been incorporated into his general function. The encroachment of inhalation upon the domain of physiotherapy, therefore, was not intentional but developed only as a means to give a full spectrum of care to the respiratory patient.

With the inhalation therapist responsible for administering the basic aids to ventilation and for maintaining the patient during acute illness, it is only reasonable that he also have at his disposal any procedures that may further aid his patient's breathing and that will permit him to continue caring for the patient during convalescense and rehabilitation. We will see that some physiotherapy is indicated as a part of pressure breathing treatments, for example; and it is not in the interest of efficiency or good medicine to make the simultaneous services of two technicians necessary when one can do the job or to send the patient back and forth between two departments when only one is needed. The greatest justification for allocating chest physiotherapy to the inhalation therapist, however, is his specialized knowledge of, as well as interest in, pulmonary physiology and mechanics. It is hoped that the future education of the inhalation therapist will involve him more deeply in the techniques of chronic care, but at this time his training should include the following physical procedures: postural drainage, chest percussion, chest vibration, cough control, acute chest compression, pursed-lip breathing, abdominal breathing, and other ventilatory exercises. These are the subjects we will discuss below, but to understand the objectives and techniques of postural drainage, the therapist must know the segmental anatomy of the lung and the spatial relationships of segments and bronchi.

INHALATION THERAPY OF CHRONIC CARE

Postural drainage

The purpose of postural drainage is to increase the removal of bronchial secretions by so positioning the patient that gravity will aid their cephalad movement. As employed by the inhalation therapist, "tipping," to use the British expression, is often an important part of an IPPB treatment. He will have frequent occasion to stop therapy, tip the patient, percuss and vibrate his chest, and then resume pressure breathing. In theory, the therapist should have the prior consent of the patient's physician to perform these added services, but in hospitals where the medical staff is properly informed in chest therapy, a reliable therapist may be permitted to use his judgment. In the sophisticated inhalation therapy department, such physiotherapy is considered not as "added services" but as much a part of patient treatment as is the use of a respirator. Before initiating drainage, the therapist must consider such factors of the patient's general condition as related diseases, other infirmities, and age; but there are few who cannot benefit from some form of this therapy. This statement does not imply that all patients given IPPB must have postural drainage; for drainage is specifically reserved for those with significant secretions that cannot be readily removed by other means. It is true, however, that IPPB will often fail to achieve its purpose if stubborn secretions are permitted to obstruct the airways, and much time and effort can be wasted on fruitless therapy.

Patients for whom postural drainage is indicated will mostly fall in the following disease categories, listed in order of frequency: obstructive bronchitis-emphysema, bronchiectasis, resolving pneumonia, lung abscess, necrotizing pneumonia. Of the patients the therapist drains, by far most will have bronchitis-emphysema; and their retained secretions will usually involve the basal segments of the lower lobes. Thus, in a general way, referring to the therapist's average daily work, postural drainage will mean positioning the patient to remove secretions from the lower lobe basal segments, and especially the posterior basal segment, either side or both. The other diseases listed above may require treatment of different segments with localization by x-ray examination or bronchography. When a physician specifically orders postural drainage, he should indicate the area to be treated. This he probably will do if the disease is other than bronchitis-emphysema, but often with the latter he will merely request "IPPB and postural drainage," which implies treatment to the posterior, lateral, and anterior basal segments bilaterally. Drainage undertaken on the therapist's initiative should be confined to these segments. There are several good manuals on postural drainage describing and illustrating in detail the many available positions and their relationship to the bronchial tree.[281-283] It would be a redundant use of time to reproduce them all on these pages, for the therapist can consult such sources and familiarize himself with all the techniques. Since our interest is in the common daily use of postural drainage, we will confine our discussion to basal segment drainage only but with some recommendations that will apply to all techniques.

Fig. 11-1 illustrates two methods of posterior basal segment drainage. Position *A* is the one preferred if the patient's condition will permit tipping him head down. There are three important points to assure effectiveness with maximum comfort. First, the angle of 45 degrees between the patient's trunk and the horizontal is relatively critical since this puts the posterior basal segment bronchus in the most favorable position for gravity drainage. Second,

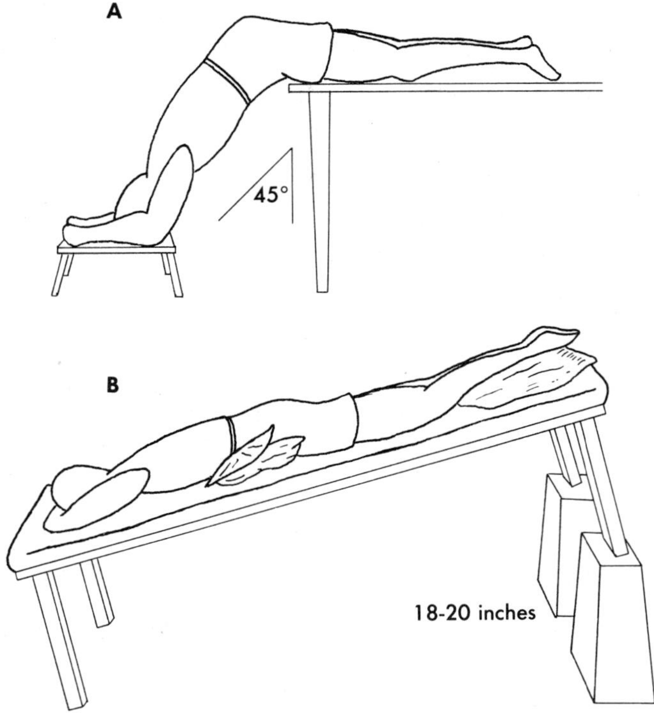

Fig. 11-1. Postural drainage, posterior basal segments. Position **A** is preferred. **B** is reserved for those for whom the head-down position is not indicated.

the back should be kept as straight as possible, avoiding a tendency to sag, for this will impair effective drainage and strain the back muscles. Third, the patient's arms should be supported or he will be unable to maintain his position with any degree of comfort; a footstool, a pile of books, or any other suitable object upon which the patient can rest his crossed arms may be used. It is not always easy to find a satisfactory surface across which the patient can lie at the desired angle. Many beds are too low or have too much give to them. If a bed is used, it should be adjustable to accommodate the patient's height and its mattress firm enough to be free of sagging. A tilt-table that will allow the entire body to be put a 45-degree angle is ideal, and this should be part of the equipment of an ambulatory-care service of the inhalation therapy department, to which many patients can be brought for therapy. Such a table must have shoulder supports to prevent the patient from sliding off its end. Sketch *B* shows an alternate technique for those patients for whom the head-down position is contraindicated. Drainage will be aided if the patient is placed in the prone position with two pillows under the hips and the foot of the bed elevated about 18 to 20 inches. The bed may be raised by blocks of suitable size under the foot legs or by an automobile jack under the foot end to which an extension angle iron has been welded to prevent rocking. Strength of the head legs must be assured, for elevation of the foot places a tremendous

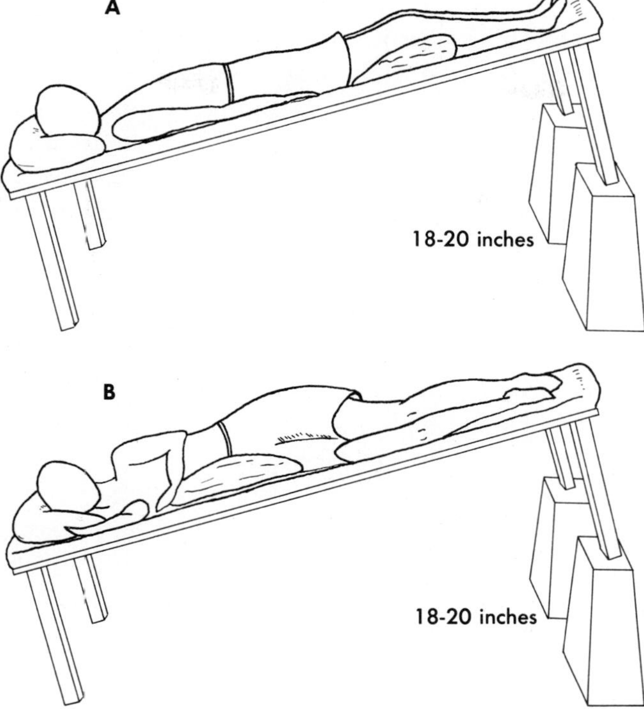

Fig. 11-2. Postural drainage. Position **A** is for anterior basal segments. **B** is for lateral basal segments.

strain on the head of the bed. This method is not quite as effective as the head-down, for the body assumes an angle of no more than about 15 degrees; but it has the advantage that it can be maintained for long periods of time. Fig. 11-2, *A* shows the position that will drain the anterior basal segment, with the foot of the bed raised 18 to 20 inches and a pillow under the knees for comfort. Fig. 11-2, *B*, demonstrates the position for lateral basal drainage, depending upon the side on which the patient is placed. A pillow or two is placed under the waist to keep the spine straight.

Judgment will determine whether all three positions should be used in sequence during any one treatment. From a practical point of view, considering the elements of time and patient fatigue, it is probably advisable to use the head-down technique whenever possible and as the first maneuver; and, if therapeutic results are satisfactory, to do no more. On the other hand, if the patient presents a particularly difficult secretion problem, it may be necessary to rotate him through a series of all three. Initially, a patient may be able to tolerate the head-down technique for only a minute, but he will soon adjust to it for as long as is necessary. When the patient is in position, the therapist should warn him not to make a deliberate effort to cough vigorously, for this will markedly raise intracranial pressure. Rather, the patient should be instructed frequently to "clear his throat" with sharp grunting sounds but with only gentle effort. This maneuver will elevate intrathoracic pressure momentarily at intervals, transmitting short bursts of high-velocity air in the bronchi to loosen and move secretions. Both the patient and the therapist should understand that the value of postural drainage is not in the immediate production of a great flow of secretions; for very often the treatment will seemingly accomplish little. Its function is to mobilize secretions intrabronchially for easier removal with a less effortful cough long after the tipping. If drainage should be effective at once, so much the better; and if it precipitates hard coughing, the patient should sit up until the cough subsides.

Chest percussion

Percussion, also known as tapping or clapping, is a technique of striking the patient's chest to loosen bronchial secretions as an aid to postural drainage. The striking force must be against the bare skin, delivered by the therapist's hand held slightly cupped with fingers and thumb closed so a cushion of air is trapped between the hand and chest wall. The therapist, holding his arm with the elbow partially flexed and wrist loose, whips his hand sharply down onto the chest over the area being drained. Best results come from using both hands alternately in rapid sequence for several seconds at a time. It is a noisy procedure, but, far from being painful to the patient, it is stimulating and the coarse vibrations set up in the thorax literally shake loose secretions. Naturally, care must be exercised by the therapist to avoid tender areas or sites of trauma or surgery. It is not a difficult technique to master, but skill and experience are needed to determine the force to use for a given chest wall thickness and to maintain a uniform blow throughout the procedure.

Chest vibration

Like percussion, chest vibration is an accompaniment to postural drainage and has the same objective as percussion but through a little different technique. In the classical maneuver, the therapist lays one hand on the patient's chest over the involved area and places his other hand on top of the first. Then, while exerting slight to moderate pressure on the chest wall, he rapidly produces an even vibratory motion of his hands. In contrast to the more violent percussion, this procedure sets up fine vibrations that are transmitted to the secretions. More effective is the use of an electric hand vibrator. This instrument not only assures prolonged uniform vibrations to loosen secretions but is also relaxing to the patient.

The combination of IPPB, postural drainage, chest percussion, and vibration can thus be considered as a treatment unit; and the physical therapy elements have proved themselves very helpful in increasing the efficiency of pressure breathing and aerosol therapy. In practice, the therapist will often start IPPB in the usual manner and then, upon noting the apparent presence of resistant secretions that the patient raises with great difficulty if at all, will stop and position the patient for drainage. He will apply percussion and vibration over the basal areas, giving the patient ample opportunity to cough as needed. Again, he will resume IPPB and so continue to alternate between pneumatic, aerosol, and physical therapy according to the results he obtains. The ability and judgment of the inhalation therapist to use such combined therapy effectively rank equally with his skill at maintaining mechanical ventilation.

Cough control

To the patient with a basically normal respiratory tract, a cough is usually a necessary nuisance that gives him relief from bronchial irritation. To the patient with chronic pulmonary disease, on the other hand, an effective cough may mean the difference between adequate and inadequate air exchange; and this he may not be able to accomplish. In general, patients who need some type of cough assistance will be found among those with (1) postoperative or posttraumatic pulmonary restriction (thoracic or abdominal), (2) postventilator weakness, or (3) air trapping. The patient with restriction, usually due to pain, has limited inspiration and is unable to generate enough propulsive power to remove secretions effectively. The therapist can help such a patient by supporting his lower thorax bilaterally with the hands. As the patient inhales, the therapist moves with the expanding chest but still maintains resistance against which the patient must work. At the limit of the patient's inspiration, the pressure exerted by the therapist gives impetus to the start of a cough, and continued compression increases the force and velocity of the exhaled air. The therapist can repeat this maneuver several times to mobilize secretions and may be able to teach some patients to do it themselves, although this is usually less effective.

The patient recently weaned from a mechanical ventilator and the patient with air trapping, as from emphysema, may have adequate inspiratory capacities but lack expulsive power for effective removal of secretions. The reasons for their problems differ, however. Prolonged assisted ventilation may allow one patient to lose tone and strength of his ventilatory muscles so that, although he can move tidal air satisfactorily, he cannot generate cough power. Also, irritation of his throat from intubation or actual laryngeal damage may limit cough. On the other hand, the patient with bronchiolar damage may have commendable vital and inspiratory capacities, but the buildup of intrathoracic pressure during cough compresses the weakened bronchiolar walls to stop the cough before it has had time to be effective. Both these patients can be taught to overcome their problems, a responsibility of the inhalation therapist when he notes that the problems exist. The therapist instructs the patients to start their coughs from a midinspiratory position rather than the usual full inspiration, which is more natural. This reduces the volume of air to be removed by the weak patient and lowers the intrathoracic pressure of the air trapper. To compensate for resultánt loss of expulsive force, the patients are then told to exhale in a rapid series of "machine gun" bursts of short, sharp coughs, repeated several times always from a midinspiratory position or even the end-expiratory resting level. This technique relieves the weak patient of the strain of a prolonged hard cough, and the staccato rhythm at a relatively low velocity minimizes airway collapse in the air-trapping patient.

Acute chest compression

Acute chest compression is related to the procedure just described for cough control, but it has a specific and often acute indication, especially in the patient with severe emphysema and air trapping. Not only may the mechanism of air trapping interfere with effective cough, as already noted, but it may place the patient's life in jeopardy. The emphysematous patient with chronic bronchial secretions may suddenly be stimulated by the need to cough, take a deep breath, start his cough, and suddenly find his airflow shut off before end-expiration. At this point he may be unable either to exhale or inhale, and his chest becomes "frozen" and immobile. He continues to strain in an attempt to move air, his neck veins distend from the intrathoracic pressure, his face becomes cyanotic, and he is suddenly in acute danger of suffocation. Fortunately, most such episodes are self-limiting, as perhaps weakness causes enough relaxation of intrathoracic pressure to permit air to move; but the experience is frightening to patient and family alike, and it severely strains the heart and subjects the brain to acute hypoxia. The inhalation therapist should be prepared to manage this event, for the overbreathing from IPPB and breathing exercises may precipitate an attack of acute air trapping. Should this happen or the patient give a history of its occurrence at home, family members should be taught how to treat it. The technique is quite simple but effective and is applied as soon as the patient's distress is seen, for, of course, he will be unable to speak. If the patient is relatively slight in stature, the therapist, standing behind him, places both hands over the lateral costal margins and lower chest and exerts a series of strong short compressions, releasing completely between each. This develops bursts of enough intrapulmonary pressure to break through airway obstruction and allow completion of exhalation. If the patient is large, with a heavy chest wall, the therapist can exert greater expulsive force by standing to the patient's side and, grasping him in a bear hug around the lower thorax, sharply squeezing him laterally against his own body. The occurrence of acute air trapping whenever an attempt is made to cough indicates the need for intensive therapy to remove offending secretions but at the same time is a warning to use caution in treatment and to try to maintain the patient's ventilation at a level of low velocity.

Pursed-lip breathing

Pursed-lip breathing is a simple maneuver that many patients learn for themselves without knowing why, but because it is so useful in breathing exercises and breath control, it should be taught to those unaware of it. Its purpose is to prevent the air trapping due to bronchiolar collapse, serving the same purpose as the retard cap on the exhalation port of the IPPB respirator, and is almost exclusively used for emphysema. The patient is instructed to purse his lips as if whistling during exhalation, controlling the velocity of his exhaled air to the slowest that is consistent with his ventilation. A variation of this, which is not really pursed-lip, consists of placing the tongue on the roof of the mouth and releasing the air slowly as if saying the letter "s." This has no inherent gain over pursing the lips and is certainly noisier. In either case, resistance of the mouth transmits back pressure throughout the bronchial tree, and its gradual release during exhalation prevents intrathoracic pressure from compressing shut those bronchioles weakened by disease. When used with the forceful abdominal-breathing exercises to be described next, the pursed-lip retard of airflow is continued to the end of the prolonged exhalation. At other times, such as during the breath control of quiet breathing or moderate exercise, the pursed-lip retard may be released at midexhalation to allow a normal terminal flow, since the naturally slowing velocity of passive end-expiration carries little risk of air trapping.

Abdominal breathing

Of the many available exercises directed toward improving the mechanics of ventilation, we will describe but four, for it is felt that these have the widest application in the general treatment of respiratory deficiencies. Many of the others are designed to improve skeletal muscle performance and posture, but we will let the therapist pursue their uses at his leisure. When we discussed the mechanics of ventilation, we learned how such pulmonary pathology as obstruction, destruction of alveoli, and air trapping upset the normal ventilatory pattern, lowering the diaphragm and effectively removing it from useful ventilation and throwing the burden of air movement on the thorax. We learned how inefficient is thoracic breathing, with its need to activate accessory ventilatory muscles, and how the subsequent distortion of a barrel chest aggravates the problem. In this section we will be interested in the patient with thoracic breathing, especially if paradoxical, for the thoracic breather is expending much more energy moving his chest wall than he would if he had only to move his more flexible abdominal wall. The additional oxygen need for the work of breathing seriously compounds the disability of his underlying disease. Abdominal-breathing exercises are designed to ease ventilatory work by gradually changing the pattern from thoracic to abdominal. This is a slow and difficult process and requires the utmost patience of the inhalation therapist. He should understand that it is often very difficult for a patient who has developed a thoracic breathing pattern to revert to abdominal; and many never do accomplish it. It is quite remarkable that what was once a natural function, when lost, is so difficult to relearn. There is no set method of teaching effective breathing, but we will present suggested techniques upon which the therapist can improve with experience and which he can modify according to need. Before starting a breathing exercise, the therapist should have the patient take two or three inhalations of a bronchodilator and permit him to relax mentally and physically. Before teaching a new exercise, he should demonstrate it plainly to the patient, explaining the purpose of each move and how best the patient can accomplish it.

Forced-exhalation abdominal breathing. The purpose of this exercise is to strengthen the contractile force of the abdominal wall muscles so that they can effectively elevate the diaphragm and empty the lungs. Although it can be done in almost any position, it is best taught in the supine with a pillow under the patient's head and his knees drawn up comfortably to relax the anterior abdominal wall. The principles of technique are illustrated in Fig. 11-3. The patient's hand is placed on his epigastrium, not to exert pressure but only to focus his attention to this area (*A*). Much of the success of therapy will depend upon the degree to which the therapist can keep the patient's mind on epigastric movement. Exercise is always started in the same manner, by exhaling from the resting level through pursed lips. At the same time the patient is instructed to pull in his upper abdomen gradually, with conscious force, prolonging exhalation as long as he can (*B*). At end-exhalation, he is told to inhale easily through his nose, letting his upper abdomen balloon out (*C*); and the cycle is repeated. From now on, however, exhalation will start from end-inspiration, and the patient is urged to let the air flow out slowly through pursed lips until near the end of normal expiration and then forcibly to contract the upper abdomen to extend expiration to its maximum.

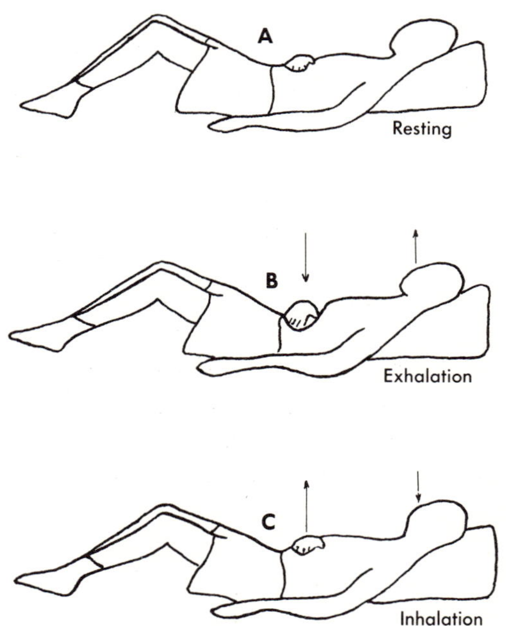

Fig. 11-3. Forced-exhalation abdominal breathing. See text for description.

He is advised to think of all his breathing as taking place in his abdomen rather than in his chest; therefore, as he fills with air, his abdomen should swell, lifting up his hand, and as he expels air, his hand should fall with his receding abdomen. During the maneuver the therapist must keep reminding the patient to concentrate on all respiratory movement as taking place in the area in contact with his hand and to disregard his chest completely. Many patients, trying hard to cooperate, will suddenly forget the sequence they were taught, contracting the epigastric wall during inhalation and attempting to relax it during exhalation, and may even stop breathing in their confusion. The therapist will find two things of help. The first is the steady repetition over several breathing cycles of "breath in, abdomen out, breath out, abdomen in" to help fix the rhythm in the patient's mind. The second is the placement of his hand over the patient's on the abdominal wall to exert gentle but firm pressure, depressing the epigastrium during the prolongation of exhalation. Much practice may be required for this seemingly simple procedure, but as proficiency is acquired, the patient is encouraged to make a positive effort to keep the chest immobile while ventilating completely with the abdomen.

If the patient has exceptionally poor coordination and is unable to achieve adequate expiratory contraction of his abdomen, the surface upon which he is lying may be tilted so that the body inclines cephalad about 20 degrees. A pillow may be used under the head, but care is taken that it does not extend beneath the shoulders. In this position the force of gravity shifts the abdominal contents against the diaphragm to assist in elevating it. This technique is useful only to get the procedure under way, for success depends upon developing sufficient abdominal strength to raise the diaphragm against gravity.

For the breathing exercise to be of value, it must be performed regularly and frequently, not just in the presence of the therapist. A regular schedule of exercise must be set up, perhaps as much as 5 to 10 minutes every hour until clinical results justify reducing it.

To vary the forced exhalation exercise, the patient may be taught to do it in the seated position, employing the added techniques of forward bending as shown in Fig. 11-4. The patient relaxes in a hard, straight-backed chair, sitting upright to commence the maneuver. With the arms hanging loosely by the side to promote relaxation of the thoracic skeletal muscles, he slowly exhales through pursed lips while slowly bending forward and retracting the upper abdomen (sketch *A*). When properly timed, flexion of the trunk should be complete at the moment of end-expiration. The body is then raised while the patient inhales through the nose, letting the abdomen distend as the lungs fill. When inhalation is completed, the patient should be back in the upright position. To aid exhalation, the forward bending uses the flexion of the trunk to compress the abdomen and elevate the diaphragm. This exercise is especially helpful to the patient when he is troubled with secretions, for it enables him to hyperventilate slightly and stimulate the mobility of his secretions for easier cough removal.

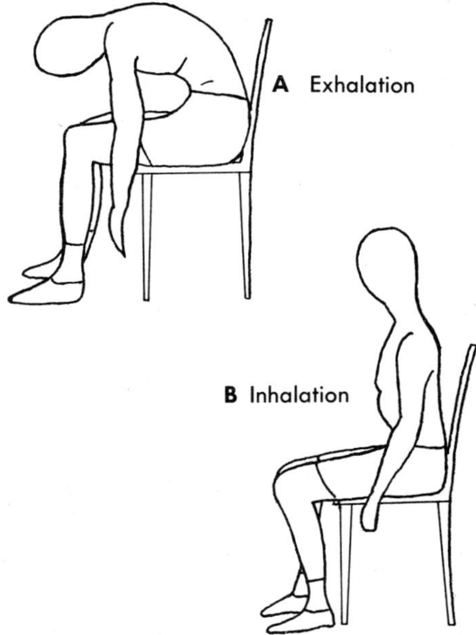

Fig. 11-4. Forced-exhalation abdominal breathing, seated. See text for description.

Forced-inhalation abdominal breathing. In contrast to forced exhalation, the physical effort in this exercise is directed toward inhalation with exhalation mostly passive. This more closely resembles the normal pattern of breathing. The patient is positioned as for forced exhalation but preferably with a 20-degree head-down tilt, and a weight of 10 to 15 pounds is placed over the midabdomen. A set of five fabric bags containing sand or buckshot is helpful, two weighing 5 pounds and three weighing 10 pounds. Since the abdominal weight will make exhalation easy for the patient, his attention is directed to strengthening his inspiratory effort. After letting his air out through pursed lips and terminally contracting his abdominal muscles, the patient is instructed to inhale through his nose, "taking air into the abdomen," with an effort forceful enough to lift the weight visibly. Because of the physical work involved, the initial time tolerated by the patient may be short, but as his performance improves, the exercise may be extended to a half hour three to four times daily. The abdominal weight is also increased in increments of 5 pounds and over a period of several weeks may reach 30 pounds. This exercise is especially useful for the patient with paradoxical breathing since it almost forces him to accept a normal breathing pattern. At the same time, the abdominal muscles are strengthened so that he can meet his ventilatory needs by this pattern. The therapist must warn the patient not to overdo the exercise, for soreness of the neglected muscles subjected to the strain of exercise is common and, if severe enough, can impede performance.

Forced-exhalation with walking. The primary objective of ventilatory exercise is to increase the patient's tolerance to physical activity, the most important of which is walking. One of his major complaints is his inability to walk comfortably, sometimes even from one room of his home to another; and going out of doors may be impossible. Improving his walking tolerance will do more to increase the patient's morale than any other therapeutic benefit. The inhalation therapist will observe that many patients who breathe with ease, resting in bed or chair, will revert to severe thoracic or paradoxical ventilation as soon as they start to walk. The purpose of the present exercise is to coordinate walking, and eventually other exertion, to the rhythm of abdominal breathing, using the prolonged phase of exhalation as the period of maximum effort. This implies that the patient has mastered the act of abdominal breathing and fully understands its purpose.

To prepare for walking exercise, the patient must practice abdominal breathing a few times in the standing position. This position, however, should not be rigidly upright but rather slightly bent forward, and although its esthetic effect may be less than desirable, it will make breathing easier. In a straight position, the abdominal muscles are under tension, as the string of a bow, but are relaxed by forward flexion and more available for controlled ventilation. The normal subject exerts and adjusts his ventilation accordingly to supply body oxygen needs, but the patient who is our present concern has limited ventilation and so must adapt his physical activity to it. This makes for an artificial and somewhat awkward relationship between breathing and walking but one that can be mastered profitably with practice. The technique is based upon establishing a ratio between a given amount of walking and the phasing of breathing, and experience has shown the following to be practical: The patient is instructed to move and breathe slowly, taking three steps during exhalation and two steps during inhalation. This does two things. It helps the patient to maintain a good ventilatory rhythm whereby exhalation exceeds inhalation, ensuring maximum air clearance of the lung; and it lets the patient perform the most exertion when it is easier, during expiration. Because this exercise is developed so that it can be done smoothly, the patient will find that his walking will consume much less energy than when his breathing was haphazard. The rationale of this technique can be explained to the patient in the following way so that he will understand the need to persist in what may seem to him at first to be a silly effort: When the normal subject is faced with a strenuous act, he first inhales, closes his glottis to hold his breath, and then contracts the necessary muscles. If the physical action is prolonged, he slowly releases his air, often in short bursts, prolonging exhalation while he continues to strain, and then takes a rapid inspiration and repeats until his effort is finished. The point to note is that maximum physical effort is expended during exhalation, not inhalation. With markedly limited ventilation, it is important that our patient with respiratory insufficiency correlate as much of his effort with exhalation as possible.

The patient who learns coordinated walking will find the technique applicable to many other activities. It will greatly help him in climbing stairs, ordinarily one of his most difficult chores, if he develops the habit of managing two or three steps during exhalation and resting during inhalation. Most emphysematous patients get extremely short of breath bending to pick up an object. This can be made much easier by exhaling slowly through pursed lips while bending and grasping the object, then inhaling while arising and lifting, much in the manner of doing the forward bending exercise in a chair.

Mobilization of the lower ribs. The final maneuver to be described is not strictly an abdominal exercise, but it is intended to augment abdominal breathing by utilizing a portion of the thorax that does not hinder ventilation. This consists of expanding and contracting the costal margin, which will give maximum mobility to the diaphragm and increase aeration of the lung bases. At first the exercise needs the help of the therapist, but later it can be self-administered. The patient will best understand the purpose of the exercise if he is introduced to it in the relaxed supine position; but the maneuver can be as well done seated. The therapist places his hands over the costal margins so that they almost cup the lower rib edges, and as the patient exhales through pursed lips, the hands follow the slightly contracting rib margins. Just before the end of exhalation the therapist exerts a forceful crescendo squeeze, holding the pressure firmly. As inhalation begins, the therapist gradually releases his manual pressure but retains some resistance to the expanding ribs. The patient is instructed to "breathe around the waist and push the hands away," to direct his attention to this area. He is also told to make an effort to squeeze in his costal edge himself while he pulls in his abdomen during exhalation. Finally, he is allowed to use his own hands to mobilize the lower ribs, and some therapists recommended the use of a swathe or a belt that the patient can use instead of his hands.

Graded exercises

Somewhat as the culmination, or end objective, of the breathing exercises just described, a system of graded exercises is used to condition the patient for prolonged activity, principally walking. As the name implies, the patient's effort is built up gradually against controlled resistance, both to minimize injury to him and to monitor his progress with objective data. A patient is ready for this aspect of rehabilitation only after maximum airway patency has been achieved and after he has mastered breath control through abdominal breathing, although it is still frequently necessary to use aerosol therapy, pressure breathing, and postural drainage in conjunction with graded exercise.

Whereas techniques in performing progressive exercises may vary, the general principles are the same. Either a treadmill or an exercising bicycle is used, the resistance of which can be adjusted. Both are satisfactory, but the treadmill has the advantage that it more closely simulates the type of physical activity we are trying to develop—walking—and we will use it in our discussion. Supplemental oxygen is usually given to the patient, at least in the early stage of therapy, so that he can withstand the stress of activity. A loosely fitting plastic mask or nasal cannula is satisfactory. Ventilatory function, blood gas, cardiac function, and any other evaluation data are obtained prior to starting the program and are repeated according to the needs of each treatment schedule. The therapist should note that walking on a treadmill is not exactly the same as walking on a stable surface because there is a certain knack to using the legs in a normal manner while the body remains in position and the underfooting moves. This should be explained to the patient and demonstrated by the therapist. The patient should step onto the treadmill mat while it is moving slowly, and although he should be allowed to place his hands gently on the safety railing, he should be instructed not to let the support bear his weight. The first exposure of the patient to exercise is tentative, to judge his response and tolerance and to teach him the proper technique. He is given oxygen and the treadmill adjusted to 0% grade and a rate not to exceed 1 mph. The therapist must give reassurance and encouragement to many patients who are initially apprehensive, and they may be told that they can step off the moving surface at any time. During the first trial the therapist must see that the patient is using his abdomen to breathe, for it is under such conditions of stress that he is apt to revert to thoracic or paradoxical breathing; and this cannot be permitted if the therapy is to be successful. Whatever program is used, graded exercises are given regularly and daily, sometimes for several weeks. The pitch of the walking surface, its speed, and the duration of exercise are increased in increments tailored to each patient; and these are good criteria for evaluating progress. For example, if a patient walks 10 minutes at 0% grade and 1 mph at one time and later walks 15 minutes at 2% grade and 1.5 mph, this represents significant improvement.

Even more important is the gradual reduction in the need for supplemental oxygen as the intensity of the exercise increases. It may seem paradoxical that increasing exercise of a patient with respiratory insufficiency should lower his oxygen requirement, but the physiologic reason for this is the foundation for this aspect of rehabilitation. We must remember that patients with impaired breathing become sedentary, suffering progressive atrophic weakness of their leg muscles from disuse; and the less efficient the work of a muscle, the greater is the consumption of oxygen for the energy expended by the muscle. To put it another way, more oxygen must be taken in by the body to supply the needs of a poorly conditioned muscle in performing a given amount of work than is required by a well-conditioned muscle. The clinical improvement from a graded exercise program is attributed to two factors. First, although pulmonary function tests may show little change, ventilatory muscle training improves the patient's pattern of breathing with better pulmonary aeration and an increased ability to satisfy the needs of exertion. Second, the physical conditioning with improved efficiency of ventilatory and leg muscles reduces their oxygen demand. Together, both factors markedly increase the amount of work produced per unit of energy expended. Finally, although strenuous exercise may be contraindicated or must be used with caution in patients with some types of heart disease, cor pulmonale is probably not a contraindication if the heart is not in frank failure. The heart strain is apparently not worsened because of the eventual reduction in metabolic oxygen demand.

The program just described must be carried out in a rehabilitation facility, of course, with elaborate equipment under the constant supervision of trained personnel. It is felt that this is the most desirable management, but there may be instances in which such supervision is not practical or possible. With proper selection, many patients can profit from a well-planned home-care program; and one of the many valuable services of the inhalation therapist is the training and follow-up supervision of patients for such programs. The home-care patient must be carefully taught the postural-drainage and breathing-exercise techniques; and it is wise also to teach these techniques to a reliable family member who may have to assist the patient. Graded exercises with oxygen can be done at home but should be attempted only if both the patient's attending physician and inhalation therapist feel the patient is responsible and intelligent enough to follow directions accurately. Home exercise can be provided by an exercise cycle, which is space saving, or by level walking, if space permits. Supportive oxygen, gaseous and liquid, is available in small enough containers to be carried by a shoulder sling. Small gaseous cylinders can be refilled from large cylinders, but there is some potential risk in this and it must be advised with caution. According to the patient's capabilities, a graded schedule of walking can be made for him, but it must be reviewed frequently for modifications and to assess its results. Experience has shown that only an exceptional and unusually motivated patient will persist in a graded exercise program at home, away from professional supervision and encouragement, for long enough periods to realize much gain from it as his primary therapy. As a follow-up to a rehabilitation area course of treatment and after the discontinuance of supportive oxygen, home exercises of the postural and kinetic types not only are valuable, but for many patients they must be continued indefinitely.

OTHER ASPECTS OF REHABILITATION

The rest of our discussion of rehabilitation will not involve the direct technical services of the inhalation therapist, but the therapist should be aware of all the efforts made on the disabled patient's behalf, for each facet of therapy or management has some influence on the others. The more each member of the rehabilitation team knows about the patient, the better able he will be to evaluate the patient's progress and his own role in it.

Psychosomatic support

The term *psychosomatic* refers to the relationship between the emotional state or outlook of an individual *(psyche)* and the physical responses of the individual's body *(soma).* Everyday life is full of such relationships, as, for example, the physical fatigue that follows a period of emotional tension; and many of them are considered part of normal human behavior. Some, however, cause or aggravate an existing, physical disability; and it is with this aspect of chronic pulmonary insufficiency that we are concerned. It is important for the inhalation therapist to realize that all his skilled technical services, as well as the best pharmacologic therapy, can be negated and a patient driven to a progressively downhill course because of an unfavorable mental attitude. Emotional instability is not unique to patients with respiratory disease alone, of course, for we frequently see severe signs of depression and hostility complicating many acute and chronic diseases. In chronic respiratory disease, however, it may be a double-edged sword; for not only can psychic disturbances affect the general well-being of the patient, but they may also directly aggravate the very defects that are responsible for his underlying disability. The ease and frequency with which emotional upsets affect the respiratory function are recognized in such commonly expressed relationships as "holding one's breath in anticipation," or being "choked up with emotion." Thus, it is not difficult to imagine that a patient with labored breathing could be made much worse by a psychic stimulus affecting his breathing.

The role of emotional and personality problems in the genesis of childhood bronchial asthma is well known, as has been extensively recorded in medical literature. It is quite probable that many instances of adult asthma, for which no specific allergic basis can be found, likewise stem from some recent or unresolved emotional conflict. The psychic element in nonasthmatic chronic pulmonary disease is probably of a different nature, although such patients, too, may have preexisting problems. Often the patient with progressive emphysema develops severe anxiety and hostility as a direct consequence of his disability. Because he is fearful of economic loss and death, he develops hostility toward his disease and often toward those with whom he comes into close contact. Patients with chronic respiratory disease are frequently seen to become acutely dyspneic during conversation that touches upon subjects arousing fear and hostility.

The therapist should not entertain the impression that all patients chronically ill with pulmonary disability are primarily neurotic or that they imagine their symptoms. From our examinations, we know the severe physical impairment of these patients; but we should also recognize that part of their symptomatology may well be due to psychosomatic influences. Unfortunately, proper attention to this side of their disability has been generally neglected, probably for two basic reasons. First, the great spurt of interest in pulmonary disease of the past two decades has centered mostly on the physiology of diseases and physical therapeutic measures. Second, short as are the facilities for chronic physical care and rehabilitation, those for mental rehabilitation have been even shorter, for psychosomatic therapy demands the services of both psychiatrists and clinical psychologists who are especially interested in the chronically disabled respiratory patient. Such therapy has been used in the management of bronchial asthma, and results justify its wider application to nonasthmatic diseases as well. No suggestions are made here as to how to include adequate psychotherapy into the overall rehabilitation program, but it should be an integral part. It is quite probable that superficial treatment might be satisfactory in the majority of cases, such as could be provided in group therapy. General observation of patients in an inhalation therapy outpatient service suggests that many derive support and encouragement by association with others; but to be most effective, this association should be professionally guided and directed. On the other hand, some would profit most from private care, in which their personal emotional conflicts could be aired and the relationship of such conflicts to their breathing explained to them. It is hoped that, as pulmonary rehabilitation becomes more definitive, some technique of psychotherapy will evolve, directed to the specific needs of the respiratory cripple.

Occupational retraining and placement

Many disabled pulmonary patients are in their economically productive years and are anxious to be self-sufficient. For them, occupational retraining and job placement are necessary ingredients of a purposeful rehabilitation program. Such a program should not be on a hit-or-miss basis but upon classifiable data, specific for each patient. Much study is yet needed to categorize occupations in terms of their energy requirements of the respiratory system and to derive simple but informative tests of the work of breathing to enable the rehabilitation team to match patients to those jobs in which they would have the greatest chance of success. Not only must the patient's physical status be considered but his education, past experience, and aptitudes as well. Obviously, this is not solely the responsibility of medicine but will require the skills of counselors trained in occupational needs, and the cooperation of business and industry in each community. These efforts have already been made in behalf of disability due to such conditions as incapacitating trauma and stroke and could readily be applied to pulmonary disability as soon as the specific needs of the latter have been classified.

Family counseling

Family counseling is included not merely to round out the program in a general way but because experience has shown its great importance in therapy. Those of us who treat patients with respiratory diseases daily become familiar with the patterns of their diseases, but among the laity there is still a considerable lack of understanding as to the extent of disability that chronic pulmonary disease can produce. Relatives often consider the patient's cough an unnecessary nuisance to them and his reluctance to be physically active a manifestation of laziness, an impression supported by his frequent healthy appearance in the resting state. The patient is acutely aware of this attitude and is hurt, discouraged, and anxious. So sensitive are many patients with chronic disability to the discrepancy between how they look and how they feel that they react very irritably to simple greetings by their medical attendants of how well they look. It is essential that members of the patient's family fully understand the nature of his disease and the extent of his disability. It must be stressed to them that there are good reasons why he can look comfortable in a chair but may not be able to walk to the next room without assistance. They must also understand the objectives of chronic care and rehabilitation, the duration of treatment, its cost and inconvenience to the family, and the probability of improvement. Because home care is usually an important part of the program, full cooperation of the family is necessary or all efforts will fail.

The first responsibility for educating the family falls to the attending physician, but the follow-up role of the inhalation therapist is equally, if not more, important. His explanation of technique and procedures to both patient and relatives can do much to ensure understanding of and cooperation with the program. Both the social worker and the respiratory-trained visiting nurse can offer valuable services by checking on the home progress and helping to correct unfavorable conditions at home that may be detrimental to the patient. In the latter category, assistance may be offered to relieve the financial problems so often found with long-term illness and advice given on more efficient arrangement of home facilities and labor-saving techniques.

We can summarize the philosophy of chronic and rehabilitative care of the pulmonary disabled patient by emphasizing the following three points: First, in contrast to the treatment of many other chronic illnesses, respiratory therapy depends to a major degree upon a well-trained technical specialist who has often followed the patient through an acute illness into the chronic state and is now available to give long-term care based on firsthand knowledge of the patient's present and future needs. The inhalation therapist is a bridge between the acute and chronic phases of the disease and makes possible a valuable continuity of treatment. Second, many of the treatment procedures can be self-administered by the patient, not only relieving the financial burden of his care but also putting upon him some of the responsibility for his own welfare and, by such a commitment, helping him to become free of complete dependence upon others. Third, for maximum rehabilitation of this ever-growing patient population, the team approach is essential. Only through the cooperative efforts of the many whose services can benefit the respiratory patient will we be able to set up a practical program that will permit us to evaluate him physiologically, socially, and economically and, on the basis of this evaluation, help him to regain optimum well-being and independence.

Chapter 12

The organization, staffing, and services of an inhalation therapy department*

It seems appropriate to close our discussion of the many things we feel a good inhalation therapist should know and be able to do by describing the structure of the unit in which he will work. There can be no blueprint of an ideal inhalation therapy department that will satisfy the needs of all hospitals; but we will make some suggestions that have been time tested by experience to serve as sort of a skeleton which can be modified for custom use. We will also have an opportunity to summarize the overall services of inhalation therapy in the general hospital and to describe personnel requirements and divisions of labor.

Hospitals have been facing an increasing load of patients with cardiopulmonary diseases over the past several years but often lacking both the physical facilities and technical personnel to provide modern care. The techniques that have evolved for the treatment of these patients require the assistance of skilled technical help, and we have already indicated that they are too detailed for the average attending physician, house physician, or nurse to supervise or administer. It was in response to this need that the technical specialty of inhalation therapy emerged to take its place in the hospital organization. Historically, the predecessor of inhalation therapy was the well-known but little regarded hospital oxygen service. However, the highly skilled offspring bears little resemblance to its humble ancestor, for during his evolution, the inhalation therapist has undergone intensive medically supervised education and training, enabling him to provide skills and services not available from any existing hospital personnel. Because of the large number of patients who can benefit from the well-organized services of inhalation therapy, it is the responsibility of every general hospital that opens its doors to the public to provide such services. The utilization of inhalation therapy services where effective departments operate is remarkable and is ample proof of their acceptance by the medical profession. After observing the growth of this technical specialty for several years and reviewing the ex-

*This chapter is an expanded version of a paper published in Hospitals, Sept 1, 1968, and is reprinted with permission.

perience of 17 hospitals with active services, we can make the conservative estimate that an efficient department in a busy general hospital will probably provide some form of inhalation therapy to about 20% of patients admitted. Let us now comment on the services, structure, operation, and size of a workable inhalation therapy department.

SERVICES OF AN INHALATION THERAPY DEPARTMENT

It is not necessary to describe in detail the services offered by inhalation therapy since we have covered their technical aspects in other chapters, but the outline below summarizes them for us in a bird's-eye view. It can be noted, however, that these services cut across established hospital departmental lines, the administrative implications of which will be mentioned later.

Inhalation therapy services

A. *Therapeutic gases*
  1. Oxygen: mask, catheter, cannula, face tent, canopy tent
  2. Helium-oxygen mixtures
  3. Carbon dioxide–oxygen mixtures

B. *Aerosols and humidity*
  1. Bronchodilators, detergents, mucolytics, proteolytic enzymes, antibiotics, steroids
  2. High humidity, aerosolized water
  3. Procurement of sputum specimens for cytologic and bacterial examination

C. *Mechanical ventilation*
  1. Intermittent positive-pressure breathing
     a. Administration of aerosols for airway patency
     b. Prevention of postoperative atelectasis
     c. Treatment of acute pulmonary edema
  2. Assisted ventilation for inadequate spontaneous breathing
     a. Continuous ventilation by pressure-regulated ventilators
     b. Monitoring by blood gas analysis, tidal volume
     c. Maintenance of airway patency by tracheobronchial aspiration
  3. Controlled ventilation for apnea
     a. Continuous ventilation by tank, volume-regulated, flow-regulated, pressure-regulated ventilators
     b. Maintenance of adequate volume, rate, pressure
     c. Maintenance of circulatory stability

D. *Physical therapy and rehabilitation*
  1. Ambulatory service for aerosol and pressure breathing treatments
  2. Postural drainage
  3. Corrective breathing exercises
  4. Oxygen-supported ambulatory exercises
  5. Integration of treatments into custom-made progressive program for home care: patient instruction, follow-up supervision

E. *Pulmonary function testing*
  1. Minimum requirement examinations for routine respiratory care
     a. Spirometry
     b. Lung volume measurements
        (1) Nitrogen-washout
        (2) Helium equilibration
     c. Arterial or arterialized blood analysis
        (1) pH
        (2) Oxygen tension
        (3) Carbon dioxide tension
  2. Selected examinations

a. Alveolar ventilation
b. Dead space volume
c. Arterial-alveolar carbon dioxide difference
e. Pulmonary diffusion measurement
f. Pulmonary compliance measurement

F. *Unclassified*
1. Emergency resuscitation
2. Extracorporeal pump operation
3. Technical assistance in cardiopulmonary research
4. Future services yet unexplored

This list is not proposed as total and definitive, for the final boundaries of inhalation therapy are far from established; and from hospital to hospital there will be variations in the number and types of services offered. The last item noted above may turn out to be the most important of all as progress in chest medicine continues. It is essential that all departments be developed with a philosophy of flexibility to allow future growth as time may dictate.

DEPARTMENTAL STRUCTURE: ADMINISTRATION AND PERSONNEL

The organization of an effective inhalation therapy department will include some or all of the following personnel: medical director(s), chief therapist (technical director), assistant chief therapist(s), night supervisor, staff therapists, ambulatory service supervisor, chief laboratory technician and technicians, instructors, and secretary(ies). Certainly, all departments will not have all of these, and there may be other job specialties according to individual hospital needs. Fig. 12-1 outlines a suggested departmental organization, showing the relationship among the components of the department and between the department and the administration. This is presented only as a possible suggestion that is flexible enough to lend itself to the needs of any general hospital.

Note that the administrative outline depicts the inhalation therapy department in three modules, as a practical method of description. Ideally, the inhalation therapy department should be an independent administrative unit with its own budget and administrative support stemming from the hospital administration. Thus, in administrative and fiscal matters, the director of the department works directly with the hospital administration. The education module applies primarily to those hospitals that intend to include in their structure an inhalation therapy school or that have departments large enough to maintain a continuing inservice educational program. The medium to small-sized community hospitals will be primarily interested in the service and laboratory functions of their inhalation therapy departments. A small hospital may be adequately served by one medical director supervising a service function and a modest pulmonary function laboratory. Where there is a larger demand upon the inhalation therapy department, there may be an effective division of labor, employing two or more associate directors. Here the duties may be divided, with one director responsible for service function

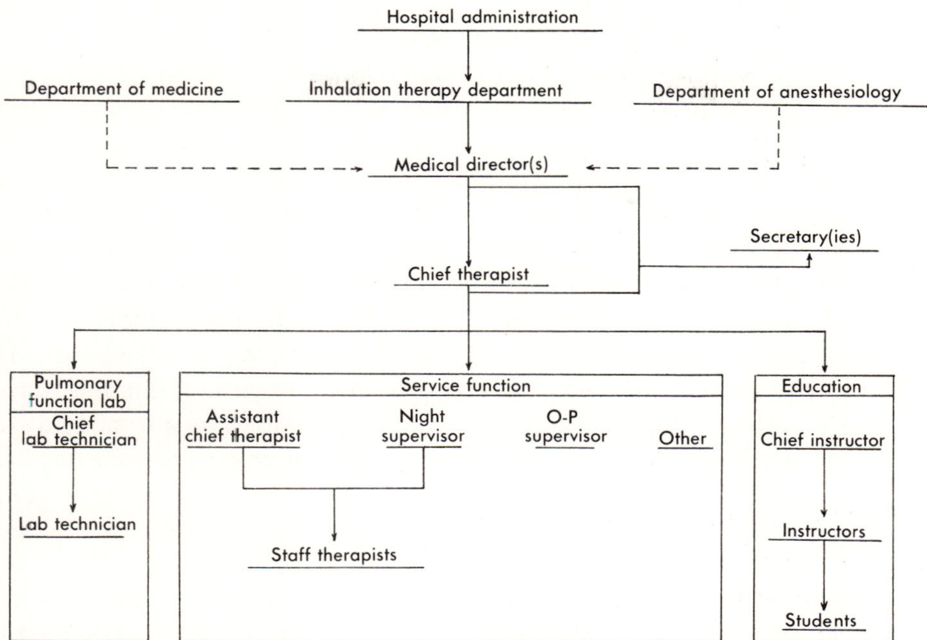

Fig. 12-1. Organizational outline for an inhalation therapy department. See text for descriptive details.

and another for the laboratory. In larger hospitals, where the work load may be exceptionally heavy, with much work being done in all three modules, the administrative and professional relationships may be varied again. In some instances it is practical to consider the service function of the inhalation therapy department, the pulmonary function laboratory, a school or other training and educational facility in inhalation therapy, and an ambulatory clinic for respiratory diseases, all as components of a larger professional unit, a section of chest diseases. Such a facility might have an overall chief of section; and the various subdivisions, their own individual directors. This arrangement most effectively combines the diagnostic and therapeutic facilities for treatment of cardiopulmonary diseases into a common unit in which administrative work is kept to a minimum and the professional cooperation and exchange of ideas make for the highest degree of patient care.

A vital subdivision of the service module is the respiratory care unit, not shown in the schematic outline since it requires no special administrative positioning. The need for such a unit has already been made clear, and it should be the direct responsibility of the inhalation therapy department. Its supervision and clinical servicing are assured through the regular departmental personnel and the pulmonary function laboratory. The only nondepartmental service needed is nursing, and this can be provided through an arrangement with the nursing service.

The success of any department will be in direct proportion to the efficiency and skill of its personnel, and in conformity with accepted terminology differentiation should be made at this time between an inhalation therapist and an inhalation therapy technician. By definition the *therapist* is a technician who has successfully passed a rigidly limiting examination given by the American Registry of Inhalation Therapists, Inc., earning him the title of "registered therapist." Eligibility for taking the Registry examination requires an academic associate degree or the equivalent of 2 years of college study, in addition to specific education in inhalation therapy acceptable to the Board of Schools for Inhalation Therapy. The *technician*, on the other hand, is one engaged in providing inhalation therapy services but who is not registered—currently a definition for the most part based on exclusion. It is expected that more specific educational criteria will be established for the inhalation therapy technician in the near future; and perhaps a qualifying examination will be provided to designate him as "certified" or some other suitable title. Theoretically the therapist is supposedly qualified for supervisory and managerial responsibilities, and the technician for patient-care services, under supervision. For the sake of simplicity, however, the term *inhalation therapist* in this text has not been so restrictive and has referred to all technical specialists in inhalation therapy, generally. Idealism must frequently give way to reality, and in view of the shortage of trained personnel, many hospitals assign duties and responsibilities based on individual abilities rather than on technical classification.

Each member of the department listed in the organizational table will be described, with emphasis on specific duties.

Medical director(s)

The decision as to whether the departmental directorship should be in the hands of one or more persons or should be full or part time is a matter to be determined by each hospital. Whatever arrangement is made at the start, the hospital can be assured that there will be an increasing amount of time demanded of the director as the department grows; and this must be taken into consideration in planning for the future. Such anticipated growth may necessitate the addition of associate directors as time goes on. The medical director must be a physician who is interested in chest diseases and who has had at least some clinical experience or training in this field. Whether his duty hours are full or part time, his responsibility as director of the department will be full time, and he must be reasonably available for consultation and advice for the safe and effective supervision of the department.

Since the medical director must be a member of the hospital staff, he will be affiliated with one of the major hospital departments. From a practical point of view, there are only two major departments that lend themselves well to affiliation with inhalation therapy—anesthesiology and internal medicine. Historically, many departments of inhalation therapy have been organized under the direction of anesthesiologists for two primary reasons: (1) the common foundation of pulmonary physiology underlying both anesthesiology and inhalation therapy, (2) the presence of anesthesiologists in the hospital for extended periods of time. They may be justly credited with much of the development of inhalation therapy into the organized specialty as it now exists. The evolution of inhalation therapy, however, has evoked some subtle changes in its function that affect its relationship to anesthesiology. Whereas the therapist of the early days of the technology performed relatively simple tasks, under the direct guidance of the medical director, the contemporary therapist is permitted a significant degree of exercise of judgment and plays an important role in patient care. Inhalation therapy, as it is now practiced, primarily directs itself to the diagnosis and treatment of medical diseases or medical complications of surgery or trauma; and to realize his full potential, the therapist must be well grounded in many aspects of clinical medicine. It is not sufficient that he merely be skilled in manual techniques, but he must understand cardiopulmonary physiology to a considerable depth and the changes in physiology wrought by disease. Such a view implies a clinical and medical orientation in the teaching and direction of inhalation therapy, most realistically provided by an internist trained in the physiologic and clinical aspect of chest diseases.

Unfortunately, there is a shortage of clinicians able or willing to undertake the supervision of an inhalation therapy department, but there is hope for an improved future supply as greater emphasis is placed upon postdoctoral training in chest disease. It should also be noted that the availability of the anesthesiologist for management of inhalation therapy is often more apparent than real. Since his first responsibility is to the operating and recovery rooms, as the work load of inhalation therapy grows, he may find himself increasingly unavailable for its supervision; and many anesthesiologists have found the extracurricular demands of the technical field an unwelcome chore. Thus, the choice of a medical director depends upon the local factor of available personnel and the objectives of inhalation therapy in the individual hospital, but a general recommendation can be made. If the treatment of cardiopulmonary disease in a given hospital is to be completely managed by each attending physician and inhalation therapy is to provide only a skilled technical service of limited scope, supervision and quality control of such services can be performed by either an anesthesiologist or an internist. If however, inhalation therapy is to function maximally, integrating diagnostic laboratory facilities, professional consultation and referral services, and outpatient and rehabilitation care, a clinically trained internist is preferred as medical director. Where the employment of a full-time department head is not feasible, some hospitals have placed the supervision of inhalation therapy in the hands of a small committee of diversified interests, thus distributing the work and covering different areas of professional responsibility.

Regardless of his disciplinary affiliation, the medical director of the department is professionally responsible for the entire function of the department. Because of this responsibility, he should be afforded considerable authority in establishing the professional policies and practices of inhalation therapy in his hospital, although any major policy involving patient care or relationship between the department and staff physicians should be approved by the hospital medical board. Such a move would ensure understanding of the policy and guarantee maximum cooperation at all levels. The major responsibilities of the medical director include the following: provision or supervision of medical care of patients with respiratory diseases, including consultation and referral, acute respiratory care, ambulatory care, and pulmonary function evaluation; establishment of departmental clinical policies and procedures; supervision of inhalation therapy school and/or inservice training and education; education of medical and nursing staffs; selection and promotion of students, trainees, and therapists; maintenance of personnel and medical records; and preparation of the departmental budget.

Chief inhalation therapist (technical director)

The efficiency of departmental operation will depend upon this key figure. The chief therapist must be well trained in all aspects of inhalation therapy and experienced in its clinical application. He must be thoroughly versed in the techniques of therapy and the function of equipment, and he must possess leadership qualities and administrative ability. Although his position will probably have more prestige if he is registered by the American Registry of Inhalation Therapists, registration alone is not sufficient, for there are many registered therapists who do not have the other necessary qualities of a chief therapist. There is no guideline to indicate the depth of experience necessary for this position, but as a generalization, it might be assumed that the average therapist would need a minimum of 3 years of practical experience in the field, following his training, to prepare him for the duties of a chief therapist. His selection must depend upon a detailed interview for an appraisal of his background as well as candid references from previous teachers and employers. Whereas the medical director is responsible for the overall policies and professional functioning of the department, the chief therapist is responsible for the daily operation of this service. His administrative authority must be well understood and completely supported by the medical director, and he is an important link between the medical director and the technical staff. Among the chief's duties are the scheduling of staff assignments; the maintenance of payroll data on all technical personnel; maintenance of statistical data for reports of departmental activity; the maintenance of an inventory of all expendable equipment and supplies; advice and assistance to technical personnel; assistance in the training of new therapists; and assistance to the medical director on special projects and in preparation of the budget.

Assistant chief inhalation therapist

One or more assistant chief therapists will be needed according to the size of the department. The assistant chief should possess technical skills similar to those of the chief therapist but does not need as much administ perience. He has a responsible double role. In the absence of therapist, he acts as the technical director of the department, but in operation he is a troubleshooter. The assistant chief supervises the service in the respiratory care unit and consults with or advises staff therapists in the management of difficult patients, especially when it is necessary to improvise techniques or equipment. He takes an active role in the training and orientation of students and new therapists, and he evaluates all new or recently repaired equipment.

Night supervisor

Functioning somewhat as an assistant chief therapist during the evening and/or night shifts, the night supervisor must be an individual with a high degree of dependability and independent action. With less teaching and equipment evaluation responsibilities than his daytime counterpart, the night supervisor must be well trained to respond to emergency situations. He supervises and assigns work to the evening- and night-shift therapists and is available to do emergency blood gases in the cardiopulmonary laboratory should the duty laboratory technician be absent or overburdened.

Outpatient supervisor

The outpatient supervisor must be a highly skilled clinical therapist, especially effective in the techniques of physical therapy of chest diseases, which include segmental postural drainage, thoracic clapping and vibration, ventilatory exercises, and walking exercises. One of his most important functions is the instruction of patients in the techniques and use of equipment for home-care programs. He takes an active part in the teaching of student therapists, since the outpatient service provides an excellent opportunity for students to learn positive-pressure, aerosol, and physical therapy techniques with patients who are not critically ill and who are generally cooperative.

Pulmonary function laboratory technicians

An experienced and well-trained inhalation therapist is especially well founded to operate a pulmonary function laboratory. His background knowledge of cardiopulmonary physiology as well as of clinical chest diseases makes the purpose of pulmonary function testing more meaningful to him than to a technician without this experience. His insight into laboratory procedures makes him a good judge of the reliability of his results and makes him better able to recognize inaccuracies or laboratory errors or inconsistencies. Also, a pulmonary function laboratory staffed with inhalation therapists has close technical rapport with the clinical inhalation therapy personnel.

The chief pulmonary function laboratory technician must know the details and techniques of all the procedures in his laboratory and be able to train or orient students or new employees. He is responsible for supervising the quality of the work done by the other technicians, the scheduling of assignments, the maintenance of laboratory records, and the maintenance of an inventory of supplies. His knowledge of equipment must be sufficient for him to recognize malfunction and know what measures are necessary for repair of equipment. He also assists the director of the department or laboratory with special projects.

The staff technicians of the laboratory must be as well versed in the procedures and techniques as the chief technician but without the administrative or supervisory experience or authority. With careful selection of personnel, it is possible to teach noninhalation therapists to perform such specific duties as blood gas analyses for part-time laboratory coverage during the off hours of nights and weekends.

Staff inhalation therapist

The staff therapists comprise the work force of the department and are expected to know their equipment in detail, including its structure, function, the indications for its use, and its physiologic effect upon the patient. They must also know at least the basic maintenance procedures for this equipment. Before a therapist is allowed to treat patients, he must understand the physiology of respiration and circulation, both normal and abnormal, as it applies to inhalation therapy, and have a good working knowledge of the diseases to which he will be exposed. The therapist will be responsible for performing all the services listed above as functions of an inhalation therapy department except for some cardiopulmonary laboratory work and specialized tasks.

Because the inhalation therapist has close and intimate patient contact, it is essential that he be able to establish a good rapport with his patients; and this requires a stable personality, a strong motivation to work with the sick, and a personal conservatism in appearance, speech, and manner. He must understand the need for tact and the principles of medical ethics since patients frequently develop a strong attachment to the therapist and often confide in him and ply him with professional questions. The skill of the therapist in managing as well as treating his patient is an important factor in the patient's response to therapy. Extreme care and screening are needed in hiring personnel for this important job.

Instructors

Even in the absence of a formal school, an inservice continuing educational program should be followed and some of the regular staff given the responsibility for the technical teaching. Instructors must be well trained and experienced and able to transmit their knowledge to others. The technical instructors are especially valuable in teaching procedures and equipment function and for supervision of the clinical application of inhalation therapy at the bedside, but other subjects may be delegated to them as their qualifications permit. An important contribution of the instructor is his evaluation of his student and his recommendation of the degree of independent action that a student can be expected to fulfill. The instructors function directly under the medical director, correlating their material with his overall objectives and reporting their findings and recommendations to him for his final action.

DEPARTMENTAL OPERATION

Distribution of services

In terms of time coverage and scope of services, local hospital needs and available personnel will be the determining factors. Ideally, all inhalation therapy services should be available 24 hours a day 7 days a week. However, the very real chronic shortage of trained inhalation therapists makes this an almost impossible task, and most hospitals find it necessary to effect a compromise between demand and supply. Every attempt should be made to complete the maximum work volume during the day shift, and for this the full cooperation of the medical and nursing staffs is essential. Physicians should be urged to order therapy in advance so that it may be scheduled at the start of each day. The chief therapist always attempts to leave flexibility in his assignments to accommodate emergencies, but this requires a careful planning of more routine work. Staff nurses are usually too confined with their own responsibilities to take an active role in inhalation therapy, but frequently private-duty nurses can assist their patients by administering therapy under the instruction and supervision of a therapist.

The provision of services during nights and weekends always presents a problem. In general, only emergency cases and patients most acutely ill are serviced during those hours, and since the inhalation therapist is a technical rather than a professional person, it is the responsibility of the attending physician and supervisory nurses to cooperate in determining those patients who need care in off-hours. There is no general rule for the classification of patients according to need for inhalation therapy services, but the following list is offered as a suggested priority scale to help medical, nursing, and inhalation therapy personnel in scheduling work assignments.

Suggested priority for inhalation therapy services

1. Emergency resuscitation
2. Continuous mechanical ventilation
3. Any intensive-care area
4. Emergency room
5. Postoperative care
6. Oxygen or humidity administration
7. Prescheduled positive-pressure breathing
8. Physical therapy

The grouping represents only a commonsense classification of the patient suffering from acute cardiorespiratory failure as most in need of attention, and the patient in a period of convalescence or rehabilitation as least in need. It is emphasized that the objective of such a priority scale is not to restrict the application of inhalation therapy services but rather to enable the department to make the maximum use of them.

Clinical experience has demonstrated the necessity of having pulmonary function evaluation facilities available wherever inhalation therapy is being utilized to its maximum potential. At the current stage of inhalation therapy as a clinical technical specialty, its techniques frequently need some physiologic evaluation to determine proper therapy. This is especially true wherever patients are being maintained on mechanical ventilation. In such circumstances it is mandatory that the physiologic status be monitored by frequent examination of arterial or arterialized blood for pH, carbon dioxide tension, and oxygen tension; and the experienced therapist will use these data along with other criteria to adjust the ventilators accordingly. Since patients in ventilatory failure are as much in need of close supervision during the night and on weekends as at other times, it is necessary that facilities for blood gas monitoring be available. The ease with which this can be accomplished will be determined by the available laboratory facilities and personnel and is another valuable service the inhalation therapist will be able to perform. It is ideal to have full-time laboratory technicians on duty around the clock 7 days a week, but often this is not feasible and a compromise schedule must be established. Sometimes the night supervisor is able to handle the necessary laboratory work during his duty hours, but if this is not sufficient, as indicated earlier, it is frequently practical to employ the part-time services of personnel who are not inhalation therapists. Although they may know little cardiopulmonary physiology, if they are receptive and learn thoroughly, they can be taught techniques of blood gas analysis and free the regular staff for service during the working day. The success of this approach depends upon careful selection, meticulous instruction, and close supervision.

Scheduling of assignments

In the role of a dispatcher, the chief therapist designates the work areas and assigns patients to the staff therapists at the beginning of the day. A zone system is usually the most effective, and with experience, most hospitals can be divided into areas according to the average work density. One therapist may be designated to circulate, helping in the busy areas, responding to emergencies, and performing such routine duties as monitoring tent oxygen concentrations, checking tanked gas contents, and examining other operating equipment. At least one therapist should rotate through an equipment-servicing detail, in which he is responsible for cleaning and sterilizing, storage, and maintenance. If local labor supply will permit, hiring nontechnical personnel for this task will free the therapist for patient care or other duties for which he is trained. Arrangements are made to give priority service to intensive-care units and the emergency room, and response to floor emergencies is standardized.

Throughout the day all calls for service are submitted to the chief therapist's office. A written record is executed to include date and time, nature of request, and its disposition; and the record is kept on file. The chief therapist is responsible for expediting service during the day's operation, shifting personnel and assignments as needed, a task difficult but critical, requiring skill and judgment.

Efficiency of communications is an important key to smooth function. Hospital paging systems are at best only partially adequate, for most have many "deaf spots," but individual paging or signal units justify their cost in time saved and, thus, numbers of patients serviced. Since most hospitals with effective departments include a therapist in their resuscitation teams, a radio page will enhance response to emergencies.

Records and accounts

Each hospital has its own record and accounting system, and only a few comments are indicated. In great vogue now are various types of computerized techniques with memory storage and retrieval capabilities, and the capacity and flexibility of these need no amplification. However, many hospitals must yet rely upon manual systems, and every attempt is made to reduce clerical work to a minimum. The use of the portable visible index-type card file enables the therapist to carry with him a record card for each patient for whom he is responsible. All treatments or services for a given day are entered on this card, and at the end of the day charge tickets are executed for each patient and submitted to the accounting office. From the accumulated patient cards, data are obtained for a statistical account of the departmental activity and transferred to a day sheet. The day sheet tabulates such items as the number of patients treated, the patient days of treatment, the numbers of individual services, and patient charges according to type of service. Each month the total of the day sheets is recorded in a monthly statistical report, which is submitted to the hospital administration, the accounting department, and the director of the department; and these reports form the basis for evaluating departmental progress. Many modifications of this system are possible, especially for recall of grouped data, and can be achieved by special filing procedures or the use of punched cards. Because each therapist must keep track of service data on patients scattered all over the hospital, it is essential that the system chosen be as simple and error-proof as possible.

In addition to accounting records, the inhalation therapy department must maintain a clinical record in each patient's chart. Simplicity is advised in the format of such a record, and a ruled sheet with a place to note date and time, room for comments, and an initial or signature column is adequate. Following each treatment, the therapist is expected to note on the sheet a comment concerning the treatment and the patient and any other information he considers relevant. This is an invaluable guide for subsequent therapists.

Professional supervision

Reference was made earlier to an important aspect of inhalation therapy when it was noted that the services of inhalation therapy extend into all major hospital divisions. As a hospital service, the department provides facilities available on the order of all staff physicians. At the same time, the services so provided are under the control of and are the responsibility of another physician, the medical director of the department. Whereas care must be taken to minimize the risk of interference with the autonomy of the attending physician by the medical director, close control of the proper use of inhalation therapy services must be assured by the director. These objectives can easily be attained by willing cooperation among hospital administration, medical staff, and the inhalation therapy department. Many therapeutic procedures can be classified as "standard," with little ambiguity as to their function and generally complete understanding of their clinical application. Among others, this group might include such services as oxygen administration, aerosols of wide acceptance, and mist therapy. The direct responsibility of the medical director in the application of these services requires little more than ensuring a smooth-running department. In contrast, the safe and effective use of some inhalation therapy techniques requires much experience as well as specific professional and technical knowledge. Especially is this true in the management of the critically ill patient in ventilatory failure, the techniques of rehabilitation and chronic care, and the interpretation of pulmonary function tests.

There are two administrative policies that can be used to handle these sensitive areas, the choice of which will depend upon each local hospital situation. First, it can be established that the use of certain specified treatments will require prior official consultation with the medical director, who will follow the patient management with the attending physician. Second, the director can be given the authority to observe closely all patients receiving the services of his department and to interfere with the management at any time his judgment determines that the best interests of a patient are not being served. The degree of sophistication of the medical staff in the management of cardiopulmonary problems will usually be the determinant of the exact supervisory program most suitable. It is strongly suggested that the following philosophical observation be accepted: At the present time, inhalation therapy is still a young and growing field, and the exact legal and moral responsibilities of an inhalation therapy director toward other physicians and their patients have not been clarified. It must be assumed that he is responsible for the actions of technicians under his jurisdiction and for the safety and efficacy of the procedures of his department. It is only just, therefore, that being asked to assume responsibility, he also be given authority to control his sphere of responsibility. Further experience will be necessary to delineate more precisely the boundaries of his position.

SIZE OF INHALATION THERAPY DEPARTMENT

Personnel and space

Any opinions concerning number of personnel, size of physical facilities, and type of equipment must be of the most general nature because of the wide variation in individual hospital needs. The following comments are based upon the experiences of, and information from, a number of selected hospitals with known active departments. Although there is no statistical significance attached to the data acquired, they were felt to have general informative value; and analysis of the data revealed better correlation of numbers of personnel and floor space with average yearly admissions than with bed capacity. The range of yearly admissions among the hospitals polled extended from 7000 to 30,000, and the number of therapists felt to be adequate averaged 1 per 1000 yearly admissions. Despite a wide spread, it is felt that this ratio is a useful guide, especially for hospitals in the initial stages of planning a department. If anything, such a figure is small, for it does not take into account the specialty positions or stratification that inevitably develop. Thus, as a department increases its scope of services, this ratio can be expected to increase.

Data on inhalation therapy floor space yielded an average of about 70 square feet of space per 1000 yearly admissions. However, the breakdown of utilization of space was not available, and it is not known, for example, how much of the reported space was used for general service areas, offices, storage, or treatment rooms. It is strongly advised that hospitals anticipating physical expansion allow extra space above the immediate needs of inhalation therapy, for it can almost be guaranteed that a growing department will find its existing facilities inadequate within 2 to 3 years.

The general service or marshaling area should be large enough to accommodate a generous working space for repair and maintenance of equipment and a convenient area for cleaning and sterilization. The location of bulk storage space is a matter of expediency, but it should be near the general area. Provisions should also be made for separate office space for the medical director, the chief therapist, and a secretary and a writing area for record-keeping duties of the staff therapists. One of the most important contributions of inhalation therapy will be denied if an adequate ambulatory-care room is not provided, preferably immediately adjacent to, but separated from, the general service area. Ideally, the space provided for pulmonary function testing should be isolated from other activities, but this can often be skillfully done by properly placed partitions in the service area or treatment room. The difficulties of incorporating new facilities into existing buildings are well recognized, and makeshift arrangements often must be made. In new construction, however, every attempt should be made to locate the general service room, the laboratory, and the respiratory-care unit in contiguous areas, with the ambulatory service as close by as possible. This will permit the maximum effective use of personnel and equipment with minimum loss of time.

Equipment

Fortunately, much equipment is disposable in nature, easing the burden of maintaining large inventories of permanent items and allowing greater flexibility in purchasing according to changes in need. Of nonexpendable therapy equipment, the largest and most expensive pieces are the ventilators and oxygen-mist tents. It is quite improper, here, to recommend specific types or brands of such equipment, for these are decisions that should be left to the chief therapist with the approval of the medical director. Departmental policy will determine whether it is in the best interest of the hospital to strive for maximum uniformity of procedure through the use of a limited variety of types or for greater flexibility with a wide variety. In general, it might be advised that an active inhalation therapy service will be able to use one to two mechanical ventilators per 1000 yearly admissions and approximately one oxygen-mist tent per 1000 admissions. The minimum equipment for the pulmonary function laboratory consists of a spirometer with facilities for measurement of lung volumes, available as a single unit if desired, and a blood gas analyzer. Before investing in large numbers of equipment, both the medical director and chief therapist of a newly developing department would be well advised to visit a few established units to observe utilization and techniques.

SUMMARY

Inhalation therapy still poses many unsolved problems, some of which have been alluded to in the foregoing text. Paramount among them is the relationship between inhalation therapy and other hospital departments and services. As it has developed, inhalation therapy has admittedly encroached on clinical areas previously in the domains of nursing, physical therapy, clinical laboratory, and even the medical house staff. Such moves have been part of the natural evolution of an emerging clinical field directing itself toward the care of a substantial group of patients who, in the past, have received all too little attention. There is a natural hesitation on the part of physicians to delegate care of their patients to technicians, of whose work the physicians themselves know so little. The medical director of the department may well feel on unsure ground when he supervises the services of his therapists to a patient on whom he has not been asked to consult. Indeed, the matter of legal and moral responsibility of the medical director is still unsettled and will probably require more experience in the field to resolve. In the meantime, cooperation among the inhalation therapy department, the hospital administration, and the medical and nursing staffs will allow the useful services of inhalation therapy to find its niche in the overall medical care program of the hospital.

Finally, we might indulge in some imaginative speculation as to what the future could hold for inhalation therapy. The rapidly increasing population is straining the ability of currently organized medicine to supply adequate medical care. The problem is not merely a quantitative shortage of personnel; but with the emergence of so many new diagnostic and therapeutic techniques, skills are needed that have not traditionally been part of medicine. This is an era of technical as well as professional specialization, and it seems almost inevitable that delivery of medical care to our society in the near future will

Table 12-1. *Inhalation therapy vs. cardiopulmonary technology*

Inhalation therapy services	*Cardiopulmonary technology services*
Pulmonary function tests Spirometry Lung volumes Blood gases *Gas therapy* Oxygen Helium-oxygen Carbon dioxide–oxygen *Aerosols and humidity* Pharmacologic aerosols Humidity and vapor Cytology specimens *Mechanical ventilation* Positive-pressure breathing Assisted ventilation Controlled ventilation Emergency resuscitation *Physical therapy* Ambulatory service Postural drainage Breathing exercises Rehabilitation exercises	*Inhalation therapy* Clinical pulmonary function tests Gas therapy Aerosols and humidity Mechanical ventilation Physical therapy and rehabilitation *Cardiopulmonary lab* Diagnostic techniques Research assistance Electronic and mechanical instrumentation Hyperbaric medicine *Cardiovascular service* Cardiac pump operation Cardiac catheterization Research assistance Electrocardiography C-V surgical technology *C-P intensive care* Technical supervision C-P resuscitation Monitoring-equipment operation

depend upon the delegation of many responsibilities to highly skilled and finely trained nonphysician specialists. One of the fastest-growing segments of medicine is that of cardiopulmonary disease, and it is in this area that the present inhalation therapist may find himself becoming a more committed part of the future medical team. With his background in cardiopulmonary physiology, his participation in laboratory diagnosis, and his intimate patient-care experience, he is a natural subject to expand into related cardiovascular fields, where technology is becoming increasingly important. Perhaps we should already be orienting our education toward the development of *cardiopulmonary technology*, which could formally extend the function of the therapist beyond his present services. This is being done on scattered individual bases in many centers; and it is quite probable that before long, inhalation therapy will be one facet of the larger technical specialty of cardiopulmonary technology, with the relationships between the suggested services of the two as shown in Table 12-1. Time will tell.

Appendixes

Appendix 1

SYSTEMS OF MEASUREMENTS AND EQUIVALENTS

I. *Scientific notation*

A. The purpose of scientific notation is to convert a large or small awkward number from its usual form to an integer between 1 and 10, multiplied by the appropriate power of 10 so its value is unchanged.

B. Tabulation of the powers of 10:

$10^0 = 1$	$10^0 = 1$
$10^1 = 10$	$10^{-1} = 1/10 = 0.1$
$10^2 = 10 \times 10 = 100$	$10^{-2} = 1/10^2 = 0.01$
$10^3 = 10 \times 10 \times 10 = 1000$	$10^{-3} = 1/10^3 = 0.001$
$10^4 = 10 \times 10 \times 10 \times 10 = 10{,}000$	$10^{-4} = 1/10^4 = 0.0001$
$10^5 = 10 \times 10 \times 10 \times 10 \times 10 = 100{,}000$	$10^{-5} = 1/10^5 = 0.00001$
$10^6 = 10 \times 10 \times 10 \times 10 \times 10 \times 10 = 1{,}000{,}000$	$10^{-6} = 1/10^6 = 0.000001$
etc.	etc.

C. General rules for writing scientific notation:

1. For a number larger than 10: Move the decimal to the position to the right of the first integer, and multiply the new number by 10 raised to the power equal to the number of places the decimal was moved. Zeros to the right of the last integer may be dropped. For example:

$$2{,}655 = 2.655 \times 10^3 \qquad 301{,}010 = 3.0101 \times 10^5$$
$$54{,}000 = 5.4 \times 10^4 \qquad 866.67 = 8.6667 \times 10^2$$

2. For a number smaller than 1: Move the decimal to the position to the right of the first integer, and multiply the new number by 10 raised to a *negative* power equal to the number of places the decimal was moved. For example:

$$0.454 = 4.54 \times 10^{-1} \qquad 0.00000703 = 7.03 \times 10^{-6}$$
$$0.00306 = 3.06 \times 10^{-3} \qquad 0.01010 = 1.01 \times 10^{-2}$$

II. *The metric system*

A. The three basic units of linear, weight, and volume measurements of the metric system are, respectively, the *meter* (m), the *gram* (gm), and the *liter*. Multiples and divisions of the units are related to one another as powers of 10. Multiples are identified by Greek prefixes, and fractions by Latin. Thus:

deca $= 10$	deci $= 10^{-1}$
hecto $= 10^2$	centi $= 10^{-2}$

kilo	$= 10^3$	milli	$= 10^{-3}$
myria	$= 10^4$	micro	$= 10^{-6}$
mega	$= 10^6$	nano	$= 10^{-9}$

B. Table of metric measurements

Linear		*Weight*		*Volume*	
kilometer (km)	m × 10^3	kilogram (kg)	gm × 10^3	kiloliter	1 × 10^3
hectometer	m × 10^2	hectogram	gm × 10^2	hectoliter	1 × 10^2
decameter	m × 10	decagram	gm × 10	decaliter	1 × 10
meter (m)		gram (gm)		liter	
decimeter	m × 10^{-1}	decigram	gm × 10^{-1}	deciliter	1 × 10^{-1}
centimeter (cm)	m × 10^{-2}	centigram	gm × 10^{-2}	centiliter	1 × 10^{-2}
millimeter (mm)	m × 10^{-3}	milligram (mg)	gm × 10^{-3}	milliliter (ml)	1 × 10^{-3}
micrometer (micron, μ*)	m × 10^{-6}	microgram (μg)	gm × 10^{-6}	microliter (μl)	1 × 10^{-6}
		nanogram (ng)	gm × 10^{-9}	nanoliter (nl)	1 × 10^{-9}
angstrom (Å)	m × 10^{-10}				

C. US customary and metric equivalents

Linear		*Weight*		*Volume*	
inch	2.54 cm	ounce (av)	28.35 gm	ounce (fl)	29.57 ml
foot	3.048 × 10^{-1} m	pound	4.54 × 10^{-1} kg	quart	9.463 × 10^{-1} liter
mile	1.609 km			gallon	3.785 liters
		gram	3.528 × 10^{-2} oz	cubic inch	16.39 ml
micron	3.937 × 10^{-5} in	kilogram	2.205 lb	cubic foot	28.32 liters
centimeter	3.937 × 10^{-1} in				
meter	39.37 in			liter	1.057 qt
kilometer	6.214 × 10^{-1} mi				61.02 in³
					3.532 × 10^{-2} ft³

D. Equations to convert between Celsius and Fahrenheit temperatures

$$°C = \frac{5\ (°F - 32)}{9}$$

$$°F = \left[\frac{9 \times °C}{5}\right] + 32$$

* The micrometer is usually called a "micron." Because mm is the abbreviation for millimeter, the micron is symbolized by the Greek letter *mu* (μ).

Appendix 2

PHYSIOLOGIC AND SELECTED PHYSICAL ABBREVIATIONS AND SYMBOLS

a = (1) Arterial blood
  = (2) Acceleration
ā = (1) Mixed arterial blood
  = (2) Mean acceleration
ATPD, ATPD = Ambient temperature and pressure, dry
ATPS, ATPS = Ambient temperature and pressure, saturated with water vapor
A = Alveolar gas
b = Blood, generally
BTPD, BTPD = Body temperature, ambient pressure, dry
BTPS, BTPS = Body temperature, ambient pressure, saturated with water vapor
B = Barometric
c = Capillary blood

C = (1) Compliance
= (2) Concentration of gas in blood
°C = Degree of temperature by Celsius scale
d = Distance covered by a moving body
D = (1) Diffusing capacity
= (2) Density
D = Dead space gas
ERV = Expiratory reserve volume
E = Exhaled gas
f = Respiratory frequency (breaths per minute)
F = (1) Fractional concentration of dry gas
= (2) Force
°F = Degree of temperature by Fahrenheit scale
FRC = Functional residual capacity
g = Acceleration due to the force of gravity
gm = Gram
IC = Inspiratory capacity
IRV = Inspiratory reserve volume
I = Inhaled gas
K = Constant of a chemical equilibrium (ie, dissociation constant of a buffer system)
°K = Degree of temperature by Kelvin scale
KE = Kinetic energy
lpm = liters per minute
L = Lung (pulmonary)
mb = Millibar
mM = Millimole ($M \times 10^{-3}$)
M = Mole(s), molar
n = Number (especially number of molecules)
nM = Nanomole ($M \times 10^{-9}$)
pH = Negative common logarithm of molar hydrogen ion concentration
pK = Negative common logarithm of a chemical equilibrium constant (ie, dissociation constant of a buffer system)
psia = Pounds per square inch, absolute
psig = Pounds per square inch, gauge
P = Gas pressure
Q = Blood volume
$\dot{Q}$ = Rate of blood flow, volume per time

R = (1) Resistance
= (2) Respiratory exchange ratio (V_{CO_2}/V_{O_2})
= (3) Universal gas constant (0.0820561)
°R = Degree of temperature by Rankine scale
RC = Respiratory center
RH = Relative humidity
RV = Residual volume
s = Distance covered by a moving body
S = Percent saturation of hemoglobin with O_2 or CO
ST = Surface tension
STPD, STPD = Standard temperature (0° C), standard pressure (760 mm Hg), dry
s = Subscript to show steady state.
t = (1) Temperature generally
= (2) Time
T = Absolute temperature
TLC = Total lung capacity
T = (1) Tidal gas
= (2) Thorax
v = (1) Venous blood
= (2) Velocity
$\bar{v}$ = (1) Mixed venous blood
= (2) Mean velocity
V = Gas volume
VC = Vital capacity
V_A = Volume of total alveolar space
V_E = Volume of exhaled gas (often used for tidal volume)
V_D = Volume of dead space
$V_{D_{alv}}$ = Volume of alveolar dead space
$V_{D_{anat}}$ = Volume of anatomic dead space
$V_{D_{phys}}$ = Volume of physiologic dead space
V_T = Tidal volume
$\mathring{V}$ = Rate of gas flow, volume per time
$\mathring{V}_A$ = Minute alveolar ventilation (1pm)
$\mathring{V}_D$ = Minute dead space ventilation (1pm)
$\mathring{V}_E$ = Volume of exhaled gas per unit of time (usually 1pm, or minute volume)

Appendix 3

ALTITUDE AND DEPTH CHARACTERISTICS OF ATMOSPHERE*

Feet	*t° C*	*Atm*	*psi*	*mm Hg*	P_{O_2}	*% O_2 Equiv*	*Density*
300,000	− 2.2	7.3×10^{-6}	1.1×10^{-4}	0.0055	1.1×10^{-4}	1.4×10^{-5}	8.57×10^{-6}
200,000	33.8	3.2×10^{-4}	4.6×10^{-3}	0.24	5.0×10^{-2}	6.6×10^{-3}	3.28×10^{-4}
100,000	−55.0	0.011	0.155	8.0	1.7	0.22	1.74×10^{-2}
90,000	−55.0	0.017	0.250	12.9	2.7	0.36	2.80×10^{-2}
80,000	−55.0	0.027	0.403	20.8	4.3	0.57	4.52×10^{-2}
70,000	−55.0	0.044	0.649	33.6	7.0	0.92	7.30×10^{-2}
60,000	−55.0	0.071	1.05	54.1	11.3	1.49	1.18×10^{-1}
50,000	−55.0	0.115	1.69	87.4	18.3	2.41	1.90×10^{-1}
40,000	−55.0	0.191	2.72	140.6	29.4	3.87	3.06×10^{-1}
35,000	−54.3	0.236	3.46	178.6	37.4	4.92	3.87×10^{-1}
30,000	−44.4	0.296	4.36	225.7	47.3	6.22	4.67×10^{-1}
25,000	−34.5	0.372	5.46	282.0	59.1	7.78	5.60×10^{-1}
20,000	−24.6	0.460	6.76	348.8	73.1	9.62	6.66×10^{-1}
15,000	−14.7	0.566	8.29	428.6	89.8	11.82	7.86×10^{-1}
10,000	− 4.8	0.690	10.11	522.9	109.5	14.41	9.22×10^{-1}
5000	5.1	0.835	12.23	632.3	132.5	17.43	1.08
0	15.0	1.000	14.70	760.0	159.0	20.95	1.25
33		2.000	29.4	1520.0	318.0	41.90	2.50
66		3.000	44.1	2280.0	477.0	62.85	3.75
99		4.000	58.8	3040.0	636.0	83.80	5.00
132		5.000	73.5	3800.0	795.0	104.75	6.25
165		6.000	88.2	4560.0	954.0	125.70	7.50
198		7.000	102.9	5320.0	1113.0	146.65	8.75
231		8.000	117.6	6080.0	1272.0	167.60	10.00
264		9.000	132.3	6840.0	1431.0	188.55	11.25
297		10.000	147.0	7600.0	1590.0	209.50	12.50

*Adapted from Dittmer, D. S., and Grebe, R. W., editors: Handbook of respiration, Philadelphia, 1958, W. B. Saunders Co.

Appendix 4

FACTORS TO CONVERT GAS VOLUMES FROM ATPS TO BTPS*

Factor to convert volume to 37° C saturated	*When gas temperature (°C) is*	*With water vapor pressure (mm Hg)† of*
1.102	20	17.5
1.096	21	18.7
1.091	22	19.8
1.085	23	21.1
1.080	24	22.4
1.075	25	23.8

*Adapted from Comroe, J. H., Jr.: Methods in medical research, Chicago, 1950, Year Book Medical Publishers, Inc., vol 2.

†H_2O vapor pressures adapted from Handbook of chemistry and physics, ed 28, Cleveland, 1944, Chemical Rubber Publishing Co., p 1802.

Factor to convert volume to 37° C saturated	*When gas temperature (°C) is*	*With water vapor pressure (mm Hg)† of*
1.068	26	25.2
1.063	27	26.7
1.057	28	28.3
1.051	29	30.0
1.045	30	31.8
1.039	31	33.7
1.032	32	35.7
1.026	33	37.7
1.020	34	39.9
1.014	35	42.2
1.007	36	44.6
1.000	37	47.0

Note: These factors have been calculated only for a barometric pressure of 760 mm Hg. Since factors at 22°C, for example, are 1.0904, 1.0910, and 1.0915, respectively, at barometric pressures of 770, 760, and 750 mm Hg, it is unnecessary to correct for small deviations from standard barometric pressure.

$$\text{Factor} = \frac{[760 - P_{H_2O} \text{ at } t_{amb}] \times 0.435}{[t_{amb} + 273]}$$

Appendix 5

TEMPERATURE CORRECTION OF BAROMETRIC READING*

Temperature (°C)	*730 mm Hg*	*740*	*750*	*760*	*770*	*780*
15.0	1.78	1.81	1.83	1.86	1.88	1.91
16.0	1.90	1.93	1.96	1.98	2.01	2.03
17.0	2.02	2.05	2.08	2.10	2.13	2.16
18.0	2.14	2.17	2.20	2.23	2.26	2.29
19.0	2.26	2.29	2.32	2.35	2.38	2.41
20.0	2.38	2.41	2.44	2.47	2.51	2.54
21.0	2.50	2.53	2.56	2.60	2.63	2.67
22.0	2.61	2.65	2.69	2.72	2.76	2.79
23.0	2.73	2.77	2.81	2.84	2.88	2.92
24.0	2.85	2.89	2.93	2.97	3.01	3.05
25.0	2.97	3.01	3.05	3.09	3.13	3.17
26.0	3.09	3.13	3.17	3.21	3.26	3.30
27.0	3.20	3.25	3.29	3.34	3.38	3.42
28.0	3.32	3.37	3.41	3.46	3.51	3.55
29.0	3.44	3.49	3.54	3.58	3.63	3.68
30.0	3.56	3.61	3.66	3.71	3.75	3.80
31.0	3.68	3.73	3.78	3.83	3.88	3.93
32.0	3.79	3.85	3.90	3.95	4.00	4.05
33.0	3.91	3.97	4.02	4.07	4.13	4.18
34.0	4.03	4.09	4.14	4.20	4.25	4.31
35.0	4.15	4.21	4.26	4.32	4.38	4.43

* From US Dept of Commerce, Weather Bureau: Barometers and the measurement of atmospheric pressure, Washington, 1941, US Govt Printing Office.

Appendix 6

FACTORS TO CONVERT GAS VOLUMES FROM ATPS TO STPD

Observed P_B	*15°*	*16°*	*17°*	*18°*	*19°*	*20°*	*21°*	*22°*	*23°*	*24°*	*25°*	*26°*	*27°*	*28°*	*29°*	*30°*	*31°*	*32°*
700	0.855	851	847	842	838	834	829	825	821	816	812	807	802	797	793	788	783	778
702	857	853	849	845	840	836	832	827	823	818	814	809	805	800	795	790	785	780
704	860	856	852	847	843	839	834	830	825	821	816	812	807	802	797	792	787	783
706	862	858	854	850	845	841	837	832	828	823	819	814	810	804	800	795	790	785
708	865	861	856	852	848	843	839	834	830	825	821	816	812	807	802	797	792	787
710	867	863	859	855	850	846	842	837	833	828	824	819	814	809	804	799	795	790
712	870	866	861	857	853	848	844	839	836	830	826	821	817	812	807	802	797	792
714	872	868	864	859	855	851	846	842	837	833	828	824	819	814	809	804	799	794
716	875	871	866	862	858	853	849	844	840	835	831	826	822	816	812	807	802	797
718	877	873	869	864	860	856	851	847	842	838	833	828	824	819	814	809	804	799
720	880	876	871	867	863	858	854	849	845	840	836	831	826	821	816	812	807	802
722	882	878	874	869	865	861	856	852	847	843	838	833	829	824	819	814	809	804
724	885	880	876	872	867	863	858	854	849	845	840	835	831	826	821	816	811	806
726	887	883	879	874	870	866	861	856	852	847	843	838	833	829	825	818	813	808
728	890	886	881	877	872	868	863	859	854	850	845	840	836	831	826	821	816	811
730	892	888	884	879	875	870	866	861	857	852	847	843	838	833	828	823	818	813
732	895	891	886	882	877	873	868	864	859	854	850	845	840	836	831	825	820	815
734	897	893	889	884	880	875	871	866	862	857	852	847	843	838	833	828	823	818
736	900	895	891	887	882	878	873	869	864	859	855	850	845	840	835	830	825	820
738	902	898	894	889	885	880	876	871	866	862	857	852	848	843	838	833	828	822
740	905	900	896	892	887	883	878	874	869	864	860	855	850	845	840	835	830	825
742	907	903	898	894	890	885	881	876	871	867	862	857	852	847	842	837	832	827
744	910	906	901	897	892	888	883	878	874	869	864	859	855	850	845	840	834	829
746	912	908	903	899	895	890	886	881	876	872	867	862	857	852	847	842	837	832
748	915	910	906	901	897	892	888	883	879	874	869	864	860	854	850	845	839	834
450	917	913	908	904	900	895	890	886	881	876	872	867	862	857	852	847	842	837
752	920	915	911	906	902	897	893	888	883	879	874	869	864	859	854	849	844	839
754	922	918	913	909	904	900	895	891	886	881	876	872	867	862	857	852	846	841
756	925	920	916	911	907	902	898	893	888	883	879	874	869	864	859	854	849	844
758	927	923	918	914	909	905	900	896	891	886	881	876	872	866	861	856	851	846
760	930	925	921	916	912	907	902	898	893	888	883	879	874	869	864	859	854	848
762	932	928	923	919	914	910	905	900	896	891	886	881	876	871	866	861	856	851
764	934	930	926	921	916	912	907	903	898	893	888	884	879	874	869	864	858	853
766	937	933	928	925	919	915	910	905	900	896	891	886	881	876	871	866	861	855
768	940	935	931	926	922	917	912	908	903	898	893	888	883	878	873	868	863	858
770	942	938	933	928	924	919	915	910	905	901	896	891	886	881	876	871	865	860
772	945	940	936	931	926	922	917	912	908	903	898	893	888	883	878	873	868	862
774	947	943	938	933	929	924	920	915	910	905	901	896	891	886	880	875	870	865
776	950	945	941	936	931	927	922	917	912	908	903	898	893	888	883	878	872	867
778	952	948	943	938	934	929	924	920	915	910	905	900	895	890	885	880	875	869
780	955	950	945	941	936	932	927	922	917	912	908	903	898	892	887	882	877	872

$$\text{Factor} = \frac{[P_{B\,abs}\text{ corrected for } t_{amb} - P_{H_2O}\text{ at } t_{amb}] \times 0.359}{[t_{amb} + 273]}$$

Appendix 7

FACTORS TO CONVERT GAS VOLUMES FROM STPD TO BTPS AT GIVEN BAROMETRIC PRESSURES

Pressure	*Factor*	*Pressure*	*Factor*	*Pressure*	*Factor*	*Pressure*	*Factor*
740	1.245	750	1.227	760	1.211	770	1.193
742	1.241	752	1.224	762	1.208	772	1.190
744	1.238	754	1.221	764	1.203	774	1.188
746	1.235	756	1.217	766	1.200	776	1.183
748	1.232	758	1.214	768	1.196	778	1.181

$$\text{Factor} = \frac{863}{[P_{B_{amb}} - 47]}$$

Appendix 8

LOW-TEMPERATURE CHARACTERISTICS OF SELECTED GASES AND WATER

Substance	*Critical Temperature*		*Critical pressure*	*Boiling point*		*Melting (freezing) point*	
	°C	*°F*	*atm*	*°C*	*°F*	*°C*	*°F*
Acetylene	36.0	96.0	62.0	− 88.5	−119.2	− 81.8	−114.6
Air	−140.7	−221.0	37.2	−194.4	−317.9	–	–
Ammonia	132.4	270.3	111.5	− 33.4	− 28.1	− 77.7	−108.0
Carbon dioxide	31.1	87.9	73.0	− 78.5	−109.3	− 56.6	− 69.9
Cyclopropane	124.7	256.4	54.2	− 32.9	− 27.2	−127.5	−197.7
Freon-12	111.6	233.6	40.6	− 29.8	− 21.6	−158.0	−252.4
Freon-14	− 45.4	− 49.9	36.8	−128.0	−198.4	−184.0	−299.2
Helium	−267.9	−450.2	2.3	−268.9	−452.1	−272.2	−455.8
Hydrogen	−239.9	−399.8	12.8	−252.8	−423.0	−259.2	−434.5
Nitrogen	−147.1	−232.6	33.5	−195.8	−320.5	−209.9	−345.9
Nitrous oxide	36.5	97.7	71.8	− 88.5	−127.2	− 90.8	−131.6
Oxygen	−118.8	−181.1	49.7	−183.0	−297.3	−218.4	−361.8
Propane	95.6	206.2	43.0	− 42.2	− 43.7	−189.9	−305.8
Water	374.0	705.0	218.0	100.0	212.0	0.0	32.0

Appendix 9

SELECTED ELEMENTS AND RADICALS: SYMBOLS, APPROXIMATE ATOMIC WEIGHTS, VALENCES

Element	*Symbol*	*Atomic weight*	*Valence*	*Element*	*Symbol*	*Atomic weight*	*Valence*
Aluminum	Al	27	+3	Chlorine	Cl	35	−1, 3, 5, 7
Argon	A	40	0	Copper	Cu	64	+1, 2
Arsenic	As	75	+3, 5	Fluorine	F	19	−1
Barium	Ba	137	+2	Helium	He	4	0
Bromine	Br	80	−1, 3, 5, 7	Hydrogen	H	1	±1
Calcium	Ca	40	+2	Iodine	I	127	−1, 3, 5, 7
Carbon	C	12	+2, 4	Iron	Fe	56	+2, 3

Element	*Symbol*	*Atomic weight*	*Valence*	*Element*	*Symbol*	*Atomic weight*	*Valence*
Krypton	Kr	84	0	Phosphrous	P	31	+3, 5
Lead	Pb	207	+2, 4	Potassium	K	39	+1
Magnesium	Mg	24	+2	Silver	Ag	108	+1
Mercury	Hg	200	+1, 2	Sodium	Na	23	+1
Neon	Ne	20	0	Sulfur	S	32	±2, 4, 6
Nitrogen	N	14	+3, 5	Xenon	Xe	133	0
Oxygen	O	16	−2	Zinc	Zn	65	+2
Bicarbonate	HCO_3		−1	Nitrate	NO_3		−1
Carbonate	CO_3		−2	Phosphate	PO_4		−3
Chlorate	ClO_3		−1	Sulfate	SO_4		−2
Hydroxyl	OH		−1				

Appendix 10

CALCULATION OF P_{CO_2} FROM H-H EQUATION

$$pH = 6.1 + \log\left[\frac{HCO_3}{\text{Dissolved } CO_2}\right]$$

$$pH = 6.1 + \log\left[\frac{\text{Total } CO_2 - 0.03\ P_{CO_2}}{0.03\ P_{CO_2}}\right]$$

$$pH - 6.1 = \log\left[\frac{\text{Total } CO_2}{0.03\ P_{CO_2}} - 1\right]$$

$$\text{antilog}\ (pH - 6.1) = \frac{\text{Total } CO_2}{0.03\ P_{CO_2}} - 1$$

$$\text{antilog}\ (pH - 6.1) + 1 = \frac{\text{Total } CO_2}{0.03\ P_{CO_2}}$$

$$P_{CC_2} = \frac{\text{Total } CO_2}{0.03 \times [1 + \text{antilog}\ (pH - 6.1)]}$$

Appendix 11

RELATION OF ARTERIAL OXYGEN SATURATION TO CAPILLARY UNSATURATION

With 15 gm% of hemoglobin and an arterial-venous oxygen content difference of 5.0 vol%, the a-v oxygen saturation difference is 24%. The arterial oxygen saturation required to produce a specific concentration, in grams percent, of unsaturated capillary blood hemoglobin can be computed by the following formula, derived below:

$$S_{a_{O_2}} = \frac{16.8 - y}{15}$$

$$(1)\ \text{Mean capillary unsaturation} = \frac{\text{Arterial unsaturation} + \text{Venous unsaturation}}{2}$$

(2) $x = S_{a_{O_2}}$ thus, $(1.00 - x)$ = arterial unsaturation

$(x - 0.24) = S_{v_{O_2}}$

$(1.00 - [x - 0.24])$ = venous unsaturation

y = gm% unsaturated hemoglobin in capillary blood

(3) Substituting in (1) above:

$$\frac{15\,(1.00 - x) + 15\,(1.00 - (x - 0.24))}{2} = y$$

(4) $15 - 15x + 15 - 15x + 3.60 = 2y$

(5) $-30x + 33.6 = 2y$

(6) $x = \dfrac{16.8 - y}{15}$

Appendix 12

ALVEOLAR AIR EQUATION

Accurate measurement of alveolar oxygen tension by direct analysis of alveolar air samples is difficult because of the inability to obtain reliable samples that are representative of all lung areas. The alveolar air equation permits calculation of a close estimation of $P_{A_{O_2}}$ if the $F_{I_{O_2}}$, $P_{a_{CO_2}}$, and respiratory exchange ratio ($\dot{V}_{CO_2}/\dot{V}_{O_2}$) are known. Its derivation is well explained by Comroe,* and need not be repeated here, but we will demonstrate its application by two examples. The equation is stated as follows:

$$P_{A_{O_2}} = F_{I_{O_2}}(713) - P_{a_{CO_2}}\left(F_{I_{O_2}} + \frac{1 - F_{I_{O_2}}}{R}\right)$$

Example 1. Calculate $P_{A_{O_2}}$ breathing room air, when $P_{a_{CO_2}} = 40$ mm Hg, and $R = 0.8$:

$$\begin{aligned} P_{A_{O_2}} &= 0.21(713) - 40\left(0.21 + \frac{1 - 0.21}{0.8}\right) \\ &= 149.73 - 40(1.198) \\ &= 149.73 - 47.92 \\ &= 101.8 \text{ mm Hg} \end{aligned}$$

Example 2. Calculate $P_{A_{O_2}}$ breathing 40% oxygen, when $P_{a_{CO_2}} = 55$ mm Hg, and $R = 0.9$:

$$\begin{aligned} P_{A_{O_2}} &= 0.40(713) - 55\left(0.40 + \frac{1 - 0.40}{0.9}\right) \\ &= 285.2 - 55(1.07) \\ &= 285.2 - 58.85 \\ &= 226.4 \text{ mm Hg} \end{aligned}$$

---

* Adapted from Comroe, J. H., Jr., et al: The lung, Chicago, 1962, Year Book Medical Publishers, Inc.

Appendix 13

BREATHING NOMOGRAM

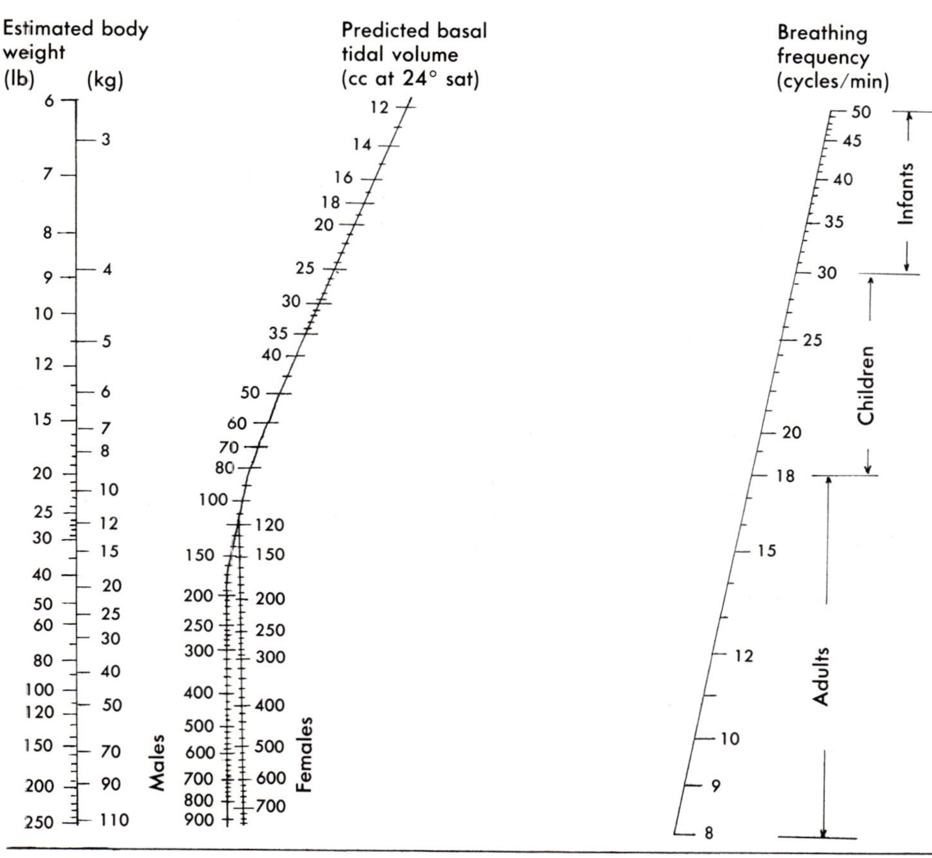

Corrections of predicted basal tidal volumes.

For patients not in coma: add 10%

Fever: add 5% for each °F above 99 (rectal)
add 9% for each °C above 37 (rectal)

Altitude: add 5% for each 2000 feet above sea level
add 8% for each 1000 meters above sea level

Intubation: subtract volume equal to one half body weight in pounds
subtract 1 cc/kg of body weight

Dead space: add equipment dead space

(Adapted from Radford, E. P., Jr.: Ventilation standards for use in artificial respiration, J Appl Physiol 7:451, 1955.)

Answers to exercises

Exercise 1-1:

(a) 1.16 gm/liter
(b) 0.759
(c) 4.64
(d) 1.25
(e) 2.855
(f) 1.455
(g) 0.428
(h) 0.553
(i) 2.12
(j) 1.45

Exercise 1-2:

(a) 1023.1 gm/cm^2
(b) 15.4 lb/in^2
(c) 14.8 lb/in^2
(d) 982.1 gm/cm^2
(e) 34.8 ft H_2O
(f) 751.2 mm Hg
(g) 30.9 in Hg
(h) 11.0 mm Hg
(i) 763.0 mm Hg
(j) 1022.0 mb

Exercise 1-3:

(a) 157.6 mm Hg
(b) 167.7 mm Hg
(c) 668.3 mm Hg
(d) 400.5 mm Hg
(e) 124.5 ft

Exercise 1-4:

(a) $P_2 = P_1V_1T_2/V_2T_1$
(b) $T_1 = T_2P_1V_1/P_2V_2$
(c) $V_1 = V_2P_2T_1/P_1T_2$
(d) $T_2 = T_1P_2V_2/P_1V_1$
(e) $n_2 = n_1P_2V_2T_1/P_1V_1T_2$

Exercise 1-5:

(a) 137.5 ml
(b) 2.54 liters
(c) 348 ml
(d) 20.9 liters
(e) 94.4 ml

Exercise 1-6:

(a) 251.6 ml
(b) 1.84 liters
(c) 59.7 m
(d) 358.3 m
(e) 2.37 liters

Exercise 1-7:

(a) $V_1 \times 726.4 \times 303/694.6 \times 303$
(b) $V_1 \times 724.7 \times 297/734.6 \times 297$
(c) $V_1 \times 724.1 \times 298/741.0 \times 293$
(d) $V_1 \times 754.2 \times 295/715.6 \times 288$
(e) $V_1 \times 763.0 \times 303/734.4 \times 297$

Exercise 2-1:

(a) 81 gm
(b) 32.7 gm
(c) 47 gm
(d) 47.3 gm
(e) 17 gm
(f) 56 gm
(g) 49.5 gm
(h) 26 gm
(i) 35 gm
(j) 29.2 gm

Exercise 2-2:

(a) 31 gm
(b) 55.5 gm
(c) 54.7 gm
(d) 51.7 gm
(e) Al = 32.1 gm; OH = 48.3 gm; Cl = 96.5

Exercise 2-3:

(a) 2 gew
(b) 0.9 gew
(c) 2.19 gew
(d) 0.193 gew
(e) 22.3 gew

Exercise 2-4:

(a) 100 meq
(b) 0.1 meq

(c) 18 meq
(d) 204 mg
(e) 1.615 gm

Exercise 2-5:

(a) 129 meq/liter
(b) 291 mg%
(c) 5.9 meq/liter
(d) 4.5 meq/liter
(e) 159 mg%

Exercise 2-6:

(a) 9 gm
(b) 1 ml
(c) 25 gm:225 gm
(d) 250 gm
(e) 2.5 M
(f) 500 ml
(g) 51.3 gm
(h) 0.5 N
(i) 100 ml
(j) 114.04 mg

Exercise 2-7:

(a) 22.5 ml
(b) 13 ml
(c) 10.14%
(d) 0.8 ml
(e) 1.5 N

Exercise 2-8:

(a) 6.42×10^{-5}
(b) 1.84×10^{-5}

Exercise 2-9:

(a) 4.12
(b) 1.52
(c) 11.29
(d) 7.99
(e) 9.06

Exercise 2-10:

(a) 6.17×10^{-4}
(b) 1.21×10^{-9}
(c) 9.77×10^{-6}
(d) 5.50×10^{-11}
(e) 2.19×10^{-7}

Exercise 3-1:

(a) 27.2 cm H_2O
(b) 4.70×10^{-2} cm (470μ)

Exercise 3-2:

$C_T = 0.18$ liters/cm H_2O

Exercise 4-1:

2.01 times as diffusible

Exercise 4-2:

(a) 7.49
(b) 7.32
(c) 6.82
(d) 53.2
(e) 22.6
(f) 23.9
(g) 35.3 33.7
(h) 31.1 29.9
(i) 13.1 12.4

References

1. Saunders, F. A.: A survey of physics for college students, New York, 1936, Henry Holt & Co.
2. Quagliano, J. V.: Chemistry, Englewood Cliffs, NJ, 1964, Prentice-Hall, Inc.
3. Armstrong, H. G.: Aerospace medicine, Baltimore, 1961, The Williams & Wilkins Co.
4. List, R. J., editor: Smithsonian meteorological tables, Washington, 1958, Smithsonian Institution.
5. Campbell, E. J. M.: The respiratory muscles and the mechanics of breathing, London, 1958, Lloyd-Luke, Ltd.
6. Sinclair, J. D.: Therapeutic exercises (Licht, S., editor), New Haven, Conn., 1961, Elizabeth Licht, Publisher.
7. Agostoni, E.: Breathlessness (Howell, J. B. L., and Campbell, E. J. M., editors), Oxford, 1966, Blackwell Scientific Publications.
8. Dejours, P.: Respiration, New York, 1966, Oxford University Press, Inc.
9. Winterstein, H.: Chemical control of pulmonary ventilation, New Eng J Med **255**:331, 1956.
10. Winterstein, H.: Chemical control of pulmonary ventilation, New Eng J Med **255**:216, 1956.
11. Best, C. H., and Taylor, N. B.: The physiological basis of medical practice, Baltimore, 1943, The Williams & Wilkins Co.
12. McDonald, J. E.: The shape of raindrops, Sci Amer **190**:64, 1954.
13. Clements, J. A.: Surface tension in lungs, Sci Amer **207**:121, 1962.
14. Avery, M. E., and Clements, J. A.: Pulmonary surfactants and atelectasis, Physiology, vol 1, March, 1963.
15. Mead, J.: Mechanical properties of the lung, Physiol Rev **41**:281, 1961.
16. Rahn, H., Otis, A. B., Chadwick, L. E., and Fenn, W. O.: The pressure-volume diagram of the thorax and lung, Amer J Physiol **146**:161, 1946.
17. Fenn, W. O.: Mechanics of respiration, Amer J Med **10**:79, 1951.
18. Comroe, J. H., Jr., et al: The lung, Chicago, 1962, Year Book Medical Publishers, Inc.
19. Comroe, J. H., Jr., et al: The lung, Chicago, 1962, Year Book Medical Publishers, Inc.
20. Black, N. H.: An introductory course in college physics, New York, 1956, The Macmillan Co.
21. Otis, A., et al: Mechanical factors in distribution of pulmonary ventilation, J Appl Physiol **8**:427, 1956.
22. Bates, D. V., and Christie, R. V.: Respiratory function in disease, Philadelphia, 1964, W. B. Saunders Co.
23. Cherniak, R. M., and Cherniak, L.: Respiration in health and disease, Philadelphia, 1962, W. B. Saunders Co.
24. Divertie, M. B., and Brown, A. L., Jr.: The fine structure of the normal alveolocapillary membrane, JAMA **187**:938, 1964.
25. Comroe, J. H., Jr., et al: The lung, Chicago, 1962, Year Book Medical Publishers, Inc.
26. Dittmer, D. S., and Grebe, R. W., editors: Handbook of respiration, Philadelphia, 1958, W. B. Saunders Co.
27. Roughton, F. J. W.: The average time spent by the blood in the human lung capillary, and its relation to the rates of carbon monoxide uptake and elimination in man, Amer J Physiol **143**:621, 1945.
28. Kleiner, I. S., and Orten, J. M.: Biochemistry, St. Louis, 1962, The C. V. Mosby Co.
29. Davenport, H. W.: The ABC of acid-base chemistry, Chicago, 1963, University of Chicago Press.

30. Dejours, P.: Respiration, New York, 1966, Oxford University Press.
31. Peters, J. P., and Van Slyke, D. D.: Quantitative clinical chemistry, Baltimore, 1931, The Williams & Wilkins Co., vol 2.
32. Refsum, H. E.: Acid-base disturbances in chronic pulmonary disease, Ann NY Acad Sci **133**:142, 1966.
33. Snively, W. D., et al: Systematic approach to fluid balance, Part 1, GP **13**:74, Jan, 1956.
34. Snively, W. D., et al: Systematic approach to fluid balance, Part 2, GP **13**:74, Feb, 1956.
35. Fordham, C. C., III, and Relman, A. J.: Mixed respiratory and metabolic acidosis, New Eng J Med **256**:698, 1957.
36. Robin, E. D.: Abnormalities of acid-base regulation in chronic pulmonary disease, with special reference to hypercapnia and extracellular alkalosis, New Eng J Med **268**:917, 1963.
37. Scher, A. M.: The electrocardiogram, Sci Amer **205**:137, 1961.
38. Bjurstedt, H.: Cardiovascular functions (Luisada, A., editor), New York, 1962, McGraw-Hill Book Co.
39. Visscher, M. B., et al: The physiology and pharmacology of lung edema, Pharmacol Rev **8**:389, 1956.
40. Egan, D. F.: Management of acute pulmonary edema, Hosp Med **2**:20, 1966.
41. Ferrer, M. I., and Harvey, R. M.: Pulmonary circulation (Adams, W. R., and Vieth, I., editors), New York, 1959, Grune & Stratton, Inc.
42. Steinborn, K. E., et al: Chronic cor pulmonale in the respiratory poliomyelitis patient, Arch Intern Med **110**:249, 1962.
43. Stuart-Harris, C. H.: Pulmonary hypertension and chronic obstructive bronchitis, Amer Rev Resp Dis **97**:9, 1968.
44. Rushmer, R. F., et al: Shock (Bock, K. D., editor), Berlin, 1962, Springer-Verlag.
45. Friedberg, C. H.: Diseases of the heart, Philadelphia, 1956, W. B. Saunders Co.
46. Bordicks, K. J.: Patterns of shock, New York, 1965, The Macmillan Co.
47. Warren, R.: Surgery, Philadelphia, 1963, W. B. Saunders Co.
48. Smith, R. E.: Outlines of internal medicine (Watson, C. J., editor), Dubuque, Ia, 1958, William C. Brown Co.
49. Rushmer, R. F.: Cardiac diagnosis, Philadelphia, 1955, W. B. Saunders Co.
50. Price, H. L.: Effects of carbon dioxide on the cardiovascular system, Anesthesiology **21**:652, 1960.
51. Hoffman, B. F., et al: Physiological basis of cardiac arrhythmias, Mod Conc Cardiov Dis **35**: 103, 1966.
52. Cherniak, R. M., and Cherniak, L.: Respiration in health and disease, Philadelphia, 1962, W. B. Saunders Co.
53. Williams, M. H., Jr.: Clinical applications of cardiopulmonary physiology, New York, 1960, Paul B. Hoeber, Inc.
54. Editorial: Hypoxemia vs. hypoxia, New Eng J Med **274**:908, 1966.
55. Barcroft, J.: Anoxemia, Lancet **2**:485, 1920.
56. Van Liere, E. J., and Stickney, J. C.: Hypoxia, Chicago, 1963, University of Chicago Press.
57. Campbell, E. J. M.: The management of acute respiratory failure in chronic bronchitis and emphysema, Amer Rev Resp Dis **96**:626, 1967.
58. Egan, D.F.: *Personal experience.*
59. Cherniak, R. M., and Cherniak, L.: Respiration in health and disease, Philadelphia, 1962, W. B. Saunders Co.
60. Shaw, D. B., and Simpson, T.: Polycythemia in emphysema, Quart J Med **30**:135, 1961.
61. Comroe, J. H., Jr.: Physiology of respiration, Chicago, 1966, Year Book Medical Publishers, Inc.
62. Filley, G. F.: Pulmonary insufficiency and respiratory failure, Philadelphia, 1967, Lea & Febiger.
63. Clements, J. A.: The lung (Liebow, A. A., et al, editors), Baltimore, 1968, The Williams & Wilkins Co.
64. Shulman, L. E.: Hypertrophic osteoarthropathy, Bull Rheum Dis **7**:135, 1957.
65. Lipman, B. S., and Massie, E.: Signs and symptoms, Philadelphia, 1957, J. B. Lippincott Co.
66. Field, A. S., Jr., and Gray, F. D., Jr.: The width of the nail fold capillary stream in clubbing, Dis Chest **41**:631, 1962.

67. Kenney, J. (Dept. of Medicine, Harvard Medical School): *Personal communication.*
68. Tappan, V., and Zalar, V.: Pathophysiology of bronchial mucus, Ann NY Acad Sci **106**:722, 1963.
69. Pratt, P. C., and Klugh, G. A.: Chronic expiratory air-flow obstruction—cause or effect of centrilobular emphysema? Dis Chest **52**:342, 1967.
70. Bouhuys, A.: Lung volumes and breathing patterns in wind instrument players, J Appl Physiol **19**:967, 1964.
71. Colp, C., et al: Diffuse emphysema as a result of non-obstructive interstitial pulmonary disease, Amer Rev Resp Dis **96**:788, 1967.
72. Gray, F. D., Jr.: Ventilation-perfusion ratios in cardiopulmonary diseases, Conn Med **31**: 338, 1967.
73. West, J. B.: Ventilation/Blood flow and gas exchange, Oxford, 1965, Blackwell Scientific Publications.
74. Dittmer, D. S., and Grebe, R. M., editors: Handbook of respiration, Philadelphia, 1958, W. B. Saunders Co.
75. West, J. B.: Ventilation/Blood flow and gas exchange, Oxford, 1965, Blackwell Scientific Publications.
76. Neuberger, H.: Condensation nuclei. Their significance in atmospheric pollution, Mechanical Engineering **70**:221, 1948.
77. Goetz, A.: The physicochemical behavior of submicron aerosols, Amer Rev Resp Dis **83**:410, 1961.
78. Brown, J. H., et al: The retention of particulate matter in the human lung, Amer J Public Health **40**:450, 1960.
79. Lovejoy, F. W., Jr., and Morrow, P. E.: Aerosols, bronchodilators, and mucolytic agents, Anesthesiology **23**:460, 1962.
80. Hatch, T. F., and Gross, P.: Pulmonary deposition and retention of inhaled aerosols, New York, 1964, Academic Press, Inc.
81. Altshuler, B., et al: Aerosol deposition in the human respiratory tract, Arch Industr Health **15**:293, 1957.
82. Dautrebande, L., et al: Lung deposition of fine dust particles, Arch Industr Health **16**:179, 1957.
83. Hayek, A.: Cellular structure and mucus activity in the bronchial tree and alveoli, Ciba Foundation symposium on pulmonary structure and function, Boston, 1962, Little, Brown & Co.
84. Hatch, T. F., and Gross, P.: Pulmonary deposition and retention of inhaled aerosols, New York, 1964, Academic Press, Inc.
85. Hatch, T. F.: Distribution and deposition of inhaled particles in the respiratory tract, Bact Rev **25**:237, 1961.
86. Dautrebande, L.: Microaerosols, New York, 1962, Academic Press, Inc.
87. Mercer, T. T., et al: Output characteristics of several commercial nebulizers, Ann Allerg **23**:314, 1965.
88. Muir, D. C. F.: Distribution of aerosol particles in exhaled air, J Appl Physiol **23**:210, 1967.
89. Keighley, J. F.: Iatrogenic asthma associated with adrenergic aerosols, Ann Intern Med **65**:985, 1966.
90. Sollman, T.: A manual of pharmacology, Philadelphia, 1957, W. B. Saunders Co.
91. Cohen, A. A., and Hale, F. C.: Comparative effects of isoproterenol aerosols on airway resistance in obstructive pulmonary disease, Amer J Med Sci **249**:309, 1965.
92. Lands, A. M., et al: The pharmacologic actions of the bronchodilator drug isoetharine, J Amer Pharm Ass (Sci ed) **47**:744, 1958.
93. El-Shaboury, A. H.: Controlled study of a new inhalant in asthma and bronchitis, Brit Med J **5416**:1037, 1964.
94. Davison, F. R.: Handbook of materia medica, toxicology, and pharmacology, St. Louis, 1949, The C. V. Mosby Co.
95. Nadel, J. A., and Widdicombe, J. G.: Mechanism of bronchoconstriction with dust inhalation, Clin Res **10**:91, 1962.
96. Dautrebande, L., et al: Effects of atropine microaerosols on airway resistance in man, Arch Int Pharmacodyn **139**:198, 1962.

97. Segal, M. S.: Advances in inhalation therapy, with particular reference to cardiorespiratory disease, New Eng J Med **231**:553, 1944.
98. Prigol, S. J., et al: The treatment of asthma by inhalation of aerosol of aminophylline, J Allerg **18**:16, 1947.
99. Horton, G. E.: The value and safety of nebulized aminophylline in acute bronchial asthma, J Tenn Med Ass **59**:239, 1966.
100. Forsham, P. H.: The adrenal gland, Clin Sympos **15**:3, 1963.
101. Kleiner, I. S., and Orten, J. M.: Biochemistry, St. Louis, 1962, The C. V. Mosby Co.
102. Williams, R. H., editor: Textbook of endocrinology, Philadelphia, 1962, W. B. Saunders Co.
103. Norman, P. S., et al: Adrenal function during the use of dexamethasone aerosols in the treatment of ragweed hay fever, J Allerg **40**:57, 1967.
104. Fisch, B. R., and Grater, W. C.: Dexamethasone aerosol in respiratory tract disease, J New Drugs **2**:298, 1962.
105. Crepea, S. B.: Inhalation corticosteroid (dexamethasone) management of chronically asthmatic children, J Allerg **34**:119, 1963.
106. Novey, H. S., and Beall, G.: Aerosolized steroids and induced Cushing's syndrome, Arch Intern Med **115**:602, 1965.
107. Linder, W. R.: Adrenal suppression by aerosol steroid inhalation, Arch Intern Med **113**: 655, 1964.
108. Cohen, B.: Acute bronchodilator properties of a steroid microaerosol, Curr Ther Res **6**:73, 1964.
109. Tainter, M. L., et al: Alevaire as a mucolytic agent, New Eng J Med **253**:764, 1955.
110. Miller, J. B., et al: Alevaire inhalations for eliminating secretions in asthma, sinusitis, and bronchiectasis of adults, Ann Allerg **12**:611, 1954.
111. Sadove, M. S., and Miller, C. E.: Postoperative aerosol therapy, JAMA **156**:759, 1954.
112. Denton, R.: Continuous nebulization therapy, Pediat Clin N Amer **1**:625, 1954.
113. Palmer, K. N. V.: The effect of an aerosol detergent in chronic bronchitis, Lancet **272-1**:611, 1957.
114. Sheffner, A. L.: The mucolytic activity, mechanisms of action, and metabolism of acetylcysteine, Pharmacotherapy **1**:47, 1964.
115. Hirsch, S. R., and Kory, R. C.: An evaluation of the effect of nebulized N-acetylcysteine on sputum consistency, J Allerg **39**:265, 1967.
116. Moser, K. M., and Rhodes, P. G.: Acute effects of aerosolized acetylcysteine upon spirometric measurements in subjects with and without obstructive pulmonary disease, Dis Chest **49**:370, 1966.
117. Thomas, P. A., and Treasure, R. I.: Effect of N-acetyl-L-cysteine on pulmonary surface activity, Amer Rev Resp Dis **94**:175, 1966.
118. Webb, W. R.: New mucolytic agents for sputum liquefaction, Postgrad Med **36**:449, 1964.
119. Mucolytic agent, Brit Med J **2**:603, Sept, 1966.
120. Anderson, G.: A clinical trial of a mucolytic agent—acetylcysteine—in chronic bronchitis, Brit J Dis Chest **60**:101, 1966.
121. Denton, R., et al: N-acetylcysteine in cystic fibrosis, Amer Rev Resp Dis **95**:643, 1967.
122. Luisada, A. A., et al: Alcohol vapor by inhalation in the treatment of acute pulmonary edema, Circulation **5**:363, 1952.
123. Limber, C. R., et al: Enzymatic lysis of respiratory secretions by aerosol trypsin, JAMA **149**:816, 1952.
124. Unger, L., and Unger, A. H.: Trypsin inhalations in respiratory conditions with thick sputum, JAMA **152**:1109, 1953.
125. Prince, H. E., et al: Aerosol trypsin in the treatment of asthma, Ann Allerg **12**:25, 1954.
126. Salomon, A., et al: Aerosols of pancreatic dornase in bronchopulmonary disease, Ann Allerg **12**:71, 1954.
127. Sherry, S., et al: Presence and significance of desoxyribose nucleotide in purulent exudate, Proc Soc Exp Biol Med **68**:179, 1948.
128. Meunster, J. J., et al: Treatment of unresolved pneumonia with streptokinase and streptodornase, Amer J Med **12**:367, 1952.
129. Craven, J. F.: Treatment of obstructive atelectasis by aerosol administration of proteolytic enzymes, J Pediat **42**:228, 1953.

130. Cliffton, E. E.: Pancreatic dornase aerosol in pulmonary, endotracheal, and endobronchial disease, Dis Chest **30**:1, 1956.
131. Lyons, H. A.: Use of therapeutic aerosols, Amer J Cardiol **12**:461, 1963.
132. Olsen, A. M.: Streptomycin aerosol in the treatment of chronic bronchiectasis: preliminary report, Proc Staff Meet Mayo Clin **21**:53, 1946.
133. Garthwaite, B., and Barach, A. L.: Penicillin aerosol therapy in bronchiectasis, lung abscess, and chronic bronchitis, Amer J Med **3**:261, 1947.
134. Eastlake, C., Jr.: Aerosol therapy in sinusitis, bronchiectasis, and lung abscess, Bull NY Acad Med **26**:423, 1950.
135. Christie, H. E., et al: Aerosol therapy for lung abscess, Canad Med Ass **62**:478, 1950.
136. Melica, A., et al: Oxytetracycline inhalation in the treatment of acute and chronic bronchial infection, G Clin Med **47**:416, 1962.
137. Naumov, G. P.: Pathologic changes in upper respiratory passages and lungs following use of antibiotic electroaerosols, Fed Proc **25**: 654, 1966.
138. Pines, A., et al: Gentamicin and colistin in chronic purulent bronchial infections, Brit Med J **2**:543, 1967.
139. Bilodeau, M., et al: Studies of absorption of kanamycin by aerosol, Ann NY Acad Sci **132**: 870, 1966.
140. Spier, R., et al: Aerosolized pancreatic dornase and antibiotics in pulmonary infection, JAMA **178**:878, 1961.
141. Egan, D.: Humidity and water aerosol therapy, Conn Med **31**:353, 1967.
142. Cushing, I. E., and Miller, W. F.: Consideration in humidification by nebulization, Dis Chest, vol 34, Oct, 1958.
143. Yue, W. Y., and Cohen, S. S.: Sputum induction by newer inhalation methods in patients with pulmonary tuberculosis, Dis Chest **51**:611, 1967.
144. Cohen, B. M., and Crandall, C.: Physiologic benefits of "thermo-fog" as a bronchodilator vehicle: acute ventilation responses of 93 patients, Amer J Med Sci **247**: 57, 1964.
145. Tomashefski, J. F., et al: An environmental contamination control unit for use during aerosol administration, Amer Rev Resp Dis **96**:1246, 1967.
146. Hensler, N., et al: The use of hypertonic aerosol in production of sputum for diagnosis of tuberculosis, Dis Chest **40**:639, 1961.
147. Lillehei, J. P.: Sputum induction with heated aerosol inhalations for the diagnosis of tuberculosis, Amer Rev Resp Dis **84**:276, 1961.
148. Umiker, W. O.: A new vista in pulmonary cytology: aerosol induction of sputum, Dis Chest **39**:512, 1961.
149. Johnson, J. R., et al: Aerosol-induced sputum: an effective, inexpensive method for nebulization of a super-heated mixture of 40 percent propylene glycol in isotonic saline, Dis Chest **42**:251, 1962.
150. Robillard, E., et al: Microaerosol administration of synthetic dipalmitoyl-lecithin in the respiratory distress syndrome. A preliminary report, Canad Med Ass J **90**:55, 1964.
151. Rosner, S. W.: Heparin administration as an aerosol, Vasc Dis **2**:131, 1965.
152. Smith, G. M., and Armen, R. N.: Pulmonary moniliasis treated by brilliant green aerosol: report of a case, Ann Intern Med **43**:1302, 1955.
153. Kass, I., et al: Treatment of bronchopulmonary moniliasis by dye inhalation, Dis Chest **21**:205, 1952.
154. Egan, D. F.: Humidity and water aerosol therapy, Conn Med **31**:353, 1967.
155. Dautrebande, L.: Microaerosols, New York, 1962, Academic Press, Inc.
156. Tovell, R. M., and Little, D. M., Jr.: The utilization of fog as a therapeutic agent, Anesthesiology **18**:470, 1957.
157. Cushing, I. E., and Miller, W. F.: Considerations in humidification by nebulization, Dis Chest **34**:388, 1958.
158. Welts, R. E., et al: Humidification of oxygen during inhalational therapy, New Eng J Med **268**:644, 1963.
159. Andrews, A. H., Jr.: Ultrasonic aerosol generator, Presbyt St Luke Hosp Med Bull **3**:155, 1964.
160. Proceedings of the First Conference on Clinical Application of the Ultrasonic Nebulizer, Somerset, Pa, 1966, DeVilbiss Co.

161. Gauthier, W. D.: Operational characteristics of the ultrasonic nebulizer, Proceedings of the First Conference on Clinical Application of the Ultrasonic Nebulizer, 1966.
162. Stevens, H. R., and Albregt, H. B.: Assessment of ultrasonic nebulization, Anesthesiology **27**:648, 1966.
163. Modell, J. H., et al: Effect of ultrasonic nebulized suspensions on pulmonary surfactant, Dis Chest **50**:627, 1966.
164. Modell, J. H., et al: Effect of chronic exposure to ultrasonic aerosols on the lungs, Anesthesiology **28**:680, 1967.
165. Allan, D.: Artificial humidification, Med Sci **17**:41, Jan, 1966.
166. Doershuk, C. F., and Matthews, L. W.: Cystic fibrosis, Postgrad Med **40**:550, 1966.
167. National Fire Protection Association, 60 Batterymarch St, Boston, Mass, 02110, Pamphlet nos. 565, 566.
168. Compressed Gas Association, 500 Fifth Ave, New York, NY, 10036: Pamphlet P-2, Characteristics and safe handling of medical gases.
169. Compressed Gas Association, 500 Fifth Ave, New York, NY, 10036: Pamphlet V-1, American Standard Compressed Gas Cylinder Valve Outlet and Inlet Connections.
170. Compressed Gas Association, 500 Fifth Ave, New York, NY, 10036: Pamphlet V-5, Diameter Index Safety System.
171. Dole, M.: The natural history of oxygen, J Gen Physiol **49**:(Suppl) 5, 1965.
172. Clamann, H. G.: Fire hazards, Ann NY Acad Sci **117**:814, 1965.
173. Cullen, J. H., and Kaemmerlen, J. T.: Effect of oxygen administration at low rates of flow in hypercapnic patients, Amer Rev Resp Dis **95**:116, 1967.
174. Massaro, D. J., et al: Effect of various modes of oxygen administration on the arterial gas values in patients with respiratory acidosis, Brit Med J **2**:627, 1962.
175. Hutchison, D. C. S., et al: Controlled oxygen therapy in respiratory failure, Brit Med J **2**: 1157, 1964.
176. Arnold, W. H., Jr., and Grant, J. L.: Oxygen-induced hypoventilation, Amer Rev Resp Dis **95**:255, 1967.
177. Fine, J., Banks, B., and Hermanson, L.: The treatment of gaseous distention of the intestine by inhalation of 95% oxygen, Ann Surg **103**:375, 1936.
178. Patz, A.: Oxygen administration to the premature infant, Amer J Ophthal **63**:351, 1967.
179. Welch, B. E., et al: Time-concentration effects in relation to oxygen toxicity in man, Fed Proc **22**:1053, 1963.
180. Doleval, V.: Voluntary tolerance of 100% oxygen, Rev Med Aeron **25**:219, 1962.
181. Weir, F. W., et al: Study of effects of continuous inhalation of high concentrations of oxygen at ambient pressure and temperature, Aerospace Med **36**:117, 1965.
182. Caldwell, P. R. B., et al: Effect of oxygen breathing at one atmosphere on the surface activity of lung extracts in dogs, Ann NY Acad Sci **121**:823, 1965.
183. Pratt, P. C.: Pulmonary capillary proliferation induced by oxygen inhalation, Amer J Path **34**:1033, 1958.
184. Nash, G., et al: Pulmonary lesions associated with oxygen therapy and artificial ventilation, New Eng J Med **276**:368, 1967.
185. Bruns, P. D., and Shields, L. V.: High oxygen and hyaline-like membranes, Amer J Obstet Gynec **67**:1224, 1954.
186. Shanklin, D. R., and Wolfson, S. L.: Therapeutic oxygen as a possible cause of pulmonary hemorrhage in premature infants, New Eng J Med **277**:833, 1967.
187. Lee, C. J., et al: Cardiovascular and metabolic responses to spontaneous and positive-pressure breathing of 100% oxygen at one atmosphere, J Thorac Cardiov Surg **53**:770, 1967.
188. Wright, R., et al: Risk of mortality in interrupted exposure to 100% oxygen: role of air vs lowered oxygen tension, Amer J Physiol **210**:1015, 1966.
189. Collis, J. M., and Bethune, D. W.: Oxygen by face mask and nasal catheter, Lancet **1**:787, 1967.
190. Hedley-Whyte, J., and Winter, P. M.: Oxygen therapy, Clin Pharmacol Therap **8**:696, 1967.
191. Buck, J. B., and McCormack, W. C.: A nasal mask for premature infants, J Pediat **66**:123, 1965.
192. Committee on Public Health: A report: effective administration of inhalational therapy

with special reference to ambulatory and emergency oxygen treatment, Bull New York Acad Med **38**:135, 1962.

193. Kory, R. C., et al: Comparative evaluation of oxygen therapy techniques, JAMA **179**:767, 1962.
194. Campbell, E. J. M.: Oxygen therapy in diseases of the chest, Brit J Dis Chest **58**:149, 1964.
195. Schiff, M. M., and Massaro, D.: Effect of oxygen administration by a venturi apparatus on arterial blood gas values in patients with ventilatory failure, New Eng J Med **277**:950, 1967.
196. Bethune, D. W., and Collis, J. M.: An evaluation of oxygen therapy equipment, Thorax **22**:221, 1967.
197. Campbell, E. J. M., and Gebbie, T.: Masks and tent for providing controlled oxygen concentrations, Lancet **1**:468, 1966.
198. Glick, R. V., and Benner, J. N.: Arterial oxygen tension during oxygen breathing, Inhal Ther **13**:31, 1968.
199. Jahn, R. E.: An examination of oxygen and carbon dioxide concentrations in adult oxygen tents, Brit J Anaesth **25**:188, 1953.
200. Plano, R. J.: Tests evaluate fire hazards of static sparks, Mod Hosp **95**:154, Sept, 1960.
201. Guest, P. G.: Oily fibers may increase oxygen tent fire hazard, Mod Hosp **104**:180, May, 1965.
202. Berry, R. C.: Safe practices in handling oxygen equipment, Hospitals **37**:376, 1963.
203. Mithoefer, J. C., et al: Oxygen therapy in respiratory failure, New Eng J Med **277**:947, 1967.
204. Levine, B. E., et al: The role of long-term continuous oxygen administration in patients with chronic airway obstruction with hypercapnia, Ann Intern Med **66**:639, 1967.
205. Eldridge, F., and Gherman, C.: Studies of oxygen administration in respiratory failure, Ann Intern Med **68**:569, 1968.
206. Egan, D. F.: Therapeutic uses of helium, Conn Med **31**:355, 1967.
207. Souadjian, J., and Cain, J.: Intractable hiccup, Postgrad Med **43**:72, 1968.
208. Fishman, A. P.: The roads to respiratory insufficiency, Ann New York Acad Med **121**:657, 1965.
209. Weiss, E. B., and Dulfano, M. J.: Controlled ventilation with intermittent positive-pressure breathing in the management of acute ventilatory failure associated with chronic obstructive pulmonary disease, Ann Intern Med **67**:556, 1967.
210. Mushin, W. W., et al: Automatic ventilation of the lungs, Oxford, 1959, Blackwell Scientific Publications.
211. Mapleson, W. W.: The effect of changes of lung characteristics on the functioning of automatic ventilators, Anaesthesia **17**:300, 1962.
212. Rattenborg, C., and de Borde, R.: Lung ventilators: function and principles, Inhal Ther **12**: 48, 1967.
213. Drinker-Collins respirator, Warren E. Collins Co., Boston, Mass.
214. Portable respirator (chest), J. J. Monaghan Co., Denver, Colo.
215. U-Cyclit chest respirator, J. H. Emerson Co., Cambridge, Mass.
216. Air-Shields respirator, Air-Shields, Inc., Hatboro, Pa.
217. Post-Operative ventilator, J. H. Emerson Co., Cambridge, Mass.
218. Engström respirator, LKB Instruments, Inc., Rockville, Md.
219. Augmentor-respirator (infant), Bourns, Inc., Ames, Ia.
220. Respiration unit MA-1, Bennett Respiration Products, Inc., Santa Monica, Calif.
221. Respirators, Mark 7, 8, Bird Corp., Richmond, Calif.
222. Respiration units PR-1, 2, Bennett Respiration Products, Inc., Santa Monica, Calif.
223. Drinker, P., and McKhann, C.: The use of a new apparatus for prolonged administration of artificial respiration, JAMA **92**:1658, 1929.
224. Sheldon, G. P.: Pressure breathing in chronic obstructive lung disease, Medicine **42**:197, 1963.
225. Bird Corporation, Richmond, Calif, Form no. 8.101 (rev 1).
226. Edwards, W. L., and Sappenfield, R. S.: Pressure-cycled ventilators and flow-rate control, Anesth Analg **47**:77, 1968.
227. Glick, R. V., and Woods, R. H.: The importance of measuring inspired oxygen concentrations during mechanical pulmonary ventilation, Inhal Ther **11**:7, Feb, 1966.

228. Bennett Respiration Products, Inc.: Bennett PR-2 respiration unit, instruction manual, form 2131 (12-64).
229. Bennett Respiration Products, Inc.: Bennett PR-2 respiration unit, trainer's script, form EA-110TS.
230. Torres, G. E., et al: The effects of IPPB on intrapulmonary distribution of inspired air, Amer J Med **29**:946, 1960.
231. Ayers, S. M., and Giannelli, S., Jr.: Oxygen consumption and alveolar ventilation during intermittent positive pressure breathing, Dis Chest **50**:409, 1966.
232. Gray, F. D., Jr., and MacIver, S.: The use of inspiratory positve pressure breathing in cardiopulmonary diseases, Dis Chest, Jan, 1958.
233. Motley, H. L.: Intermittent positive pressure breathing therapy, Inhal Ther, vol 7, Feb, 1962.
234. Werko. L.: Influence of positive pressure breathing on the circulation in man, Acta Med Scand (Suppl 193), 1947.
235. Opie, L. H., et al: Intrathoracic pressure during intermittent positive-pressure respiration, Lancet **1**:911, Apr, 1961.
236. Coonse, G. K., and Aufrance, O. E.: The relation of the intrapleural pressure to the mechanics of the circulation, Amer Heart J **9**:347, 1934.
237. Printzmetal, M., and Kounts, W. B.: Intrapleural pressure in health and disease and its influence on body function, Medicine **14**:457, 1935.
238. Christie, R. V., and McIntosh, C. A.: The measurement of intrapleural pressure in man, and its significance, J Clin Invest **13**:279, 1934.
239. Kilburn, K. H., and Sicker, H. O.: Hemodynamic effects of continuous positive and negative pressure breathing in normal man, Circ Res **8**:660, 1960.
240. Bashour, F. A., et al: Effect of intermittent positive pressure breathing on the cardiac output and the splanchnic blood flow, Inhal Ther **13**:47, 1968.
241. Ashbaugh, D. G., et al: Acute respiratory distress in adults, Lancet **2**:319, 1967.
242. Sladen, A., et al: Pulmonary complications and water retention in prolonged mechanical ventilation, New Eng J Med **279**:448, 1968.
243. Murdaugh, H. V., et al: Effect of altered intrathoracic pressure on renal hemodynamics, electrolyte excretion, and water clearance, J Clin Invest **38**:834, 1959.
244. Drury, D. R., et al: The effects of continuous pressure breathing on kidney function, J Clin Invest **26**:945, 1947.
245. Henry, J. P., and Pierce, J. W.: Possible role of cardiac atrial stretch receptors in induction of changes in urine flow, J Physiol **131**:572, 1956.
246. Weg, J. G.: Prolonged endotracheal intubation in respiratory failure, Arch Intern Med **120**:679, 1967.
247. Kuner, J., and Goldman, A.: Prolonged nasotracheal intubation in adults versus tracheostomy, Dis Chest **51**:270, 1967.
248. Garzon, A. A., et al: Influence of cannula size on resistance to breathing through tracheostomies, Surg Forum **14**:219, 1963.
249. Greene, N. M.: Fatal cardiovascular and respiratory failure associated with tracheotomy, New Eng J Med **261**:846, 1959.
250. Yanagisawa, E., and Kirchner, J. A.: The cuffed tracheotomy tube, Arch Otolaryng **79**:80, 1964.
251. Meyer, J. A.: Tracheotomy care, Int Anesth Clin **4**:675, 1966.
252. Gunn, I. P., et al: Expiratory resistance of oxygen catheters in patients with tracheostomies, JAMA **193**:737, 1965.
253. Decancq, H. G., Jr.: Tissue "snowplowing": a post-tracheostomy complication, Amer J Dis Child **108**:94, 1964.
254. Bendixen, H. H., et al: Respiratory care, St. Louis, 1965, The C. V. Mosby Co.
255. Head, J. M.: Tracheostomy in the management of respiratory problems, New Eng J Med **264**:587, 1961.
256. Nelson, T. G., and Bowers, W. T.: Tracheostomy—indications, advantages, techniques, complications, and results, JAMA **164**:1530, 1957.
257. Cullen, J. H.: An evaluation of tracheostomy in pulmonary emphysema, Ann Intern Med **58**:953, 1963.

258. Feldman, S. A., editor: Tracheostomy and artificial ventilation, London, 1967, Edward Arnold (Publishers) Ltd.
259. Engstrom, C., and Herzog, P.: Ventilation nomogram for practical use with the Engstrom respirator, Acta Chir Scand (Suppl 245), 1959.
260. Engstrom, C., et al: Ventilation nomogram for the newborn and small children to be used with the engstrom respirator, Acta Anaesth Scand **6**:175, 1962.
261. Radford, E. P., Jr.: Ventilation standards for use in artificial respiration, J Appl Physiol **7**:451, 1955.
262. Merck manual of therapeutics and materia medica, Rahway, NJ, 1940, Merck & Co., Inc.
263. Dittmer, D. S., and Grebe, R. M., editors: Handbook of respiration, Philadelphia, 1958, W. B. Saunders Co.
264. Growth charts used by Children's Hospital Medical Center, Boston, Mass. Courtesy H. C. Stuart, Dept of Maternal and Child Health, Harvard School of Public Health, Boston.
265. Avery, M. E.: The lung and its disorders in the newborn infant, Philadelphia, 1964, W. B. Saunders Co.
266. Holt, L. E., Jr., and McIntosh, R.: Diseases of infancy and children, New York, 1940, D. Appleton-Century Co.
267. Cooke, R. J.: The biologic basis of pediatric practice, New York, 1968, McGraw-Hill Book Co.
268. Bendixen, H. H., et al: Impaired oxygenation in surgical patients during general anesthesia with controlled ventilation, New Eng J Med **269**:991, 1963.
269. Egan, D. F.: *Personal experience.*
270. Cherniak, R. M., and Hakimpour, K.: The rational use of oxygen in respiratory insufficiency, JAMA **199**:178, 1967.
271. Drinker, P., et al: A constant ratio air-oxygen mixer, JAMA **202**:531, 1967.
272. Smith, A. C.: Effect of mechanical ventilation on the circulation, Ann NY Acad Sci **121**:742, 1965.
273. Stamm, S. J.: Reliability of capillary blood for the measurement of P_{O_2} and O_2 saturation, Dis Chest **52**:191, 1967.
274. Hackney, J. D., and Collier, C. R.: Practical system for determining ventilatory function, JAMA **192**:16, 1965.
275. Wright respirometer, Anesthesia Associates, Inc., Hudson, NY.
276. Monitaire, ventilation monitor, Monitor Instrument Co., Inc., Hamden, Conn.
277. D. H. Taylor solid state IPPV monitor, Respiratory Function Labs, Inc., Syracuse, NY.
278. RETEC automatic respirator, RETEC, Inc., Portland, Ore.
279. Angrist, S.W.: Fluid control devices, Sci Amer **211**:81, Dec, 1964.
280. Reba, I.: Applications of the Coanda effect, Sci Amer, June, 1966.
281. Thacker, E. W.: Postural drainage and respiratory control, London, 1963, Lloyd-Luke, Ltd.
282. Physiotherapy Dept, Brompton Hospital, London: Physiotherapy for medical and surgical thoracic conditions, 1967.
283. Dept of Physical Medicine and Rehabilitation, University of Minnesota Medical School, Minneapolis: Techniques of bronchial drainage, 1967.

Index